INTRODUCTORY
NUTRITION

INTRODUCTORY
NUTRITION

Helen Andrews Guthrie

B.Sc., M.S., Ph.D.

Associate Professor of Foods and Nutrition,
The Pennsylvania State University,
University Park, Pennsylvania

SECOND EDITION

WITH 119 ILLUSTRATIONS

The C. V. Mosby Company

SAINT LOUIS, 1971

SECOND EDITION

Copyright © 1971 by
The C. V. Mosby Company

Third printing

Previous edition copyrighted 1967

Printed in the United States of America

Standard Book Number 8016-1999-8

Library of Congress Catalog Card Number 76-138540

Distributed in Great Britain by Henry Kimpton, London

Preface

THE PREFACE TO THE FIRST EDITION indicated that the presentation had been prepared for the new kind of student entering college, one who had graduated from high school well prepared for the serious study of elementary nutrition. Although the approach used in that edition did not presuppose formal training in physiology and biochemistry, it did take into account the experience most high school students had had in dealing with the concepts of the biological and physical sciences. It was assumed that the students using the book had the capacity and the desire to achieve some in-depth appreciation of nutritional processes. To aid the students, basic concepts from the related sciences were outlined in the first chapter, and a glossary and a list of terms and meanings of prefixes and suffixes were included in the Appendix.

Experience has shown that the scope of this book is suited to the capabilities of such a student with no college training in science. It has also become evident that the level of presentation is equally valuable and suited to the needs of the student with a more sophisticated background. To reflect this usefulness to a wider audience, a change of title was considered. However, since the primary purpose of providing an in-depth introduction to the principles of nutrition to students at all levels of competence remains unchanged, the original title has been retained in the hope that the content, rather than the title, will determine its acceptance.

I hope that in mastering the material presented, the student will become a discerning consumer of nutrition information, with a comprehension of the basic principles adequate to enable him to discriminate the scientific from the pseudo-scientific and fact from fallacy in the vast literature of both the lay and the scientific press. In addition to developing his own understanding of nutrition, the student should be adequately prepared to interpret his knowledge of nutrition for the general public.

Another purpose of this book is to create awareness of the importance of nutrition in such a way that the student himself will be motivated to apply this knowledge in establishing good eating habits. It is also hoped that some students will be stimulated to continue the study of nutrition to acquire the level of competence needed to qualify them for the many challenging career opportunities in the field. The recent interest in the broad social and political implications of adequate nutrition has greatly expanded the horizons of the professional nutritionist.

An assessment of the advances in our knowledge of nutrition in the four years that have elapsed since the first edition indicates that nutritional biochemists, cell biologists, and physiologists have made significant contributions to our knowledge of metabolic processes. Many of their findings are beyond the scope of this presentation, but we have attempted to interpret those of greatest significance in the application of nutritional principles to the practical task of feeding people. For the most part, however, we have drawn on the studies of clinical nutritionists, who have focussed on the questions of metabolism and nutrient needs of the total organism. Many of them have emphasized the role of social, economic, and psychological factors as well as physiological and biochemical factors involved in the availability and utilization of nutrients. Again, as in the first edition, I have chosen to include mention of some of the more recent nutritional concepts and theories, with full recognition that they may need to be modified and perhaps even deleted from future editions.

The inclusion of a new final chapter dealing with the questions of hunger and malnutrition as national and international concerns reflects a growing interest in the social implication of sound nutrition. Recognition of the effect that even moderate degrees of undernutrition may have on mental as well as physical health and development points to the availability and safety of the food supply as crucial factors in national planning. At the same time, a sizeable portion of the population and certain of the readers of this book are being called upon to cope with the equally complex problems of overnutrition.

To an even greater extent than was true in the first edition, this edition was possible only through the encouragement and cooperation of a great many individuals, including the students and colleagues whose constructive criticism led to the clarification of many points, the scientists who consented to have their work reproduced or quoted, and the persons who helped with the clerical and other time-consuming aspects of preparing a manuscript. Again, my husband and three children have remained patient and supporting and should be given major credit for making this venture a reality.

Helen Andrews Guthrie

Contents

vii

viii Contents

PART I

Basic principles of
NUTRITION

1 | *Introduction*

The science of nutrition has been defined in many ways. Most simply it has been expressed as the science of nourishing the body properly or the analysis of the effect of food on the living organism. Yudkin chooses to define nutrition as the relationship between man and his food and implies the psychological and social as well as the physiological and biochemical aspects. Others have chosen to define it as a science devoted to the determination of the requirements of the body for food constituents both qualitatively and quantitatively and to the selection of food in kinds and in quantity to meet these requirements. The Council on Foods and Nutrition of the American Medical Association elaborates still further in declaring nutrition as "the science of food, the nutrients and other substances therein, their action, interaction, and balance in relation to health and disease and the processes by which the organism ingests, digests, absorbs, transports, utilizes and excretes food substances." Regardless of the basic definition, persons studying nutrition agree that they are concerned with the changes that occur in food and the way in which the body uses it from the time food is ingested until it is eventually incorporated into the body tissues, participates in biological reactions, or is excreted from the body. This includes the study of digestion, absorption, and transportation of nutrients to the cells and their metabolism within the many types of body cells. In addition, nutritionists are becoming increasingly concerned with the factors that determine what a person chooses to eat.

The nutrients in food with which nutrition is concerned are those chemical components of the food that perform one of three roles in the body: supply energy, regulate body processes, or promote the growth and repair of body tissue.

The science of nutrition is a relative youngster in the scientific community, having been recognized as a distinct discipline only in 1934 with the organization of the American Institute of Nutrition. By its very nature, a science relying on the techniques of the chemist and biologist, nutrition had to await the development of these other branches of science. Nutrition, like other sciences, does not stand alone. It draws heavily on the basic findings of chemistry, biochemistry, microbiology, physiology, medicine, and, most recently, cellular biology. In turn, it also contributes to these fields of scientific investigation.

HISTORICAL BACKGROUND

Although the organized study of nutrition has been confined to the twentieth century, there is evidence of a long-standing curiosity about the subject. A few well-conceived nutritional experiments were performed earlier, but these stimulated little interest. Schneider has very aptly divided the history of nutrition into three eras: the *naturalistic era* (400 B.C.-A.D. 1750), the *chemical-analytical era* (1750-1900), and the *biological era* (1900 to present). Running concurrently with the latter from 1955 to the present could be added the *cellular* or *molecular* era, in which emphasis has been directed to the study of nutrition within the highly organized individual cells.

Although no attempt will be made to discuss all the findings of each era, we will mention a few highlights to give some picture of the extent of the knowledge of nutrition in each stage.

Naturalistic era. During the naturalistic era people had many vague ideas about food, most of which revolved around taboos, magical powers, or medicinal value. Just as millions do today, early man considered food essential for survival and made little discrimination about the relative value of different foods. In Biblical times Daniel observed that men who ate pulse and drank water thrived better than did those who ate the king's food and drank wine. Hippocrates, the father of medicine, in his discussion of food in health and disease in 400 B.C. considered food one universal nutrient. He believed that weight loss during starvation was caused by insensible perspiration. By the sixteenth century a doctrine of diet and longevity had been well established.

In the early seventeenth century an Italian physician, Sanctorius, curious about the fate of food in the body, weighed himself before and after each meal. His only explanation of his failure to gain weight commensurate with the amount of food taken in was that there must be weight loss in insensible perspiration. It was during this period that such men as Harvey and Spallanzani, with their interest in circulation and digestion, made observations that eventually facilitated the study of nutrition. At the end of this era the first controlled nutrition experiment was carried out in 1747 by a British physician, Lind, who attempted to find a cure for scurvy by treating twelve sailors ill with the disease with six different substances. He determined that either lemon or lime juice was effective, while the others, such as oil of vitriol, seawater, or vinegar, were ineffective in curing this scorbutic condition.

Chemical-analytical era. The chemical-analytical era in the study of nutrition was initiated by Lavoisier, who became known as the father of nutrition. His work involved the study of respiration, oxidation, and calorimetry—all concerned with the use of food energy. His work with guinea pigs on the rate of uptake of oxygen with and without food and during work was the first investigation of the question of energy. Black and Priestley also contributed to the growing knowledge of respiration and energy metabolism. All these men worked in the eighteenth century.

Early in the nineteenth century, methods for determining carbon, hydrogen, and nitrogen in organic compounds were developed. Analyses of foods for these elements led Liebig to suggest that the nutritive value of foods was a function of its nitrogen content. He also postulated that an adequate diet must provide plastic foods (protein) and fuel foods (carbohydrate and fat). Dumas, a French chemist, tested this hypothesis during a siege of Paris in 1871. His efforts to produce a synthetic milk of carbohydrate, fat, and protein in the proportions believed to be found in cow's milk proved unsuccessful, and the infants to whom he fed it died. Dumas logically concluded that milk must contain some unknown nutritive substance.

A similar conclusion was reached in 1881 by Lunin, who found that mice fed a diet of purified casein (a protein), milk sugar (a carbohydrate), milk fat, and the inorganic ash from milk died, while those who were fed milk thrived. Between then and 1906 there were reports of twelve experiments on the use of purified diets in the feeding of animals. All led to essentially the same conclusion that the addition of "astonishingly" small amounts of natural foods was necessary to promote growth and to maintain health in the animals. Obviously food contained more than carbohydrate, fat, protein, and mineral ash, but the nature of the other substances remained a mystery. In spite of these findings the United States Department of Agriculture steadfastly maintained until 1910 that carbohydrate, fat, and protein were the only nutrients essential in the human diet.

By 1912 it had been well established that there was an additional dietary essential besides carbohydrate, fat, protein, and mineral ash. Funk, recognizing that this dietary component was essential to life *(vita)* and believing it to be *amine* or nitrogen containing, introduced the term *vitamine* to describe this elusive dietary factor. McCollum's work at the University of Wisconsin showing that some fats such as butter contained this essential growth factor, whereas others such as lard did not and Eijkman's observations that a water-soluble substance in rice bran prevented beriberi, a disease common in the Orient, made it clear that at least two vitamins, fat-soluble A and water-soluble B, were essential. By 1920 it was established that all vitamins did not contain nitrogen and the final "e" was dropped to obtain the term *vitamin,* which is still used.

In spite of the relatively slow communication in this period, scientists in Europe, Asia, and North America made rapid progress in identifying essential dietary components. Many times discoveries were made almost simultaneously by scientists working independently and in widely separated laboratories. The concept that diseases such as beriberi, scurvy, rickets, and pellagra, previously considered to be caused by toxic substances or to be infectious in nature, were in reality the result of an absence of nutrients needed in very small amounts did much to stimulate the attempts to identify the nature of these dietary essentials.

Biological era. The early part of the biological era was characterized by the discovery of many factors with vitamin-like properties. It soon became clear that there were several components of both fat-soluble A and water-soluble B. By 1940 four fat-soluble and eight water-soluble vitamins had been identified as essential elements of the human diet, and several others had

been identified for various species of animals. The chemical structure of each had been established, many had been synthesized, and knowledge of their biological roles was accumulating rapidly. Since 1940 only two essential vitamins, folic acid and vitamin B_{12}, have been identified. The emphasis in nutrition research has changed from a search for essential dietary components to a study of the interrelationship between nutrients, their precise biological roles, and the determination of human dietary requirements. More recently, interest has been directed toward the problems of nutrition education as the result of the widening gap between our theoretical knowledge of nutrition and its application in the improvement of nutritional status.

During this same period the noncombustible component, or mineral ash, of the diet was being studied, and it too proved to be a complex mixture of elements—seventeen of which have been established as dietary essentials for human beings. The essentiality of several others is still uncertain. Here again there was evidence of involved interrelationships among mineral elements; some were capable of replacing others, whereas a high intake of one could cause the excretion of another.

Cellular or molecular era. Since 1955 the development of the electron microscope, the ultracentrifuge, microchemical techniques, and the use of radioactive isotopes, has made it possible to study the nutritional needs and metabolism of the individual cells and even the subcellular components, or organelles, of the cell. At the present time a vast body of information is accumulating, which is leading to a more complete understanding of the intricacies of cell structure and the complex and vital role that nutrients play in the growth, development, and maintenance of the cell. Nourishment of the cell is basic to the nourishment of the collection of cells known as tissue, and this in turn is basic to the nourishment of organs of the body and ultimately of the whole complex body. Thus a defect in nutrition at the cellular level can adversely affect the health of the whole body. The study of the cell has stimulated interest in the role that genetics may play in influencing the nutritional needs of the organism.

Present status. We now find ourselves, less than a hundred years after the first studies that showed that more than carbohydrate, fat, and protein were necessary for normal growth and development, with a vast, complex, and rapidly expanding knowledge of at least thirty-five nutritional principles that must be supplied by food for normal body functioning. The absence of any one of these, regardless of the amount needed, can have a profound effect on the functioning of the whole body.

Although it is now twenty-three years since the discovery of the last vitamin, nutrition is a vital, exciting field in which new information is being accumulated at a phenomenal pace. The contributions of the nutritionist alone have been many and significant, but when one integrates with these the related findings of the biochemist, the physiologist, the biologist, and the physicist, one realizes that understanding the complexity of the process of nourishing the body is a challenging frontier of science that is only beginning to be explored.

The fact that scurvy, rickets, beriberi, pellagra, and kwashiorkor, all nutritional deficiency diseases, can be found in affluent and developing countries alike is stark evidence of our failure to apply what nutrition information we do have.

Many new approaches to the study of nutrition are emerging. The interaction of nutrition and genetics in the developmental process is providing an explanation for some congenital abnormalities and metabolic defects. The role of nutrition in brain development, behavior, resistance to infection, and stress and the role of environmental factors such as pollution on nutrition are but some of the newer concepts

being explored. As the biochemist becomes more concerned with the fine points of metabolism and less and less with the total organism, the nutritionist is turning much of his attention to the integration of the theoretical knowledge from many fields of study and to the application of this to the maintenance of health and the prevention and treatment of disease. Iatrogenic nutrition, which is concerned with nutritional disease resulting from the activities of a physician in treating a patient with drugs, surgery, or therapeutic diets, represents another new area of interest.

The rate at which the time, effort, and money expended on nutrition research increased after the concept of vitamins was first postulated can be judged by the number of scientific publications in the field. In 1913 there were four publications, all by Casimir Funk; by 1920 the number had risen to 73; and in 1930, 724 articles appeared. In 1970 a review of current literature on one of the vitamins, vitamin B_{12}, listed over 1300 references on this one topic. At least ten scientific journals are devoted entirely to reporting findings of nutrition research. In 1971 over 4000 papers dealing directly or indirectly with subjects of significance in nutrition will be presented at a single scientific meeting. The large number of investigators who consider nutrition their major interest is obvious from the number of members in scientific organizations devoted to nutrition and from their attendance at professional meetings. The Institute of Nutrition, whose membership is restricted to scientists who have made an outstanding contribution to the field, has over 1300 members. The year 1968 saw the beginning of a surge of public interest in nutrition in the United States. This was the result of the realization that hunger and malnutrition existed in the midst of plenty. The first White House Conference on Food, Nutrition, and Health, which convened in 1969, represented a concern on the part of the federal

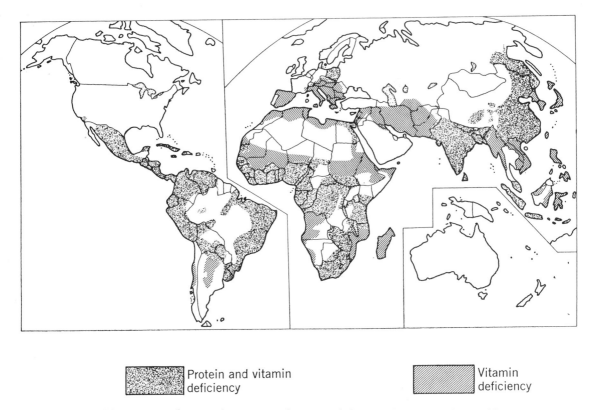

Protein and vitamin deficiency   Vitamin deficiency

Fig. 1-1. Distribution of protein- and vitamin-deficiency diseases in the world.

government that the problem be identified and that steps be taken to alleviate it.

The importance that political leaders attach to nutrition is best illustrated by the fact that the first agency authorized within the United Nations was the Food and Agricultural Organization, commonly known as FAO. In 1944 it was charged with the responsibility of devising ways to improve the nutritional status of the world's population as one of the major pathways to peace. Since then interest in international nutrition problems has increased rapidly. Numerous conferences are devoted to discussion of efforts to improve the nutritional status of the expanding populations of developing countries. The necessity of making maximum use of indigenous food products to provide a level of nutrition capable of supporting health and promoting individual productivity is an ever-present challenge to nutritionists. The worldwide incidence of nutritional deficiency diseases indicates the scope of the problem (Fig. 1-1).

IMPORTANCE OF GOOD NUTRITION

Before launching on an intensive study of the individual nutrients, the student of nutrition may legitimately ask, "What evidence is there that nutrition makes a difference?"

Although a comprehensive review of studies in this area is well beyond the scope of this text, a few examples may serve to illustrate the point.

A change from the use of poorly refined brown rice to more highly refined white rice with its improved keeping qualities occurred in the Philippines and other rice-eating countries around the turn of the century. With this change there was a marked increase in the incidence of the disease beriberi, which first was believed to be caused by a toxic substance in rice and later was attributed to unsanitary milling conditions. By 1935, however, an antiberiberi factor in rice bran had been identified, establishing that beriberi was the result of a lack of a nutrient that was apparently removed in the milling process. It became known as thiamin. Once this vitamin had been synthesized and was available commercially, the Philippine government and the Williams Waterman Fund backed a study of rice enrichment to determine the effect of adding thiamin back to the rice. People on one half of the island of Bataan ate rice enriched with thiamin, whereas those on the other half ate the unenriched milled white rice. After nine months of rice enrichment 90% of the population that had previously shown mild or definite signs of the disease were improved and the death rate had dropped by two thirds. At the end of the second year there were no deaths at

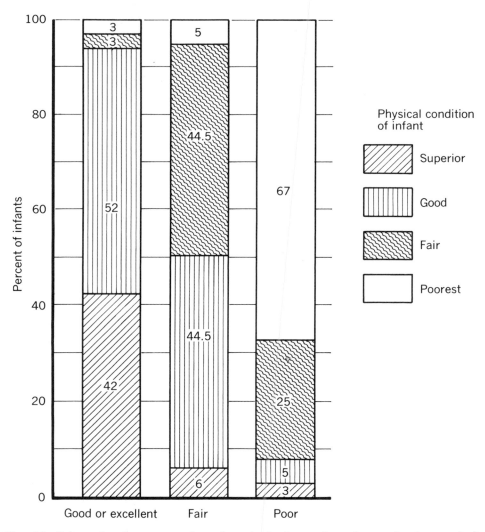

Fig. 1-2. Relationship between quality of mother's diet and condition of infant at birth. (Adapted from Burke, B. S.: J. Nutr. **38**:453, 1949.)

all from beriberi, indicating fairly clearly that the addition of a nutrient brought about a general improvement in the health and marked decrease in beriberi.

In 1946 Burke, working with patients at the Boston Lying-In Hospital at Harvard, studied the relationship between the quality of the diet of the mother during pregnancy and the health of the infant at the time of birth. Of the infants born to mothers whose diet was rated good or excellent, 94% were judged in superior or good physical condition at the time of birth, and only 6% were rated in fair or poor condition. Conversely, when the diet was assessed as poor, only 8% of the infants received a superior or good rating, whereas 92% were judged in fair or poor condition. These observations are illustrated in Fig. 1-2. Since people change food habits slowly even under conditions of high motivation such as pregnancy, the dietary ratings undoubtedly reflected longstanding patterns of eating rather than those that prevailed during pregnancy. Failure of subsequent studies to show such a clear-cut relationship may reflect an overall improvement of the diet of mothers as our knowledge of nutrition increases.

The reduction in the incidence of simple goiter experienced in Michigan after an intensive educational campaign on the use of iodized salt is further evidence of the differences between poor and adequate nutrition in respect to one nutrient. In a thirty-year period there was a drop from 47.2% to 1.4% in the reported cases of endemic goiter. Similarly, the addition of fluorine to drinking water has resulted in a 50% to 70% reduction in the incidence of tooth decay.

In Newfoundland a nutritional survey in 1945 revealed a high incidence of subclinical evidence of nutritional deficiency, such as rough dry skin, cracks in the corner of the lips, and soft bleeding gums. This was attributed to suboptimal intakes of the B vitamins, vitamin A, and ascorbic acid. A program of enriching flour with thiamin, riboflavin, niacin, and iron and enriching margarine with vitamin A resulted in a marked reduction in these conditions.

The change in stature of children in the United States that has occurred in the past few decades has been in part attributed to improved nutrition. There is ample evidence that children are heavier and taller than their parents. For instance, Philadelphia schoolchildren in first through fifth grades in all socioeconomic groups averaged 3 inches taller and 3 pounds heavier in 1951 than in 1925. In 1880, 5% of male college freshmen were over 6 feet tall, whereas in 1955, 30% reached this stature. Nutrition has undoubtedly contributed to this gain, but one must also keep in mind advances in other areas of medicine that have reduced the incidence of infection and other deterrents to maximum growth at an early age. Adult heights have not shown a comparable increase. The question is now being raised as to whether these increases in growth rate are necessarily desirable. Evidence from animal studies indicates a decrease in life-span among animals fed at a level to stimulate early and rapid growth. On the other hand, women over 5 feet 4 inches tall, possibly the better nourished members of the population, were found to have fewer complications during pregnancy and easier deliveries than did those under 5 feet tall.

HOW THE BODY USES FOOD

Food fulfills many roles for the individual. Its psychological value, its social significance, and its satiety value are more likely determinants of when, how much, and what foods are consumed than are nutritional considerations.

The role of food to which our interests will be directed primarily, however, is that of nourishing the body. Food chosen wisely provides all the nutrients essential for the normal functioning of the body. If food is not properly chosen, there will be a deficiency of one or more of the essential nutrients. An essential nutrient is considered one that must be provided to the organism by food, since it cannot be synthesized by the body at a rate sufficient to meet its needs. Nutrients essential for one species may not be essential for another.

Although we have a rapidly expanding body of information on the biological role of and the need for specific nutrients, the long-established broad classification of the function of nutrients in the body is still valid. The major functions are to supply energy, to promote growth and repair of body tissues, and to regulate body processes.

The nutrients that perform these functions may be divided into six main categories: carbohydrate, lipid, protein, minerals, vitamins, and water. Following is a classification of the nutrients in each of these broad groupings.

Carbohydrate
   Glucose

Fat or lipid
   Linoleic acid

Protein
   Amino acids*
      Leucine   Phenylalanine
      Isoleucine   Threonine
      Lysine   Trytophan
      Methionine   Valine
   Nonessential nitrogen

Minerals
      Calcium   Zinc
      Phosphorus   Manganese
      Sodium   Copper
      Potassium   Cobalt
      Sulfur   Molybdenum
      Chlorine   Iodine
      Magnesium   Chromium
      Iron   Fluorine
      Selenium

*Vitamins**
   Fat-soluble vitamins
      A   E
      D   K

---
*Chemical formulas are shown in Appendix H.

Vitamins—cont'd
   Water-soluble vitamins
      Thiamin   Pyridoxine
      Riboflavin   Cobalamin
      Niacin   Pantothenic acid
      Biotin   Ascorbic acid
      Folacin

Water

The nutrients listed are absolutely essential to human growth and maintenance. Some nutrients are present in a wide variety of foods in nature and there is little likelihood of deficiency occurring. On the other hand, some are distributed in a very limited number of foods and will be present in less than optimal amounts if the variety of foods in the diet is limited.

It is clear from the following classification of nutrients according to functions that some, such as protein, perform all three functions, whereas some of the minerals are involved in two functions, and vitamins, directly, only in one. A nutrient that performs only one function is equally as essential as one involved in all three functions.

Source of energy
   Carbohydrate
   Lipid
   Protein
   Minerals*
   Vitamins*

*Growth and maintenance
   of tissue*
   Protein
   Mineral elements
   Vitamins*
   Water*

*Regulation of body
   processes*
   Protein
   Mineral elements
   Vitamins
   Water

---
*These play an indirect role, since they are necessary to catalyze the use of the nutrients directly involved.

The amount of each of the essential nutrients needed for normal body functions bears no relationship to its importance in the diet. In the adult male, needs vary from $5 \mu g. \left(\frac{5}{28,000,000} \text{ ounce} \right)$ of cobalamin (vitamin B_{12}) to 65 gm. (2 ounces) of protein to as much as ¾ pound of carbohydrate, depending on his energy needs. A deficiency of a nutrient needed in extremely small amounts may precipitate more severe symptoms more rapidly than a deficiency of one needed in much larger amounts. Figs. 1-3 and 1-4 show effects of a severe or prolonged lack of a nutrient. It was the search for a cause and cure of diseases such as these that stimulated much of the early research in nutrition.

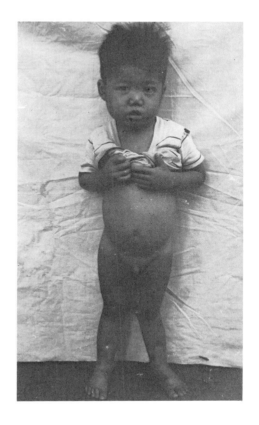

Fig. 1-3. Hidden hunger. This child, 4 years of age, looks plump enough. Closer inspection shows pitting edema of the legs caused by dietary protein deficiency and low serum albumin level. This is kwashiorkor (without dermatosis). The child is also dull, apathetic, potbellied, and has ophthalmic xerosis and Bitot's spots on the conjunctiva of both eyes. (Courtesy WHO Regional Office, Manila.)

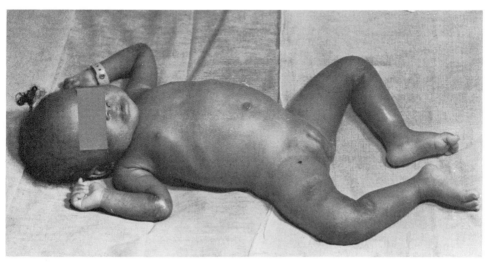

Fig. 1-4. Case of infantile scurvy caused by a lack of ascorbic acid (vitamin C). Note typical frog position, swelling of right thigh, and hyperpigmentation of skin. (From Ossofsky, H. J.: Amer. J. Dis. Child. **109:**173, 1965.)

Table 1-1. *Extent of body reserves of nutrients*

Nutrient	Time required to deplete reserves
Amino acids	Few hours
Carbohydrate	13 hours
Sodium	2-3 days
Water	4 days
Fat	20-40 days
Thiamin	30-60 days
Ascorbic acid	60-120 days
Niacin	60-180 days
Riboflavin	60-180 days
Vitamin A	90-365 days
Iron	125 days (women)
	750 days (men)
Iodine	1000 days
Calcium	2500 days

One factor that influenced the ease with which nutritional factors were identified was the rapidity with which body reserves are depleted in times of dietary deficiency. Table 1-1 shows that the time varies from a few hours in the case of labile amino acids, which the body has virtually no capacity to store, to about sixty days for many water-soluble vitamins, to seven years for calcium. The major site of storage differs with the nutrient—liver for iron, vitamin A, and carbohydrate, the adrenal gland for vitamin C, and bone for calcium. For some nutrients there is no storage site. In these cases, deficiency symptoms will become evident once the individual cells have become depleted of the nutrient.

The elucidation of the role of individual nutrients was further complicated by the interrelationship and interdependence that exists among the nutrients. For instance, the need for thiamin (vitamin B_1) is a function of the amount and kind of carbohydrate in the diet, the absorption of calcium is dependent on a supply of vitamin D, vitamin E protects vitamin A, and the nature and amount of fat in the diet affects the vitamin E requirement. Current re-

search is bringing forth even more evidence of the complexity of these interrelationships. Manipulation of one dietary component may lead to changes in the utilization or need of many others. Hence the evaluation of the results of manipulating one dietary factor depends on knowledge of the status of all other dietary factors.

BASIC CONCEPTS FROM RELATED SCIENTIFIC FIELDS

Although this treatment of introductory material basic to the understanding of nutrition does not presuppose any previous training in the related fields of biochemistry, physiology, and cellular biology, certain concepts from these fields will facilitate the understanding of the processes involved in nourishing the body. They are well within the grasp of any college student and will be presented here as an elementary review for those with previous instruction in these fields and as the bare fundamentals for those unfamiliar with the subject matter.

Physiology. Before the cells, the smallest structural units of the body, can receive nourishment, the food taken into the body in a complex state must undergo many changes to reduce it to a form in which it can be transported to and used by the cells. These changes occur primarily in the digestive tract of the body (Fig. 1-5). The digestive tract is essentially a tube passing through the center of the body; until food passes through the walls of this tube, it is, from a physiologic standpoint, still outside the body. The walls of the intestines regulate not only the form in which nutrients enter the body but also the amounts.

The process of digestion is accomplished by mechanical and chemical processes. Mechanically, food is broken down into small pieces by the action of chewing in the mouth. This increases the surface area on which the enzymes of the digestive juices can act. As the food mass passes down the digestive tract, peristalsis, the churning ac-

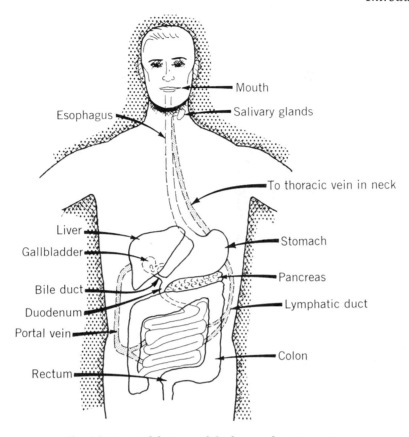

Fig. 1-5. Essential features of the human digestive system.

tion resulting from the contraction and relaxation of the very muscular wall of the tract, reduces the size of food particles still further and mixes them thoroughly with digestive juices.

Chemically the character of ingested food is changed by the action of digestive enzymes secreted in the salivary juice in the mouth, the gastric juice in the stomach, and the pancreatic juice, the intestinal juices, and the bile secreted into the small intestine. In addition, it now appears that some digestion, known as membrane digestion, occurs within the wall of the small intestine. Together these digestive juices provide all the enzymes necessary to prepare food for use by the body.

Once the food has been changed chemically into the simple form so that it is in the form in which the body can use it, it passes through the wall of the intestinal tract into the blood or lymph, by which it is carried to the body cells. Most absorption occurs through walls of the small intestine, but some also occurs in the stomach and large intestine, and a very little in the mouth. For some nutrients the passage through the intestinal wall is by diffusion, for others by osmosis, and for many by *active transport,* a process that requires energy and often a special carrier. In any case, the nature and amount of food that enters the body from the digestive tract is regulated in the intestinal wall.

After the digested food has passed through the wall of the digestive tract, it is picked up by one of two circulatory systems of the body—the arteriovenous, or

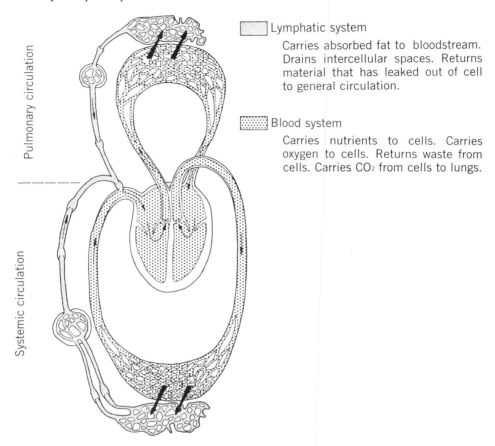

Pulmonary circulation

Systemic circulation

Lymphatic system

Carries absorbed fat to bloodstream. Drains intercellular spaces. Returns material that has leaked out of cell to general circulation.

Blood system

Carries nutrients to cells. Carries oxygen to cells. Returns waste from cells. Carries CO_2 from cells to lungs.

Fig. 1-6. Two circulatory systems, the blood and the lymphatic, are related in this schematic diagram. Oxygenated blood is pumped by the heart through a network of capillaries, bringing oxygen and nutrients to the tissue cells. Venous blood returns to the heart and is oxygenated in the course of the pulmonary (lung) circulation. Fluid and other substances seep out of the blood capillaries into the tissue spaces and are returned to the bloodstream by the lymph capillaries and larger lymphatic vessels. (From Mayerson, H. S.: Scient. Amer. **208**:80, June, 1963.)

blood, system or the lymphatic system. The relationship of these two systems is illustrated in Fig. 1-6. Nutrients that enter the arteriovenous system are carried by the portal vein to the liver, where they are released into the general circulatory system. In the circulatory system they are distributed through the arteries and very small blood vessels, the capillaries, and finally to the extracellular fluid bathing each individual cell of the body. Nutrients, primarily fats and fat-soluble nutrients that enter the lymphatic system (an auxiliary circulatory system that serves primarily to collect body fluids), bypass the liver and enter the general arteriovenous circulation at a point in the neck just before the blood enters the heart. From this point they are distributed to the cells in the same way as are nutrients that passed through the liver. It is from the extracellular fluids bathing the cells that the cell obtains the nutrients it needs. In this case the cell membrane acts as a selective barrier to the entrance of material into the cell.

The waste products of cellular metabolism are released into the extracellular fluid, enter the bloodstream, and are eventually excreted from the body, primarily through the lungs and kidneys.

The lungs serve as the main excretory organ for carbon dioxide and for much of the water. The kidney acts as a very efficient and selective filtering system for the bloodstream. It is capable of concentrating in the urine waste products of metabolism, such as creatinine and urea, and excreting them. It will also allow excesses of such nutrients as water-soluble vitamins to leave the body. However, for nutrients such as glucose, which the body needs to conserve, the kidney will resorb practically all that is present in the blood filtered through it. In the case of some other nutrients it will resorb the amounts needed to maintain normal blood and tissue levels and will release the rest. It is very sensitive to the needs of the body and will regulate the nature and amount of the metabolites excreted in response to the many regulatory forces that influence it. Some nutrients are also lost from the body through the skin—either in perspiration or in the sloughing of epithelial cells or the loss of hair and nails. Cells lining the intestinal tract are completely replaced every three to four days, the old ones being excreted in the feces. Fecal excretions may also contain nutrients that are part of the digestive juices, which are not reabsorbed. A determination of the kinds and amounts of nutrients lost from the body through any or all of these pathways sheds much light on the need for various nutrients and the way in which they are changed in the body.

Biochemistry. The nature of the nutrients and the chemical changes that occur in them from the time they are taken into the body until they are built into body tissue, are used, or are excreted is part of the subject matter of biochemistry—the chemistry of living material. All biological compounds contain the elements carbon and hydrogen, practically all contain oxygen, and they may have nitrogen, sulfur, or other inorganic elements.

Basic to any understanding of biochemistry is knowledge of the chemistry of carbon compounds. Carbon, an element capable of reacting with both positively and negatively charged elements, *always* has a valence of four, which means that there are four places on a carbon atom to which some other element is attached:

$$(1-\overset{\overset{4}{|}}{\underset{\underset{2}{|}}{C}}-3)$$

If two adjacent carbon atoms are unsaturated or do not have anything to attach to their carbon bonds, they will join together, forming what is known as a double bond:

$$(1-\overset{\overset{4}{|}}{C}=\overset{\overset{4}{|}}{C}-3)$$

This is a relatively unstable bond that is easily broken to two single bonds if some elements become available to attach to the bonds. Compounds that contain double carbon bonds are active chemically, since they are receptive to the addition of other elements.

In general, however, carbon compounds are relatively inert, reacting very slowly with each other, with water, and with oxygen.

About 99% of the body is made up of biological material whose basic chemical structure involves carbon compounds. These range from simple 2-carbon compounds such as acetic acid to the extremely large molecules of hormones and enzymes containing several hundred carbon atoms linked together in a straight chain, a branched arrangement, or a three-dimensional molecule. Some compounds are biologically active, undergoing constant and sometimes very rapid change, whereas others are relatively inert, changing slowly. A portion of the study of nutrition involves studying the nature and extent of the changes and the way in which various nutrients are involved in these changes. The biological material enters the body as carbohydrate, fat, protein, or vitamins and eventually is excreted through the lungs as carbon dioxide and water and in the urine as a variety of substances. The time elapsing between these two extremes may be a matter of seconds or a matter of years. In the interval they may be subjected to a few minor biochemical changes or a series of very complex biochemical actions and interactions. Thus, when we refer to changes involving a single carbon unit such as a methyl group (CH_3), we are speaking of one small molecule or a small portion of a molecule; when we talk of a long-chain carbon unit such as a peptide chain or a fatty acid, we may be referring to a large portion of a biological compound.

Biochemical compounds are subject to the same fundamental reactions that inorganic compounds undergo. Thus biochemical substances such as carbohydrate may unite with oxygen in a process called *oxidation* or combustion. The removal of a hydrogen atom has the same effect and is another way in which oxidation can occur. On the other hand, if hydrogen is incorporated, the substance is said to have been reduced or to have undergone hydrogenation. The removal of oxygen is also a reducing reaction. A compound that has been either reduced or oxidized will have physical, chemical, or biological properties that differ from the original compound. Nutritionally, the value of a nutrient may be completely destroyed or reduced by either oxidation or hydrogenation; in some cases the biological value of a nutrient is unaffected and in others it is enhanced.

In biochemical compounds the presence of an OH, or hydroxyl group, in a terminal position identifies the compound as an alcohol (comparable to hydroxide in inorganic compounds). When this is oxidized, it forms an aldehyde, —CHO, which can be further oxidized to an acid in which the terminal group is —COOH. This conversion of alcohol to aldehyde to acid by oxidation may be reversed by reduction reactions.

Other biochemical reactions to which a student of nutrition may be exposed are deamination, the removal of the amino group (NH_2) from a compound; transamination, the transfer of NH_2 from one compound to another; and transmethylation, the transfer of a methyl group (CH_3).

Cellular biology. The smallest unit of body structure is the cell, which occurs in many sizes and shapes in the body. Fig. 1-7 shows various types of cells that have specific characteristics, depending on the particular tissues of which they are a part. Discovery of the electron microscope has allowed scientists to determine a very definite structure within individual cells, indicating a high degree of organization of subcellular particles, or organelles. The use of the ultracentrifuge and various microchemical techniques has made possible the determination of the biochemical makeup of these organelles and has indicated definite biochemical specialization in these small subcellular units. Even the cell membrane has been determined as a highly structured, complex, and functional unit of the cell. Since many of the advances in nutrition are the result of the study of cellular nutrition and since popular publications are using these findings with increasing frequency, a familiarity with cell structure seems desirable for a student of nutrition. Just as there is no typical human, there is no typical cell. Each varies according to its function. Fig. 1-8, however, is a representation of the essential features of most cells.

Among the main organelles, or functional units, of the cell is the cell membrane, composed of protein and fat, which regulates the uptake of material from the external environment of the cell, the extracellular fluid. It also governs the release of material, either newly synthesized material or waste products from the cell. In a sense, it is the "doorkeeper" of the cell. Within the cell is

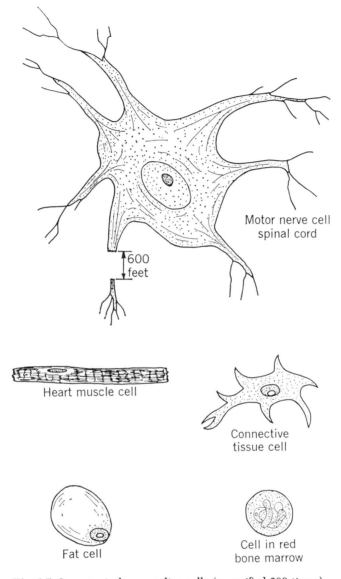

Motor nerve cell
spinal cord

600
feet

Heart muscle cell

Connective
tissue cell

Fat cell

Cell in red
bone marrow

Fig. 1-7. Some typical mammalian cells (magnified 200 times).

a mass of material, the cytoplasmic matrix, within which are several highly organized areas.

The mitochondrion, another double-membraned structure within the cell, contains upward of 500 enzymes involved in the release of energy from energy-yielding nutrients. Its vital role in energy metabolism has led to its designation as the powerhouse of the cell. The number of mitochondria within a cell varies, depending on the function of the cell, but in very active cells, such as those of liver or heart muscle, there may be as many as 1000.

Lysosomes contain the digestive enzymes of the cell and serve to digest particles that may enter the cell in a form that must be changed before they can be used. Lyso-

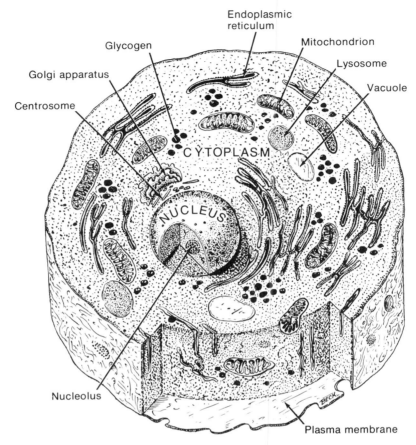

Fig. 1-8. Diagrammatic representation of a typical cell. (From Tuttle, W. W., and Schottelius, B. A.: Textbook of physiology, ed. 16, St. Louis, 1969, The C. V. Mosby Co.)

somes are capable of digesting complex substances in the cytoplasm of the cell and releasing them as their simple components into the cytoplasm again. If released from their membranes, the enzymes of the lysosomes are capable of digesting the cell itself. This occurs at the death of the cell.

Throughout the cytoplasm is a network of canals, some of which are lined with small granules. The canals are known as endoplasmic reticulum and serve as communication channels within the cell and between cells. The small granules are microsomes, or ribosomes, in which the synthesis of protein within the cell occurs. Those with ribosomes attached are identi-

fied as rough endoplasmic reticulum, whereas those without the protein-synthesizing mechanism are known as the smooth endoplasmic reticulum. The latter may be involved in hormone synthesis.

In the center of the cell, separated from the cytoplasm by a membrane, is the nucleus. The nucleus contains the genetic information that allows the cell to reproduce in the pattern of the parent cell. The code contained in the genetic material deoxyribonucleic acid (DNA), is transmitted through the nuclear membrane to the ribosomes by another nucleic acid, messenger ribonucleic acid (RNA), produced in the nucleolus of the nucleus.

SELECTED REFERENCES

Crane, R. K.: A perspective of digestive-absorptive function, Amer. J. Clin. Nutr. **22**:242, 1969.

Goldblith, S. A., and Joslyn, M. A., editors: Milestones in nutrition, Westport, Conn., 1964, AVI Publishing Co.

Goldsmith, G. A.: Clinical nutritional problems in the United States today, Nutr. Rev. **23**:1, 1965.

Griffith, W. H.: Food as a regulator of metabolism, Amer. J. Clin. Nutr. **17**:391, 1965.

Hegsted, D. M.: Nutritional requirements in disease, J. Amer. Diet. Ass. **56**:303, 1970.

Hurley, L. S.: Nutrients and genes: interactions and development, Nutr. Rev. **27**:3, 1969.

King, C. G.: Notes on the history of nutrition in America, J. Amer. Diet. Ass. **56**:188, 1970.

McCollum, E. V.: A history of nutrition, Boston, 1957, Houghton Mifflin Co.

Ross, M. L.: The long view, J. Amer. Diet. Ass. **56**:295, 1970.

Schneider, H.: What has happened to nutrition? In Ingle, D. J., editor: Life and disease, New York, 1963, Basic Books, Inc., Publishers.

Sebrell, W. H.: Changing concepts of malnutrition, Amer. J. Clin. Nutr. **20**:653, 1969.

Todhunter, E. N.: Development of knowledge in nutrition. I. Animal experiments. II. Human experiments, J. Amer. Diet. Ass. **41**:328, 335, 1962.

Todhunter, E. N.: Some classics of nutrition and dietetics, J. Amer. Diet. Ass. **44**:100, 1964.

Todhunter, E. N.: The evolution of nutrition concepts, J. Amer. Diet. Ass. **46**:120, 1965.

Youmans, J. B.: Changing face of nutritional diseases in America, J.A.M.A. **189**:672, 1964.

Yudkin, J.: Disagreement, Nutr. Today 3(3):25, 1969.

2 | Carbohydrate

Carbohydrate, an energy-yielding nutrient, is the largest single component, aside from water, of most diets, about two thirds of a pound of carbohydrate being present in a 2400-kilocalorie (kcal.) diet. Carbohydrates are identified by most people as starches and sugars. They provide slightly less than half the calories in the typical American diet. Carbohydrates make up about three fourths of the plant world on which animal life depends for food. In the last sixty years the total consumption of carbohydrate in the United States has declined by at least 25%. At the same time, the consumption of sugar has increased by 25%, which means, of course, that sugar represents an increasing proportion and starch a decreasing proportion of the carbohydrate intake.

Since carbohydrate foods are easy to grow, can be stored with a minimum of deterioration, and have a high energy yield per unit of land, they are relatively inexpensive sources of energy. As a result, when the amount of money available for food is restricted, the proportion of carbohydrate foods in the diet increases. Although refined carbohydrates contribute little other than calories to the diet, the less refined products may make substantial contributions of other nutrients.

Carbohydrate was one of the first nutrients to be chemically identified, yet only now is evidence appearing to indicate that it is essential in human nutrition. It is a compound composed of the three elements carbon, hydrogen, and oxygen. The ratio of hydrogen to oxygen in all carbohydrates is 2 to 1, the same ratio found in water—hence the term *carbohydrate*. In simple carbohydrates there are equal numbers of carbon and oxygen atoms ($C_nH_{2n}O_n$); for complexes of two or more simple carbohydrates there is one less oxygen atom than carbon atoms ($C_n[H_2O]_{n-1}$). It is as carbohydrate that green plants store the energy they derive from the sun.

SYNTHESIS

Plants with green leaves are able to trap the radiant energy of the sun and through a process known as photosynthesis store it as chemical energy. This process is essential for the continuation of life. As shown in Fig. 2-1, the carbon dioxide of the atmosphere and water from the soil are picked up by the plant and combined in the presence of chlorophyll, the magnesium-containing pigments of plants, to form an energy-rich carbohydrate—either starch or sugar. In some plants, such as potatoes, wheat, and rice, the carbohydrate is in the form of starch; in others, such as sweet peas, bananas, cherries, and sugar beets, it is in the form of sugar. In peas and corn, carbohydrate is stored initially as sugar and is changed to starch as the seed matures. The sweetness of carrots also declines as the sugar in the root is converted to starch with aging. On the other hand, starch in fruits such as bananas, apples, and pears is converted to sugar during the ripening process. Regardless of the form in which it is stored or whether it is stored in the root, leaf, seed, or fruit of the plant, carbohydrate represents the reserve of energy for the plant.

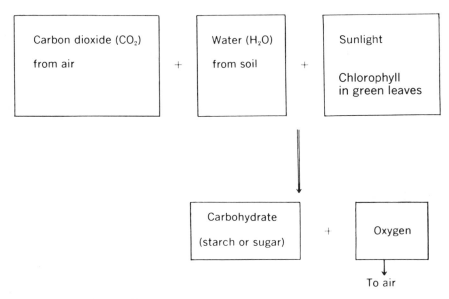

Fig. 2-1. Process of photosynthesis.

CLASSIFICATION

Monosaccharides. The simplest structural unit of carbohydrates is a monosaccharide. This is the chemical building block from which all more complex carbohydrates are built. Most of the monosaccharides are also known as hexoses, since they are composed of a 6-carbon chain to which hydrogen and oxygen atoms are attached as hydrogen or hydroxyl (OH) groups. There are three monosaccharides of importance in nutrition—*glucose, fructose,* and *galactose.* A fourth, *mannose,* has limited significance in human nutrition, since it is found in food to a limited extent and only in poorly digested complexes. It has been used, however, in intravenous feedings. All hexoses contain the same number and kinds of atoms—6 carbon atoms, 12 hydrogen atoms, and 6 oxygen atoms ($C_6H_{12}O_6$). They differ from one another only in the way in which the hydrogen and oxygen atoms are arranged around the chain of carbon atoms. The differences in monosaccharides can be observed from the following formulas:

O ‖ C—H | H—C—OH | HO—C—H | H—C—OH | H—C—OH | H—C—OH | H	H | H—C—OH | C=O | HO—C—H | H—C—OH | H—C—OH | H—C—OH | H	O ‖ C—H | H—C—OH | HO—C—H | HO—C—H | H—C—OH | H—C—OH | H	O ‖ C—H | HO—C—H | HO—C—H | H—C—OH | H—C—OH | H—C—OH | H
Glucose	*Fructose*	*Galactose*	*Mannose*

(Boxed areas are where structure differs from glucose.)

These different arrangements of atoms within the carbohydrate molecule account for the variation in sweetening power, solubility, and other properties of the different monosaccharides. One method of identifying sugars involves passing a beam of polarized light through a solution of the sugar. On the basis of its effect on polarized light, glucose, which causes the light to rotate to the right, has been named dextrose. A fructose solution, on the other hand, causes polarized light to rotate to the left. Hence fructose is known as levulose.

Monosaccharides occur in fruits and in some vegetables, accounting for 1% to 16% of their weight. Both glucose and fructose are found in honey. Fructose is present in many syrups. It is found in fetal blood and amniotic fluid but otherwise does not occur in animal tissue. So far no food has been found that contains galactose. It does occur as a component of the more complex carbohydrates in milk and the seed coat of legumes. Monosaccharides are usually derived from the digestion, or breakdown, of more complex carbohydrates.

Glucose is sometimes referred to as blood sugar, since it is the only carbohydrate found in the general circulation of the body, where it occurs in both the blood plasma and the red blood cells. The total amount of glucose in blood and extracellular tissue is estimated at 17 gm. in an adult male. Normal fasting blood glucose levels are about 100 mg. per 100 ml. of blood. The level usually rises following a meal and falls gradually until it hits the fasting level, which is usually associated with the onset of hunger. When levels rise above 160 mg. per 100 ml., the condition is known as hyperglycemia; when they fall below 80 mg., hypoglycemia results. If blood glucose levels get so high that the kidney, which normally prevents the loss of sugar from the body, cannot resorb it, sugar appears in the urine. This occurs in diabetes mellitus.

Glucose can be reduced to an alcohol sugar, sorbitol. Sorbitol, with a sweetening power equivalent to glucose, has been used in some weight-reducing aids on the theory that the body cannot utilize it. It now appears the body can use it, but because of the slow rate at which it is absorbed, it helps keep blood sugar levels high after a meal and delays the onset of hunger sensations. It has been found in many fruits and vegetables.

Mannitol, another alcohol sugar used as a drying agent in some foods, has a sweetening power similar to glucose, but because it is only partially absorbed yields only half as many calories per gram as other carbohydrates. It is found in pineapple, olives, asparagus, carrots, and sweet potatoes.

Some 5-carbon sugars, pentoses, are found occasionally in plants but do not represent an appreciable source of dietary carbohydrate. Ribose, arabinose, and xylose are the most common. In the body, ribose is part of some vital body compounds, such as the riboflavin-containing enzymes and nucleic acids in the nucleus and cytoplasm of the cell. The body can produce ribose from glucose and so does not depend on a dietary source of 5-carbon sugars to form the essential nucleic acids.

Disaccharides. More common in foods are the disaccharides, which are each composed of two monosaccharide units. When two monosaccharides are joined to form a disaccharide, one molecule of water is split off. Conversely, when a disaccharide is broken into its two component monosaccharide units, as occurs in digestion, a molecule of water must be added in a process known as hydrolysis. Thus we have a reversible reaction (see top of p. 23).

The most common disaccharide, *sucrose,* a combination of glucose and fructose, is a familiar item in the diet. Granulated sugar is 100% sucrose. Brown sugar, the slightly less refined, more flavorful product of either beet or cane sugar, is 97% sucrose. The

$$C_6H_{12}O_6 \quad + \quad C_6H_{12}O_6 \quad \xleftarrow{\hspace{1cm} (1) \hspace{1cm}} \quad C_{12}H_{22}O_{11} \quad + \quad H_2O$$

Monosaccharide + Monosaccharide $\xrightarrow{\hspace{1cm} (2) \hspace{1cm}}$ Disaccharide + Water

(1) *Hydrolysis*
(2) *Synthesis*

world consumes 30 million tons of sucrose a year, two thirds of it coming from sugar cane and one third from beet sugar. Both cane and beet sugars yield far more calories per acre of land than any other crop. The consumption of sucrose in the American diet continues to increase and is believed to be a contributing factor to the high incidence of tooth decay.

Lactose, which accounts for one tenth of the total dietary carbohydrate, is a combination of glucose and galactose. It is found only in milk, where it makes up half the total solids. Sometimes known as milk sugar, it was first identified in 1633 and is the major source of the monosaccharide galactose. In the intestine certain microorganisms cause the production of lactic acid from any unabsorbed lactose. This increased acidity in the lower intestinal tract creates a medium in which the organism *Lactobacillus bifidus* grows to produce the *bifidus factor* believed to be beneficial to very young infants in preventing the growth of the less desirable bacteria that cause intestinal putrefaction. This factor is found primarily in the intestines of breast-fed infants, and its presence has been identified as one of the advantages of breast-feeding infants over bottle-feeding. Evidence has been compiled that a relatively soluble calcium-lactose complex increases the extent to which calcium is absorbed or that lactose increases the permeability of the intestinal membrane to ions such as calcium. Whatever the mechanism, it is interesting to note that the best source of lactose and of calcium in the diet is the same food—milk.

Maltose, the third disaccharide, is found in germinating cereals. It is composed of two molecules of glucose.

All members of the monosaccharide group and disaccharide group are considered sugars, as indicated by the suffix *-ose.*

Sugars differ in their sweetening power, as shown in Table 2-1. The sweetening power of sugar parallels its solubility. Fructose, with the greatest sweetening power, is most soluble and therefore difficult to crystallize from a solution and to obtain in crystalline form. This makes it useful in syrups but also means that the small amount of fructose available in crystalline form is expensive. Lactose, which is relatively insoluble, is difficult to incorporate in a solution and hence is not practical as a sweetening agent for liquids.

Polysaccharides. The third group of carbohydrates, the polysaccharides, are much more complex and are considered starches rather than sugars. They represent about half of the dietary carbohydrate. They are composed solely of glucose units linked together in long chains. A polysaccharide may contain as many as 2000 glucose units, which may be in one long chain (an amylose) or in a branched arrangement (an amylopectin), as illustrated:

$$G\text{—}G\text{—}G\text{—}G\text{—}G\text{—}G\text{—}G\text{—}G\text{——}G_n$$

Amylose

$$
\begin{array}{c}
G\text{—}G\text{—}G\text{—}G\text{—}G\text{————}_n \\
\quad\ G \qquad\qquad G \\
G \qquad\qquad\quad G \\
\qquad\qquad\qquad G\text{————}_n
\end{array}
$$

Amylopectin

Table 2-1. Comparison of physical properties of carbohydrates (relative values)

Monosaccharides	Sweetening power	Soluble	Rate of absorption
Hexoses			
Glucose	74	Yes	100
Fructose	173	Yes	30
Galactose	32	Yes	110
Mannose			10
Alcohol sugars			
Sorbitol	54	Yes	
Mannitol		Slightly	
Pentoses			
Ribose	—	Yes	
Xylose	40	Yes	15
Arabinose	—	Yes	9
Disaccharides			
Sucrose	100	Yes	
Lactose	16	Yes	
Maltose	33	Yes	
Polysaccharides			
Starch		No	
Dextrin		Slightly	
Glycogen		No	
Cellulose		No	

The number of glucose units and their arrangement within the molecule determine the characteristics of the starch. Each plant deposits a starch characteristic of its species. Granules of potato starch can thus be distinguished from granules of rice, wheat, cassava, corn, or any other starch by microscopic examination of the shape and size of the granule. In addition, each of these starches has unique properties in regard to solubility, thickening power, and flavor. Nutritionally the body does not discriminate among starches but is able to break them all into their component glucose units for absorption and utilization by the body cells.

The animal stores a limited amount of carbohydrate as the polysaccharide *glycogen*. It is stored primarily in liver and muscle, the only two animal tissues, aside from milk and blood, that contain carbohydrate. The adult male stores only about ¾ pound of glycogen—¼ pound as liver glycogen and ½ pound as muscle glycogen. The energy thus stored represents only enough energy to last an adult male about half a day. When excess calories are consumed in the form of carbohydrate, the capacity of the liver and muscle to store glycogen may increase as much as 100%. This is the basis of the recommendation by athletic coaches that sprinters and others who need a large amount of energy in a short period of time can increase their glycogen reserves by first depleting them and then eating substantial amounts of carbohydrate before a competition. Reserves are depleted when a diet low in carbohydrate is consumed during a period of high-energy needs. Adipose or fat tissues may show evidence of increased carbohydrate content under such circumstances, but they will soon convert it to fat for more permanent storage in these tissues. There is virtually no glycogen in liver or muscle as they are eaten, since most is converted into lactic acid at the time of slaughtering.

Dextrin, another nutritionally important

Table 2-2. Carbohydrate content of foods*

Food	Total carbohydrate	Fiber
	gm./100 gm. food	
Sugar, granulated	99.5	0
Sugar, brown	96.4	0
Cornstarch	87.6	0.1
Raisins	77.4	0.9
All-purpose flour	76.1	0.3
Macaroni, dry	75.2	0.3
Chocolate fudge	75.0	0.2
Maple syrup	65.0	—
Enriched white bread	50.5	0.2
Whole wheat bread	47.7	1.6
Muffins	42.3	0.1
Rice, coated	24.2	0.1
Macaroni, cooked	23.0	0.1
Potatoes, baked	21.1	0.6
Bananas	22.2	0.5
Ice cream	20.6	0.8
Lima beans, cooked	19.8	1.8
Corn, cooked	18.8	0.7
Grapes	15.7	0.6
Apple, not pared	14.5	1.0
Ginger ale	8.0	—
Beans, green	7.1	1.0
Cabbage	5.4	0.8
Beef liver	5.3	0
Whole milk	4.9	0
Oysters, raw	3.4	0
Pears, cooked	2.0	0.6

*Based on Watt, B. K., and Merrill, A. L.: Composition of foods—raw, processed and prepared, U. S. Department of Agriculture Handbook No. 8, Washington, D. C., 1963, U. S. Department of Agriculture.

polysaccharide, is the slightly soluble product resulting from the initial breakdown of a starch when the very long glucose chains are split into shorter chains by the orderly removal of maltose units. This may be accomplished by enzymes, as occurs during digestion, or by action of dry heat on starch, such as in toasting bread or browning flour. In either case the resulting dextrin is sweeter and more soluble than the original starch. A starch hydrolysate, dextromaltose, is often used in infant feeding, since it helps prevent the formation of a heavy curd in the infant's stomach and does not ferment readily.

Cellulose, which is also composed of many glucose units linked in a slightly different manner from starch units, is an important dietary constituent. It accounts for 50% of all carbon in vegetables and is the most abundant organic compound in the world. Cellulose is the structural framework of plant tissue, and the body lacks the enzyme necessary to break its monosaccharide linkages. This indigestible residue then contributes bulk to the diet and is important in maintaining intestinal motility. A minimum of 100 mg. of fiber per kilogram of body weight per day is needed to stimulate normal intestinal motility and to favor normal elimination. Ruminants have a bacterial enzyme system capable of fermenting cellulose linkages, which explains their ability to exist on grasses and forage crops composed largely of cellulose, whereas human beings cannot. This fermentation produces short-chain fatty acids used for energy and a useless gas, methane. Table 2-2 includes the fiber content of several foods. Newer procedures for determining fiber indicate that actual values may be several times as high as these currently accepted figures. If the cellulose content of the diet is very high, it may have an adverse effect on the absorption of other nutrients by speeding the passage of food through the intestinal tract. Methyl cellulose, a synthetic product, is being used commercially in the preparation of low-calorie products. It can be used to simulate foods such as mayonnaise, cookies, or candy without providing energy.

Related carbohydrates. Mucopolysaccharides and mucoproteins are a group of compounds that are extremely important body constituents; they occur in the body but are not found in food. Mucopolysaccharides are complex combinations of two or more compounds, one of which is a carbohydrate. Many consist of loose combinations of amino sugars with protein. Some of the common mucopolysaccharides are hyaluronic acid, present in the fluid lubricating the joints and the vitreous humor of the eyeball; chondroitin sulfate in cartilage, skin, and bone; heparin, an anticoagulant; and keratosulfate, found in hard structures such as nails. Mucoproteins such as the protein in eggs and some hormones are more tightly bound polysaccharides and proteins.

DIGESTION

Before carbohydrate can fulfill its established roles in the body it must be con-

verted into sufficiently small units to pass through the walls of the intestine into the bloodstream. The monosaccharides are the only units that normally cross the intestinal membrane. The process by which complex carbohydrates are reduced to their component monosaccharide units is digestion. Virtually all these changes are brought about by starch-splitting enzymes—*amylases*.

The amylases are present in three digestive juices—the saliva in the mouth and the pancreatic and intestinal juices in the small intestine. The salivary amylase of the saliva, which mixes with the food in the mouth, acts on the starch in a slightly alkaline medium to convert it to simpler carbohydrates, usually dextrins. If it remains in contact with the saliva sufficiently long before being acidified by the hydrochloric acid secreted in the stomach, the starch may be split as far as the disaccharide maltose. As much as 75% of potato starch may be digested by salivary amylase before it is inactivated by gastric acidity. Virtually no digestion of starch occurs in the stomach, which possesses no starch-splitting enzyme. Some sucrose, in the presence of hydrochloric acid secreted in the stomach, may undergo acid hydrolysis to glucose and fructose. From the stomach the digestive mass passes to the small intestine, where alkaline secretions neutralize the hydrochloric acid and create the slightly alkaline medium necessary for the action of the starch-splitting enzymes secreted into the small intestine. Pancreatic amylase attacks complex carbohydrates and converts them into the disaccharide, maltose. The final conversion of sucrose to fructose and glucose is accomplished by intestinal sucrase, of maltose to two glucose molecules by intestinal maltase, and of lactose to glucose and galactose by intestinal lactase. The long-standing belief that these enzymes act within the intestinal cavity is now being questioned. Evidence is appearing to indicate that these enzymes are not secreted into the intestinal cavity but remain in the

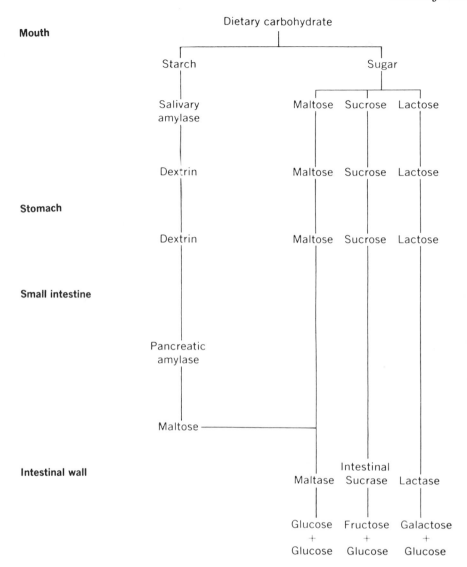

Fig. 2-2. Summary of digestion of carbohydrate.

membrane of the cells lining the intestinal cavity, where they accomplish the ultimate conversion of the disaccharides to the monosaccharides.

The digestibility of carbohydrates varies with the source but ranges from 90% to 98% for most foods. The digestion of carbohydrate is summarized in Fig. 2-2.

ABSORPTION AND TRANSPORTATION

Monosaccharides pass freely across the walls of the villi, the small fingerlike projections lining the intestinal tract, but the rate varies with the sugar. Galactose is absorbed slightly faster than glucose, whereas fructose is absorbed at less than half the rate. The rate of absorption tends to decrease with time, to increase with increase in concentration of the carbohydrate solution, and to increase in the presence of the hormones insulin, secreted by the pancreas, and thyroxin, secreted by the thyroid glands. From the intestinal wall the monosaccharides accumulate in the small blood vessels that eventually carry them to the portal vein. This large blood vessel carries the absorbed monosaccharides to the liver where two paths may be followed by the monosaccharides glucose, fructose, and galactose. They may all be converted into glycogen up to the capacity of the liver to store glycogen, or the galactose and fructose may be converted to glucose and along with the absorbed glucose may be released to the bloodstream to be carried to various cells of the body. In muscle cells some glucose may be stored as muscle glycogen. Most glucose, however, will be used as an immediate source of energy for the cells. The nerve and lung cells depend entirely on glucose as a source of energy, since they are unable to utilize other energy-yielding nutrients.

METABOLISM

The liver releases carbohydrate as glucose to the bloodstream at a rate to maintain a minimum level of 100 mg. of glucose per 100 ml. of blood. After a meal, the level of glucose may rise considerably above this but drop again as it is withdrawn by the cells. The difference between blood sugar levels in arterial and venous blood, Δ-glucose, is believed to influence the appetite-regulating mechanism, the hypothalamus of the brain. A small difference, representing depletion of blood glucose reserves, triggers the appetite. A large difference, showing an available supply of blood sugar, leads to a depressed appetite.

Glucose released from the liver is carried by the bloodstream to all tissues of the body. Here the individual cells take up the glucose through a carrier system in the cell membrane. Once within the cell, the glu-

cose is oxidized to pyruvic acid. Then in the mitochondrion the energy stored in the carbohydrate is released to supply energy for the many needs of the body, such as heat, muscle contraction, synthesis of essential compounds, and conduction of nerve impulses. Within the mitochondrion are concentrated the many enzymes necessary for the orderly and slow release of energy from glucose in the form of adenosine triphosphate (ATP). Once the energy of glucose has been released, the other end products of carbohydrate metabolism, carbon dioxide and water, are released from the cell and are eventually excreted from the body.

STORAGE

When carbohydrate is supplied in the diet and monosaccharides are absorbed beyond the body's immediate needs for energy and its capacity to store glycogen, they cannot be excreted but must be converted into a form in which to be stored in the body. The body has an unlimited capacity to store fat. It also has the ability to convert extra carbohydrate into fat. This conversion of glucose to fatty acids occurs primarily in the microsomes of the liver. The glucose molecule is broken down into 2-carbon fragments that are then synthesized into fatty acids. These are transported in the bloodstream to the adipose tissue cells, where they combine with a 3-carbon compound, glycerol, also derived from glucose, to form fat.

The digestion and metabolism of carbohydrate is summarized schematically in Fig. 2-3. It is clear that carbohydrate in food can be used in one of three ways in the body:

1. Metabolized or oxidized immediately as a source of energy
2. Converted into glycogen and stored as liver glycogen or muscle glycogen when carbohydrate intake exceeds the amount needed immediately for energy

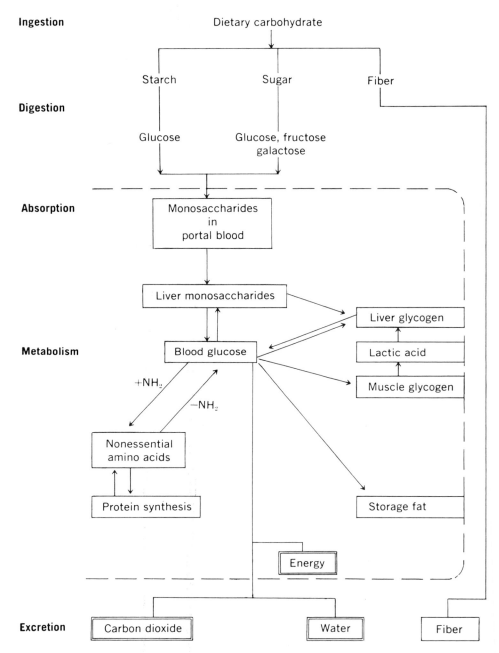

Fig. 2-3. Summary of carbohydrate digestion and metabolism. Double-boxed items are end products of metabolism. Changes within dotted line occur after absorption and before excretion.

3. Converted into fat and stored as a reserve of energy as fat in regular cells or in special adipose cells when the carbohydrate intake exceeds the amount needed immediately for energy and when the limited glycogen reserves are saturated

The eventual end products of carbohydrate metabolism are carbon dioxide, water, and energy. The period of time elapsing between the intake of carbohydrate and its excretion as carbon dioxide and water may range from a few minutes to a few hours to several months.

FUNCTIONS

Source of energy. The major function of carbohydrate is as a source of energy. This function is not unique to carbohydrate, although carbohydrate is the least expensive source of energy. Nervous tissue and lung tissue can use only glucose as a source of fuel, but since glucose can be produced from part of the fat molecule and from some amino acids in a process called *gluconeogenesis,* even these tissues can get along without dietary carbohydrates. When blood glucose levels fall, the brain is deprived of glucose, its only source of energy, and reacts by firing off uncontrolled and uncoordinated impulses that produce the symptoms of convulsions.

The amount of energy provided by carbohydrate is almost constant for all forms. One gram of carbohydrate provides 4 kcal. of energy regardless of the source—starch, sugar, monosaccharides, or disaccharides. In the typical American diet in 1966 carbohydrate provided slightly less than 50% of the total calories. The proportion from starches has declined from 31% to 24%, and that from sugar has increased between 1930 and 1962. The amount of carbohydrate tends to increase with a decrease in the amount of money available to spend on food, since it is a much less expensive source of calories than protein or fat. In some countries, such as Japan and Indonesia, where rice or cassava is the staple in the diet, as much as 80% to 85% of the calories come from carbohydrate. At the other extreme, carbohydrate provides only 8% of the energy in the high-fat diet of Eskimos. Since the caloric value of carbohydrate is the same from all sources, when a sauce can be thickened with half as much cornstarch as wheat starch it will have half the calories from starch. Similarly a sugar with high sweetening power will contribute the same degree of sweetness with less sugar and fewer calories than one of low sweetening power. Conversely, the use of a starch with a low thickening power and a sugar with a low sweetening power may help step up the caloric value of a diet without appreciably changing its character.

Dietary essential—an unexplained role. Although carbohydrate can be replaced by fat and protein as a source of energy, recent evidence indicates that a diet devoid of carbohydrate produces many undesirable symptoms. Persons on a diet of protein and fat very rapidly develop the same symptoms as persons on a starvation regimen. They lose very large amounts of sodium, are unable to prevent the breakdown of body protein except at very high levels of protein intake, and develop ketosis from the accumulation in the blood and urine of abnormal products of fat metabolism by the second day of a carbohydrate-free diet. The subjects all experience loss of energy and fatigue. All these undesirable results of a lack of carbohydrate in the diet are reversed by the addition of carbohydrate, which would indicate that carbohydrate is a dietary essential. No evidence has been compiled whether the need is for any carbohydrate, specifically for one group such as monosaccharides, disaccharides, or polysaccharides, or for a specific carbohydrate. Persons on a diet lacking in carbohydrate experience as rapid a loss of weight as do persons subjected to total starvation. It should be pointed out, however, that diets are seldom devoid of carbohydrate and that intakes as low as 60 gm. will prevent these undesirable symptoms.

Carbohydrates or products derived from them also serve as precursors of vital body compounds, such as nucleic acids and connective tissue matrix.

FOOD SOURCES

Carbohydrate is found almost exclusively in foods of plant origin. Milk, with its high lactose content, is the only important source of animal carbohydrate. Human milk contains considerably more lactose (7%) than cow's milk (4.8%). Eggs contain a very small amount, and scallops and oysters are the only other animal tissues that contain carbohydrate. The small amount in the liver is almost all converted to pyruvic and lactic acids during the slaughtering process.

Table 2-2 shows some typical sources of carbohydrate. The figures for total carbohydrate include the utilizable sugars and starches and the nondigestible cellulose, or fibers. The values for fiber content represent the best currently available but may be low. When tables of food composition are used to determine the utilizable carbohydrate in the diet, the values for fiber should be subtracted from those for total carbohydrate.

It is noted that some foods, such as sugar and cornstarch, are high in carbohydrate. Others, such as the potato and rice, commonly considered carbohydrate foods, contain a much lower percentage of carbohydrate. Most of the caloric content of the foods listed in Table 2-2 is derived from carbohydrate.

The range in the amount of carbohydrate in fruits and vegetables is evident. Persons who must regulate the carbohydrate content of their diets are well aware of the classification of fruits and vegetables into exchange lists based on the carbohydrate content. The amounts of the different foods with equivalent amounts of carbohydrate are included so that a person can make substitutions.

Carrageenin, or Irish moss, is a polysaccharide that cannot be utilized by the human. Because of its ability to absorb water, it is a useful ingredient for several synthetic foods such as imitation milk.

DIETARY REQUIREMENTS

Since the body can function with considerably less carbohydrate than is present in most diets, it has been impossible to establish a dietary standard for carbohydrate. Diets low in or devoid of carbohydrate are so unpalatable that there is little likelihood of their being consumed for any appreciable length of time. In addition, the fact that carbohydrate is the most economical source of calories leads to its use in sufficient quantities to ensure at least a minimum intake. The Food and Nutrition Board of the National Research Council recommends an intake of 100 gm. of carbohydrate per day to prevent the undesirable consequences of a lower intake, such as ketosis, excessive breakdown of protein, and other undesirable metabolic responses.

ABNORMALITIES OF METABOLISM

There are several pathological conditions under which people have difficulty utilizing carbohydrate. The most common is diabetes, in which a person suffers from a relative lack of the hormone insulin. Whether this is due to a decreased production of insulin by the pancreas or an excess of an insulin inhibitor in the blood, the cell cannot pick up and utilize carbohydrate from the bloodstream at a normal rate. Other people may lack the enzyme necessary to convert galactose to glucose in the liver. Galactose then appears as an abnormal constituent of the blood and the condition is known as galactosemia. This may also occur when the intake of galactose is extremely high. Weight loss, vomiting, and mental retardation are some of the consequences of galactosemia. The lack of an enzyme needed to release stored glycogen from the liver leads to glycogen storage disease.

In the past few years, evidence has accumulated showing that many Orientals, American Indians, and Negroes do not produce the enzyme lactase and as a result may not be able to tolerate the lactose in milk. Whether this deficiency results when the young child, deprived of milk after weaning, has no need for lactase and hence ceases to produce it or whether this is a genetically determined trait in which adults regardless of diet fail to produce the enzyme is still debatable. It is possible, however, that the bulk of the world's adult population cannot tolerate milk. Symptoms of lactose intolerance tend to appear in adolescence and the early twenties. They include abdominal cramps, diarrhea, and flatulence.

CARBOHYDRATE AND DENTAL HEALTH

Carbohydrate is often implicated in the etiology of dental caries. In preeruptive stage when the tooth is forming and is being nourished through the bloodstream, carbohydrate has little direct effect on the tooth quality. However, if the carbohydrate in diet replaces protective foods that carry nutrients such as calcium, vitamin D, and vitamin C, which are necessary for normal tooth formation, they indirectly have an adverse effect on the health of the tooth before eruption.

In the posteruptive stage when the tooth is exposed to the oral environment and has only limited systemic connection, carbohydrate assumes importance. It has been established that before tooth decay occurs, there must be present microorganisms and food for the microorganisms—carbohydrate. A carbohydrate in solution that does not adhere to the tooth surface causes relatively little harm. However, a carbohydrate-rich food, such as toffee or caramel, that tends to adhere to the tooth surface provides the food needed by the organisms to

produce the acid that ultimately facilitates the solution of tooth enamel, with resultant decay of a caries-susceptible tooth. In dental health the form of the carbohydrate is equally as important as the amount.

Carbohydrate has less detrimental effect on tooth health if it is followed by liquids or other detergent foods, such as apples, that tend to remove the carbohydrate from the tooth surface.

CARBOHYDRATE AND ATHEROSCLEROSIS

Recent research to identify a dietary factor involved in atherosclerosis, now a leading cause of death in the United States, has suggested that both the kind and amount of carbohydrate in the diet may be important factors. To date the evidence is far from conclusive but suggests that high intakes of sucrose are associated with a higher incidence of atherosclerosis, possibly through its effect in stimulating high blood triglyceride levels. Only individuals with certain genetic characteristics are susceptible. There is insufficient evidence to indicate that the quantity of simple sugar in the American diet has any effect on serum lipid levels.

SUGAR SUBSTITUTES

In attempts to reduce the caloric value of foods without sacrificing their palatability, considerable use has been made of nonnutritive sweeteners. Saccharin, discovered in 1879, was popular for a considerable period of time but had the disadvantage that it could not be used in any appreciable amounts or in cooked products because of an undesirable aftertaste. Both sodium and calcium cyclamates, discovered in 1937, became widely accepted, but in 1969 their use was prohibited on the basis of evidence that they are potential carcinogens and could cause chromosomal damage. The limitations of these two products, which are ten and one hundred times as sweet as sugar, respectively, has prompted a search for a safe alternative. A dipeptide of aspartic acid and phenylalanine, both amino acids from protein, is 250 times as sweet as sugar. Three different chemicals derived from the rind of oranges and grapefruit and belonging to a group of substances known as bioflavonoids also show promise as acceptable sweeteners without caloric value.

ALCOHOL (ETHANOL)

Ethyl alcohol, produced from the fermentation of glucose in the presence of enzymes in yeast and in the absence of oxygen, accounts for an average energy intake of 76 kcal. per day for all Americans. Since many persons do not use alcohol, for those who do the contribution of this nutrient to the energy intake may reach as high as 10% of the total caloric intake. For this reason it is appropriate that a student of nutrition have an understanding of its metabolism.

Absorption and metabolism

Ethanol is a small, neutral, water-soluble molecule that does not require digestion. It is absorbed by diffusion throughout the length of the gastrointestinal tract. As much as 80% of the intake is absorbed in the small intestine immediately after leaving the stomach. There is no upper limit on the rate of absorption, and the absorbed alcohol, being water soluble, immediately disperses throughout the body fluids. Its concentration in any one tissue parallels the water concentration of the tissue. Thus a large amount of absorbed alcohol is found in the blood and relatively little in adipose tissue and bone. Little alcohol is excreted. Less than 5% is lost through the kidney and lungs. However, since the amount in the expired air and in the urine is in equilibrium with that in the blood, it is possible to use a measure of alcohol content of these as a legally valid measure of alcohol content of the blood. A blood concentration of 0.1% is considered a maximum,

and a level of 0.15% is evidence of intoxication.

The metabolism of alcohol begins in the liver and kidney, which contain the enzyme alcohol dehydrogenase necessary to convert the alcohol to the form in which it can be used in the same way that carbohydrate and fatty acids are used as a source of energy. Since skeletal muscles lack this enzyme, the metabolism of alcohol cannot be initiated there, but once the intermediate has been formed, muscle tissue as well as all other tissues can use it as an energy source. It is possible that alcohol could be converted to fat and stored, but in general it is metabolized immediately to carbon dioxide, water, and energy in preference to fatty acids and glucose. By sparing these energy sources, ethanol can contribute to positive caloric balance. The brain also contains some alcohol dehydrogenase to metabolize sufficient alcohol to make local adjustments to regulate neural effects of alcohol.

Alcohol contributes 7 kcal. of energy per gram or 5.6 kcal. per milliliter. Thus 1 fluid ounce of 100-proof alcohol (50% alcohol) contains 12 gm. of alcohol, which contribute 84 kcal. of energy. Similarly, 12 ounces of beer with an alcohol content of 3% or 4 ounces of wine with a 12% alcohol content contribute 80 kcal. to the energy pool. Individuals vary greatly in the rate at which they metabolize alcohol, but for most people it ranges between 100 and 200 mg. per kilogram of body weight per hour. This is equivalent to one fifth of a gallon of 100-proof whiskey per day for a 154-pound man. The rate of metabolism does not respond to the need for calories and thus exercising will not speed up the oxidation of alcohol.

The consumption of alcohol in excessive amounts can lead to severe liver damage and the accumulation of fat in liver tissue. In cases in which alcohol consumption does not lead to a decreased intake of other nutrients, the liver is generally protected against damage.

SELECTED REFERENCES

Bayless, T. M., and Huang, S.: Inadequate intestinal digestion of lactose, Amer. J. Clin. Nutr. **22:**250, 1969.

Goodhart, R. S.: Cyclamate sweeteners in the human diet—a scientific evaluation, North Chicago, 1968, Abbott Laboratories.

Hardinge, M. G., Swarner, J. B., and Crooks, H.: Carbohydrates in foods, J. Amer. Diet. Ass. **46:**197, 1965.

Harper, A. E.: Carbohydrates. In Food yearbook of agriculture, Washington, D. C., 1959, U. S. Department of Agriculture.

Hodges, R.: Present knowledge of carbohydrate, Nutr. Rev. **24:**65, 1966.

Krehl, W. A.: The nutritional significance of the carbohydrates, Borden Rev. Nutr. Res. (No. 6) **16:**85, 1955.

Passmore, R.: Carbohydrate, the Cinderella of nutrition: In Wolstenhome, G. E. W., and O'Connor, M.: Diet and bodily constitution, Ciba Foundation Study Group No. 17, London, 1963, J. & A. Churchill, Ltd.

Price, J. M., Biava, C. G., Oser, B. L., Vogin, E. E., Sreinfeld, J., and Ley, H. L.: Bladder tumors in rats fed cyclohexamine or high doses of a mixture of cyclamates and saccharin, Science **167:**1132, 1970.

Review: Carbohydrate, digestion and absorption, Nutr. Rev. **21:**279, 1963.

Stevens, H. A., and Ohlson, M. A.: Estimated intake of simple and complex carbohydrates, J. Amer. Diet. Ass. **48:**294, 1966.

Victor, M.: Alcohol and nutritional diseases of the nervous system, J.A.M.A. **167:**65, 1958.

Westerfeld, W. W., and Schulman, M. P.: Metabolism and the caloric value of alcohol, J.A.M.A. **170:**197, 1959.

Fats or lipids

Lipids, the most concentrated energy-yielding group, are familiar items in the diet. The term *fat* is commonly used instead of the more correct term *lipid*. Both terms are used to identify fats and oils found in food. The visible fats, such as butter, margarine, vegetable fat, and the layer of fat on meat, account for only 40% of the fat in the American diet. The remaining 60% is present as invisible fat—that marbled throughout meat fibers, in egg yolk, homogenized milk and milk products, nuts, and whole-grain cereals.

The fat content of the American diet has been increasing steadily. In 1910 it was estimated that fat provided 32% of the calories available in the food supply. By 1930 the figure had risen to 35% and in 1966 had reached 41%. Since there are sizeable losses of fat in cooking, the amount actually ingested will be less than that available. About two thirds of available fat comes from animal sources and one third from vegetable sources, primarily vegetable oils. The kind and amount of fat consumed by an individual will be influenced by many social, cultural, economic, geographical, racial, and technological factors. For instance, the Japanese have a relatively low intake compared to the Italians, as do low-income families compared to those with high incomes, people in tropical regions compared to those in arctic regions, and older people compared to younger.

At the same time that the total amount of fat in the diet has been increasing to the current level of 145 gm. per person per day, there have been changes in the character of the fat consumed. The use of fats of animal origin has declined, whereas that of fats of vegetable origin has increased. The use of nondairy coffee whiteners and whipped toppings made with vegetable oils in place of cream and the use of margarine in place of butter accounts for a large part of this shift.

CHEMICAL COMPOSITION

Like carbohydrate, lipid is composed of three elements—carbon, hydrogen, and oxygen. It differs from carbohydrate, however, since it contains a much lower ratio of oxygen to carbon and hydrogen. This means that less of the fat molecule is composed of oxidized carbon and hydrogen so that there is a greater potential for the release of energy when these elements are oxidized within the body cells.

Biochemically all food fat is composed of a molecule of glycerol to which is attached from one to three fatty acid molecules. The structure of glycerol, a 3-carbon alcohol, is as follows:

$$
\begin{array}{c}
H \\
| \\
H-C-OH \\
| \\
H-C-OH \\
| \\
H-C-OH \\
| \\
H
\end{array}
$$

The glycerol portion of the molecule is common to all fats. The fatty acids attached to it vary in kind and number. Fatty acids, as they occur in food, are straight-chain carbon compounds the majority of which have an even number of carbon atoms, a methyl (CH_3) group at one end, and a carboxyl group (COOH) at the other. Thus a simple fatty acid could be represented as follows:

$$CH_3—CH_2—CH_2—CH_2—CH_2—COOH$$

A general formula for fatty acids is $CH_3—(CH_2)_n—COOH$, where *n* may be any even number from 2 to 24. Most natural fats contain a predominance of long-chain fatty acids with 16 to 18 carbon atoms. Medium-chain fatty acids with from 8 to 12 carbon atoms and short-chain fatty acids with 2 to 6 carbons occur less frequently. For instance, milk has 4%, butter 8%, and coconut oil 10% medium-chain fatty acids. Short-chain fatty acids are more soluble and more easily absorbed and transported in the blood than long-chain fatty acids.

Fatty acids are attached to the OH portion of the glycerol molecule through the OH of the carboxyl end of the fatty acid. Water is split off, leaving the fatty acid attached through the remaining oxygen.

In addition to varying in chain length, fatty acids may vary in the extent to which they are saturated with hydrogen atoms. In a saturated fatty acid each carbon atom in the chain has 2 hydrogen atoms attached to it—the maximum it can hold. In some fatty acids, referred to as monounsaturated fatty acids, 2 adjacent carbon atoms will each lack 1 hydrogen atom. Since they each then have an unsaturated bond, they become attached to each other through a second bond and the linkage is called a double bond. If a double bond occurs in two or more places in the chain, the resulting fatty acid is called a polyunsaturated fatty acid (PUFA). If saturated fatty acids predominate in a fat, the fat will have a higher melting point and will more likely be solid at room temperature than if unsaturated fatty acids predominate. This is due to the the fact that the straight chains can fit together very closely. The character of the fat formed will also be influenced by whether or not the fatty acid bends at the double bond or remains in a straight chain. Monounsaturated fatty acids represent 40% of total dietary fat, polyunsaturated 12%, and saturated 37%. The relative amount of polyunsaturated fatty acids and saturated fatty acids in food is expressed by the P/S ratio. The P/S ratio of the American diet is gradually increasing and has been estimated to be as high as 0.33. This suggests that approximately one third of dietary fatty acids are polyunsaturated. By adding hydrogen to a fat, it is possible to change the degree of saturation of the fatty acids present and in this way to modify and control the characteristics of the fat. This process of hydrogenation of liquid fats is widely used in the food industry. Not only does it change the physical characteristics of the fat, it also increases its stability, since an unsaturated double bond increases the susceptibility of the fat to oxidation.

The most common saturated fatty acids in foods are butyric (4 carbons), palmitic (16 carbons), and stearic (18 carbons); monounsaturated fatty acids are predominantly oleic with 18 carbons and one double bond. Linoleic acid with 18 carbons and two double bonds is the most common polyunsaturated fatty acid. It represents 75% of the fatty acids in safflower oil, 54% in corn oil, and 2% in butter.

It is obvious that all fats are not alike—butter fat has characteristics different from those of beef fat, chicken fat, and corn oil. Each animal has a fat that is characteristic of its own species. Chicken fat can readily be distinguished from the more solid beef fat and this in turn from the hard white mutton fat. It is possible to modify the character of fat of a nonruminant by modifying its diet, and animal breeders take advantage of this to market the type of fat the consumers want. For instance, pigs fed peanuts produce a soft greasy fat that is less acceptable in some areas and more acceptable in others than the harder fat resulting when a corn diet is fed. Fats formed from carbohydrate are more likely to be saturated and hence firmer than those from protein and fat.

The different characteristics of fats are the result of the kinds and number of fatty acids and their arrangement in the fat. These may vary in the length of the carbon chain from a 4-carbon chain to a 26-carbon chain and may be either saturated, mono-unsaturated, or polyunsaturated. In addition to the type of fatty acids incorporated in a fat molecule, the number of fatty acids influences the character of the fat. Over 98% of the fat found in food and 20% of that in liver and blood is composed of triglycerides, fats in which the glycerol molecules have fatty acids attached in all three possible positions. These three fatty acids may be all the same, as in simple triglycerides, all different, or two alike, although most fats contain at least two different fatty acids and are known as mixed triglycerides. All triglycerides within a single food fat are not necessarily the same. For instance, 140 fatty acids have been identified in milk fat, making possible 125,000 different triglycerides. Most food fats contain at least eight to ten different fatty acids. When two or more fatty acids appear in a fat molecule, the order in which they are arranged affects the character of the fat. The remaining 2% of the fat in foods is composed of monoglycerides, glycerol to which only one fatty acid is attached; diglycerides, glycerol to which two fatty acids are attached; and phospholipids, glycerol with a phosphate and nitrogen-containing substances replacing one of the fatty acids of a triglyceride.

The general formula for glycerides may then be written as follows (FA represents a fatty acid):

$$
\begin{array}{c}
\text{H} \\
| \\
\text{H—C—OH} \\
| \\
\text{H—C—OH} \\
| \\
\text{H—C—O—FA}_1 \\
| \\
\text{H}
\end{array}
$$

Monoglyceride

$$
\begin{array}{c}
\text{H} \\
| \\
\text{H—C—OH} \\
| \\
\text{H—C—O—FA}_1 \\
| \\
\text{H—C—O—FA}_2 \\
| \\
\text{H}
\end{array}
$$

Diglyceride

$$
\begin{array}{c}
\text{H} \\
| \\
\text{H—C—O—FA}_1 \\
| \\
\text{H—C—O—FA}_2 \\
| \\
\text{H—C—O—FA}_3 \\
| \\
\text{H}
\end{array}
$$

Mixed triglyceride

CLASSIFICATION

Fats are frequently identified as saturated or unsaturated, depending on the degree of saturation of the fatty acids present. These terms are only relative, as a triglyceride that is completely saturated or completely unsaturated is very rare. Likewise the general designation of animal fats as saturated fats and vegetable fats as unsaturated fats is not a valid classification. Most food fats have eight to ten fatty acids, some of which will be saturated and some unsaturated. Unsaturated fatty acids tend to produce a fat with a lower melting point that is liquid at room temperature. Conversely, saturated fatty acids tend to raise the melting point and result in a fat more solid at room temperature. Most vegetable oils are relatively high in monounsaturated and polyunsaturated fatty acids, and most animal fats are relatively high in saturated fatty acids. Exceptions are poultry and fish fats, which contain highly unsaturated fatty acids, and coconut oil, which is composed of saturated fatty acids but is liquid because it has a predominance of short-chain fatty acids.

Vegetable oils, such as cottonseed, peanut, corn, safflower, and soybean, are considerably less expensive than animal fats.

They can be economically and effectively changed to fats with more plastic qualities by the process of hydrogenation, in which hydrogen is introduced into the fat molecules to saturate the carbon atom with hydrogen and to eliminate the double bond. Margarine and vegetable shortenings are examples of vegetable oils that have been changed by saturating at least some of the unsaturated double bonds with hydrogen to produce fats with the desired physical characteristics. The hydrogenation process can be controlled to give a fat with specific characteristics. Competition among processors to produce the most acceptable product is evident in current advertising. As a result of hydrogenation the consumption of vegetable fats is rising, whereas that of animal fats is declining. About 3 billion pounds of hydrogenated fats are consumed in the United States each year.

PHYSICAL PROPERTIES

Fat is insoluble in water but soluble in fat solvents such as ether, chloroform, or benzene. Fats are less dense than water and so will rise to the surface of any aqueous mixture. Emulsified fats, in which fat globules are in finely divided form and are kept separated from one another by an emulsifying agent, are prevented from coalescing or fusing together to form large globules. The dispersed fat in homogenized milk is an example of an emulsified fat. Egg yolk fat is a naturally emulsified fat.

Fat is not affected by temperatures normally used in food preparation; however, heating at high temperatures, often indicated by the smoking of the fat, leads to the decomposition of fatty acids and the production of acrolein from glycerol. Acrolein has a very pungent acrid fume that is extremely irritating to the nasal passages and the gastrointestinal tract. Fats are also subject to oxidation. Natural fats containing unsaturated fatty acids are very susceptible to oxidation, especially in the presence of catalysts such as iron. When they are low in antioxidants, which retard oxidation, they become rancid because of the production of peroxides of fatty acids, a major cause of spoilage in fats. Fats may also become unpalatable because of their tendency to absorb odors and flavors.

DIGESTION

Before fat can enter the general circulation to be transported to the tissues, it must be broken down chemically into molecules sufficiently small to pass into the cells of the membranes lining the gastrointestinal tract. In most cases, fat is reduced to fatty acids and glycerol, but a few monoglycerides with short-chain fatty acids can be absorbed.

Digestion of fat begins in the stomach, but only a small fraction occurs there. The enzyme gastric lipase, a component of the gastric juice secreted from the wall of the stomach, is able to break naturally occurring emulsified fat, such as that in egg yolk and homogenized milk, into fatty acids and glycerol. It is unable to attack the larger particles of unemulsified fat found in meat, butter, and salad oils. Fatty acids liberated at this stage may be exchanged in the stomach or intestine with fatty acids of other triglycerides to modify the makeup of ingested fat. Long-chain fatty acids are more likely to be reincorporated into triglycerides than are short-chain fatty acids as the synthesis and hydrolysis of fat occur simultaneously.

In the small intestine the bile secreted by the gallbladder acts on the larger fat molecules to break them into many smaller fat particles. This emulsification, the result of reducing surface tension on fat molecules, increases the surface area on which the digestive enzymes can act, reduces the distance through which enzymes must penetrate, and prevents the coalescing of fat molecules. Once the fat molecules are in a sufficiently finely divided form, they are acted upon by both pancreatic lipase and intestinal lipase. In both cases the enzymes

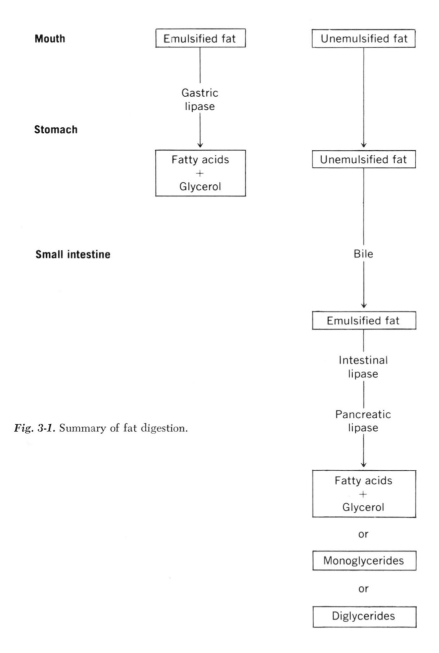

Fig. 3-1. Summary of fat digestion.

split the fat molecule by enzyme hydrolysis, involving the addition of water as each fatty acid is split off from the glycerol core. The breakdown of fat progresses from triglycerides to diglycerides to monoglycerides and finally to the complete separation of fatty acids from glycerol. At any one time during digestion, fat exists as a complex mixture of triglycerides, diglycerides, or monoglycerides and fatty acids, with virtually all being changed to the more soluble monoglycerides, glycerol, and fatty acids before absorption.

Most fats are between 95% and 100% digestible. The extent of digestion depends on the length of the fatty acid chain and the number and arrangement of fatty acids in the molecule. Hydrogenation will decrease digestibility only if it is carried far enough to produce significant amounts of saturated fatty acids. The changes occurring during fat digestion are shown in Fig. 3-1.

ABSORPTION AND TRANSPORTATION

The divided or digested fat molecules are taken up from the gastrointestinal tract as separate molecules of fatty acids and glycerol and as monoglycerides, diglycerides, and triglycerides. About 30% of the free fatty acids with less than 12 carbon atoms and glycerol are absorbed directly into the bloodstream to be carried by the portal vein to the liver. As soon as they pass into the mucosal cells of the lining of the intestine, many of the remaining free fatty acids with more than 12 carbon atoms unite with a different molecule of glycerol or with a monoglyceride to form fats either as monoglycerides, diglycerides, or triglycerides. About 70% of absorbed fat is resynthesized to form triglycerides. These then enter the lacteals (fat-collecting ducts for lymph) that finally carry the fat to the lymphatic system. The lymphatic system, which is concerned primarily with collecting body fluids and returning them through the tho-

racic duct to the general circulatory system, is illustrated in Fig. 1-6. The fat molecules absorbed through the lacteals are transported as microscopic fat particles called chylomicrons. These are stabilized combinations of 99% fat with 1% protein that are more soluble than fat and therefore more easily transported in the blood. Fat collected in the lymphatic ducts empties into the general circulation in the neck region and from there is circulated to all body cells. The presence of the chylomicrons in the blood gives a milky or turbid appearance to the blood that disappears gradually as the fat is removed by organs and tissues. Some fatty acids that do not recombine with glycerol are transported bound to plasma albumin.

Factors affecting absorption. Absorption of fat will be decreased when there is increased motility in the gastrointestinal tract. This decreases the time during which fat is in contact with digestive juices and with the walls of the intestinal tract through which it is absorbed. Absence of bile to emulsify fat or of fat-splitting enzymes also decreases absorption, resulting in undigested fat in the feces—a condition known as steatorrhea. Longer-chain fatty acids are less well absorbed than those with shorter chains, and saturated fatty acids less well than unsaturated ones.

METABOLISM

Lipids that have been removed from the blood as it passes through the liver and other tissues are hydrolyzed, or split, into fatty acids and glycerol by cellular lipases. The fatty acids soon reappear in the blood as free fatty acids as components of lipoproteins, the soluble combination of a fat with a protein. These lipoproteins, which can be low-density substances with 10% protein and 90% fat or high-density substances with 45% protein and 55% fat, facilitate the transport of fat throughout the body.

Fat is removed from the blood lipoproteins by various tissues and meets one of two fates. It can be oxidized (burned) through a series of complex biochemical reactions to form carbon dioxide, water, and energy, or it may be stored in the fat depots of each cell or in special adipose (fat) cells for future use as a source of energy. Some fat will be used by the mammary gland during lactation in the production of milk. Fat is the only source of energy used by heart muscle.

When the body has need for the energy reserves, the fat stored as triglycerides is hydrolyzed by lipases within the cell to fatty acids and glycerol. The fatty acids leave the cell, become bound to the protein albumin in the bloodstream, and are carried to the tissues requiring energy. Since these fatty acids have not recombined with glycerol, they are known as nonesterified fatty acids (NEFA). There is about 1% NEFA to 99% albumin. The glycerol core of the stored triglycerides is oxidized as a carbohydrate within the adipose cell.

The digestion and metabolism of fat is

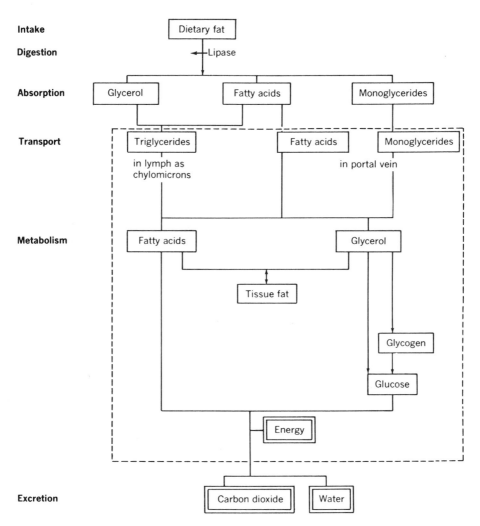

Fig. 3-2. Summary of fat digestion and metabolism. Double-boxed items are end products of metabolism. Changes within dotted line occur after absorption.

summarized in Fig. 3-2. This indicates that ingested fat available to the cells as fatty acids and glycerol follows one of three paths during metabolism:

1. Both fatty acids and glycerol are metabolized immediately as a source of energy in all tissues except the central nervous system.

2. Glycerol and fatty acids combine to form fat, which is stored as a reserve of energy.

3. Glycerol is converted into glucose and then is metabolized in the same way as a source of energy, converted into glycogen, or converted into fat. Fatty acids are metabolized as a source of energy.

FUNCTIONS IN DIET

Source of energy. Fat serves as a concentrated source of energy. Each gram of fat, whether animal or vegetable, liquid or solid, provides 9 kcal. per gram—two and one-fourth times as much energy as an equal weight of either carbohydrate or protein. Fat represents the form in which the animal stores excess energy; thus the amount of fat in an animal product is determined by the energy balance of the animal. Practically all animal foods contain some fat. Even relatively lean steak is 28% fat, which contributes 70% of its energy.

Satiety value. Fat tends to leave the stomach relatively slowly, being released approximately 3½ hours after ingestion. This delay in the emptying time of the stomach helps to delay the onset of hunger pangs and contributes to a feeling of satiety after a meal. The presence of fat in the duodenum stimulates the release of a hormone in the stomach, which in turn inhibits hunger contractions. Because of its high caloric value, fat is frequently reduced and visible fats virtually eliminated from diets suggested for weight control. Current research shows that the inclusion of some fat—whole milk, butter on vegetables and bread, or oil on salads—increases the satiety value of low-calorie diets so that they are

more easily adhered to. This more than compensates for the concentrated caloric content of the fat. Currently, moderate-fat reducing diets are considered more successful than low-fat diets.

Carrier of fat-soluble vitamins. Among the dietary essentials are four fat-soluble vitamins—vitamins A, D, E, and K. Dietary fat serves as a carrier for these nutrients or their precursors. Thus the elimination of fat from the diet leads to a reduced intake of these nutrients. Fat also appears necessary for the absorption of vitamin A precursors from nonfat sources such as carrots. Similarly, anything that interferes with the absorption or utilization of fat, such as an obstruction of the bile duct or rancidity of fat, depresses the availability of the fat-soluble vitamins.

Source of essential fatty acids. Among the fatty acids is a polyunsaturated fatty acid, linoleic acid, that is effective in curing the dermatitis and restoring the growth of young animals fed a diet devoid of or very low in fat. Because it cannot be produced by the body, linoleic acid is considered an essential fatty acid (EFA). Two closely related fatty acids—linolenic acid, an 18-carbon acid found in vegetable fats, and arachidonic acid, a 20-carbon polyunsaturated fatty acid found in some animal tissues—can be synthesized from linoleic acid. Since the body can synthesize them, they are not considered essential fatty acids even though they perform some of the same functions as linoleic acid. Linolenic acid is effective in restoring growth but has no antidermatitis effect, whereas arachidonic acid will cure dermatitis but will not promote growth. The relationship between these three is shown in Table 3-1.

The essential fatty acids are metabolized more slowly than the nonessential saturated fatty acids. In an EFA deficiency, changes occur in the structure and enzyme function within the mitochondrion of the cell. There is some evidence that EFA's are precursors of a group of substances, known as pros-

Table 3-1. Relationship of related fatty acids to linoleic acid

Fatty acid	Structure	Biological role	Sources
Linoleic	18 carbons	Growth factor	Vegetable
↓	2 double bonds	Antidermatitis factor	Seed oils
Linolenic	18 carbons	Growth factor	Soybean oil
⇕	3 double bonds		
Arachidonic acid	20 carbons	Antidermatitis factor	Animal fat
	4 double bonds		

Table 3-2. Fat and fatty acid composition of 100 gm. of selected foods*

Food	Total fat (gm.)	Saturated fatty acids (gm.)	Unsaturated fatty acids Oleic (gm.)	Linoleic (gm.)
Coconut oil	100	86	7	—
Corn oil	100	10	28	53
Soybean oil	100	15	20	52
Olive oil	100	11	76	7
Safflower oil	100	8	15	72
Peanut oil	100	18	47	29
Mayonnaise	79.9	14	17	40
Butter	81	46	27	2
Bacon, broiled	52	17	25	5
Peanut butter	50.6	9	25	14
Cream cheese	37.7	21	12	1
Beef, rib, raw	37.4	18	16	1
Cheddar cheese	32.2	18	11	1
Ham	23	4	5	1
Chicken, raw	17.1	5	6	3
Avocado	16.4	3	7	2
Egg, cooked	11.5	4	5	1
Tuna, canned, drained	8.2	3	2	2
Milk, whole	3.7	2	1	Trace

*From Watt, B. K., and Merrill, A. L.: Composition of foods—raw, processed and prepared, U. S. Department of Agriculture Handbook No. 8, Washington, D. C., 1963, U. S. Department of Agriculture.

taglandins, that function in many of the metabolic processes involved in the control of blood pressure, muscular contractions, and enzyme and hormone metabolism.

Saturated fatty acids have no EFA activity and may increase the need for EFA as does an increase in dietary cholesterol. Young animals need more EFA than older animals, males more than females, and diabetics and persons with hypothyroidism more than persons under normal metabolic conditions. Needs also increase in pyridoxine deficiency. The needs for essential fatty acids are usually met when 2% of the total calories are provided by linoleic acid. Linoleic acid is present in highest concentrations in vegetable oils, with some, such as corn oil, soybean oil, and safflower oil, containing over 50% linoleic acid. Lesser and variable amounts are present in hydrogenated fats or spreads made from these oils. Most diets provide many times the minimum EFA requirements. The fatty acid composition of some representative fats is given in Table 3-2. EFA deficiency occurs most frequently in bottle-fed infants fed a nonfat milk formula. The essential fatty acids requirement of infants has been set at 3% of the total calories. This is easily met by breast milk, in which 6% to 9% of the calories come from linoleic acid.

With the increasing use of vegetable oils rather than animal fats in the American diet the amount of EFA is increasing.

Palatability. The role of fat in contributing to the palatability of food is appreciated best by those forced to exist on a low-fat diet. The use of fat for frying food, as a spread, as a base for salad dressing, and as a flavor adjunct for vegetables does much to improve the taste appeal of our meals. Many substances responsible for the flavors and aromas of food are fat soluble. Thus fat generally contributes to the acceptability of our meals. It has also been suggested that fat in the diet stimulates the flow of digestive juices.

ROLE IN THE BODY

Energy reserve. Body fat represents the primary form in which energy is stored in the body. Since it is an essential constituent of the cell membrane, all tissues contain some fat. In addition, the body has a group of specialized cells, called adipose cells, whose main function is the storage of fat that exceeds the capacity of regular cells. Although the number of cells may increase in the adult in response to a need for more storage sites for fat, there is considerable evidence that the number of adipose cells is determined within the first few years of life. If this is the case, the amount of fat stored will be a function of the extent to which the adipose cells are saturated with fat rather than of the rate of increase in number of cells. Once fat has been formed and deposited in the adipose tissues, the body has no way of excreting it. Thus the only way in which body fat can be reduced is by oxidizing or burning it as a source of energy when caloric intake is less than caloric expenditure. A certain amount of body fat, about 18% to 20% of body weight for women and 15% for men, is considered normal and desirable. Reserves of fat in excess of this represent first overweight and in extreme cases obesity with all the physical, physiological, and aesthetic disadvantages associated with the latter.

Body regulator. As an essential constituent of the membrane of each individual cell, fat helps regulate the uptake and excretion of nutrients by the cell.

Insulation. Deposits of fat beneath the skin (subcutaneous fat) serve as insulating material for the body, protecting it against shock from changes in environmental temperature. Here again a certain minimum layer is desirable to prevent excessive heat loss from the body, but too thick a layer slows down the rate of heat loss during hot weather, with resultant discomfort to the individual. Thick subcutaneous fat layers impede physical movement and present many aesthetic problems.

Protection of vital body organs. The fat deposits that surround certain vital organs and that are the last depots to be reduced when there is a caloric deficit serve to hold them in position and to protect them from physical shock. The kidney and heart are protected in this way.

FOOD SOURCES

The amount of fat in representative foods is shown in Table 3-2, which also indicates the amount present as saturated and unsaturated fatty acids. Some advertisers are making use of a P/S ratio to identify the nature of the fat in their product. They assume that a high P/S ratio is desirable because of some evidence that polyunsaturated fatty acids inhibit cholesterol formation more than do other fatty acids. Special margarines now on the market have a P/S ratio of 1.0 to 2.4 compared with 0.2 to 0.5 for regular margarines. In the hydrogenation of polyunsaturated fatty acids, essential fatty acids may be converted into monounsaturated acids that lack the effectiveness of the essential fatty acids. In addition, the double bond sometimes shifts so that the common *cis* form is changed to the less well utilized *trans* form of the acid. These may constitute up to 40% of the fatty

acids in margarines. Until we have access to more precise information on the chemical nature of the hydrogenated fats in margarines, it is difficult to assess or to predict the effect of these on metabolism.

In checking the linoleic acid content of vegetable oils, it is obvious that coconut oil, chocolate, and palm kernel oils contain virtually no EFA. On the other hand, wheat germ oil and walnut oil contain 57% to 73% linoleic oil respectively. Poultry and game are good sources of EFA.

It is also difficult to present precise data on the fatty acid composition of animal fats because of the differences that will result from variations in the diet of the animal.

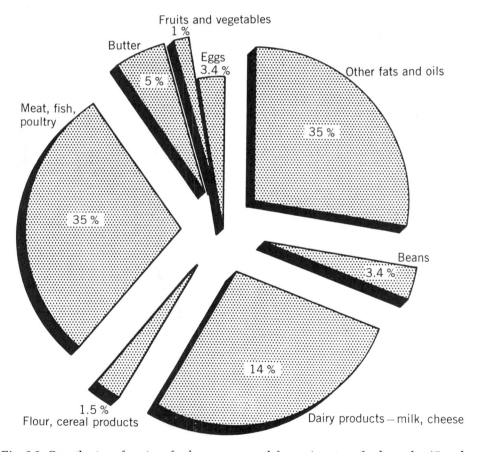

Fig. 3-3. Contribution of various food groups to total fat in American food supply. (Based on Contribution of major food groups to nutrient supplies available for civilian consumption, National Food Situation No. 130, 1969.)

The method of food processing and storage may also have an effect on the fatty acid composition of the food as it is consumed.

The percentage of calories contributed by fat tends to be relatively high in most animal foods. In whole milk with 3.2% fat, 53% of the calories come from fat; in cheese with 32% fat, 68%; in beef with 28% fat, 83%; and in frankfurters containing 27% fat, 70%.

Vegetable foods contain less fat. Whole-grain cereals have about 2% to 9% fat, mainly in the germ. The fat in seeds ranges from 4% in corn to 17% in soybeans. Peanuts have 48% fat, and pecans have 41%. Avocado with 16% and ripe olives with 30% are the only fruits with any appreciable fat.

Based on its nutrient composition, bacon is correctly designated as a fat food rather than a protein food. It contains 69% fat in raw form and 52% fat when cooked, although the latter figure varies with the extent of cooking.

Fig. 3-3 shows the contribution of various food groups to the total fat in the American food supply.

Because of the frequent suggestion in popular literature that mineral oil be substituted for vegetable oils in salad dressings, it is appropriate to mention it although it has no nutritional value. It is a hydrocarbon, a by-product of the oil-refining process. The body possesses no enzymes capable of digesting it so that it passes through the digestive tract unchanged, acting as a lubricant and contributing no calories to the body's energy pool. Unfortunately however, it acts as a solvent for the fat-soluble vitamins, which are then excreted along with the mineral oil. Since the low-calorie homemade mineral oil salad dressings are generally used on vegetable greens, one of our best sources of vitamin A, its use in the diet should be discouraged.

DIETARY REQUIREMENTS

Aside from the need for a dietary source of linoleic acid, the human does not require fat in the diet. A diet providing 2% of its calories from linoleic acid meets this requirement. However, as a concentrated source of energy, fat is important in allowing us to meet our energy requirements without eating large quantities of food. The current practice of obtaining as much as 40% of the calories from fat is being questioned because of the prevalence of excessive calorie intake and the possibility of an adverse effect of high-fat diets in arteriovascular diseases. Nutritionists suggest that an intake of fat providing 25% to 30% of the calories is more compatible with good health.

Modification of dietary fat intake may be desirable in several conditions. In gallbladder disease, the amount of bile secreted is limited, and it may be necessary to restrict the total to as little as 10% of the calories from fat or to substitute emulsified fats for nonemulsified ones. Medium- and short-chain fatty acids can be absorbed in the absence of bile. In addition, they are transported through the portal vein to the liver, where they are usually metabolized as a source of energy, instead of being incorporated into tissue lipid. As a result, they can be used in the treatment of steatorrhea without requiring the reduction in the total amount of fat in the diet. Some disorders of absorption, such as sprue or ileitis (inflammation of the ileum), inhibit the absorption of fat, and the usual manifestation of this is the appearance of as much as 60 gm. of fat in the stools compared to normal levels of 2 to 5 gm. Until the cause of the problem can be corrected, the person is given as much fat as he can absorb, since a restriction limits caloric intake and the absorption of fat-soluble vitamins. Hyperlipidemia, in which levels of certain fat constituents of the blood are elevated, may call for a restriction in either the kind or amount of dietary fat. Some types of hyperlipidemia do not respond to dietary changes and can be treated only with drugs.

The necessity of restricting fat intake in such conditions as hepatitis, cirrhosis, and jaundice is now questioned.

RELATIONSHIP TO HEART DISEASE

The discussion of the relationship of dietary fat and atherosclerosis in an elementary text can be legitimately questioned. However, since the topic is being widely discussed in popular literature, it seems appropriate to include a statement of the current interpretation of the question. This is done with the full recognition that scientific thinking on the topic may have changed direction completely in the necessary time lapse between the preparation of the manuscript and publication of the textbook.

Interest in a possible relationship between dietary factors and the incidence of heart disease was triggered by the observation that persons who suffered heart attacks almost always had above-normal levels of blood cholesterol. Cholesterol, a fat-related compound that is present in many animal foods and that the body can also synthesize, was shown to be a major constituent of the atherosclerotic plaques or precipitates that form on the inside of some blood vessels, eventually narrowing the passage to the point that if a clot forms, it closes the vessel entirely. It was also noted that the incidence of heart disease is higher in populations that derive a higher percentage of their calories from saturated fat than it is in populations that consume less saturated and more unsaturated fats.

Efforts to lower blood cholesterol levels by dietary manipulation were made after studies on rabbits, in which a restriction of dietary cholesterol results in lower levels of cholesterol in the blood. In human beings, however, control of dietary cholesterol by restricting the amount of cholesterol-containing foods such as eggs, meat, and liver led neither to lowering of blood cholesterol levels nor to a reduction in heart disease. The reason became clear when it was learned that the body can synthesize in the liver as much as 2 gm. of cholesterol from fat, carbohydrate, and protein in the diet whenever the amount of these in the diet exceeds the body's need for energy. This is considerably more than the 0.5 gm. provided from a normal diet. Since a certain amount of cholesterol is essential for the synthesis of sex hormones, for the transport of essential fatty acids, and as a constituent of the skin and covering of nerve fibers, it must be considered a normal body constituent.

Attention was next focused on the nature of fat in the diet with the observation that persons who consumed liquid fats or oils rather than solid fats have lower blood cholesterol levels than those who eat more solid animal fats. Since liquid fats differ from solid fats primarily in the proportion of PUFA they contain, emphasis in dietary treatment shifted toward an increased use of vegetable oils high in PUFA. This dietary modification when PUFA provided about half the dietary fat did indeed lead to a reduction in blood cholesterol levels but not to concurrent reduction in heart disease. Vast research has shown that dietary patterns and habits are reflected in blood cholesterol levels, but the need for reducing blood cholesterol has not been established.

Interest shifted to a search for another fat-related component of the blood that may reflect a tendency toward atherosclerosis. It was found that heart disease occurred only in persons who had a high blood cholesterol level coupled with a high blood triglyceride level. Triglycerides appear in the blood after a diet high in fat, but their presence also reflects the synthesis of fat from excess carbohydrate or excess protein. Carbohydrate in the form of sugar rather than the more complex starches is more likely to stimulate cholesterol synthesis. This situation is most likely to occur when caloric intake exceeds outgo and carbohydrate intake is high. It would appear, then, that modifying the diet to limit the carbohydrate and substituting polyunsaturated fats for saturated fats would be most likely to reduce both the triglyceride and cholesterol content of the blood, especially if accompanied by a control of caloric intake and the maintenance of optimum body weight. Such a regimen is not universally effective, however.

Knowledge of the dietary factors involved and the balance that exists among these factors in the development of atherosclerosis is at present far from conclusive. It is believed that any drastic modification of the American diet on the basis of current information would be unwise except perhaps for middle-aged men with high blood cholesterol and triglyceride levels, with a family history of heart disease, and who are working under emotional tension—the type of person most likely to suffer from atherosclerosis. On the other hand, there would be no harm and possibly there would be benefits (1) if the amount of fat in the diet were reduced from the present level of 40% of total calories to perhaps 25% of calorie intake and (2) if the amount of dietary cholesterol were reduced and polyunsaturated fat substituted for some of the saturated fat in the diet. Techniques for identifying those persons in whom dietary restrictions are most likely to result in change in blood lipids are now available.

SELECTED REFERENCES

Council of Foods and Nutrition, American Medical Association: Regulation of dietary fat, J.A.M.A. **181**:441, 1962.

Food and Nutrition Board: Dietary fat and human health, Publication No. 1147, Washington, D. C., 1966, National Academy of Sciences–National Research Council.

Hansen, A. E., Stewart, R. A., Hughes, G., and Soderkjelm, L.: Role of linoleic acid in infant nutrition, Pediatrics **31**:171, 1963.

Holt, P. R.: Dietary triglyceride composition related to intestinal fat absorption, Amer. J. Clin. Nutr. **22**:279, 1969.

McGandy, R. B., Hegsted, D. M., and Stare, F. J.: Diet, fat, carbohydrate and atherosclerosis, New Eng. J. Med. **277**:242, 1967.

Mead, J. F.: Present knowledge of fat, Nutr. Rev. **24**:33, 1966.

Pollock, H.: The genesis of atherosclerosis, Bull. N. Y. Acad. Med. **40**:204, 1964.

Scheig, R.: Absorption of dietary fat: use of medium-chain triglycerides in malabsorption, Amer. J. Clin. Nutr. **21**:300, 1968.

Scheig, R.: What is dietary fat? Amer. J. Clin. Nutr. **22**:651, 1969.

4 | *Protein*

The term *protein,* meaning to take first place, was introduced by Mulder, a Dutch chemist, in 1838. He attributed it to a nitrogen-containing constituent of food that he believed to be of prime importance in the functioning of the body and without which life is impossible. Although it is now difficult to maintain that protein is more important than other nutrients, it is unlikely that Mulder had any conception of the extremely important roles this group of compounds plays in the body or of the number and complexity of the protein components of the body and of food. We now have evidence that protein is a constituent of every living cell. Half the dry matter of an adult is protein. One third is in muscle, one fifth in bone and cartilage, one tenth in skin, and the rest in other tissues and body fluids. All enzymes are protein in nature. Many hormones are either protein or protein derivatives. Viruses are proteins. The nucleic acids in the cell nucleus responsible for the transmission of genetic information in cell reproduction often occur in combination with protein as nucleoproteins. The only body constituents that normally contain no protein are urine and bile. In the absence of protein there is a failure in body growth, followed by a loss of already established body tissue. Proteins as part of every body enzyme and many hormones are vital in the regulation of body processes. When the needs for growth and repair of tissue have been met, any remaining protein is used as a source of energy, a rather expensive one, however.

Early in the twentieth century, with the availability of methods of analyzing for protein by determining the nitrogen in food and tissues, there was widespread interest in protein nutrition and especially in qualitative differences in proteins. The most significant work was done by Folin, who differentiated between *endogenous* and *exogenous* protein metabolism. He showed that endogenous metabolism (the metabolism of body proteins) is reflected in the excretion of a nitrogen-containing substance, creatinine, which remains a fairly constant indicator of body mass and basal energy expenditure. On the other hand, the metabolism of the exogenous dietary protein results in the excretion of urea, which fluctuates with dietary intake.

With the discovery of vitamins in the period between World Wars I and II, emphasis in nutrition research shifted toward a clarification of their role and structure. Again, however, in the early 1950's interest in protein was revived. Several factors were responsible for this:

1. Recognition of a widespread protein deficiency disease, kwashiorkor, which plagues a large segment of the world's population, especially young children in developing countries
2. Availability of radioactive isotopes, which made possible investigations of a scope not previously possible
3. Recognition of blood and plasma transfusions as means of saving lives

Current interest in protein nutrition is evident from the vast literature on the subject in scientific journals and books.

CHEMICAL COMPOSITION

Proteins are extremely complex substances made up of many amino acids, the structural units of protein. These are the basic units from which protein is synthesized and into which it is converted in the course of digestion. The twenty different naturally occurring amino acids that have been identified as the building blocks for body proteins are listed in Table 4-1. Chemically the amino acids are composed of a carboxyl group (COOH), a hydrogen atom (H), an amino group (NH$_2$), and

an amino acid radical (R) attached to a carbon atom as shown below:

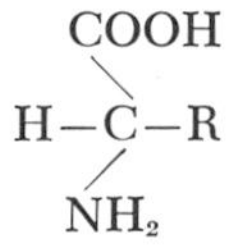

$$COOH$$
$$H-C-R$$
$$NH_2$$

The nitrogen of the amino group is unique to protein and represents an average 16% of the amino acid molecule, ranging from 15% in milk protein to 17% in cereals and 18% in nuts. Because of the constancy of nitrogen in protein, most studies of protein metabolism can be based on ni-

Table 4-1. Amino acids in food and body tissue

Classification	Amino acid
Naturally occurring amino acids Essential for all human beings*	Isoleucine Leucine Lysine Methionine Phenylalanine Threonine Tryptophan Valine
Essential for infants	Histidine
Nonessential	Glycine† Glutamic acid Arginine‡ Aspartic acid Proline Alanine Serine Tyrosine Cysteine Asparagine Glutamine
Related compounds sometimes classified as amino acids	Hydroxyglutamic acid Hydroxylysine Hydroxyproline Thyroxin Norleucine Cystine

*Chemical formulas are shown in Appendix H.
†Essential for chicks.
‡Essential for birds.

trogen determinations. The carboxyl group, the amino group, and the hydrogen atom are common to all amino acids. It is the nature of the *R group* that distinguishes one amino acid from another. *R* varies from a single hydrogen (H) atom as found in glycine, the simplest amino acid, to longer carbon chains of 1- to 7-carbon atoms. Those in which the carbon atoms are arranged in a hexagon rather than a straight-line (benzene ring) are called aromatic amino acids. Tyrosine and phenylalanine are examples. Others, such as cysteine and methionine, also contain sulfur. Arginine, histidine, and tryptophan contain a second nitrogen atom and are thus called dibasic amino acids. Otherwise the amino acids differ from one another only in the number of carbon atoms and the arrangement of the hydrogen and oxygen atoms attached to them in the characteristic radical (R).

SYNTHESIS

Proteins are built when amino acids join together in a long chain. This peptide chain is so named because the chemical bond that holds two amino acids together is called a *peptide bond.* An amino group of one amino acid joins with a carboxyl group of the next with the release of one molecule of water. Conversely, when we break the peptide linkage, as in digestion, water must be added before the amino acids can be split apart in either acid or enzyme hydrolysis. This is illustrated in Fig. 4-1. Proteins, as found in nature, consist of many amino acids linked together. The characteristics

of the protein are determined not only by which amino acids are used and the number of times they are repeated but also by the order in which they are joined together. Since each amino acid may be used any number of times in any relation to other amino acids, the possibility for the formation of different proteins becomes enormous. It is analogous to the number of words of fifty or more letters that could be made from an alphabet of twenty letters with no apparent limitations on the order in which they may be joined. In addition, the spatial arrangement of the amino acid chain, whether coiled, folded, or straight, influences manyfold the properties of the resulting protein and the possibilities of the number of proteins. It is unlikely that anywhere near the theoretical number of proteins exists in nature, but we have evidence that a great many do. The human body contains hundreds of different proteins, some of which contain as many as 200 amino acids. It is estimated that the liver cell alone contains a thousand different enzymes, each of which is a protein. In addition, each species builds proteins characteristic of itself. Thus, although the hemoglobin protein of a horse resembles that of a duck or a dog or a human being, they differ sufficiently that they cannot be interchanged with one another. In fact, the protein of one species is frequently toxic to another if introduced into the other before being hydrolyzed into its constituent amino acids. This, of course, makes transfusion of blood from one species to another impos-

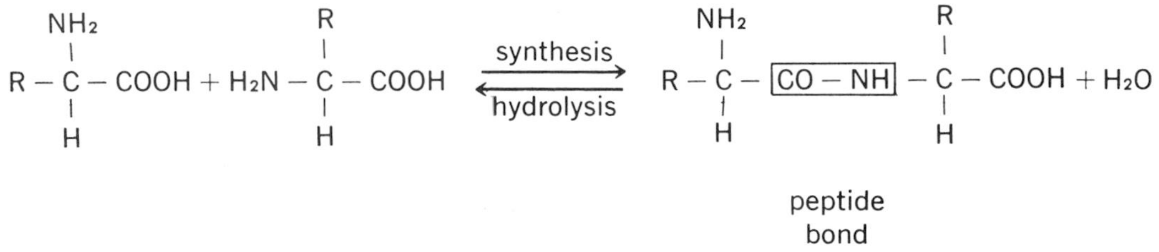

Fig. 4-1. Synthesis and hydrolysis of a dipeptide.

sible. These slight differences in hemoglobin from one species to another can be used as a basis for identifying the source of a blood sample.

Only in the last two decades have analytical techniques enabled us to determine the amino acid composition of a protein. It was even later before scientists could establish the order in which amino acids occur in a peptide chain. Now further advances have allowed us to determine the spatial relationship of the amino acids in a protein molecule. Myoglobin, consisting of one hundred fifty amino acid units representing nineteen different amino acids, is considered a simple protein and was the first for which the complete composition and structure was known. It was elucidated in 1961. Since then rapid progress has been made in determining the amino acid com-

position and sequence in many of the proteins that had previously been purified.

In 1969 two groups of scientists almost simultaneously announced the synthesis of the enzyme ribonuclease. The complexity of the structure of this enzyme is depicted in Fig. 4-2. They used different methods and produced slightly different forms of the same enzyme, accomplishing after fifty years of work what the ribosome of the cell accomplishes in 1 to 3 minutes. It is inevitable that the synthesis of other enzymes will follow rapidly, opening up a whole new area of nutritional investigation.

One of the long-term goals of biologists, nutritionists, and biochemists has been to determine how the cell knows which protein to build, that is, the kind and order and number of amino acids to incorporate when building new protein. This goal was

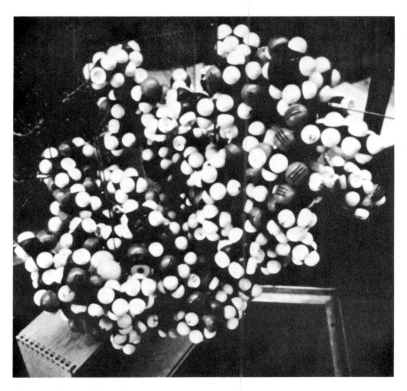

Fig. 4-2. Ribonuclease—three-dimensional structure. (Courtesy Dr. H. W. Wyckoff; from Denkewalter, R. G., and Hirschmann, R.: Amer. Sci. **57:**389, 1969.)

reached in 1962 when Watson and Crick showed that the pattern for protein synthesis was present in the substance DNA (deoxyribonucleic acid), the gene in the nucleus of the cell. The pattern is transferred to the ribosomes, the protein-synthesizing mechanism in the cytoplasm, by another nucleic acid, RNA (ribonucleic acid), known as messenger RNA. The ribosome is able to pick up amino acids carried to it by yet another form of RNA called transfer RNA and to incorporate them in a protein molecule in a prescribed order dictated indirectly from DNA through messenger RNA. Research findings announced in 1970 suggest that in the case of viruses the pattern for protein synthesis may be passed from RNA to DNA. The code or codes for specific amino acids have now been identified. With this information, geneticists may be able to change the message and hence the amino acid sequence in a protein. This offers much promise in the control of genetic defects that result in the production of a defective protein, usually an essential enzyme.

FOOD AS A SOURCE OF AMINO ACIDS

The ultimate value of a food protein to the body lies in its amino acid composition. Actually it is the amino acids that are the essential nutrients rather than the protein. Many foods commonly designated as proteins are more accurately called protein-rich foods, and their nutritive value lies in the amino acid composition of their various proteins. Some foods, such as gelatin, contain only one protein, but many have more than one. For example, hemoglobin, myoglobin, elastin, and collagen are all found in meat; casein and lactalbumin are found in milk.

Plants are able to build protein by fixing the element nitrogen from the soil and incorporating it in the amino acid and then in the protein molecule. Bacteria are able to utilize atmospheric nitrogen, but animals have no capacity to utilize the element nitrogen. They must depend on amino acids manufactured by plants, on proteins made by herbivorous animals, or on the limited capacity of bacteria in their gastrointestinal tracts to synthesize amino acids.

CLASSIFICATION

Amino acids. From a functional nutritional standpoint amino acids are classified into two groups—essential (indispensable) and nonessential (dispensable). An essential amino acid is one that cannot be synthesized by the body *at a rate* sufficient to meet the needs for growth and maintenance. In the classification in Table 4-1 it is seen that eight of the twenty amino acids are essential and must be provided by the diet. There is strong evidence that histidine is also essential for infants. Other species may require other amino acids. If sufficient nitrogen is available, the human being can synthesize the other twelve amino acids needed to build body proteins. The nitrogen used in the synthesis of nonessential amino acids and referred to as nonessential nitrogen may come from other nonessential amino acids or an excess of essential amino acids. In addition, there is some evidence that the human, like many animals, can make use of a limited portion of nitrogen provided by nonprotein nitrogen such as urea for the synthesis of nonessential amino acids. Amino acids from food that serve as a source of nitrogen for the synthesis of other amino acids undergo a process called *transamination*, in which the amino group is transferred to another substance, often a carbohydrate derivative, to form the required amino acid. Since the body must obtain this nitrogen from food, nonessential nitrogen is now considered a dietary essential.

Protein. Proteins in food are classified on the basis of their amino acid content. Although there is an overlap in the classification, it provides a simple basis on which to

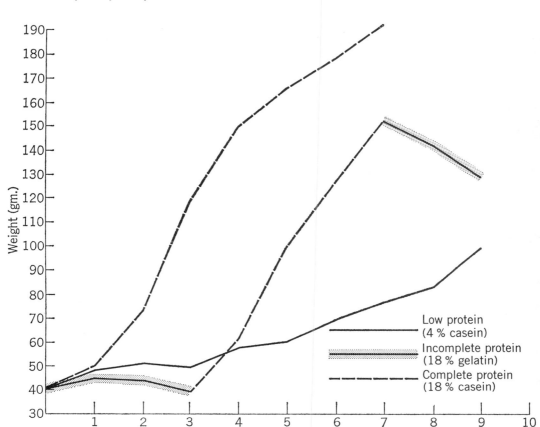

Fig. 4-3. Effect of complete, partially complete, and incomplete protein on growth of weanling rats.

evaluate protein quality. Proteins that contain all essential amino acids in proportions capable of promoting growth when they are the sole source of protein in the diet are described as complete proteins, good-quality proteins, or proteins of high biological value. They contain about 50% essential and 50% nonessential amino acids. All animal proteins except gelatin, which lacks both tryptophan and lysine, are complete proteins. Incomplete proteins, poor-quality proteins, or proteins of low biological value are those that lack one or more essential amino acids and hence are unable to provide all the amino acids for the synthesis of body proteins. When they are the sole source of protein in the diet, no new tissue

can be formed, nor can worn-out tissue be replaced. An animal on such a diet loses weight rapidly. All vegetable proteins except nuts are incomplete proteins. It is possible to simulate a complete protein by supplying simultaneously two vegetable proteins that supplement or complement one another or to supplement an incomplete protein with a small amount of animal protein. For instance, a combination of wheat lacking in lysine and corn lacking in tryptophan would provide a mixture containing all essential amino acids. Similarly, a small amount of milk taken with a wheat cereal would provide the missing amino acid and would enhance the biological value of the wheat protein. Some proteins that con-

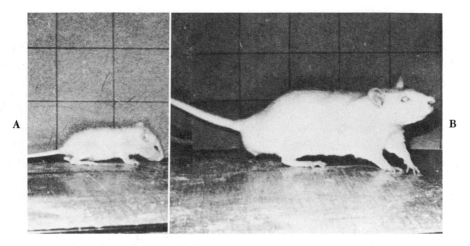

Fig. 4-4. Nine-week-old weanling rats. Rat **A**, raised in litter of 16, was fed a diet with 3% casein after weaning and weighed 19 gm. Rat **B**, raised in litter of 8, was fed diet with 18% casein after weaning and weighed 311 gm.

tain all essential amino acids but a relatively small amount of one have sufficient amino acids to repair body tissue if they are the sole source of dietary protein, but they do not have enough to promote growth. They are designated as partially complete proteins. The amino acid present in the smallest amount relatively is called a *limiting amino acid.* Arginine is the limiting amino acid in casein, and methionine is the one in fish and eggs. Lysine is the amino acid most often lacking in vegetable protein and methionine the next most limiting, although it does vary from one protein to another. A complete protein functions as a partially complete protein when it constitutes a small portion of the diet.

Fig. 4-3 shows the results of feeding complete, partially complete, and incomplete proteins to rats, and Fig. 4-4 shows 9-week-old littermates raised on a 3% and an 18% protein diet, respectively, for nine weeks.

FUNCTIONS

Although we must rely on protein-rich foods as a source of amino acids, it is the eight essential amino acids that are the ultimate nutrients for the body. It is the type and amounts of amino acids provided by the dietary protein that determine how effectively the body can perform the functions for which amino acids are needed. The needs for amino acids fall into five broad categories:

1. *Essential for growth.* Before cells can synthesize any new protein, they must have available the eight essential amino acids, plus sufficient nitrogen to incorporate with other materials to form the nonessential amino acids. Some amino acids are required to replace tissue that is constantly being broken down. If these are not available, there will be a loss of total body protein that will eventually result in loss of weight and emaciation. For growth to occur, amino acids must be present in amounts over and above those needed for maintenance. The growth of some tissues calls for specific amino acids, such as the sulfur-containing amino acids characteristic of hair, skin, and nails.

Gain in body weight per se is not an adequate criterion of protein nutrition. Pups fed a diet with a wheat protein, gluten, as the source of protein gained as much weight as a group receiving egg protein.

However, they were obese and inactive and had delayed skeletal development, whereas egg-fed pups were lean and active and had gained three times as much body protein. Rats will gain more weight on egg diet than on gluten diet, indicating that there is a correlation between weight gain in rats and tissue protein synthesis. Rather than store fat if the dietary amino acid pattern does not lead to protein synthesis, they reduce their food intake. A protein of high quality will yield maximum growth on a relatively low intake, after which weight gain per unit of protein drops and the efficiency with which protein is used also falls.

When normal body tissue fails to respond to a diet lacking in one or more amino acids, it has been found that tumor or abnormal tissue growth also subsides. This points to some hope that nutrition therapy, along with other forms of treatment, may prove useful in controlling tumor growth. If the nutrient is not available or its uptake by the cell is controlled, growth should be retarded.

2. *Formation of essential body compounds.* Hormones such as insulin, adrenaline, and thyroxin have been identified as protein substances. Every body cell contains many different enzymes, each catalyzing a specific reaction. All enzymes so far identified are protein. Coenzymes necessary for the action of enzymes have a protein structure usually associated with a specific vitamin. Hemoglobin, the substance in blood responsible for its oxygen and carbon dioxide–carrying properties so vital in respiration, is a protein complex. The amino acid tryptophan acts as a precursor to niacin, itself having a regulatory function as a vitamin.

The formation and replacement of these vital body compounds have high priority within the body and will suffer only in severe protein deprivation. Some tissue enzymes may be reduced 10% to 20% during protein depletion, those of brain being resistant to change and those of kidneys,

skeletal muscle, and spleen showing some reduction.

3. *Regulation of water balance through the maintenance of oncotic pressure.* The distribution of fluids on either side of a cell membrane is regulated by the osmotic pressure exerted by electrolytes and the oncotic pressure exerted by protein. Since plasma protein cannot penetrate the capillary membrane, it remains in the bloodstream when the hydrostatic pressure in the capillaries forces the plasma into the interstitial spaces to nourish the cells. When the oncotic pressure exerted by the plasma proteins exceeds the lowered hydrostatic pressure, the fluid is drawn back into the blood. In a protein deficiency the plasma albumin level drops, reducing the oncotic pressure to the point where the fluid is not drawn back and accumulates in the interstitial spaces. Under these conditions a soft spongy tissue, described as edematous, results and the animal suffers from edema, an early sign of protein deficiency. The restoration of normal plasma protein levels with an adequate dietary intake restores normal fluid balance, the fluid being withdrawn from the intercellular spaces to restore the blood volume.

4. *Maintenance of body neutrality.* Proteins are considered amphoteric substances, or buffers, capable of reacting with either acids or bases. Their presence in the blood helps prevent the accumulation of too much acid or base, either of which would interfere with normal body functioning. When an excess of base occurs, the protein acts as an acid by combining with the base to neutralize it and to prevent it from contributing to the alkalinity of the blood. Conversely, when excess acid appears in the body fluids, the proteins of the blood act as a base to neutralize it. Thus plasma protein performs an important function in helping to maintain body neutrality essential to normal cellular metabolism.

5. *Stimulation of antibody formation.* The antibodies of the body responsible for

its ability to combat infection are protein substances. The increased susceptibility to infection noted in low-protein diets is attributed to a lower level of antibodies capable of combatting the infective agents.

The ability to detoxify toxic material in the body is controlled by enzymes that are protein in nature. In protein depletion the ability to counteract the toxic effect of chemicals is reduced, rendering persons less resistant to certain poisons or drugs.

DIGESTION

Before protein can be absorbed through the wall of the intestine into the bloodstream, which carries it to the intercellular fluids that in turn bathe the individual cells, it must be broken down into its simplest structural blocks, the constituent amino acids. It now appears that two amino acids linked together as a dipeptide may enter the absorbing cells of the intestine. There, however, they must be broken into their constituent amino acids before passing into the bloodstream through the capillary wall into the intercellular spaces and eventually into the cell. This involves breaking the peptide linkages by which the amino acids are joined.

There are no protein-splitting enzymes in the saliva, and so the first attack made on the peptide linkages of the complex protein is in the stomach. Here in the acid media of the gastric contents, gastric protease (pepsin), the protein-splitting enzyme of the gastric juice, attacks specific linkages in the peptide chain remote from the ends and reduces it to shorter units of amino acids, known as peptones and peptides. From the stomach the partially digested proteins pass into the small intestine, where the acid is neutralized and the mixture becomes slightly alkaline. The pancreatic juice contains a protein-splitting enzyme, pancreatic protease or trypsin, which attacks very specific protein linkages—those involving carboxyl groups of lysine and arginine —but different ones from those attacked by gastric protease. The resulting shorter fragments may contain two amino acids (dipeptides) or three (tripeptides) but may also be more complex. The intestinal juice also secreted into the intestine contains enzymes capable of breaking the short protein fragments into their component amino acids. Two groups of enzymes attack the ends of the peptide chains—one, known as carboxypeptidase, attacks the carboxyl end; the other, an aminopeptidase, the amino end, releasing amino acids until only two remain joined as dipeptides. This final bond is broken by the action of dipeptidases—enzymes whose unique function is to separate two amino acids. The action of the dipeptidases may occur within the intestinal wall rather than in the intestinal lumen. All the protein-splitting enzymes are hydrolytic in that they require water to free the amino acids. This is a reversal of the process of synthesis, in which the amino acids are joined together with the release of one molecule of water for each linkage formed. Protein digestion is summarized in Fig. 4-5.

The apparent digestibility of protein based on differences between dietary nitrogen and fecal nitrogen is about 92%, but the fact that a variable amount of fecal nitrogen comes from intestinal cells and digestive enzymes makes true digestibility difficult to determine.

ABSORPTION

The amino acids formed in the process of digestion are in sufficiently simple form chemically to pass from the wall of the intestinal tract into the bloodstream either by diffusion or by the energy-requiring process of active transport. They are carried by the portal vein to the liver, where they are released into the general circulation and carried to the various tissues and cells. Vegetable proteins are less well absorbed than animal proteins, a difference that is only partially explained by the high fiber content of vegetables.

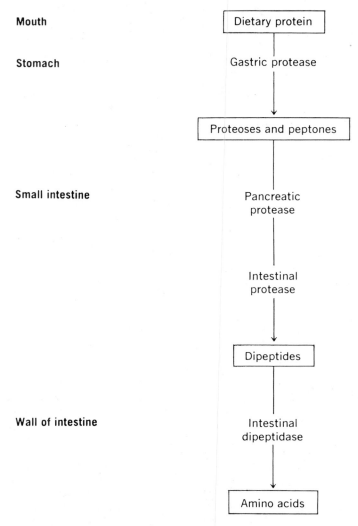

Mouth

Stomach

Small intestine

Wall of intestine

Fig. 4-5. Summary of protein digestion.

METABOLISM

The amino acids are taken up by the individual cells that use them in the synthesis of a specific protein. If the cell is to synthesize a protein, all the essential amino acids needed for its structure must be provided simultaneously. If they are not available, the cell will release the other essential amino acids, and no protein will be formed. In addition to the essential amino acids that the cell cannot manufacture, many nonessential amino acids are provided from the bloodstream. The cell will pick up at the same time any of the nonessential amino acids needed or, if they are not available in the amino acid pool, will synthesize them, using the nitrogen of other amino acids. It is conceivable that every cell is not capable of synthesizing all twelve indispensable amino acids but may rely on those synthesized by other cells and released into the amino acid pool of the bloodstream. For some particular cells, then, there may be more than eight essential amino acids. Although very complex, the whole process of protein synthesis is very rapid, sometimes taking only minutes.

Amino acids not needed by any of the body cells for building new protein will be released and returned to the liver, where the nitrogenous group will be removed in a process called *deamination*. The nonnitrogenous residue enters the metabolic cycle for carbohydrates and fats and will either be oxidized to provide energy or will be converted into fat and stored as an energy reserve. The nitrogen portion undergoes a series of chemical changes and is converted into urea by the liver and excreted by the kidney in the urine. Since the kidney is called upon to excrete this urea as metabolic waste, when protein is consumed in excess of needs for building body tissue and essential body compounds, a high protein intake, especially when fluid intake is low, may tax the capacity of the kidney to excrete waste.

An amino acid that, after deamination, is treated as a carbohydrate is described as a *glucogenic* amino acid. One that is metabolized as a fatty acid is referred to as a *ketogenic* amino acid.

Early concepts of protein metabolism maintained that body proteins were relatively static. However, once radioactive isotopes became available, it was soon demonstrated that body proteins are in a state of dynamic equilibrium with a constant interchange of nitrogen from one tissue to another and between newly absorbed and older amino acids. Tissue proteins are continually being broken down and resynthesized—contributing to and taking away from the metabolic pools of amino acids to which dietary proteins also contribute. Although there is no major storage site for extra protein, the size of the liver will increase when protein is available, and some tissue proteins, such as plasma albumin, represent labile protein reserves. In a de-

ficiency of either quantity or quality of dietary protein, storage protein is broken down to provide amino acids for more vital uses in the body. Plasma globulin levels, however, are maintained in periods of protein depletion, although they may be metabolically active at the time albumin levels are being depleted. Liver, gastric mucosa, pancreatic, muscle, and skin proteins can be used as labile reserves of amino acids, but the protein of the brain is resistant to change. The labile protein reserves, which can be reversibly depleted and repleted, comprise up to 25% of total body protein, and the amino acid pool represents about 0.5 gm. of nitrogen per kilogram of body weight. The total amount of protein in the body does not change as long as the body is in nitrogen equilibrium, but the rate of turnover of body protein varies from tissue to tissue. Some, such as the gut, pancreas, and liver, exhibit a very rapid amino acid turnover, whereas muscle and collagen turn over their amino acids more slowly. The rate of turnover in all tissues tends to decrease when dietary protein is limited. The half-life of total body protein is estimated at 80 days, and the rate of synthesis of protein in the adult man at 0.3 gm. per kilogram of body weight per day.

Under certain conditions amino acids tend to accumulate in specific tissues. For instance, insulin stimulates uptake of amino acids in muscle cells, estradiol stimulates uptake in the uterus, and both epinephrine and a growth hormone increase muscle uptake.

The digestion and metabolism of protein is summarized diagrammatically in Fig. 4-6. It is clear that dietary protein available to the cells as amino acids may be used in several ways.

1. If the caloric intake is adequate, amino acids are used for synthesis of protein as far as is needed.

2. If caloric intake is insufficient to meet energy needs *or* if more amino acids are available than are needed for synthesis of

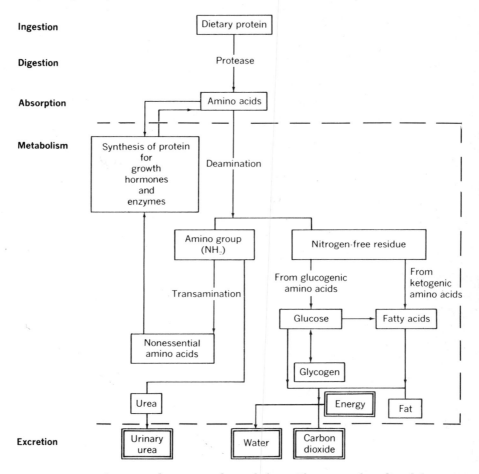

Fig. 4-6. Summary of protein digestion and metabolism. Changes within dotted lines occur after absorption and before excretion. Double boxes = end products.

protein *or* if all the essential amino acids are not present simultaneously, amino acids are deaminated, with the amino group being excreted as urea and the nonnitrogenous fraction being used as a source of energy.

3. If glucogenic amino acids (those capable of forming glucose) are deaminated they are converted into glucose and then are metabolized as glucose, that is, used as an immediate source of energy, stored as glycogen, or stored as fat.

4. If ketogenic amino acids (those capable of forming fatty acids directly) are deaminated, they are converted into fatty acids and either are used directly as a

source of energy or are converted into triglycerides and stored as fat.

The end products of protein metabolism are carbon dioxide, water, energy, and nitrogenous products in the urine. As with carbohydrates, the time elapsing between ingestion and excretion may vary from a few minutes to several months, depending on the intermediary steps involved and the stability of the protein.

FACTORS AFFECTING PROTEIN UTILIZATION

Amino acid balance. Equally important as the presence of all essential amino acids for protein synthesis is the balance of amino acids available to the cell. The pattern, or balance, of amino acids in egg protein is considered excellent for growth. Deviations from such a balance of amino acids results in less efficient growth response. It has been suggested that the limiting factor in the biological value of a protein is as frequently the pattern as the quantity of the essential amino acids. One of the hazards of supplementing a low-protein diet with a single amino acid is that an imbalance in the amino acid pattern of the total diet, which would occur if too much were added relative to the others present, may depress rather than improve the growth response. The growth depression noted in the addition of a single amino acid to low-protein diets is not present when a high-protein diet is supplemented. Apparently the dietary imbalance is reflected in a proportionately high level of the amino acid in the plasma that seems to interfere with the passage of the amino acid into the cell and the ability of the cell to synthesize tissue protein.

Caloric value. The protein content of the diet cannot be adequately evaluated without a consideration of the caloric content. As the caloric value of the diet drops below a certain critical point, the retention of nitrogen drops, indicating that part of the protein was deaminated and used for energy purposes. If caloric level is adequate, the level of protein utilization depends on the protein needs and the quality of the protein.

Immobility. The ability to synthesize protein is influenced by activity. It has been observed that bedridden patients, especially older people, experience a negative nitrogen balance even when dietary protein seems adequate. Protein tissue lost in febrile illness is regained at a slower rate than that at which it is lost. In studying protein metabolism in infants, Stearns found it necessary to limit the periods of observation to a maximum of three days, since further physical restraint decreases the efficiency of protein utilization.

A healthy individual in bed at rest loses nitrogen at a rate of 12 to 18 gm. per day.

Injury. Increase in nitrogen excretion after injury is well documented. It may reach as high as 20 gm. of nitrogen on a normal food intake. The use of high protein intakes immediately after injury neither prevents nor reverses the nitrogen loss. The losses are recovered once healing begins.

Emotional stability. Abnormal emotional stresses such as fear, anxiety, or anger increase the secretion of adrenaline, which in turn causes a series of changes that result in loss of nitrogen. Students lose nitrogen under the stress of examinations, as do persons experiencing severe pain, those whose work requires them to reverse normal night and day patterns, or those experiencing personal anxieties. Stress of a cold also increases nitrogen excretion.

NITROGEN BALANCE STUDIES

Practically all proteins have a constant and equal percentage of nitrogen—16%. It does vary slightly in a few proteins, depending on their amino acid content, but it is sufficiently close that scientists have been able to use the relatively simple Kjeldahl determination of nitrogen as indicative of protein. Since nitrogen accounts for 16% of the protein molecule, values for nitrogen can be multiplied by 6.25 (100/16) to give protein values. Thus studies of nitrogen metabolism have become the basis for assessing protein metabolism. The few vitamins and the nucleic acids that contain nitrogen have so little that it does not appreciably affect the results.

Nitrogen balance studies, which involve a determination of the nitrogen content of all food intake compared to the amount of nitrogen excreted, have provided us with basic information on the overall gain or loss of body protein. They do not, however, give information on changes among tissues. Most nitrogen is excreted either in the urine or feces. Urinary nitrogen represents

Table 4-2. Coefficient of digestibility of representative proteins

Food	Coefficient of digestibility
Eggs	97
Meat, fish	97
Milk	97
Wheat (70% to 74% extraction)	89
Fruits	85
Rice	84
Wheat cereals	79
Legumes (peas, beans, etc.)	78
Oatmeal	76
Root vegetables	74
Other vegetables	65

both endogenous nitrogen from the breakdown of body tissue and exogenous nitrogen, which represents that from digested and absorbed amino acids in excess of the body's need to build or repair body tissue or vital body compounds. In both cases the nitrogen is that which has been removed from the absorbed amino acids so that the rest of the protein molecule can be used as a source of energy. Exogenous nitrogen will appear in the urine when protein intake exceeds the body's need for protein, when caloric intake is insufficient to meet needs of the body, or when the protein does not contain enough of the essential amino acids to allow the body to synthesize protein to replace that lost through the breakdown of body tissue. The small and fairly constant percentage of ingested nitrogen, which appears in the feces and represents undigested protein, amounts to about 8% of the total intake, although this varies with the source of protein. Table 4-2 gives the coefficient of digestibility of various proteins. Some nitrogen is also lost in perspiration and the sloughing of cells, such as the cuticle and from the surface of the body, but the difficulties involved in measuring this loss and the fact that it is likely an insignificant amount relative to the total urinary and

fecal loss have not warranted its determination. Losses that range up to 0.56 gm. per square meter of body surface do assume greater importance when nitrogen balances are done in a tropical climate. Errors in nitrogen balance studies tend to overestimate intake and to underestimate excretion.

When nitrogen intake equals nitrogen excretion, the individual is said to be in nitrogen equilibrium. This indicates that the protein intake is sufficient to take care of replacing and repairing body tissue but that no growth or increase in body tissue is occurring. This is a condition that should prevail in any adult who is receiving at least the minimum protein needed. It also occurs at any level above minimum where no growth is occurring. When nitrogen intake exceeds nitrogen excretion, positive nitrogen balance prevails. Under these conditions growth occurs. Tissue or vital body compounds are being built at a rate faster than that at which they are being destroyed. Positive nitrogen balance should prevail throughout the period of childhood and adolescence and during pregnancy and lactation. It will also occur in recovery from an illness in which protein has been lost. Nitrogen excretion in excess of intake, negative nitrogen balance, means that body tissue is wearing out or breaking down at a rate faster than it is being repaired. It occurs not only when protein intake is low but also when calories are restricted. This is an undesirable situation, reflecting wasting of body tissue and loss of body protein. There is some evidence that individuals adapt to low protein intakes, since low levels of intake that produce a negative balance when fed after a higher intake may eventually be sufficient to establish nitrogen equilibrium as the body adjusts toward more efficient use of the amount available. Fig. 4-7 shows the amount of nitrogen needed to maintain body tissue and the amount needed to meet requirements for growth with increasing age. In infants almost equal amounts are needed for growth

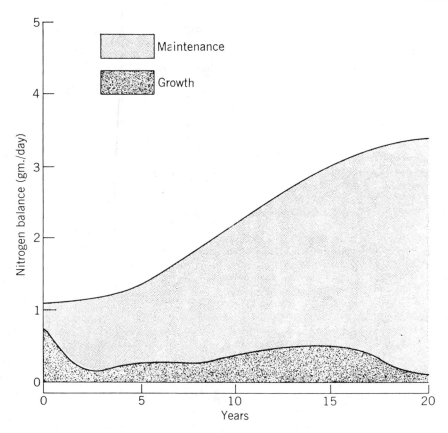

Fig. 4-7. Amounts of nitrogen needed for maintenance and growth of boys at various ages. (Adapted from Allison, J. B.: Trans. N. Y. Acad. Sci. **25**:293, 1963.)

Table 4-3. Summary of significance of nitrogen balance data

Condition	Measurement	Significance
Positive nitrogen balance	N intake > N excretion	Growth
Nitrogen equilibrium	N intake = N excretion	Maintenance and repair of tissue
Negative nitrogen balance	N intake < N excretion	Wasting of body, loss of weight

and maintenance, but in older persons the proportion needed for maintenance increases and that for growth decreases until adulthood, when virtually none is used for growth. An unexplained retention of nitrogen above that needed for repair of tissue has been observed in many adults. It has been designated as nitrogen needed for adult growth, although the nature of the need remains obscure.

Nitrogen balance studies yield information only on total protein mass and give no indication if a shift in body proteins from one tissue to another is occurring. For instance, plasma albumin levels may drop in an individual in nitrogen equilibrium, indicating that this labile nitrogen pool has been depleted to meet needs of another tissue. Thus it is possible for a suboptimal level of protein nutrition to prevail before it is manifest in negative nitrogen balance.

The significance of nitrogen balance data is summarized in Table 4-3.

DETERMINATION OF MINIMAL NEEDS

Nitrogen balance studies have been used to determine both minimum total protein and essential amino acid needs. In this technique the subject is fed progressively lower levels of nitrogen in successive balance periods, usually of 3 to 7 days' duration. As long as the individual is in nitrogen equilibrium, he is getting enough total protein, or if one amino acid is being tested, he is getting a sufficient amount of that amino acid. The point at which his nitrogen balance becomes negative is that at which his needs exceed his intake. His minimum protein need falls between the lowest point in which he was in equilibrium and the level at which his balance is negative. It is possible to arrive at a more precise figure by gradually increasing the protein in successive balance periods until the individual is again in equilibrium. By using this technique, it has been established that the requirements for the essential amino acids are surprisingly low. It is also evident that there are wide individual differences in needs for amino acids, as for other nutrients. There is still much controversy over proposed values. In addition to the minimum amounts proposed for these amino acids, there must be sufficient nonessential nitrogen to allow for the synthesis of nonessential amino acids. With the recognition that the body needs amino acids, nitrogen, and organic acids rather than protein as such for protein synthesis, the term *protein requirement* is becoming outmoded. How-

ever, in the following discussion of requirements we will think of the amount of protein necessary to provide the amino acids and nitrogen needed by each group.

DIETARY REQUIREMENTS

Estimates of desirable protein intakes may be obtained in two ways. They may be based on observations of the minimum amount of protein that will promote growth in children and maintain nitrogen balance in adults. Alternatively, they may be based on calculations of the losses of nitrogen that occur through the urine and feces on a protein-free diet together with allowances for losses through the skin, sweat, and loss of cells and amounts needed to take care of the increase in body mass during growth. This latter method was used by the Food and Nutrition Board of the National Research Council in arriving at the recommended dietary allowances (RDA).

The Food and Nutrition Board calculated that losses of endogenous nitrogen in the urine amounted to 2 mg. per basal kilocalorie of energy expenditure (Chapter 5); in the feces, 0.4 mg.; and through the skin and for growth of hair and nails, 0.8 mg. This is a total of 3.2 mg. of nitrogen per basal kilocalorie. Since protein is 16% nitrogen, the replacement of this much nitrogen would require an intake of 20 (3.2 × 6.25) mg. of protein per basal kilocalorie. Since these figures were based on average losses, adjustment had to be made to take into account the variations that could be expected within a population group. Assuming that the needs of almost all people would fall within two standard deviations of the average, they added an additional 30% to take into account those people with the largest needs. Since the biological value of the protein in the average diet cannot be assumed to be 100, a further adjustment had to be made to reflect the lower biological value of the diet, which was arbitrarily set at 70. Thus the estimate of 20 mg. for the average person using a high-quality protein must be increased by 6 mg. (30%) to take into account individual variation and by a further factor of 100/70 to adjust for biological value for a recommendation of 38 mg. per basal kilocalorie. Since basal energy requirement is 1 kcal. per kilogram of body weight per hour, the protein requirement becomes 38 mg. × 24 (hr.) per kilogram of body weight, or 0.9 gm. per kilogram of body weight. This figure was used to arrive at all the recommendations for periods when growth is not normally occurring.

In figuring the needs during growth, they assumed that increase in body weight was 18% protein and added an appropriate figure based on observations of growth rate.

The Food and Agricultural Organization in setting practical protein allowances came up with a comparable figure of 0.71 gm. of protein of high biological value per kilogram of body weight. They believed this would meet the needs of all but a small segment of the population. They suggested that estimates of needs during growth should be based on intakes observed to be compatible with growth rather than on estimations derived by the factorial method used by the National Research Council.

For protein diets of different biological value and different coefficients of digestibility, the requirement can be calculated.

For infants and children experiencing a rapid increase in body weight, much of which is bone and muscle growth, the recommended levels of protein intake are considerably higher per unit of body weight. Intakes of 2.2 gm. per kilogram of body weight are proposed for the first 2 months, 2 gm. from 2 to 6 months, and 1.8 gm. from 6 to 12 months of age.

Minimum protein level needed by infants will usually be reached when protein provides 6% of the caloric intake. For breast-fed infants this amounts to 1.5 to 2.5 gm. per kilogram.

In periods from 1½ to 3 years of age,

increase in muscle accounts for half the weight gain. The amount needed to ensure normal growth is again a function of the biological value of the protein in the diet as well as the individual characteristics of the infants.

Up to 9 years of age the skeleton grows faster than the body as a whole so that protein needs are proportionately high. As legs grow in length and the center of gravity becomes farther from the floor, more muscles must be developed to maintain posture and to permit activity.

For adolescents the recommendation is that 15% of the calories be provided by protein. Since protein has a physiological fuel value of 4 kcal. per gram, a person needing 2800 kcal. should receive 420 from protein, or 105 gm. of protein. This is in excess of the RDA of 65 gm. One of the important considerations in establishing recommended levels for adolescents is an evaluation of the level that produces a healthy adult.

During pregnancy the NRC suggests intakes that are increased 10 gm. This is used not only for the growth of the fetus but also for the growth of the placenta, mammary glands, and other tissue reserves for lactation. A 7-pound baby has 1 pound of protein, acquired primarily in the last half of pregnancy. This growth calls for 4 to 6 gm. of protein per day above maintenance requirements. Restriction of protein in the mother's diet leads to the birth of shorter, lighter infants. Two thirds of the protein in the diet of pregnant women should be of high biological value. In lactation the requirement is raised by 20 gm. The production of 850 ml. of mature human milk with a protein content of 1.2% involves the synthesis of 10 gm. of milk protein, mostly lactalbumin.

A comparison of protein standards recommended by various groups is given in Table 4-4.

Amino acids. In the determination of the requirements of essential amino acids based

Table 4-4. Comparison of protein standards for selected age groups (in grams)

	NRC recommended allowances*	Canadian dietary standards†	FAO‡	Nutrient allowances, United Kingdom§
Adult men (70 kg.)	65	48	0.71/kg.	75
Adult women (58 kg.)	55	39	0.77/kg.	55
Pregnancy	+10	+9	+6 gm./day	60
Lactation	+20	+23	+15 gm./day	68
Children 1– 3 years	25	17	1.06/kg.	20-35
3– 6 years	30	20	0.97/kg.	40
6– 8 years	35	24	0.92/kg.	45
8–10 years	40	30	0.86/kg.	53
Adolescent 14–18 years (boy)	60	45	0.84/kg.	75
14–18 years (girl)	55	41	0.84/kg.	58

*Food and Nutrition Board: Recommended dietary allowances, ed. 7, Publication No. 1694, Washington, D. C., 1968, National Academy of Sciences—National Research Council.
†Dietary standards for Canada, Canadian Bulletin on Nutrition, vol. 6, No. 1, March, 1964 Rev. 1968.
‡Joint FAO/WHO Expert Group: Protein requirements, FAO Nutrition Meeting Report Series No. 37, Rome, 1965, p. 49.
§Department of Health and Social Security, Recommended intakes of nutrients for the United Kingdom, Reports on Public Health and Medical Subjects No. 120, London, 1969, Her Majesty's Stationery Office.

Table 4-5. Minimal amino acid requirements

	Infants (mg./kg.)*	Adult female (mg./day)†	Adult male (mg./day)†
Isoleucine	126	450	700
Leucine	150	620	1100
Lysine	103	500	800
Methionine	45‡	350	200‡
Phenylalanine	90§	220	300§
Threonine	87	305	500
Tryptophan	22	157	250
Valine	105	650	800
Histidine	34	—	—

(Suggested adult protein intake is 0.52 gm. per kilogram per day.)

*Holt, L. E., Gyorgy, P., Pratt, E. L., and Wallace, W. M.: Protein and amino acid requirements in early life, New York, 1960, New York University Press.
†Food and Nutrition Board Committee on Amino Acids: Evaluation of protein nutrition, Publication No. 711, Washington, D. C., 1959, National Academy of Science–National Research Council.
‡In presence of adequate tyrosine.
§In presence of adequate cystine.

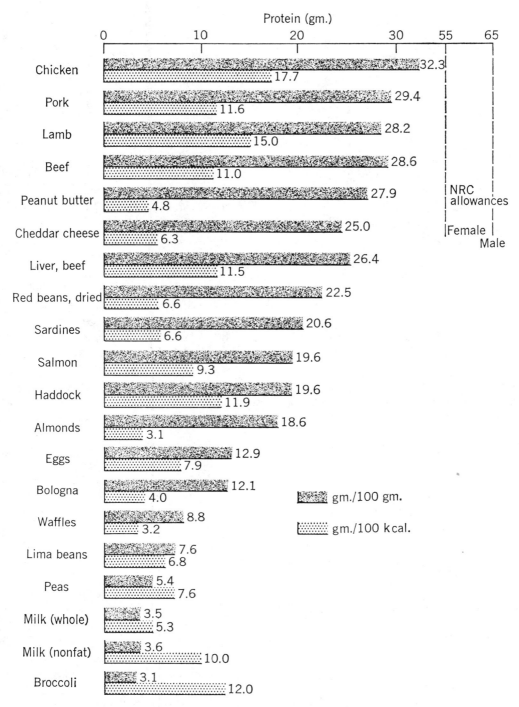

Protein (gm.)

Chicken	32.3 / 17.7
Pork	29.4 / 11.6
Lamb	28.2 / 15.0
Beef	28.6 / 11.0
Peanut butter	27.9 / 4.8
Cheddar cheese	25.0 / 6.3
Liver, beef	26.4 / 11.5
Red beans, dried	22.5 / 6.6
Sardines	20.6 / 6.6
Salmon	19.6 / 9.3
Haddock	19.6 / 11.9
Almonds	18.6 / 3.1
Eggs	12.9 / 7.9
Bologna	12.1 / 4.0
Waffles	8.8 / 3.2
Lima beans	7.6 / 6.8
Peas	5.4 / 7.6
Milk (whole)	3.5 / 5.3
Milk (nonfat)	3.6 / 10.0
Broccoli	3.1 / 12.0

NRC allowances — Female — Male

▓ gm./100 gm.

░ gm./100 kcal.

Fig. 4-8. Protein contribution of 100 gm. and 100 kcal. portions of some representative foods. (Based on Watt, B. K., and Merrill, A. L.: Composition of foods—raw, processed and prepared, U. S. Department of Agriculture Handbook No. 8, Washington, D. C., 1963, U. S. Department of Agriculture.)

on nitrogen balance studies, amino acids must be provided in purified form and the level of all amino acids as well as that of nonessential nitrogen must be carefully controlled. The technique is costly and time consuming. The results of experiments to assess the amino acid needs of infants, adult men, and adult women have not been accepted uncritically. The currently accepted standards are given in Table 4-5, although it is recognized that further work will undoubtedly lead to modifications.

FOOD SOURCES

Some of the major food sources of protein and their contribution to the total protein requirement are shown graphically in Fig. 4-8. Values are expressed in terms of 100 gm. of the food and 100 kcal. It must be remembered that the ultimate value of a protein-rich food to the diet is determined by its amino acid pattern. Generally speaking, proteins of animal origin have a better distribution of amino acids than do those of vegetable origin, but within each group there is a wide range in biological values.

The effect of heat on the utilization of dietary protein has been the subject of much research. The results of such studies have not been conclusive, however. The peak level of amino acids in the blood after the ingestion of overheated pork was not reached for 5 hours, indicating slow digestion of the protein. Weight gain was reduced 22% on overheated pork. When soybeans were fed, moderate heating of the beans increased plasma amino acid levels, whereas overheating reduced them. The beneficial effects of heating were believed to be caused by greater ease in the release of the limiting amino acid methionine. On the other hand, the protein of wheat and oats is adversely affected by heat, as is that of nine out of seventeen legume seeds tested. The amount of heat used in the preparation of evaporated and dried milks seems to improve the digestibility and utilization of the protein. When heat does decrease the nutritive value of proteins, the effect seems to be caused by a reduction in hydrolysis of heated proteins by digestive enzymes, indicating that heating has produced complexes resistant to the action of digestive enzymes. If heating affects the *rate* of release of amino acids from a protein, it could affect the nutritive value that is dependent on the release of all amino acids simultaneously.

Some protein-rich foods such as peanuts cannot be eaten raw as they contain either toxic substances or enzymes that must be destroyed before they are of value to the human body. Some are susceptible to the growth of toxic molds.

Since protein-rich foods are one of the most expensive items in the average diet, it is helpful to have information on the cost of similar amounts of protein from various sources. Such information is provided in Table 4-6, which shows the cost of one third of a day's allowance of protein for the adult male—22 gm. In interpreting this data it must be kept in mind that they are based on average prices in April, 1970, and may not be accurate at any specific date in the future, especially in the light of seasonal variations in costs of products such as eggs and pork. They are presented only to give some concept of relative costs. Many of the foods represented make significant contributions of other nutrients as well.

In assessing the value of a day's diet, it is important to look at the distribution of dietary protein throughout the day's meals. Generally it is recommended that at least one third of the protein be from animal sources of high biological value. The typical American diet is more likely to contain 60% to 80% animal protein. But if this is not distributed so that the amino acid composition of each meal is adequate through some complete protein or a mixture of vegetable proteins that supplement one another, the individual will be unable to use protein as a body builder and will be forced to

Table 4-6. Cost of one-third daily recommended allowance of protein for an adult male, based on average retail prices in Pennsylvania in April, 1970

Cost of portion providing 22 gm. protein	Food	Amount (lb.) to be purchased to provide 22 gm. protein	kcal.
<10 cents	Dry beans	0.22	339
	Nonfat dried milk	0.13	220
10 to 20 cents	Cottage cheese	0.36	173
	Cornmeal	0.61	1007
	Pork liver	0.24	143
	Cheddar cheese	0.19	343
	Tuna fish	0.20	152
	Rice	0.72	1186
	Enriched white bread	0.56	683
	Peanut butter	0.19	502
	Hamburger	0.23	187
	Eggs, large	0.42	276
	Chicken	0.30	118
20 to 30 cents	Fresh whole milk	1.38	407
	Veal cutlet	0.25	177
	Haddock fillet	0.26	93
	Chuck roast	0.28	385
	Frozen peas	0.90	302
30 to 40 cents	Frankfurters	0.39	157
	Canned lima beans	1.18	380
	Bologna	0.40	552
>40 cents	Bacon, sliced	0.58	1749
	Ham, sliced	0.36	428
	Lamb chops	0.34	390

deaminate it for use as a source of energy. Traditionally we do use complete protein to supplement incomplete protein in the diet. The use of milk with cereal, cheese with macaroni, meat with rice, and peanut butter with bread are examples of these complementary relationships. The increasing use of dried milk solids in commercially baked bread has a supplementary effect on the amino acid pattern of the wheat protein and improves the biological value of the bread protein. Any baked flour product such as muffins or waffles will have the protein quality of the flour enhanced by the egg protein.

The efforts of some commercial interests to promote the addition of lysine to bread and flour in the United States are likely not justified, since there is no evidence of a lysine deficiency in the American diet. In addition, recent studies suggest that protein quality may be depressed rather than increased if the level of one amino acid is increased out of proportion to the others. Amino acid supplementation of a low-quality protein may be justified when it is a staple item in a total diet of low biological value, but not when protein quality is high.

The relative contribution of various food groups to the protein in the American diet is shown in Fig. 4-9 and trends in the contribution of various food groups to total protein intake in Fig. 4-10.

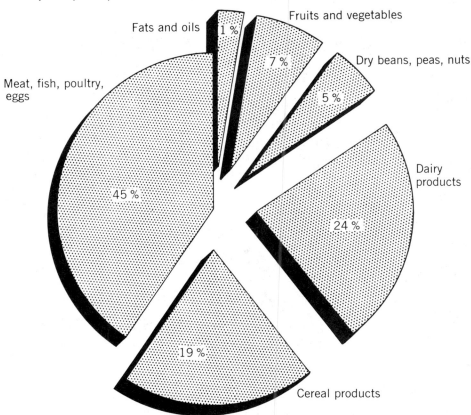

Fig. 4-9. Contribution of food groups to protein content of the American food supply. (Based on Contribution of major food groups to nutrient supplies available for civilian consumption, National Food Situation No. 130, 1969.)

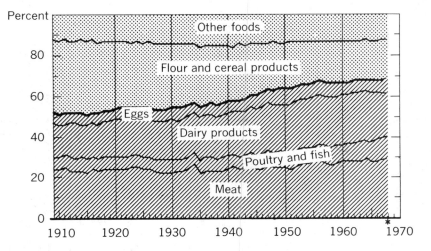

Fig. 4-10. Trends in the contribution of various food groups to the protein content of the American diet from 1910 to 1968. Sources of protein, per capita civilian food supply. *Total animal sources. (From 1968 preliminary data, Agricultural Research Service, U. S. Department of Agriculture, 1969.)

EVALUATION OF PROTEIN QUALITY

Since the amino acid content of a protein as well as the total amount of protein in the diet determines the value of the protein, the problem of measuring the relative value of various proteins as dietary constituents is complex. Both biological and chemical methods of evaluating protein quality have been tried.

A widely used index is the biological value (BV). This is a measure of the relationship of protein retention to protein absorption on the assumption that more will be retained when the essential amino acids are present in sufficient quantity to meet the needs for growth. The biological value is assessed by determining the nitrogen in the food intake and the urinary and fecal excretions. Urinary nitrogen includes that from absorbed amino acids that have been deaminated, and fecal nitrogen represents that which was unabsorbed, plus that from any cells that may have sloughed off the lining of the digestive tract or digestive enzymes that have not been themselves digested and reabsorbed. The formula for determining biological value becomes the following:

$$BV = \frac{\text{Dietary N} - (\text{Urinary N} + \text{Fecal N})}{\text{Dietary N} - \text{Fecal N}} \times 100$$

A protein with a biological value of 70 or more (that is, 70% of the intake of nitrogen is retained) is considered capable of supporting growth, assuming that the caloric value of the diet is adequate. Dietaries with a biological value of less than 70 are less capable of supporting growth through the use of more of that protein. This index may be applied to single proteins, single foods, or combinations of protein in foods. The biological value of representative proteins is given in Table 4-7. In testing for the biological value of a protein, it is necessary to feed it at the level needed for maintenance or slightly below so that it will be used with maximum efficiency.

Since the BV is based only on the

Table 4-7. Biological value of representative proteins

Food	Biological value
Egg	100
Milk	93
Rice	86
Fish	75
Beef	75
Casein	75
Corn	72
Cottonseed flour	60
Peanut flour	56
Wheat gluten	44

amount of nitrogen absorbed, it does not take into account differences in digestibility from one protein to another. The measurement of protein quality by an index known as *net protein utilization* (NPU) has been introduced to express in a single measurement both the digestibility of the protein and the biological value of the amino acid mixture absorbed from the intestine. NPU = N retained/N intake and can be represented by BV × digestibility.

The protein efficiency ratio (PER) is the simplest method of determining protein quality, since it requires no chemical analyses. It merely requires calculating the weight gain of a growing animal in relation to its protein intake when calories are adequate and the protein source is fed at an adequate level for a sufficiently long period of time to assess the protein. It is based on the assumption (which may be in error) that weight gain of a growing animal is in proportion to gain in body protein.

In addition to the biological methods of evaluating protein quality, there are several chemical methods that are based on the determination of the amino acid pattern of a particular food and a comparison of this to a reference protein. In 1957 the FAO proposed a reference protein based on the amino acid requirements of man but in 1965 decided to abandon its use in favor of an amino acid pattern of whole egg or

Table 4-8. *Selected essential amino acid patterns**

| Amino acid | A/E ratio: mg/gm. total essential amino acids | | | |
	1957 FAO provisional pattern	Cow's milk	Human milk	Hen's egg (whole)
Isoleucine	134	127	132	129
Leucine	152	196	184	172
Lysine	134	155	128	125
Total "aromatic" amino acids	178	197	226	195
Phenylalanine	89	97	114	114
Tyrosine	89	100	112	81
Total sulfur-containing amino acids	133	65	87	107
Cystine	62	17	43	46
Methionine	71	48	44	61
Threonine	89	91	99	99
Tryptophan	45	28	34	31
Valine	134	137	147	141

*From Joint FAO/WHO Expert Group: Protein requirements, WHO Techn. Rep. Ser. 301, 1965.

human milk as a standard. Chemical scores based on these standards are in closer agreement with the biological indices of protein quality. To obtain a chemical score, the amount of each essential amino acid is expressed as a ratio of total essential amino acids in the test protein. This is compared to similar calculation for the reference protein to yield a score that reflects the extent of the deviation of the most limiting amino acid. Chemical scores do not take into consideration imbalances in amino acid patterns, and they do not consider differences in absorption of amino acids. Both these factors could account for discrepancies between results from biological and chemical evaluation of protein quality.

The amount of each essential amino acid in relation to the total essential amino acids in the various proposed reference proteins is shown as the A/E ratio in Table 4-8.

The fact that so many standards for evaluating protein quality have been and are being proposed is evidence that we lack any single satisfactory standard. Many based on biological assays are more costly and time consuming than chemical analyses of amino acid composition. However, protein metabolism is apparently so complex that a determination of chemical makeup of a protein gives only limited information on the manner in which the animal may utilize it. Similarly, proteins that can effectively repair body tissue may have limitations as a source of growth protein.

KWASHIORKOR

The importance of protein in world nutrition has been emphasized in the last two decades with the identification of the condition *kwashiorkor* as a protein-deficiency disease. This condition occurs primarily among children between the ages of 2 and 5 years when they are weaned from mother's milk to a diet of starchy cereal pastes practically devoid of protein. Fig. 1-3 shows a child with kwashiorkor. This term, which was applied by the Ga tribe in Ghana to a sickness of a weanling child, means literally "first-second." It was appropriate because the first child developed it within 3 or 4 months after being abruptly weaned from the breast on the arrival of the second child. This corresponds to the time when milk, his only source of good-quality protein, is removed. Kwashiorkor is considered the major nutrition problem in the world today; many infants are dying as a result of it, and untold numbers are suffering from subclinical symptoms of the disease and increased susceptibility to infection. In kwashiorkor there is a deficiency in quality and quantity of dietary protein in the presence of adequate calories. *Marasmus* is the term applied to the condition resulting from a caloric deficit that is usually accompanied by a protein deficiency. The term *protein-calorie malnutrition* (PCM) is being widely used and reflects the fact that they are seldom discrete syndromes.

The main clinical symptoms of kwashiorkor are as follows:

1. Failure to grow in both weight and length, with weak, thin, and wasting muscles
2. Mental changes manifest as irritability and apathy
3. Edema—the accumulation of fluid in the tissues, causing them to be soft and spongy, especially in the lower half of the body
4. Skin changes, especially in the lower part of the body, including abnormal color in some areas, lack of color in others, and drying and peeling of the skin resulting in the formation of ulcers
5. Changes in hair, which becomes sparse and loses its pigmentation or takes on a characteristic reddish color
6. Loss of appetite, vomiting, and diarrhea
7. Enlargement of the liver
8. Anemia

The ability of the child to combat infection is very low and death is usually attributed to an infection, such as measles or pneumonia, that would not normally be fatal.

Unfortunately many children with kwashiorkor are never given medical help or are brought in for treatment only when the disease is well advanced. The most helpful diagnostic sign is a change in serum albumin levels, but this change does not occur in the very early stages of the condition. If diagnosed early enough, prekwashiorkor, which could be identified if the growth of the child were plotted regularly, can be treated simply by improving the amount and quality of protein in the diet. The treatment must also take into account the anorexia or loss of appetite that is common. However, in more advanced cases, extreme care must be taken to compensate for the low potassium levels that usually accompany low protein intake. Nonfat milk has been the most successful therapeutic food. It is diluted at first and increased in strength gradually until full strength can be tolerated. Once the edema has been eliminated and blood potassium levels have been restored, whole milk or nonfat milk with coconut and corn oil added are necessary to provide sufficient calories to stimulate growth.

The most promising attack on the problem of kwashiorkor is one of prevention, which implies the use of a diet adequate in good-quality protein and calories. Most attempts to provide sufficient animal protein are impractical where there is limited land available and where the cost of animal protein is economically out of reach of most of the population. The situation will become progressively worse as population pressures increase. The one inexpensive source of animal protein that has promise is fish, but problems of preservation in tropical climates limit the extent to which this is exploited.

Efforts are being encouraged to provide a palatable low-cost food with an adequate balance of amino acids that can be made from indigenous plant substances for use in the postweaning diet of infants to supplement the basic cereal diet. Since no one plant protein provides a desirable balance for mammalian needs, a search for such a mixture of plant proteins has been the incentive for much research. One promising effort has been that of the Institute of Nutrition in Central America and Panama, commonly referred to as INCAP. They have succeeded in producing a mixture of 58% ground maize and sorghum, 36% cottonseed flour, 3% torula yeast, 1% $CaCo_3$ and vitamin A. It is sold under the name of Incaparina and has been widely accepted for use as a relatively low-bulk beverage or gruel at a cost of less than 4 cents per day. This mixture provides the critical pattern of amino acids required for child growth and at the same time corrects the nutrient deficiencies that usually accompany kwashiorkor—vitamin A, riboflavin, calcium, niacin, and potassium. Other combinations of leaf protein and legumes available in other regions such as Lebanon and India have been developed and show promising results.

Some efforts have been made to enrich, or to fortify, cereals with the limiting amino acids, such as adding lysine to wheat, lysine and threonine to rice, and lysine, threonine, and methionine to barley. This has not proved practical, as it only improves the quality of the protein and does not solve the problem of the low protein intake. In addition, only methionine and lysine are sufficiently low in cost to begin to be economically feasible. The possibility of creating an imbalance in the amino acid pattern by the addition of too much of the limiting amino acid is another reason for caution.

A third approach has been to supplement basic cereal diets with small amounts of animal protein. The addition of 20% nonfat milk powder or 10% fish flour to a maize and pea mixture produces a protein equal to milk in nutritive value. The de-velopment of protein concentrates that can be incorporated into basic cereal products has been encouraging. Fish flour, with a protein content of 85% and produced from small fish that normally have no commercial value, is acceptable when it has been defatted and deodorized. Concentrates from coconut seed press cakes, other seed kernels, and cottonseed are inexpensive and promising as a partial solution to the problems of protein malnutrition. Care must be taken to exclude any toxic substances that are naturally present or that develop during processing.

Plant geneticists have succeeded in developing a type of corn with a protein of greatly improved nutritive value. The "miracle rice," a high-yield variety with a short growing period and a high resistance to disease, shows great promise in increasing the amount of rice available in southeast Asia. Many commercial companies are investigating the potential of soybean-based beverages for increasing protein consumption in developing countries. The possibility of using chlorella, a microscopic plankton that abounds in the sea, and a protein produced by bacteria from petroleum also are being studied experimentally.

In addition to having a protein content of high biological value, any food that will provide any hope for meeting the nutritional needs in developing countries must meet certain other criteria. It must be locally available or capable of being produced locally, must be within economic reach of the segment of the population needing it, must have long storage life under hot humid conditions, and must be easily transported; it must also have acceptable characteristics of taste, odor, and physical properties. On the other hand, if it is too popular it may become a prestige food in the culture and be consumed by the ranking adult males rather than by children and pregnant women whose needs are greatest. The food must be free from toxic and deleterious effects in the form proposed and must not be currently used to a maximum as human food. Many foods, or combination of foods, have been suggested, but at present, in addition to fish flour, the most promising appear to be soy products with a protein value of 25%, peanut flour, sesame flour, cottonseed flour, oil seed cakes, and coconut protein. Algae and yeast, although theoretically good sources, have not proved sufficiently palatable for human use. Others have been eliminated because of their unknown nutritive value, the uneconomical aspects of their production, a limited production of the raw material, or the presence of a toxic substance.

ABNORMALITIES IN AMINO ACID METABOLISM

Some infants are born with an inability to produce the enzymes necessary for phenylalanine metabolism. These children need a small amount of this essential amino acid for protein synthesis but have no ability to metabolize the rest, with the result that phenylalanine and some of its partially oxidized derivatives accumulate in the blood and urine. They have an adverse effect on nervous tissue and the resulting condition, known as phenylketonuria (PKU), is characterized by mental retardation. Early diagnosis is crucial to successful treatment in which a diet very low in phenylalanine is indicated.

A similar failure to metabolize leucine and valine is reflected as maple sugar urine disease, so named because of the characteristic odor of the urine. Failure to metabolize histidine appears related to speech defects. Up to 250 other inborn errors of metabolism involving other enzyme defects have also been reported.

SELECTED REFERENCES

Allison, J. B., and Fitzpatrick, W. H.: Dietary proteins in health and disease, Springfield, Ill., 1960, Charles C Thomas, Publisher.

Allison, J. B., and Wannemacher, R. W., Jr.: The concept and significance of labile and over-all protein reserves of the body, Amer. J. Clin. Nutr. 16:445, 1965.

Committee Report: Assessment of protein nutritional status, Amer. J. Clin Nutr. 23:807, 1970.

Denkewalter, R. G., and Hirschmann, R.: The synthesis of an enzyme, Amer. Sci. 57:389, 1969.

Food and Nutrition Board: Meeting protein needs of infants and children, Publication No. 943, Washington, D. C., 1961, National Academy of Sciences–National Research Council.

Food and Nutrition Board: Evaluation of protein quality, Publication No. 1100, Washington, D. C., 1963, National Academy of Sciences–National Research Council.

Harper, A. E.: Some implications of amino acid supplementation, Amer. J. Clin. Nutr. 9:533, 1961.

Hegsted, D. M.: Amino acid fortification and the protein problem, Amer. J. Clin. Nutr. 21:688, 1968.

Hegsted, D. M.: Minimum protein requirements of adults, Amer. J. Clin. Nutr. 21:352, 1968.

Holt, L. E., Jr., Halac, E., Jr., and Kadji, C. N.: The concept of protein stores and its implication in the diet, J.A.M.A. 181:699, 1962.

Joint FAO/Who Expert Group: Protein requirements, WHO Techn. Rep. Ser. 301, 1965.

Miller, D. S., and Payne, P. R.: The assessment of protein requirements by nitrogen balance. Proc. Nutr. Soc. 28:225, 1969.

Schrimshaw, N. S.: Nature of protein requirements; ways they can be met in tomorrow's world, J. Amer. Diet. Ass. 54:94, 1969.

Spencer, R. P.: Intestinal absorption of amino acids. Current concepts, Amer. J. Clin. Nutr. 22:292, 1969.

5 | *Energy balance*

ENERGY SOURCES

The energy value of the diet is provided entirely by its carbohydrate, fat, and protein (and alcohol) components. These may make up from 4% of foods such as lettuce to 100% of foods such as sugar, salad oil, and dry gelatin. The remaining portion of the food consists of water, cellulose, minerals, and vitamins, none of which yields energy. In the typical American diet, carbohydrate provides 50% to 60% of the energy; protein, 10% to 15%; and fat, 35% to 45%. The source of energy in diets varies with many factors—agricultural, cultural, social, and economic. For instance, in rice-eating countries, carbohydrate makes a much larger contribution, and in countries with emphasis on dairying, protein assumes greater importance. Italians, with the extensive use of cooking oil, derive more energy from fats. In America the trend is toward greater use of protein and a concurrent decrease in carbohydrate consumption with an increase in the amount of money available for food.

Unit of measurement

The energy value of a food is expressed in terms of a unit of heat, a *kilocalorie* (kcal.)* This represents the amount of heat required to raise the temperature of 1 kg. (slightly over 1 quart) of water 1° C. Although this unit is correctly designated as a kilocalorie to distinguish it from the smaller unit, a calorie (0.001 kcal.), used

---

*The American Institute of Nutrition has endorsed a proposal that the *joule* (4.18 kcal. = 1 joule) be adopted as the unit of energy in nutrition.

in most physical and chemical measurements, many nutrition sources still refer to it as the Calorie or even calorie, assuming that it is a sufficiently standardized term in nutrition that no distinction need be made. It will undoubtedly be some time before the term *calorie,* as used in popular literature, will be replaced by the more correct *kilocalorie.* Indeed, to do so may introduce undue confusion to a topic that is freely discussed but only vaguely understood by the general public.

A concept of the amount of energy or heat available from foods may be obtained by noting that 2 tablespoons of sugar provide 100 kcal., enough heat to raise the temperature of slightly over 4 cups of water from 0° C. (freezing) to 100° C. (boiling), assuming a high degree of efficiency in the conversion of energy. One tablespoon of fat or 4½ cups of shredded cabbage have a similar energy potential. In the body much of the energy obtained from food is converted into mechanical, osmotic, and chemical energy as well as heat. The ability of the animal to release this energy depends on the presence of minerals and vitamins which, along with enzymes, catalyze the many and complex chemical changes in the simple energy-yielding nutrients, glucose and fatty acids, until the energy is converted into a high-energy compound, ATP. In this form it is available in slowly regulated amounts for use within the cell. The final steps in transfer of energy to ATP take place almost exclusively in the mitochondrion of the cell. It is used, however, in virtually all organelles of the cell for the synthesis of complex substances from simple nutrients and for all metabolic reactions that require energy.

DETERMINATION OF ENERGY VALUES
Direct calorimetry

Much of our information on the energy value of foods is obtained by *direct calorimetry*. The instrument used for this is the *bomb calorimeter*, a highly insulated, compact, boxlike container about 1 cubic foot in size. The essential features of a bomb calorimeter are shown in Fig. 5-1. A dried sample of food is completely burned in the oxygen-rich environment within the container, and all the heat produced is absorbed by a weighed amount of water surrounding the platinum combustion chamber. The change in temperature of this fluid surrounding the combustion chamber is measured. Since the amount of heat required to change the temperature of a certain volume of water is known, the amount of heat required for the observed change can be readily calculated. Because the bomb is sufficiently well insulated that no heat exchange takes place with the environment, the heat necessary for the increase in water temperature must be derived from the dried sample of food, which is completely burned to release all its energy. A single bomb calorimeter determination takes about 20 minutes but must be preceded by very precise weighing and careful drying of the sample.

Heat of combustion

The energy value of a sample of food determined in a bomb calorimeter is known as the *heat of combustion*, the maximum amount of energy, measured as heat, that the sample is capable of yielding under conditions providing for complete burning or oxidation.

As explained more fully in Chapter 14, when purified samples of carbohydrate, fat, and protein are burned in the bomb calorimeter, the amount of heat produced will vary slightly with the source and chemical composition of the nutrient, but values of 4.1 kcal. per gram of carbohydrate, 9.45 kcal. per gram of fat, and 5.65 kcal. per gram of protein are generally considered representative of the carbohydrate, fat, and protein found in the American diet.

The heat of combustion represents the energy produced by the oxidation of the carbon molecule to carbon dioxide, the hydrogen to water, and the nitrogen of protein to nitrous oxide. The body is capable of releasing this energy potential of carbon through a process of *decarboxylation*, or removal of carbon dioxide and of hydrogen through a series of reactions referred to as *coupled oxidative phosphorylation*. It cannot, however, release the energy potential of nitrogen. Thus the heat measured in the bomb calorimeter from the oxidation of nitrogen is not available when protein is utilized in the body. It is necessary then to subtract the amount of heat representing the oxidation of nitrogen from the total heat of combustion of protein in estimating the amount available to the body. The oxidation of nitrogen accounted for 1.3 kcal. of the 5.65 kcal. per gram of protein, leaving a potential of only 4.3 kcal. per gram of protein available to the body.

Coefficient of digestibility

Since the body is not 100% efficient in digesting (preparing food for absorption), in absorbing, or in metabolizing nutrients, if one wishes to determine the amount of energy available to the body from an energy-yielding nutrient, one must take into account the extent to which the ingested nutrient is available to the cells. The extent of digestion varies from one nutrient to another and is also influenced by the nature of the food in which it is found. However, to calculate the potential energy from carbohydrate, fat, and protein, representative *coefficients of digestibility* expressing the percentage of the nutrient

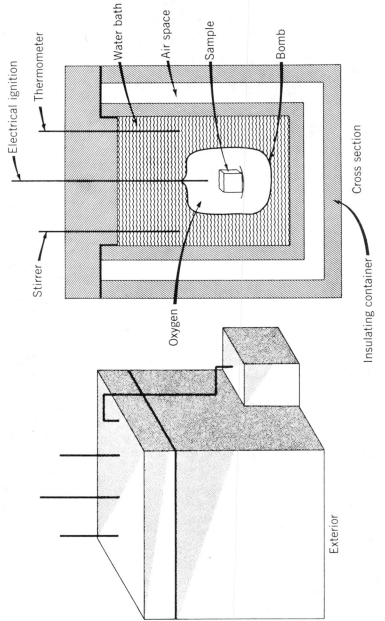

Electrical ignition

Thermometer

Water bath

Air space

Sample

Bomb

Stirrer

Oxygen

Cross section

Insulating container

Exterior

Fig. 5-1. Essential features of a bomb calorimeter. Exterior and cross section are shown.

ultimately available are used. For carbohydrate, which is 98% digested, fat, 95% digested, and protein, 92% digested, the coefficients of digestibility are 0.98, 0.95, and 0.92, respectively. Although nutritionists are well aware that these factors may not be accurate for any one food, they do represent the best currently available factors to apply to the energy-yielding nutrients in the American diet to calculate the *physiological fuel value,* or the amount of potential energy available from a diet. It has been observed that other factors would be more appropriate for use in diets of other countries where the composition of the diet and its digestibility may be different.

Physiological fuel value

The calculation of the physiological fuel value of the three energy-yielding groups is summarized in Table 5-1.

The factors 4, 9, and 4, representing the amount of energy available to the body per gram of carbohydrate, fat, and protein in the diet, are widely used in nutrition and dietetics. Although they may be influenced by many variables and their use may lead to some inaccuracies, they represent a useful tool in calculations involving energy values of diets.

Indirect calorimetry, or oxycalorimetry

The energy value of a substance may also be obtained by indirect calorimetry,

in which the oxygen used in burning the samples and the carbon dioxide produced are measured. Results obtained in the *oxycalorimeter* correspond closely to those from the bomb calorimeter, but oxycalorimetry is seldom used.

ENERGY VALUE OF FOODS

A determination of the fuel value of a food may be made in two ways: by analysis or by calculation based on its carbohydrate, fat, and protein content.

Direct calorimetry

The bomb calorimeter is used in determining the caloric value of a food by direct calorimetry. A weighed sample of food or mixture of foods is dried to a constant weight, burned in the bomb calorimeter, and the amount of heat given off measured directly. The values obtained in this way represent the heat of combustion of the food and not its physiological fuel value. They are from 7% to 10% higher, depending on the percentage calories from protein. The more protein, the greater the error.

Proximate composition

For most foods we now have analytical data for *proximate composition*—the percentage of carbohydrate, fat, protein, and water found in a typical sample of the food. If less precise data on the energy

Table 5-1. Calculation of physiological fuel value of nutrients

	kcal./gm.		
	Carbohydrate	Fat	Protein
Heat of combustion	4.1	9.45	5.65
Energy from combustion of nitrogen unavailable to the body	—	—	1.3
Net heat of combustion	4.1	9.45	4.35
Coefficient of digestibility	0.98	0.95	0.92
Physiological fuel value	4.0	9.0	4.0

Table 5-2. Calculation of energy value of a food from proximate analysis

Nutrient	Percent in food	Amount in 100 gm. (gm.)	Energy value per gram (kcal.)	Energy value of 100 gm. (kcal.)
Carbohydrate	21.4	21.4	4	85.6
Fat	9.2	9.2	9	82.8
Protein	5.5	5.5	4	22.0
Total energy				190.4

Table 5-3. Amount of food needed to provide 100 kcal., the size and caloric value of an average serving*

Food	Average serving	kcal. per serving	Amount to provide 100 kcal.
Lettuce	¼ head	7	4½ heads
Cabbage	½ cup	12	4 cups
Asparagus	6 spears	20	30 spears
Carrots	1 medium	20	5 medium
Sugar	1 tablespoon	50	2 tablespoons
Bread	1 slice	60	1⅔ slices
Apple	1 medium	70	1½ apples
Egg	1 large	80	1¼ large
Banana	1 medium	85	1⅙ medium
Nonfat milk	1 cup	90	1 cup +
Potato	1 medium	90	1 large
Pear	1 medium	100	1
Dates	4	100	4
Butter	1 tablespoon	100	1 tablespoon
Mayonnaise	1 tablespoon	110	1 tablespoon
Salad oil	1 tablespoon	125	⅘ tablespoon
Whole milk	1 cup	165	⅝ cup

*From Nutritive value of foods, Home and Garden Bulletin No. 72, Agriculture Research Service, Washington, D. C., 1964, U. S. Department of Agriculture.

value of a food is needed, this method is quicker and less costly than the use of the bomb calorimeter. For example, from tables of food composition we may learn that a particular food contains 9.2% fat, 21.4% utilizable carbohydrate, and 5.5% protein—the only energy-yielding nutrients in food. To calculate the energy value of 100 gm. of the food, the procedure shown in Table 5-2 would be used.

From the information that the food sample provided 190.4 kcal. per 100 gm. or 1.9 kcal. per gram, one can readily calculate the energy value of a food sample of any size. Also knowing the total carbohydrate, fat, or protein content of the diet, one can readily determine the percentage of total calories contributed by any one food group. In fact, knowing the sample size and any three of the four variables, carbohydrate, fat, protein, and total energy, it is possible to calculate the unknown factor.

Table 5-4. Effect of method of
preparation on energy value of an
average serving of a single food

Food	kcal.
Apple	70
Applesauce	185
Baked apple	225
Apple Betty	350
Apple pie	330
Apple pie a la mode	440
Potato (1 medium)	
Boiled	90
Mashed with 1 teaspoon butter	120
Baked (served with 1 pat butter)	140
French fried	155
Creamed	200

Table 5-5. Caloric value of 100 gm.
portions of food*

Food	Caloric value per 100 gm.
Lettuce (½ cup)	14
Asparagus (6 spears)	20
Cabbage (1 cup shredded)	24
Carrots (1½)	31
Nonfat milk or buttermilk (⅖ cup)	36
Milk (3.7% fat; ⅖ cup)	66
Peas (⅝ cup)	68
Potato (1 small)	76
Lamb (1 serving)	197
Chicken (1 serving)	208
Pork (1 serving)	236
Bread (4 slices)	250
Dates	274
Sugar (½ cup)	400
Butter (7 tablespoons)	716
Mayonnaise (7 tablespoons)	718
Salad oil (7 tablespoons)	884

*From Watt, B. K., and Merrill, A. L.: Composition of foods—raw, processed and prepared, U. S. Department of Agriculture Handbook No. 8, Washington, D. C., 1963, U. S. Department of Agriculture.

Variation in energy value

The energy value of a particular food is a function of its carbohydrate, fat, and protein composition in relation to cellulose and water. Foods with a high percentage of fat are concentrated sources of calories, as are foods with a low water content. Since small amounts of them are required to yield a relatively large number of calories, they are often erroneously considered "fattening" foods. It is true that it is easier to eat excess calories from foods low in water or high in fat content, but the foods themselves are not to be condemned as fattening. It is only the total diet that can be described as fattening and only then when its energy value exceeds the need of the individual for energy.

Table 5-3 presents the amounts of various foods required to provide 100 kcal. and also the size and caloric value of an average serving. It is evident from the bulk of food required that if one wishes to increase his caloric intake, foods from the bottom of the list should be chosen. Conversely, if one wishes to restrict caloric intake, more satisfaction in terms of bulk in the stomach and the amount of chewing

required will be obtained from using foods from the top of the list. It may be noted that items high in calories, such as sugar, flour, butter, and cheese, are often used to enhance the palatability of foods relatively low in calories. Examples of the effect of methods of food preparation on the caloric value of a food is shown in Table 5-4.

The relationship between the weight of a food and its caloric value is evident in Table 5-5. Foods low in water and high in fat have a high caloric value, and those low in fat but high in water and cellulose are lower in calories.

BODY'S NEED FOR ENERGY

An individual's need for energy is a function of several factors, each of which can be estimated and will be discussed separately—basal metabolism, nature and extent of activity, and the effect of food. All are a function either directly or indirectly of a person's size, a larger person always having higher requirements than a smaller person.

ENERGY EXPENDITURE
Basal metabolism

Basal metabolism, which represents the minimum amount of energy for internal work needed to carry on the vital body processes, is an expression of the energy needs during physical, emotional, and digestive rest. These vital processes, without which life is impossible, include respiration, circulation, glandular activity, cellular metabolism, and maintenance of muscle tonus and body temperature. It is well known that the rate of respiration will be increased during strenuous exercise or in the absence of sufficient oxygen, as occurs at high altitudes. These changes are a response to a need for oxygen in the cells. On the other hand, a certain minimum respiratory rate is necessary to provide sufficient oxygen to maintain life at a minimum level of cellular respiration, a rate that differs from one individual to another. In measuring basal metabolic energy needs, we include the amount of energy needed to carry on this minimum rate of respiration. Similarly, a minimum rate of circulation must be maintained to carry oxygen and nutrients to the cells and waste products away from the cells. The energy required for this minimum rate of circulation compatible with life is included in a basal metabolism determination. As long as life continues, glands, such as the thyroid, the adrenals, the pancreas, and the pituitary, produce and secrete hormones that control the level and nature of cellular metabolic activity. The synthesis and secretion of these substances into the bloodstream require energy. No matter how relaxed the person may be, there is still a state of muscular contraction or muscular elasticity. If not, the body would become a shapeless mass of protoplasm. The energy required to maintain this muscle tonus is also measured when basal metabolic needs are assessed. In addition, metabolic processes, such as the uptake of nutrients, the synthesis of new compounds, the excretion of waste, and the maintenance of internal environment of the cells, many of which require energy, are constantly going on as long as the cell is living. The minimum amount of energy to maintain this cellular activity is also included in basal metabolism. Energy to maintain the nervous system is also included.

Measurement of basal metabolism

Basal metabolism can be measured in two ways—by direct or indirect calorimetry. A third test, a clinical test of the protein-bound iodine (PBI) on a blood sample, will give relative but not exact energy costs.

Direct calorimetry. Direct calorimetry involves the measurement of the heat given off by the body in a respiration chamber, a small insulated room that operates on the same principle as the bomb calorimeter. By measuring the change of temperature of a known volume of water circulating in pipes in the top of the chamber, it is possible to determine the amount of heat produced by a subject inside it. In addition, a measurement is often made of the exchange of carbon dioxide and oxygen that takes place. This allows the calculation of a respiratory quotient (RQ), as follows:

$$\frac{CO_2 \text{ expired}}{O_2 \text{ consumed}}$$

From this one can determine whether carbohydrate, fat, or protein was burned. This is a useful piece of information in certain clinical situations. If carbohydrate is the sole source of fuel, the RQ is 1, indicating that one volume of carbon dioxide is produced from every volume of oxygen used in respiration. Fat has an RQ of 0.7; protein, approximately 0.8, depending on

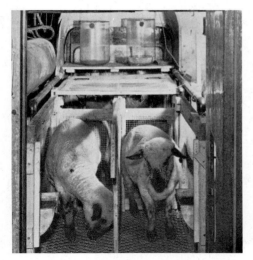

A

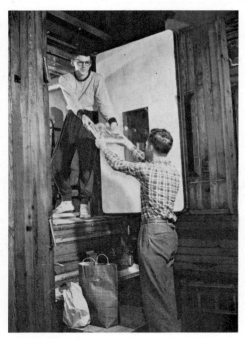

B

Fig. 5-2. **A,** Four sheep in the Armsby calorimeter participating in a metabolism experiment in animal nutrition for which the chamber was originally designed. **B,** Two men entering the same calorimeter to participate in a 72-hour metabolism study, after its conversion for use with human subjects in the 1950's. In both photos note the thickness of the walls with intervening air spaces. (Photographs by R. Beese; courtesy Dr. G. Barron, The Pennsylvania State University.)

the amino acid mixture; and mixtures of carbohydrate, fat, and protein have intermediate values. Under basal conditions the RQ is usually 0.82. If the test is conducted under basal metabolic conditions, the heat produced represents the minimum energy need of the individual. Since the cost of operating a respiration calorimeter is high and there are few available, it is used only under carefully controlled experimental conditions. Fig. 5-2 shows subjects entering one of the few respiration calorimeters in the world. This one is located at The Pennsylvania State University.

A modification of the respiration chamber, the metabolic chamber, measures the heat given off by the subject by means of thermocouples and heat-exchange disks attached to the skin. Any changes in temperature are recorded on instruments outside the chamber. Both the chambers can be used for determinations of basal energy needs and also permit the assessment of energy costs of activities that can be performed in a limited space. Fig. 5-3 illustrates the use of one type of metabolic chamber.

Indirect calorimetry. Indirect calorimetry is a much simpler method in which the oxygen consumption is measured to determine basal metabolism. For many years the Benedict Roth respiration apparatus was the standard machine used for this purpose. It is a closed-circuit system in which the subject receives his oxygen only from a measured source of pure oxygen and exhales into a container in which the carbon dioxide and water are removed and the remaining oxygen recirculated. By measuring the difference in the oxygen level in the container before and after the standard 6-minute test, one can calculate the amount of oxygen consumed. Since the use of 1 liter of oxygen represents 4.82 kcal., it is possible to calculate the caloric equivalent of a known volume of oxygen. It has been shown that open-circuit indirect calorimetry is equally valid. It involves

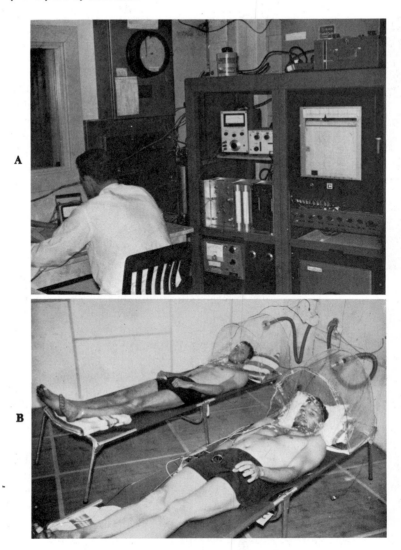

Fig. 5-3. A, Technician at control panel outside metabolic chamber at the Human Performance Laboratory at The Pennsylvania State University, monitoring the oxygen consumption, carbon dioxide excretion, and changes in surface temperature of subject in chamber behind glass. **B,** Subjects in metabolic chamber in which the effect of environmental temperature changes on oxygen consumption and skin temperature are being determined. (Photographs courtesy Public Relations Department, The Pennsylvania State University.)

the use of room air and a determination of the amount of oxygen removed from it during a test period. A measured amount of atmospheric air is breathed from a closed container and the exhalations are passed over soda lime, which removes the carbon dioxide. The amount of carbon dioxide re-moved from the exhaled air is readily measured by weighing the soda lime container before and after the test and can be used along with oxygen figures as a basis for standardized calculations of the energy used during that period. The open-circuit method is less costly and reduces the possibility of stimulation in metabolism from the use of pure oxygen.

A determination of the energy required for basal metabolism must be made when the subject is using a minimum amount of energy for respiration, circulation, glandular activity, and maintenance of muscular tonus and virtually none for nonvital functions such as digestion, absorption, the increase in muscle tonus arising from fear or anger or other emotional states, from an uncomfortable physical environment, or from physical exertion. To achieve these conditions, the subject must be lying down, preferably immediately after a night's sleep, awake, in an environment of a comfortable temperature and humidity, in a postabsorptive state (at least 12 hours since the last meal), and at a normal body temperature. Since cellular respiration in skeletal muscle accounts for the greatest part of the oxygen consumption, it is especially important that the subject be muscularly relaxed. In some tests, drugs have been used to reduce mental and muscular tension to a minimum.

The third, a method of estimating basal metabolic needs, the protein-bound iodine test on a blood sample, will be discussed in Chapter 8.

Estimation of basal energy needs

Basal metabolic tests have yielded sufficient data so that it is now possible to estimate basal energy needs from body measurements of height and weight. For persons of average body build an estimate based on body weight—1 kcal. per kilogram of body weight per hour—gives a value that corresponds well to those obtained on actual basal metabolic tests. But when this formula is applied to persons whose body build deviates from standards either in the direction of obesity or leanness, it is less satisfactory, apparently because the simple measurement of body weight does not reflect body composition. A better indication of basal metabolism

can be obtained by calculating the metabolic, or fat-free, size of the body, sometimes called biological body weight or metabolic body size. It is obtained by calculating the body weight in kilograms to the 0.75 power. This metabolic body size for different body weights is given in Table 5-6. Basal energy needs are then calculated as 70 (weight in kilograms$^{3/4}$). This amounts to about 1.3 kcal. per kilogram of fat-free weight per hour. Estimates of basal metabolism obtained this way correspond very closely to those obtained on the basis of body surface area, which has long been considered the most satisfactory body measurement on which to base predictions of basal energy needs. Body surface area reflects the rate of heat transfer from the body and corresponds very closely to the level of active metabolic tissue. Heat production per unit of surface area is almost the same for all animals under basal conditions. In general, about 82% of the energy from the metabolism of glucose and fatty acids is converted into heat. Of this, 85% is lost through the skin, the remainder through the lungs, urine, and feces. The use of body surface area as a standard is limited because of a lack of precise methods of estimating this measurement. Metabolic body size, however, is being used with increasing frequency as a basis for predicting both basal metabolism and total energy needs.

For most people actual basal metabolic needs fall within 10% (plus or minus) of the predicted values. When deviations occur, they are expressed as a percentage of predicted values, such as −12 or 12% below. Deviations may be attributed to one or more of the factors discussed below. The resting metabolic rate (RMR) is now being used in estimating total energy requirements. It is generally about 10% above basal energy requirements and represents the minimum energy needs for the night and for the periods of the day when there is no exercise and no exposure to cold. It in-

Table 5-6. Body weights in kilograms (kg.) and kg.[3/4]

	kg.	kg.[3/4]		kg.	kg.[3/4]
Infants	4	2.8	Males	35	14.4
	7	4.3		43	16.8
	9	5.2		59	21.3
Children	12	6.1		67	23.4
	14	7.2		70	24.2
	16	8.0	Females	44	17.1
	19	9.1		52	19.4
	23	10.5		54	19.9
	28	12.2		58	21.0

*From Food and Nutrition Board: Recommended dietary allowances, ed. 7, Publication No. 1694, Washington, D. C., 1968, National Academy of Sciences–National Research Council.

cludes energy costs from the specific dynamic effect of meals.

Factors affecting basal energy needs

Body composition. Although all body tissue is metabolically active, undergoing constant breakdown and repair, some tissues experience these changes much more rapidly than others. Muscle and glandular tissues are relatively active, consuming large amounts of oxygen per unit of weight in their normal functioning. On the other hand, bones and adipose tissue, although far from static, are relatively inactive tissues and require less oxygen to maintain normal metabolic activity. If we compare two men weighing 180 pounds, one 60 inches tall and the other 72 inches tall, we are comparing a short stocky person with less muscle and more fat to a tall thin person whose weight is composed of less fat and more muscle. The latter person would have a higher basal metabolic energy need, since the muscle tissue requires more oxygen than the adipose tissue. The difference in body composition is reflected in body surface area measurements or in the measurement of metabolic body size—weight in kg[3/4].

Body condition. A person in good physical condition usually has developed more muscle tissue than one who has not had as much exercise. If we compare two men, both 180 pounds in weight and both 68 inches tall, one of whom is an accountant, in an essentially sedentary occupation, and the other a stockman, an occupation calling for physical activity, we would find that the weight of the sedentary individual represents less muscle and more fat than that of the physically active person. The former's basal metabolic needs would be lower.

Sex. Differences in body composition between a male and female of the same age, height, and weight have been documented. Women characteristically develop more adipose tissue and less musculature than men. This is reflected in a basal metabolic rate for women 5% lower than for men.

Hormone secretions. The secretions of the ductless glands, the thyroid and the adrenal, have more influence on basal energy needs than any single factor. In fact, any marked deviation from predicted basal energy needs is usually attributed to an oversecretion or undersecretion of the thyroid gland, although it is not the only possible cause. Hypothyroidism, with a below-normal secretion of thyroxin, the iodine-containing hormone of the thyroid gland, may be reflected in a basal metabolic rate depressed as much as 30%. This means that the energy required for vital body functions is 30% below that for a person with normal thyroid activity. This depressed secretion can be counteracted by the careful use of thyroid extract available only under medical supervision. Conversely, hyperthyroidism, characterized by an above-normal thyroxin secretion, may elevate basal metabolism as much as 50% to 75%. Under such conditions a person would have an energy requirement for basal needs alone 50% to 75% above predicted levels. Hyperthyroidism is more difficult to correct. Drugs that interfere with the production of thyroxin or the uptake of iodine, an essential part of the thyroxin hormone, are sometimes used, are very difficult to control. Partial thyroidectomy (removal of part of the thyroid gland) has been tried, as has a limitation in the iodine intake to reduce the amount of raw material available for thyroxin synthesis. Deviations in basal metabolism from predicted levels in excess of 20% are almost always indicative of disturbed thyroid function. The very high basal metabolic rate due to excess thyroxin production is characteristic of *exophthalmic goiter* or *hyperthyroidism.*

The secretion of the adrenal gland, adrenaline, is produced in response to intense emotional stimuli, such as anger or fear. The stimulation in metabolism resulting as more adrenaline is produced is intense but of short duration, often returning to normal levels in 2 or 3 hours.

Sleep. Measurements and estimates of basal metabolism are made, assuming the individual is awake but muscularly and emotionally relaxed. During basal metabolic tests involving the use of special breathing apparatus, it is essential that the subject be awake. During sleep, however, an individual achieves a greater degree of muscular and emotional relaxation, which causes a further drop in energy needs to 10% below waking levels. However, the energy savings due to relaxation in sleep may be counteracted by the energy expended in motion during sleep so that the values obtained from basal metabolism may well be applicable over a 24-hour period, eliminating any necessity to correct for a saving in sleep in estimating energy needs.

Age. The basal metabolic rate per unit of body surface changes with age. The rate is high at birth, increases up to 2 years of age, and then declines gradually except for a rise at puberty. In males it ranges from 53 kcal. per square meter at 6 years to 41 at 20 years to 34 at 60 years of age. There is a similar gradual decline in basal energy needs for women except during pregnancy and lactation. The decline in energy needs between ages 25 and 35 amounts to only 35 kcal. per day for a 60 kg. person, but between ages 25 and 55 it amounts to a more significant 145 kcal. A person who fails to adjust his caloric intake to this reduced need will experience a slow and insidious gain in weight.

Pregnancy. During the last few weeks of pregnancy there is an increase in basal metabolism of 22% to 28% above-normal values. This represents the high metabolic activity of the fetus and placenta. Basal metabolic needs early in pregnancy are increased by only 6%.

Previous nutritional status. Basal energy studies in persons who have been subjected to prolonged caloric undernutrition usually yield values below predicted levels. This apparently reflects the body's efforts to conserve energy when calories are restricted. Although the effect of starvation is not a significant factor among American people, it may explain the ability of persons in areas of chronic undernutrition to maintain their body weight on less than predicted caloric intakes.

Body temperature. Since heat acts as a catalyst to almost all chemical reactions, it is not surprising to find that basal metabolism increases with an increase in body temperature. An increase of 1° F. in body temperature leads to an average increase of 7% in basal metabolism, although increases as high as 15% have been observed.

Environmental temperature. Lowest basal metabolism readings are obtained at an environmental temperature of 26° C., or 78° F., with higher readings being reported at both higher and lower environmental temperatures. A temporary decrease in environmental temperature, not compensated for by additional clothing, will cause

shivering and a temporary increase in basal metabolic needs.

• • •

In summary, then, although many factors, such as body composition, hormonal secretions, sleep, and previous nutritional status, may influence basal metabolism, for most persons an accurate estimate of needs can be made on the basis of body surface

Table 5-7. Energy cost of activities exclusive of basal metabolism and influence of food*

Activity	kcal./kg./hr.	Activity	kcal./kg./hr.
Bicycling (century run)	7.6	Piano playing (Liszt's "Tarantella")	2.0
Bicycling (moderate speed)	2.5	Reading aloud	0.4
Bookbinding	0.8	Rowing in race	16.0
Boxing	11.4	Running	7.0
Carpentry (heavy)	2.3	Sawing wood	5.7
Cello playing	1.3	Sewing, hand	0.4
Crocheting	0.4	Sewing, foot-driven machine	0.6
Dancing, foxtrot	3.8	Sewing, motor-driven machine	0.4
Dancing, waltz	3.0	Shoemaking	1.0
Dishwashing	1.0	Singing in loud voice	0.8
Dressing and undressing	0.7	Sitting quietly	0.4
Driving automobile	0.9	Skating	3.5
Eating	0.4	Standing at attention	0.6
Fencing	7.3	Standing relaxed	0.5
Horseback riding, walk	1.4	Stone masonry	4.7
Horseback riding, trot	4.3	Sweeping with broom, bare floor	1.4
Horseback riding, gallop	6.7	Sweeping with carpet sweeper	1.6
Ironing (5-pound iron)	1.0	Sweeping with vacuum sweeper	2.7
Knitting sweater	0.7	Swimming (2 mph)	7.9
Laundry, light	1.3	Tailoring	0.9
Lying still, awake	0.1	Typewriting rapidly	1.0
Organ playing (30% to 40% of energy hand work)	1.5	Violin playing	0.6
Painting furniture	1.5	Walking (3 mph)	2.0
Paring potatoes	0.6	Walking rapidly (4 mph)	3.4
Playing Ping-Pong	4.4	Walking at high speed (5.3 mph)	9.3
Piano playing (Mendelssohn's songs)	0.8	Walking downstairs	†
Piano playing (Beethoven's "Apassionata")	1.4	Walking upstairs	‡
		Washing floors	1.2
		Writing	0.4

*From Taylor, C. M., and McLeod, G.: Rose's laboratory handbook for dietetics, ed. 5, New York, 1949, The Macmillan Co., p. 18.
†Allow 0.012 kcal. per kilogram for an ordinary staircase with 15 steps without regard to time.
‡Allow 0.036 kcal. per kilogram for an ordinary staircase with 15 steps without regard to time.

area or metabolic body size. For many people, especially those engaged in sedentary or moderate activity, basal energy needs account for 50% to 70% of their total caloric requirements.

Activity

The energy required for physical activity above the needs for basal metabolism is a function of the type of activity, the duration of activity, and the size of the individual performing it. Since 75% of the energy expended in most activities is involved in moving the body, it has become common practice to base estimates of energy needs for activity on body weight. As a result, tables such as Table 5-7, giving the energy costs of various activities per unit of body weight, have traditionally been used in estimating energy costs. Although some workers have published tables of energy costs of activity based on the type of activity irrespective of the size of the individual (Table 20-3), most workers continue to base estimates on body weights. Tables of energy costs represent our best available estimates, but before using them, one should be aware of the limitations in their usefulness.

First, people differ from one another in the efficiency with which they perform a particular activity, either through training or innate ability, so that the actual costs may vary considerably from estimates. Calculations show that a 90 kg. person will use 50% more energy in performing the same task for the same length of time than will a 60 kg. person, and the former's needs would be calculated to be the same as a 60 kg. person carrying a 30 kg. (66-pound) load on his back. In neither case would the differences be this great because of efficiencies affected by the distribution of the weight over the whole body.

Second, while many activities, such as walking, swimming, or bicycling (which involve moving the body) do require an energy expenditure proportional to body size, others, such as knitting, writing, and piano playing, will likely not vary with body size but rather will require about the same amount of energy for all persons.

Third, since many of the values were based on a very few determinations or were extrapolated from data on similar activities, they should not be considered precise. For that reason the student is cautioned against attributing too much precision to calculations based on them. It should also be recognized that the energy expenditure attributable to the activity itself may represent a very small portion of the total energy used during the time, since a much larger portion may be used for basal metabolism.

Once the limitations are recognized, tables of energy costs can be useful tools in nutrition studies.

Many people are disillusioned to find the relatively small amount of energy expended in performing various activities. For instance, the energy cost of walking 3 miles in 1 hour is only 2 kcal. per kilogram of body weight above maintenance requirements. Thus a 60 kg. (132-pound) person will expend only an additional 120 kcal. or 96 kcal. more than sitting in such an activity. Even 1 hour of skating will involve only 210 kcal. for this same person, while bicycling requires 150 kcal. over basal. The Canadian dietary standard suggests that light work, such as cooking, typing, or golfing, involves an average expenditure of 1.1 kcal. per minute, while moderately heavy work, such as gardening, carpentry, and swimming, costs 2.6 kcal. per minute. Heavy work, such as farm chores, lumbering, or mountain climbing, costs 2.8 kcal. per minute and very strenuous work, 5.1 kcal. These are proposed in addition to the needs for basal metabolism independent of body size.

Disillusioning as it may be, it has been established that mental effort causes virtually no increase in energy requirements. The 3% to 4% increase sometimes recorded has been attributed to the increase in muscle tension rather than to brain cell activity.

The decline in caloric requirements for activity that occurs with aging is proportionately greater than the decline in basal energy requirements. It decreases at 3%, 6%, 13.5%, 21%, and 31% of that at age 25 with each succeeding decade.

To estimate the caloric needs of an individual for activity, it is necessary to keep an accurate record of all activity for a specified period of not less than 24 hours. Activities are then grouped to determine the total time spent in a particular activity according to groupings given in Table 5-7. If a particular activity is not listed, a reasonable estimate can be made by classifying it with one involving a similar degree of muscular exertion. Using the energy cost factors from Table 5-7, caloric costs per kilogram for each activity can be calculated and totalled. The day's energy requirement for all activity is obtained by multiplying this total by the body weight in kilograms. The number of kilocalories needed to take care of a day's activity vary greatly from one individual to another, but for a sedentary or moderately active person usually represent from 33% to 50% of the basal energy needs. For active and very active persons, the needs for activity may equal or exceed basal energy needs.

FAO has used the formula 10.88 (weight in kilograms) + 236 to express the energy needs for activity. The Canadian dietary standards use the values 23 kcal. per unit of metabolic body size for a sedentary person, with an additional 23 kcal. for light activity, 55 for moderate activity, such as gardening or making furniture, 80 for heavy activity, such as farm chores, lumbering, or active participation in competitive sports, and 107 for extremely heavy activity. These values are over and above the needs for basal metabolism.

Effect of food

It has been recognized for some time that the ingestion of food causes an increase in energy needs not only for the digestion, absorption, and transportation of the nutrients but also as a result of a general stimulation in metabolism that follows the ingestion of food. This effect has been referred to as the *specific dynamic effect* of food. Experiments designed to determine the exact magnitude of this effect have produced no conclusive results. It is still generally believed that the effect of food amounts to about 10% of the total energy needed for basal metabolism and activity. In the case of a diet where protein provides almost all of the calories, this stimulation in metabolism rises as high as 30%.

The stimulating effect of the high-protein diet has been attributed to the stimulating effect of some amino acids and to the heat resulting from the deamination of protein or the synthesis and excretion of urea.

Since the effect of food represents an increase in energy expenditure, it must be added to the basal needs and activity needs in calculating the total energy needs. If this factor were not considered, a diet providing only sufficient calories for basal and activity needs would lead to an inadequate caloric intake with subsequent weight loss.

Estimation of total energy needs

The method used to estimate total caloric needs depends on the degree of accuracy desired. For the most precise determination it is necessary to carry out an actual basal metabolism test and to evaluate the energy cost of activity by having the subject breathe into a portable gas meter apparatus worn on his back for all activities. This expensive method is used mainly for research purposes.

Factorial method. More easily used and less expensive, but also less precise, is the *factorial method* of estimating caloric needs. It involves estimating basal metabolism from surface area measurements or metabolic body size, activity needs from accurate activity records, and an additional factor for the effect of food. The factorial

Table 5-8. Factorial estimation of total energy needs

Subject: male	Weight: 60 kg.	Height: 70 in.	Age: 35

Basal metabolism: 1 kcal./kg./hr.

1 kcal. $\times$ 60 $\times$ 24		=	1440 kcal.

OR

$$70 \,(Wt._{kg})^{3/4} = 70 \times 60^{3/4} = 70 \times 22 = \qquad 1540 \text{ kcal.}$$

Activity needs

Activity	Time (hr.)	Energy cost kcal./kg./hr.	Energy cost kcal./kg.
Dressing	1.5	0.7	1.05
Sitting	6.0	0.4	2.4
Skating	0.5	3.5	1.7
Walking (3 mph)	2.0	2.0	4.0
Standing relaxed	1.0	0.5	0.5
Typing	4.0	1.0	4.0
Sleeping	8.0	—	—
Playing piano	0.5	2.0	1.0
Walking upstairs	4 flights	0.036*	0.14
Walking downstairs	4 flights	0.012*	0.04
			14.83
Energy cost of activity = 14.83 kcal. $\times$ 60			889
Total energy cost for basal metabolism and activity			2329 or 2429
Specific dynamic effect (10%)			232 or 242
Total energy requirement			2561 or 2671

*Allowance per kilogram for ordinary staircase (15 steps) regardless of time.

method for estimating caloric needs is outlined in Table 5-8, using either body weight or metabolic body size for estimating basal needs.

Rule of thumb. For a quick estimate of energy needs the United States Department of Agriculture suggests multiplying body weight in pounds by a factor determined by the type of physical activity in which the individual is engaged. These factors are 14 for sedentary, 18 for moderately active, and 22 for very active women. For men, values of 16, 21, and 26 are used. The limitation in this method lies in the subjective judgment of the nature of a person's physical activity. The most common error is to confuse the terms *busy* and *active*. A typical college student may be very busy but very sedentary at the same time. A busy but sedentary person needs fewer calories than a physically active individual.

Canadian and FAO dietary standards. The Canadian dietary standards estimate total energy needs on the basis of metabolic body size. Their formula is 116 (weight in kilograms$^{0.75}$). The Food and Agricultural Organization of the United Nations (FAO) has also developed a formula from which they believe one can arrive at a figure representing the energy requirement. For men they use 0.95 (815 + 36.6 [weight in kilograms]). The formula for women is 0.95 (580 + 31.1 [weight in kilograms]). Both these are very close to recommended levels of caloric intake in the United States.

NRC recommended allowances. The Food and Nutrition Board of the National Research Council has established the caloric allowances they believe provide sufficient energy to maintain body weight or rate of growth at levels most conducive to well-being for practically all healthy individuals. Recognizing the many factors that influence caloric requirements, they have expressed their recommendations for a reference man or woman and have then indicated a basis for making adjustments.

As reference individuals they chose 22-year-old persons living in a temperate zone with a mean environmental temperature of 20° C. (68° F.), and who are engaged in occupations neither sedentary nor involving hard physical labor but requiring moderate physical activity. For the reference woman weighing 58 kg. (128 pounds) the allowance is set at 2000 kcal. and for the 70 kg. (154-pound) man at 2800 kcal., but the values are planned primarily for assessing needs of groups rather than individuals.

Adjustment for age. Increasing age is accompanied by decreased caloric expenditures because of the progressive reduction in basal metabolic rate and usual decline in physical activity. Although there may be wide individual differences in the extent to which needs for activity are reduced with age, a decrease in total caloric needs of 5% between 22 and 35, 3% per decade between ages 35 and 55, 5% per decade from ages 55 to 75, and 7% after age 75 is proposed as typical.

Adjustment for body size. A basic principle in physics states that the amount of work required to move a mass is proportional to the size of the mass. In assessing human energy requirements it is assumed that 75% of the energy expenditure is directly proportional to body size and 25% is independent of body weight. On this basis, formulas for caloric needs of RMR + 13 (weight in kilograms) for men and RMR + 7 (weight in kilograms) for women 22 years

of age have been developed to reflect the effect of body size on energy needs. The use of these formulas indicates a change of 80 to 100 kcal. for every 5 kg. (11-pound) deviation from the weight of the reference man or woman. The effects of body weight and age in caloric allowances are shown in Table 5-9.

Adjustment for climate. The mean environmental temperature, 20° C. (68° F.), is used in estimating caloric needs. It is applicable to persons living in most parts of the United States, since modern technology in the form of air-conditioning and central heating has provided means of protecting persons against extremes of temperature. In temperatures below 14° C. an increase of 5% to 7% should be made to take care of the increased energy cost of work and the extra energy expended in carrying more clothing or the shivering that occurs if clothing is inadequate to protect the person. Persons who perform physical activity at temperatures over 30° C. (80° F.) have an increased caloric need of 0.5% for each degree increase in environmental temperature. For others the tendency to restrict activity at higher temperatures counteracts the increase in needs resulting from the increase in body temperature and basal metabolic rate, which increases the cost of maintaining body temperature.

Adjustment for activity. The allowances have been established for a moderately active individual. As the degree of activity increases, the caloric cost of the activity rises proportionately but even with heavy labor caloric requirements seldom increase more than 25% above those for the reference man or woman. In the urban United States, energy requirements are more likely to be below these recommended values due to the relatively sedentary life that is characteristic of the era of television.

Needs for pregnancy. Total energy needs during pregnancy represent normal needs, plus those to meet increase in basal metabolism and the demands for the growth of

Table 5-9. Adjustment of caloric (kcal.) allowances° for adult individuals of various body weights and ages (at a mean environmental temperature of 20° C. [68° F.], assuming light physical activity)[1]

Body weight		RMR† at age 22	Age‡		
kg.	lb.		22	45	65
Men					
50	110	1540	2200	2000	1850
55	121	1620	2350	2150	1950
60	132	1720	2500	2300	2100
65	143	1820	2650	2400	2200
70§	154	1880	2800	2600	2400
75	165	1970	2950	2700	2500
80	176	2020	3050	2800	2600
85	187	2110	3200	2950	2700
90	198	2210	3350	3100	2800
95	209	2290	3500	3200	2900
100	220	2380	3700	3400	3100
Women					
40	88	1280	1550	1450	1300
45	99	1380	1700	1550	1450
50	110	1460	1800	1650	1500
55	121	1560	1950	1800	1650
58§	128	1620	2000	1850	1700
60	132	1640	2050	1900	1700
65	143	1740	2200	2000	1850
70	154	1830	2300	2100	1950

[1]From Food and Nutrition Board: Recommended dietary allowances, ed. 7, Publication No. 1694, Washington, D. C., 1968, National Academy of Sciences–National Research Council.
*Kcal. allowance (males) = (RMR + 13 wt.) × (percent adjustment for age); kcal. allowance (females) = (RMR + 7 wt.) × (percent adjustment for age); wt. = weight in kilograms. Values are rounded to the nearest 50 kcal.
†RMR = resting metabolic rate, approximately 10% above the metabolic rate measured under basal conditions.
‡Age adjustments:

Age	Adjustment (percent of kcal. allowance at age 22)
22-35	100-95
35-45	95-92
45-55	92-89
55-65	89-84
65-75	84-79
75-85	72

§Reference man and woman.

the fetus, placenta, and mammary glands. During the last trimester when about two thirds of fetal growth occurs, the daily need increases by about 200 kcal., depending on the extent to which normal activity is decreased during pregnancy. It is estimated that 40,000 kcal. are needed to take care of the increased energy needs for the full gestation period of 40 weeks. Although the hazards of excessive weight gain during pregnancy, such as toxemia of pregnancy and complications during labor, have been known for some time, it is now recognized that the hazards of an inadequate weight increase may be equally as great, prematurity being most common. Caloric intake during pregnancy should lead to a weight gain of 22 to 30 pounds. The need for other nutrients is proportionately higher, necessitating care in the selection of additional calories.

Needs for lactation. The increase in energy required for the secretion of milk amounts to 600 kcal. for the milk and an additional 400 kcal. to produce the milk during the first four months of lactation. The amount, of course, varies with the volume of milk secreted, approximately 120 kcal. being needed for the secretion of 100 ml. of milk. The National Research Council recommends a caloric intake of 1000 kcal. above normal energy requirements.

Needs for infants. Growth necessitates a relatively high energy intake per unit of body weight to take care of the needs for maintenance, activity, and rapid increase in body tissue. The energy needed to meet the needs for growth fluctuates widely over even short periods of time. It must be recognized that there are wide individual differences at this age because of variations in activity patterns as well as rate of growth. Infants who cry a great deal have needs in excess of more tranquil infants.

For infants the requirement at birth of 120 kcal. per kilogram is decreased to 100 kcal. per kilogram at the end of 1 year.

CALORIC IMBALANCE

One of the major nutritional problems in the United States today is that of maintaining caloric balance. This is a problem at all stages of the life cycle but especially among adults, for whom patterns of eating and activity developed early in life are major factors in the cause and control of weight problems. As long as caloric intake is equal to caloric expenditure, there should be no change in body weight. As soon as caloric intake deviates from caloric expenditure, calories are either derived from body stores to meet a deficit or are added to body stores in cases of a surplus. Persons whose intake constantly exceeds their expenditure

are soon conscious of the storage of calories in the form of body fat, reflected as a gain in body weight. Persons whose intake is inadequate to meet their needs experience a weight loss as energy reserves are depleted to meet their needs. In either case a state of malnutrition exists, and the problems can be equally severe on either side of the balance. Those whose caloric intakes are inadequate are the forgotten group among our malnourished, partly because they fail to recognize their state as an undesirable deviation from a normal state and partly because social pressures on this group are not sufficient to motivate them to make an adjustment. On the other hand, those who accumulate excess poundage are confronted with a barrage of panaceas, miraculous and otherwise, to help them make the necessary weight loss painlessly. This group is in jeopardy not only because of the hazards of being overweight but also because of the potentially dangerous weight-reducing aids to which they may unwittingly subject themselves.

To simplify an extremely complex situation, for every 3500 kcal. deficit in the diet, 1 pound of body fat will be oxidized or lost, and for approximately 3500 kcal. in excess of needs, the weight will increase 1 pound, representing storage of 1 pound of fat or adipose tissue, which is approximately 65% fat and 35% water. It does not matter whether the imbalance is one of 700 kcal. for each of 5 days or 10 kcal. for 350 days; the end result is the same.

The ease with which some people maintain caloric equilibrium is evidenced by the number of persons who maintain the same weight year after year. The fact that about 25% of the population are considered overweight, in most cases because of an excess accumulation of fatty tissue, indicates that a large number of people fail to make the necessary adjustment.

The storage of calories will result from an excessive caloric intake or a depressed need for calories, either of which leads to a caloric imbalance. The causes, which may be many, are discussed in Chapter 20. It may be hereditary, in which case the sensitivity of the hypothalamus, the area of the brain that regulates appetite, is reduced to the point where overeating will occur before the message to stop eating is relayed through the hypothalamus in the brain. Psychological factors may lead to overeating; the pleasure derived from eating compensates for unpleasant aspects of a personal adjustment. A reduction in physical activity that accompanies increasing age or the laborsaving conveniences of the push-button age when eating practices remain the same as in an era of greater physical effort creates an imbalance. Environmental factors, such as the availability of food, the economic ability of many to buy all the food desired, the pressures of the host who sees food as an expression of hospitality, or the laden tables traditional in many cultures, create situations that tax an individual's ability to regulate intake. Physiological factors, such as a depressed basal metabolic rate resulting from decreased secretion of thyroxin, may also be a contributing cause.

That individuals differ in the efficiency with which they utilize food has been suggested for some time. Recent evidence indicates that the frequency of feedings is an influencing factor. The larger the number of meals into which a day's food intake is divided, the less likely the person is to store fat. Efforts to show that the primary source of calories—carbohydrate, fat, or protein—influences the utilization of calories have indicated that there is no difference.

Regardless of the cause of a person's failure to maintain his desired body weight—physiological, psychological, hereditary, or environmental—successful treatment involves decreasing the caloric intake to a level below caloric expenditure. Many dietary aids that may act as appetite depressants, stimulate metabolism, increase water loss through excessive perspiration or increased urinary output, and depress utilization by speeding passage of food through the intestinal tract are constantly presented to the public. Some have value to some people; many are harmless but useless; and the Food and Drug Administration is constantly on guard to protect the public against harmful aids.

Equally as often, the public is given a diet designed to solve all their weight problems. The rate at which these diets appear and the diversity of ideas presented make it impossible to evaluate them individually. A few criteria may provide a basis for judging each new diet as it appears.

1. The diet must be deficient in calories. This can be determined only by comparing the caloric value of the diet with a reasonable estimate of the individual's needs. A diet that shows a deficit for one person does not necessarily do so for others. A daily deficiency of 500 kcal. will lead to a deficit of 3500 in a week, which should result in the loss of a pound of body weight. The tendency of the body to replace this fat with water temporarily often masks the loss of fat and is a source of discouragement to the reducer. If the regimen is continued sufficiently long, the total predicted loss eventually occurs.

2. The diet should be adequate in all other nutrients except calories. Although this criterion is difficult to check precisely, a fairly good indication may be gained by checking the diet to see that it includes servings from each of the four major food groups, each of which must be present if a diet is to approach adequacy in most nutrients. There should be at least two servings each from milk and dairy products; fruits and vegetables; cereal products; and meat, fish, poultry, or eggs. At a level of 1400 kcal. it is possible with a careful choice of foods to achieve a diet that meets the National Research Council recommended allowances for all nutrients. As the calories drop, it is increasingly difficult to choose

an adequate diet, and if energy intake is restricted to less than 1000 kcal., the diet should be supplemented with a protective level of the minerals and vitamins likely to be lacking in the diet.

3. The diet should have satiety value. Diets containing moderate amounts of fat and high levels of protein delay the onset of hunger pangs for a longer time than isocaloric diets composed primarily of carbohydrate. It is easier to adhere to a diet of high satiety value than to one that leaves the stomach rapidly.

4. A diet should be one that can be adapted readily from family meals and that can be obtained in public eating places. Any diet that sets the dieter apart from others with whom he eats or imposes extra preparation on the person preparing meals is less likely to be followed than one that allows a person to eat inconspicuously with the family or friends in all social situations.

5. The diet should be reasonable in cost. If it makes use of seasonal foods and staple dietary items, it will be more acceptable than one that calls for expensive, out-of-season, unfamiliar foods.

6. It should be one that can be adhered to for a sufficient period of time to achieve the desired weight loss. It is recommended that except in extreme obesity the rate of weight loss not exceed 1 to 1½ pounds per week. Thus a person wishing to lose 20 pounds should try to accomplish this over a period of at least fifteen weeks. Crash diets, which limit the dieter to a restricted list of foods, such as cottage cheese and peaches or steak, eggs, and tomatoes, are not only nutritionally inadequate but also are so monotonous that their psychological appeal lasts only a short time. It is almost impossible for a person to remain on such a limited selection of foods to achieve the desired weight loss.

7. Most important of all, if the dieter is to achieve long-term success, the diet should represent a sufficient departure from his former pattern of eating that he will be retrained in a new set of eating habits to which he can expect to adhere, with slight modifications, as a maintenance diet for a lifetime. The failure of the once-popular liquid formula diets to achieve any permanent weight loss can be attributed partly to their failure to substitute a new socially acceptable pattern of eating for the old one that led to the weight gain.

SELECTED REFERENCES

Buskirk, E. R.: Problems related to the caloric cost of living, Bull. N. Y. Acad. Med. **36**:63, 1960.

Food and Agricultural Organization: Calorie requirements, FAO Nutr. Stud. No. 15, 1957.

Food and Nutrition Board: Recommended dietary allowances, ed. 7, Publication No. 1694, Washington, D. C., 1968, National Academy of Sciences–National Research Council.

Kleiber, M.: The fire of life, an introduction to animal energetics, New York, 1961, John Wiley & Sons, Inc.

Symposium on energy balance, Amer. J. Clin. Nutr. **8**:527, 1960.

Wait, B., Blair, R., and Roberts, L. J.: Energy intake of well-nourished children and adolescents, Amer. J. Clin. Nutr. **22**:1383, 1969.

6 | *Mineral elements*

It had been demonstrated in the middle of the nineteenth century that a mixture of the known constituents of food—the proximate principles, carbohydrate, fat, protein, and water—was not capable of supporting growth. Scientists then looked to the noncombustible fraction, or the mineral ash, of food for a clue to the growth-promoting properties of natural food absent in the synthetic mixtures. Since the mineral residue when added to a synthetic diet did not stimulate growth or prevent death in animals, it did not arouse much interest in the 1880's. It has since, however, been shown to be composed of many mineral elements that play vital roles in human nutrition.

Distribution

The elements carbon, hydrogen, and oxygen, the components of carbohydrate, fat, and protein (all of which can be oxidized to carbon dioxide and water), and the nitrogen of protein, together with water comprise 96% of the body weight. The remaining 4%, about six pounds in the adult male, is made up of many mineral elements. Approximately seventeen of these different mineral elements have been proved essential in human nutrition. However, an analysis of mineral ash may reveal an additional twenty or thirty present because of contamination from the environment—the soil, air, or water—or possibly because of an unestablished but essential role.

Essential elements

The list of essential elements continues to grow with the development of sensitive techniques for studying their metabolism. For instance, chromium, which only a few years ago was considered a contaminant, is now known to perform an essential function.

It has been observed that the body has mechanisms for controlling the absorption of essential elements and can excrete them in the urine, bile, and other intestinal secretions. There appears to be no comparable mechanism for controlling the absorption and excretion of nonessential elements. Minerals occur in the body in combination with organic compounds as the iron in hemoglobin, with other inorganic ions as the calcium phosphate of bone, or as free ionized ions, such as the calcium in the intercellular fluids.

Progressive refinement in the techniques used to study mineral metabolism—spectroscopy, colorimetry, the use of radioactive isotopes, and flame photometry—has made possible studies of progressively smaller concentrations of minerals in biological tissue and has helped elucidate roles for mineral elements that have established their essential nature. A mineral is considered essential if there is a demonstrable improvement in the health and growth of the animal upon addition of the mineral to a purified diet, if the removal of the element from a diet containing adequate but not toxic amounts of all other dietary essentials results in clear-cut evidence of deficiency symptoms, and if a low intake can be correlated with subnormal levels of the element in blood or other tissues. Even when it is determined that an element is a part of an essential enzyme system, it must still be established that the reaction cannot be catalyzed by some other means. The presence of a reserve or pool of the element that is influenced by hormones or other substances is considered further evidence of a biological role.

Classification

The essential mineral elements are often grouped as macronutrient elements, those present in relatively high amounts in animal tissue, and micronutrient elements, or trace elements, present as less than 0.005% (50 ppm) of the body weight, as presented in Table 6-1. It is entirely possible that with

the increasingly sensitive analytical techniques available, biological roles will be discovered for at least some of the elements in the last group.

Although most of the elements listed are also essential for plant growth, some, such as cobalt, sodium, and iodine, are not essential. They do, however, occur in foods of plant origin to become a major source of these elements in the human diet. The amount of a mineral element in an animal tissue reflects the amount present in the plants it eats, and this in turn is a function of the amount of the element present in the soil and the extent to which the plant con-

Table 6-1. Classification of mineral elements

Classification	Elements	Percent of body weight
Macronutrient elements essential for human nutrition (> 0.005% body weight or 50 ppm)	Calcium	1.5-2.2
	Phosphorus	0.8-1.2
	Potassium	0.35
	Sulfur	0.25
	Sodium	0.15
	Chlorine	0.15
	Magnesium	0.05
Micronutrient elements essential for human nutrition (< 0.005% body weight)	Iron	0.004
	Zinc	0.002
	Selenium	0.0003
	Manganese	0.0002
	Copper	0.00015
	Iodine	0.00004
	Molybdenum	
	Cobalt	
	Chromium	
	Fluorine	
Elements for which essentiality has not yet been established, although there is evidence of their participation in certain biological reactions	Vanadium	
	Barium	
	Arsenic	
	Bromine	
	Strontium	
	Cadmium	
	Nickel	
Elements found in the body but for which no metabolic role has been elucidated	Gold	
	Silver	
	Aluminum	
	Tin	
	Bismuth	
	Gallium	
	Lead	

centrates it. The presence of some of these elements in animal tissue may represent contamination from the environment.

The complex interrelationships that exist among the mineral elements as they function in the body suggest a discussion of the general functions of minerals. Some elements have been studied extensively and will be discussed individually. The ones on which the most information has been acquired are those most likely to be lacking in the diet and for which specific deficiency conditions have been recognized. This does not minimize the role of the other mineral elements, which are equally as important in maintaining normal body function.

General functions of mineral elements

Maintenance of acid-base balance. The tremendous number of biological reactions that take place within the cell can occur only in a very specific internal environment. Just as the enzymes of the digestive juices require a specific acidity or alkalinity, the enzymes that work within the cells can perform their task only when the fluid in the cells is essentially neutral in reaction. Anything that changes the reaction or pH of the cell environment may inactivate or change the level of activity of the cellular enzymes. Inactivation of the enzymes results in cellular starvation and death of the cell. Among the many factors that influence the reaction of the cell is the nature of the minerals available to it from the extracellular fluids.

Some minerals are acid forming, since, when in solution, they form an acid medium. These elements are chlorine, sulfur, and phosphorus. The acid-forming properties of a food are determined by the components of its noncombustible mineral ash and not by the presence of organic acids. The latter may give food an acid taste but are generally oxidized to form carbon dioxide, water, and energy. Thus they do not influence acid-base balance.

The acid-forming elements predominate in foods containing protein, such as meat, fish, poultry, eggs, and cereal products. These, in turn, are designated as acid-forming foods.

Mineral elements that are basic, or alkaline, in solution are calcium, sodium, potassium, and magnesium. These elements tend to predominate in fruits and vegetables. Thus even citrus fruits, such as grapefruit, lemons, and oranges that have an acid taste because of the presence of organic acids, are base forming, since their organic acids are metabolized and the mineral ash predominates in potentially basic or alkaline elements. A few foods, such as cranberries, rhubarb, cocoa, and tea, are acid-forming because they contain acids the body cannot metabolize—benzoic, oxalic, and tannic acid. The acid potential of these overbalances the alkalinity of the base-forming mineral elements.

Neither milk, which contains an internal balance of base-forming calcium and acid-forming phosphorus, nor pure carbohydrates and fats, which contain virtually no minerals, influence the acid-base balance of the body.

Most mixed diets contain a slight surplus of acid-forming mineral elements, but the body has mechanisms by which it can counteract this potential acidity. The excretion of carbon dioxide through the lungs and of a slightly acid urine through the kidneys rids the body of excess acid and helps maintain the neutrality of its internal environment. However, strict vegetarians who consume a diet with a predominantly basic residue, persons on an extreme high-protein diet with a predominately acid residue in the mineral ash, and those who make frequent use of sodium-containing antacids, which create an alkaline balance, may tax the body's ability to maintain neutrality. The maintenance of body neutrality is so important to the survival of body cells that there are several ways in which an excess acid or excess base can be neutralized.

The blood contains buffers, such as carbonates, phosphates, and proteins, that can react with either excess acid or excess base to prevent them from influencing the reaction of the blood and hence that of the fluids bathing the tissues. Bone can also release phosphates to act as buffers to remove hydrogen ions from surrounding fluids. If the buffers cannot take care of excess base, a reserve acid (carbonic acid) can be formed from carbon dioxide and water of metabolism, which are normally excreted. This acid then neutralizes excess alkali-forming elements and prevents alkalosis. Similarly, excess acid may be neutralized by a reserve base formed from the

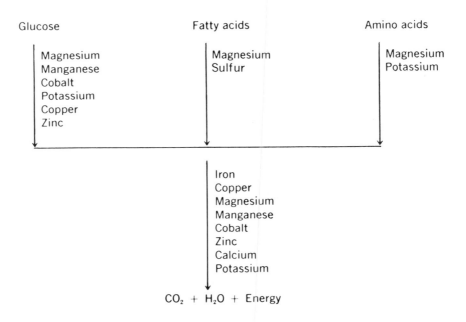

CATABOLISM

Glucose

| Magnesium
| Manganese
| Cobalt
| Potassium
| Copper
| Zinc

Fatty acids

| Magnesium
| Sulfur

Amino acids

| Magnesium
| Potassium

| Iron
| Copper
| Magnesium
| Manganese
| Cobalt
| Zinc
| Calcium
| Potassium

CO_2 + H_2O + Energy

ANABOLISM

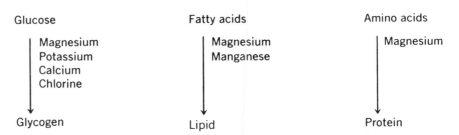

Glucose

| Magnesium
| Potassium
| Calcium
| Chlorine

Glycogen

Fatty acids

| Magnesium
| Manganese

Lipid

Amino acids

| Magnesium

Protein

Fig. 6-1. Role of minerals as catalysts to biological reactions.

NH$_2$ from deamination of protein and water. This prevents acidosis. With all these mechanisms for coping with a diet that produces an excess of either base-forming or acid-forming elements, an upset in acid-base balance can seldom be caused by dietary factors alone. However, diets that have either a predominately acid or predominately alkaline ash may be prescribed in the treatment of certain conditions.

Catalysts for biological reactions. Mineral elements are catalysts for many biological reactions. As such they are not part of the initial compounds or the end products but must be present for the reaction to take place. Minerals that catalyze the action of many of the body's enzymes sometimes serve as the vital link between an enzyme and its substrate. They catalyze many of the separate steps involved in the catabolism of carbohydrate, fat, and protein to carbon dioxide, water, and energy and in the anabolism, or synthesis, of fat and protein. The synthesis of essential body compounds such as hemoglobin depends on the presence of several mineral elements other than those that may become a part of the substance. The clotting of blood depends on the catalytic effect of calcium.

Fig. 6-1, which is by no means a complete tabulation, indicates the role of minerals in the metabolism of carbohydrate, fat, and protein in the body. It is obvious that many reactions are mineral dependent and that some of the elements listed are involved at several different stages.

The transport of substances across biological membranes, as in absorption of nutrients from the gastrointestinal tract or uptake of nutrients by the cell, is often a mineral-dependent reaction. For instance, calcium facilitates the absorption of cobalamin, or vitamin B$_{12}$, and magnesium and sodium facilitate the absorption of carbohydrate. Several digestive enzymes are activated by minerals, as in the case of activation of pancreatic lipase by calcium and magnesium. Chromium catalyzes the attachment of insulin to the cell wall.

Components of essential body compounds. Many of the hormones, enzymes, and other vital body compounds that are synthesized in the body and regulate its functioning contain minerals as integral parts of their structure. In the absence of the required mineral, the body will be unable to produce adequate amounts of the essential substance.

The production of thyroxin, which regulates energy metabolism, depends on an adequate supply of iodine to the thyroid gland. The production and storage of insulin, which regulates carbohydrate metabolism, usually involves zinc. Hemoglobin, essential for the transport of oxygen to and carbon dioxide from the cells, is an iron-containing compound. Chlorine must be available for the production of hydrochloric acid for secretion into the stomach to create the acid environment necessary for the action of digestive enzymes in the stomach.

Minerals are an integral part of many enzymes in the body. These mineral-containing enzymes are sometimes designated as "metalloenzymes," since if the metal is removed, the enzyme loses its effectiveness. To cite but a few examples: both copper and iron are part of the enzyme cytochrome oxidase involved in the release of energy; molybdenum is part of xanthine oxidase needed to release liver stores of iron for use by other tissues, and zinc is part of a protein-splitting enzyme, carboxypeptidase, secreted in the intestinal juice.

In addition to the carbon, hydrogen, oxygen, and nitrogen that are part of the vitamins most essential for body functioning, some, such as thiamin with sulfur and cobalamin with cobalt, have minerals as integral parts of their structure.

Maintenance of water balance. Water, which comprises approximately 72% of the fat-free weight of the body and 60% of the total body weight, may be considered to

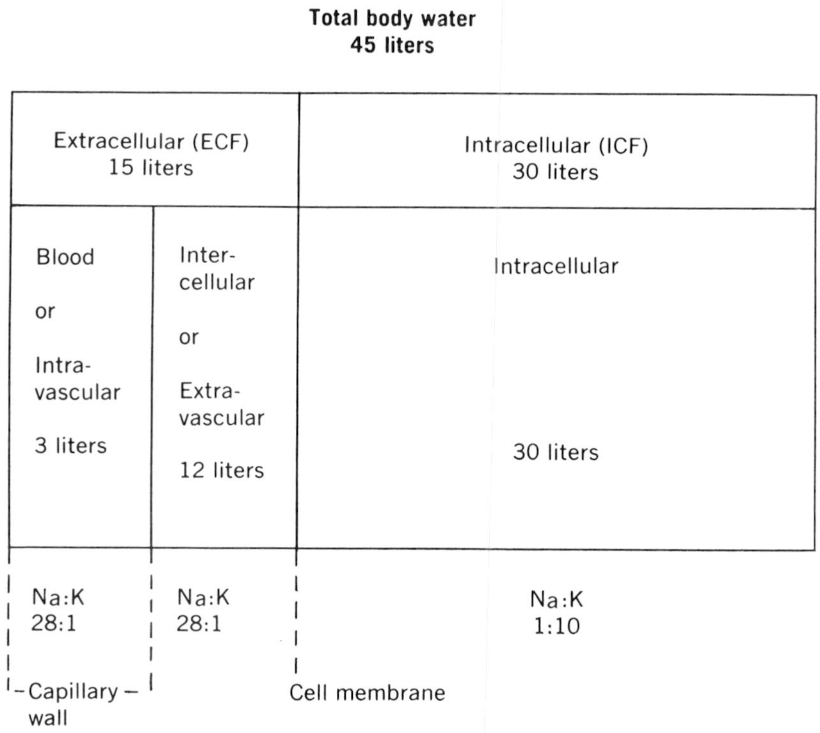

**Total body water
45 liters**

Extracellular (ECF) 15 liters		Intracellular (ICF) 30 liters
Blood or Intra-vascular 3 liters	Inter-cellular or Extra-vascular 12 liters	Intracellular 30 liters
Na:K 28:1	Na:K 28:1	Na:K 1:10
–Capillary– wall		Cell membrane

Fig. 6-2. Diagrammatic representation of three major fluid compartments of the body. A fourth division, the transcellular fluid compartment, is a subdivision of extracellular fluid and includes water in collagen, connective tissue, bone, synovial fluid, vitreous humor, and digestive secretions.

be present in three "compartments" in the body, each of which is separated from the other by a semipermeable membrane across which there is a free exchange of fluid. The compartmentalization is shown diagramatically in Fig. 6-2. The intravascular compartment includes the fluid in all parts of the vascular system—arteries, veins, and capillaries. The walls of the vascular system separate the intravascular fluid from the intercellular, or extravascular, fluid that bathes the individual cells and tissues and provides the external environment from which the cells are nourished. The fluid or nutrients in the intercellular compartment must cross the cell membrane to enter the cell and to become a source of nourishment for the cell. The intercellular compartment acts as a buffer area; its volume will change to prevent changes in the volume of either the intravascular or intracellular fluid. The term transcellular fluid has been applied to a fourth compartment—fluids such as the synovial fluid lubricating joints and the vitreous humor of the eyeball—but these represent a very small portion of total body water and are not usually involved in fluid shifts.

The movement of fluid from one compartment to another is governed to a large extent by the concentration of minerals on either side of the membrane separating the compartments. Mineral elements in body fluids occur primarily as salts. However, these salts in solution dissociate into their component ions, one of which will have a positive charge and the other a negative charge. These charged ions are known as electrolytes and account for much of the osmotic pressure of the body fluids. As the concentration of electrolytes increases, the osmotic pressure increases. Whenever the osmotic pressure of the fluid on one side of a semipermeable membrane becomes higher than that on the other, fluid is drawn from the side of the membrane with the lower concentration of electrolytes to that with the higher concentration until the osmotic pressure on each side is equalized. When the same number of molecules and ions per exact volume of fluid is present on either side of the membrane, the osmotic pressures are the same and the amount of fluid on either side remains relatively constant.

Under most circumstances the body is able to prevent a shift in electrolyte concentrations so that there is no marked change in water balance between compartments. However, in some cases the homeostatic mechanisms of the body are taxed, resulting in a noticeable change in salt and hence electrolyte concentration in one of the fluid compartments. For instance, when the sodium intake exceeds the ability of the kidney to excrete it, the level of sodium in the blood and in the intercellular fluid increases. Since the cells cannot function in such a hypertonic environment, a series of changes occur to restore normal electrolyte levels. The thirst center is stimulated to increase the water intake, and at the same time fluid is withdrawn from the cells to dilute the intercellular fluid. This causes an increase in the volume of blood and intercellular fluid. The former results in an elevated blood pressure and the latter in the accumulation of fluid in the intercellular spaces to produce a soft, spongy, edematous tissue. Conversely, if sodium levels fall, there is a contraction of blood volume, a drop in blood pressure, a decrease in intercellular fluid, and fluid is restored to the cells.

When sodium is lost from the extracellular compartment, as it may be following excessive perspiration, potassium is pumped out of the cells to replace the lost sodium and to establish electrolyte balance. At the same time some water leaves the cell. Loss of water and potassium from the cell produces symptoms of weakness in the subject so common in heat prostration.

The mineral elements within each compartment vary, sodium being present in higher concentrations outside the cell, and potassium within the cell. Chlorine, which crosses the cell membrane easily, quickly establishes an equilibrium between the cell contents and the extracellular fluid.

Transmission of nerve impulses. Minerals play a vital role in the mechanism by which nerve impulses are conducted along nerve fibers. A nerve impulse is essentially an electrical stimulus that passes through a nerve fiber. During excitation or stimulation of nerve fibers the permeability of the membrane of nerve cells changes, allowing sodium to enter the cell more freely and potassium to leave. This creates a temporary change in the electrical charge on the membrane. This in turn changes the permeability of the next segment of the membrane, which changes the electrical charge again, and the message is passed down the membrane. It is, then, the exchange of sodium and potassium ions across the cell membrane that is responsible for the transmission of a nerve impulse. Anything that changes the mineral concentration of the fluids bathing nerve cells may interfere with their ability to transmit nerve impulses.

The transmission of a nerve impulse from one nerve cell to another is dependent on the presence of acetylcholine at the junction of the two fibers. The release of this compound is regulated by calcium.

Regulation of contractility of muscles. The muscles of the body are constantly bathed in a fluid—the interstitial fluid. For normal functioning of these muscles in contraction and relaxation, the composition of the interstitial fluid must represent a certain balance between elements that tend to stimulate muscular contraction, such as calcium, and those that exert a relaxing effect, such as sodium, potassium, and magnesium. This balance is steadfastly maintained under normal conditions. An upset in this balance is usually caused by the effect of the parathyroid hormone on the calcium levels. A drop in calcium levels without a concurrent decrease in the levels of the relaxing elements leads to a state of spasmodic contractions known as tetany. Conversely, an increase in calcium levels relative to the relaxing elements produces a state of tonic contractions known as calcium rigor.

During muscular contraction there is a release of potassium from the muscle cell, which is subsequently restored during the resting period. This seems to indicate an essential role for potassium in muscular contraction.

Growth of body tissue. Some mineral elements such as calcium and phosphorus occur in large concentration in bones and teeth and can rightly be considered as building constituents of body tissue. An absence of these raw materials will be reflected as stunted growth or in the development of tissue of inferior quality. Indirectly many minerals are involved in the growth process through their catalytic action on many reactions involved in the synthesis of body compounds or in the release of energy.

In the following chapters the macronutrients will be discussed first, after which a more detailed presentation of the information available on the most extensively studied microelements will be given.

SELECTED REFERENCES

Camien, M. N., Simmons, D. H., and Gonick, H. C.: Critical reappraisal of "acid-base" balance, Amer. J. Clin. Nutr. 22:786, 1969.

Council on Foods and Nutrition: Some inorganic elements in human nutrition, Symposium, Chicago, 1955, American Medical Association.

Hoekstra, W. G.: Recent observations on mineral interrelationships, Part I, Fed. Proc. 23:1068, 1964.

Wacker, W. E. C.: Metalloenzymes, Fed. Proc. 29:1462, 1970.

7 | *Macronutrient elements*

CALCIUM

Calcium is a relatively inert inorganic mineral element usually associated with bone and tooth formation. The use of the term calcification to describe the process by which these structures assume strength and rigidity has tended to reinforce ideas of the importance of calcium in bone formation. Calcium does play an important role in this process, but it is only one of many nutrients necessary for effective bone and tooth formation. In addition, the role of calcium in bone and tooth formation is only one of several of its vital biological functions. Although many writers have chosen to discuss calcium and phosphorus together because of their intimate relationship in bone and tooth development, we will emphasize their unique and independent roles by discussing each separately.

Distribution

The adult body contains between 1.5% and 2% of its weight as calcium. Of this 850 to 1400 gm. in the adult body, 99% is present in hard tissues, bones, and teeth. The remaining 10 gm., about one third of which is loosely bound to protein, is broadly distributed in the extracellular fluids and in the intracellular material of soft tissue, where it is vital to normal cell functioning. Much of the calcium in soft tissue is concentrated in muscle, although the membrane and cytoplasm of every cell contain some. The roles of calcium in these are so important that calcium will be mobilized from bones to maintain a functional level.

Although specific deficiency symptoms can rarely be attributed to a lack of dietary calcium, we do have concrete evidence of several specific roles of the mineral in body metabolism. The great reserve of calcium in the skeleton, which can be released to meet the needs of extracellular and soft tissues, and the mechanisms by which the body adapts to low dietary intakes by absorbing more and excreting less calcium have minimized the effects of intakes below the recommended allowances. Only when the mobile reserves of calcium in the bone have been depleted will changes resulting from a lack of calcium be apparent in other tissues. Because of the limited distribution of calcium in foods, intakes below recommended levels are frequently recorded but cannot be assessed on the basis of changes in tissue calcium levels. X-ray films of the wristbone can identify changes in bone density after as much as 30% bone calcium has been withdrawn.

Functions

Bone formation. Early in fetal development a strong but flexible protein (collagen) matrix, or pattern, for bone is formed. It bears the same general shape as the mature bone but lacks strength and rigidity. The matrix remains rather flexible until after birth, possibly to facilitate the birth process. This bone matrix is composed of fibers of the protein collagen embedded in a gelatinous *ground substance* composed of mucopolysaccharides, a relationship that apparently is responsible for the ability of the bone to calcify. Shortly after birth this matrix becomes strong and rigid, primarily as the result of the deposition and growth of calcium crystals in a process known as *ossification* or *calcification*. Since calcium and phosphorus are the predominate mineral elements in these crystals of the physiologically stable compound hydroxyapatite, an adequate supply of both minerals must be present before they can precipitate from the fluids surrounding the bone matrix to grow in the bone tissue.

Calcification apparently occurs when the product of the level of calcium and inorganic phosphorus in the blood and extracellular fluids exceeds 30, as follows: that is, milligrams of phosphorus × milligrams of calcium per 100 ml. of blood > 30.

However, since normal blood serum is usually supersaturated with both calcium and phosphorus, it appears that some other factor is necessary to facilitate the calcification process. The theory that the increase in the enzyme alkaline phosphatase associated with bone growth facilitates calcification by freeing more phosphate from organic compounds is being questioned. Instead, it is being postulated that phosphatase either functions in collagen formation or destroys a substance that would normally inhibit calcification.

The shaft of the long bones becomes rigid and strong, capable of supporting the weight of the body before the infant begins to walk, sometimes as early as 8 months of age. Throughout the entire growth process there is a constant lengthening of this bone shaft as the formation of new collagen matrix is followed by its calcification. The ends of the long bones retain a porous crystalline structure, known as the *trabeculae*. The trabeculae contain a high proportion of red marrow and a liberal supply of calcium, which can be readily mobilized to maintain the critical blood calcium levels when dietary levels drop. Only when calcium reserves in the trabeculae have been depleted will decalcification of other parts of the bones occur. Under these conditions

the pelvis and the spine are the first to release calcium.

During growth and throughout adult life there is a constant remodeling and reshaping of the bone in response to changing stresses from the weight of the developing body. This constant deposition and resorption of bone is the result of the activity of osteoblasts (bone-forming cells) and osteoclasts (bone-destroying cells) in the bone surface. In the adult 20% of bone calcium is resorbed and replaced each year; every five years the calcium in the bone has been completely replaced. In adults approximately 600 to 700 mg. of calcium are deposited each day in newly formed bone, replacing that which has been resorbed. The knowledge of this dynamic or changing state of bone metabolism was possible only with the use of radioactive isotopes of calcium that could be traced in their path through the body. About one third of the calcium in the adult bone appears to be in equilibrium with that in the extracellular fluids; the rest is in a more stable complex.

The amount of calcium needed to meet demands for bone growth varies with the rate of skeletal development. The increase in calcium content of the body from 0.8% of body weight at birth (about 28 gm.) to 1.7% at maturity (about 1200 gm.) represents an average daily increment of 165 mg. with a reported range of 70 to 400 mg., depending on the stage of bone growth. Maximum needs occur between 13 and 14 years of age, when the body acquires about 90 gm. of calcium per year, representing an increase of about 300 to 400 mg. per day in body calcium. The rate at which body calcium accumulates with age is shown in Fig. 7-1. The need for calcium reflects growth in body height rather than body weight.

In addition to calcium and phosphorus, vitamin A, magnesium, manganese, choline, vitamin C, vitamin D, and protein all affect bone growth.

Tooth formation. The mineral of dentin

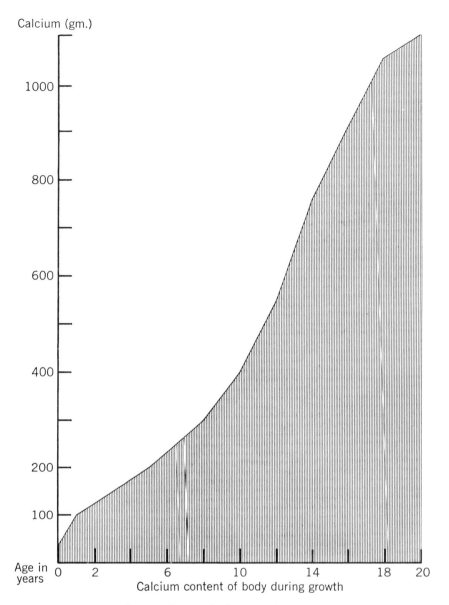

Calcium (gm.)

Age in years

Calcium content of body during growth

Fig. 7-1. Rate of accumulation of calcium in the body during growth.

and enamel is the same hydroxyapatite found in bones, but the crystals are more dense and the water content lower. The protein in enamel is keratin, whereas that in dentin is collagen. In contrast to bones, which are relatively active metabolically, teeth undergo an almost imperceptible change once they have erupted into the oral cavity. The slow rate of exchange be-

tween the tooth calcium and that of the body is confined almost entirely to the dentin layer, although evidence is accumulating to suggest that there may be some microchemical reaction involving calcium exchange between the tooth enamel and saliva that is accentuated once tooth decay has been initiated.

Calcification of deciduous teeth begins

by the twentieth week of fetal life, although it is completed only shortly before eruption into the oral cavity. Permanent teeth begin to calicify when the child is between 3 months and 3 years of age, whereas wisdom teeth, the last to erupt, may not begin to calcify until the eighth to tenth year of life. A full complement of adult teeth contains only 11 gm. of calcium, or about 1% of total body calcium.

Since teeth do not have the ability to repair themselves once they have erupted, there is no further need for a dietary source of calcium to maintain or repair teeth. A deficiency of calcium during the formative period for teeth may be reflected as a weakness in structure with increased susceptibility to tooth decay even though the teeth appear normal histologically. As in the case of bone, the integrity of tooth structure involves many nutrients in addition to calcium.

Growth. Although failure in growth is not a specific response to a dietary calcium deficiency, the observation that the stature of some persons, such as Orientals raised on a diet traditionally low in calcium, is frequently shorter than that of persons of the same race raised in a part of the world where the diet is adequate in calcium has led to the suggestion that calcium is necessary for normal growth. Since diets low in calcium also are frequently low in protein and since protein is a specific growth fac-

tor, it is difficult to argue that a lack of calcium is a primary cause of growth failure, although it may be a contributing factor.

Blood-clotting. The role of calcium in the blood-clotting mechanism is one of the more clearly understood of its functions. Once cells have been injured, ionized calcium, representing about half the total blood calcium, stimulates the release of thromboplastin from the blood platelets. Thromboplastin in turn catalyzes the conversion of prothrombin, a normal blood constituent, to thrombin. Thrombin then aids in the polymerization of fibrinogen to fibrin, the clot. The process is illustrated in Fig. 7-2. A schematic representation of the blood-clotting mechanism shows that calcium must be present to initiate a series of changes needed for the formation of the clot. Under normal conditions blood calcium levels are maintained at a sufficiently high level to facilitate the blood-clotting process so that an increase in dietary calcium will have little direct effect on blood-clotting time.

Catalyst for biological reactions. Calcium is vital to normal body functioning through its role as a catalyst in many biological reactions. The absorption of cobalamin (vitamin B_{12}) through the intestinal wall is dependent on calcium. The fat-splitting enzyme of pancreatic lipase is activated by calcium, as are many of the enzymes involved in the release of energy

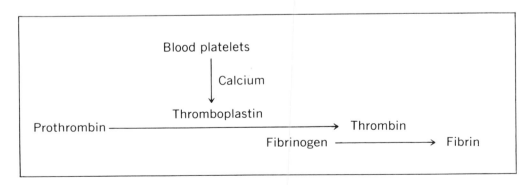

Fig. 7-2. Schematic representation of blood-clotting mechanism.

from carbohydrates, fat, and protein. In addition, the formation and breakdown of acetylcholine, the substance necessary for the transmission of an impulse from one nerve fiber to the next, is dependent on calcium. The level of calcium needed to facilitate these reactions will be maintained at the expense of skeletal calcium so that, as in blood-clotting, the level of dietary intake will not have a direct effect on these reactions.

Regulation of permeability of cell membrane. Calcium occurs in the cell membrane closely bound to the fat-related substance lecithin. Here in an antagonistic relationship with other ions it governs the permeability of the cell membrane to various nutrients and thus controls the uptake of nutrients by the cell. In much the same way it plays a role in the contraction and relaxation of muscle fibers and the transmission of nerve impulses.

Regulation of strontium uptake. With the increased amounts of strontium 90 available to humans and animals as a result of radioactive fallout, the possible protective value of a high-calcium diet in preventing the uptake of strontium has received much attention. Although similar chemically, calcium and strontium behave differently physiologically. The uptake of strontium by the body is often undesirable, since it can replace calcium in bone formation, where it may continue to cause irradiation. Present evidence indicates that if sufficient calcium is available, the body will preferentially absorb calcium by a factor of 9:1, but if less calcium is available, strontium will be taken up and will become an undesirable substitute for calcium in many compounds. The body also excretes strontium in preference to calcium in the urine, and preferentially transfers calcium to milk and across the placental barrier to the fetus. Thus, when dietary calcium is high, the body absorbs less strontium and excretes more, reducing the amount retained by the body compared to conditions of limited calcium intake. The relative value of calcium from various sources in protecting against strontium uptake is being investigated.

Absorption

In comparison with the rat, which can absorb 100% of dietary calcium, the human is very inefficient, absorbing a maximum of 40% to 60% under optimal conditions and greatest need. Normally an absorption of 20% to 30% of ingested calcium is considered good, and frequently it is as low as 10%. Most of this occurs in the upper three fourths of the small intestine, where the digestive mass is likely to be more acid. Here calcium is absorbed either by active transport, an energy-requiring process, or by passive diffusion, in which absorption occurs when calcium goes from an area of high concentration (intestine) to one of lower concentration (the blood). Before being absorbed, calcium must be separated from any complex in which it may occur in food and must be ionized. Whatever food calcium is unabsorbed passes on through the digestive tract and is excreted as exogenous fecal calcium.

The efficiency with which calcium is absorbed is a function of many factors, some of which favor and some of which depress it. Under any set of conditions there are wide individual differences in the efficiency of calcium absorption. Age has little effect.

Factors favoring calcium absorption

Vitamin D. The effectiveness of vitamin D in facilitating the uptake of calcium from the intestine has been recognized since the early 1920's, but only recently has there been any evidence about its mode of operation. DeLuca has now shown that vitamin D catalyzes the synthesis of a protein carrier in the mucosal cells of the intestinal wall. Calcium then attaches to this carrier, which is specific for calcium, and is transported across the intestinal membrane to the blood. When vitamin D is present, calcium is absorbed throughout a greater length of the intestine than when it is absent; thus more calcium will be absorbed before the food moves on to the colon, where no absorption occurs.

Acidity of digestive mass. Calcium is more soluble in acid and hence is more readily absorbed from an acid than from an alkaline medium. Since calcium is absorbed primarily from the small intestine, in which the contents must be rendered slightly alkaline before the intestinal enzymes can function, anything that increases the acidity of the digestive mass entering from the stomach and prolongs the time before the acid is neutralized should increase the possibility of calcium absorption. Hydrochloric acid normally secreted in the stomach is responsible for the acidity of the contents of the digestive tract as it enters the small intestine. When hydrochloric acid secretion is reduced, as it often is in old age, calcium absorption may be depressed. This may be partially compensated for by an increased intake of foods rich in ascorbic acid, which helps keep calcium ionized. The increase in calcium absorption noted on diets high in protein has been attributed by some to the action of the amino acids, the products of protein digestion, in forming a soluble complex with calcium to facilitate its absorption, or to preventing its precipitation as an insoluble complex. Although we have no explanation of why it is effective, there is experimental evidence to show that a high intake of the amino acid lysine will increase calcium absorption as much as 50%.

Lactose. There is ample evidence that the absorption of calcium is improved in the presence of the disaccharide lactose, with reports of increases ranging from 15% to 50%. Attempts to explain this effect on the basis of changes in the growth of microorganisms in the lower gastrointestinal tract, its slower rate of absorption, or changes in the acidity of intestinal contents as a result of the fermentation of lactose to lactic acid have failed. It has been suggested that the beneficial effects are caused by the formation of a soluble sugar-calcium complex in the intestine that keeps the calcium in a form in which it can be transported to and possibly across the intestinal wall. This complex also prevents the precipitation of calcium as an insoluble and hence unabsorbable complex as the contents of the gastrointestinal tract change from acid to alkali in the intestine. A relatively high ratio of lactose to calcium is necessary to form the soluble complex. Other sugars, such as the 5-carbon monosaccharide ribose and the 6-carbon monosaccharide fructose, also enhance calcium absorption, but lactose is the most effective. The benefits of obtaining calcium from milk, a food also high in lactose, are obvious.

Calcium to phosphorus ratio. The relationship between calcium and phosphorus levels in the diet plays an important role in the absorption of both. A dietary ratio of 1 part of phosphorus to 1 part calcium promotes the highest level of absorption. An upset Ca/P ratio is unlikely to occur on a normal diet so that its effect is of theoretical rather than practical interest, although it has been used in experimental diets to study calcium metabolism. For infants a Ca/P ratio of 1.5:2 is recommended.

Fat. The evidence of the effect of fat on calcium absorption is somewhat contradictory. Some research indicates an improved absorption resulting from the slower passage of food through the digestive tract.

The Food and Nutrition Board of the National Research Council concludes, however, that in high-fat diets the formation of insoluble soaps of fatty acids and calcium results in steatorrhea (fatty stools) and a concurrent reduction in calcium absorption. Studies with infants show that the use of whole cow's milk results in a lowering of calcium absorption.

Emotional stability. The efficiency with which the food calcium is absorbed can be influenced by the emotional stability of the individual. In one study a group of emotionally distressed young women were found to require a higher intake of calcium to maintain calcium balance than a comparable group of happy relaxed women. Another study of calcium metabolism of college men indicated a lowered absorption and increased excretion under conditions of stress such as examinations.

Need for calcium. The extent to which calcium is absorbed may be influenced by the body's need for calcium. During pregnancy and lactation and during adolescence, when needs are greater, absorption rates as high as 60% of ingested calcium have been observed. Similarly, on consistently low calcium intake the body is able to compensate by absorbing a high percentage. When the demands for calcium are lower, a smaller portion of the ingested calcium will be absorbed.

Factors depressing calcium absorption

Oxalic acid. Oxalic acid is an organic acid found in several fruits and vegetables, such as rhubarb, spinach, chard, and beet greens. It combines in the digestive tract with calcium to form an insoluble complex, calcium oxalate, from which the calcium cannot be released for absorption. In most foods containing oxalic acid, there is also present sufficient calcium to tie up all the oxalic acid, leaving no surplus to bind calcium from other foods eaten at the same time. There is no evidence, for instance, to suggest that the oxalic acid of spinach will interfere with the absorption of the calcium in milk taken at the same time. The presence of 5% to 6% unbound oxalic acid in lower grades of cocoa led to reservations about the use of chocolate milk for children. Early misgivings were based on results of studies on rats, in which the addition of a low-grade cocoa to the diet caused as much as a 27% depression of calcium utilization. More recent work on college women at the University of Illinois showed

that women could tolerate a maximum of one ounce of cocoa without nausea—an amount that could not be shown to cause any significant depression in calcium utilization on either a low or high calcium intake. Comparable studies have not been done on children, but one would expect results comparable to those on women, indicating no reason for condemning chocolate milk on the basis of decreased calcium utilization.

Phytic acid. Another organic acid, phytic acid, found predominately in the outer husks of cereals, has been shown to lower utilization of calcium by binding it in an insoluble complex. Studies comparing the utilization of calcium on diets containing comparable amounts of farina, low in phytic acid, and oatmeal, high in phytic acid, show up to 33% poorer utilization on the oatmeal diet. The human being lacks the enzyme phytase, which some species have, to hydrolyze the phytate group and to release the calcium. Only in cases where the consumption of calcium-rich foods is in conjunction with foods high in phytic acid would this inhibitory effect become a practical problem. There is evidence, too, of a rapid adaptation to diets of high phytic acid so that the depressing effect of phytic acid on calcium absorption is minimized.

Increased gastrointestinal motility. Anything that increases the rate of passage of food through the intestinal tract decreases the absorption of calcium by reducing the time in which the contents of the intestinal tract are in contact with the intestinal wall. Laxatives and foods high in bulk may have this effect.

Lack of exercise. Persons who receive little exercise and bed-ridden persons who are essentially immobilized experience a loss of bone calcium and a reduced ability to replace it. This may be a cause, or at least a complicating factor, in the decalcification of bone so often experienced by older people. Evidence now indicates that it is the lack of weight on the legs rather than immobility per se that causes negative calcium balance during bed rest. Although the explanation of this is disputed, it is postulated that either the lack of weight on the legs or the decrease in vascularity accompanying the reduced muscle contraction leads to a decrease in stimulus for bone formation.

• • •

The factors affecting calcium absorption are summarized as follows:

> Factors favoring absorption
>> Adequate vitamin D
>> Acidity of digestive mass
>> Calcium to phosphorus ratios of 1:1
>> Need for calcium
>
> Factors depressing absorption
>> Oxalic acid
>> Phytic acid
>> Increased gastrointestinal motility
>> Emotional instability
>> Presence of dietary fat

Metabolism

Once calcium has been absorbed through the wall of the intestine, it is transported in the blood plasma and released to the fluids bathing the tissues of the body. From there the cells pick up whatever calcium is needed for their normal functioning and growth. Some calcium becomes a part of the digestive secretions into the stomach and intestine. Much of this calcium is reabsorbed, but endogenous fecal calcium amounts to about 130 mg. regardless of dietary intake. As the blood plasma is filtered through the kidney, about 99% of the calcium is resorbed and the remaining 1% is excreted in the urine. This usually amounts to 100 to 175 mg. per day and represents 20% to 25% of the dietary intake.

As indicated earlier, most of the absorbed calcium is used in the calcification of bones to give strength and rigidity. The deposition of calcium in the bones is facilitated by vitamin D and the enzyme phosphatase.

The calcium in the blood is in equilibrium with bone calcium, about one third of which is available to provide calcium to maintain blood calcium levels of from 7 to 10 mg. per 100 ml. If blood calcium falls below 7 mg.%, the parathyroid gland secretes a hormone, parathormone, that stimulates the release of some of the exchangeable calcium from the bone. This usually occurs as the result of the release and metabolism of some of the carbohydrate in the bone to citrate and lactate, in which the bone calcium is soluble. This in turn increases the level of calcium in the blood and intercellular fluids to the point at which it again is adequate for normal blood coagulation, the transmission of nerve impulses, and the contraction of muscles. At the same time the parathyroid stimulates the release of stored calcium, it causes the kidney to resorb more of the calcium, which might normally be excreted in the urine, and it stimulates a greater absorption of calcium from the gastrointestinal tract. When blood levels return to normal, the secretion of the parathyroid returns to normal. Opposing the action of parathormone is a second hormone, *calcitonin,* a polypeptide with thirty-two amino acids, which is formed in the ultimobranchial glands of the thyroid gland. It is secreted when blood calcium levels become elevated and acts to lower both calcium and phosphate levels by inhibiting bone resorption. Thus the parathyroid gland, through its effect directly or indirectly on the secretion of these two hormones, is responsible for maintaining the level of calcium in the blood within the very narrow limits demanded by the body.

The regulatory effect of the parathyroid hormone is integrated with the action of vitamin D, which also stimulates the absorption of calcium from the intestinal tract, increases the retention of calcium by the kidney, and allows the parathormone to act to release bone calcium to maintain blood levels. An excess of vitamin D will stimulate the decalcification of bone and will produce high blood calcium levels. An excess of vitamin D may lead to decalcifica-

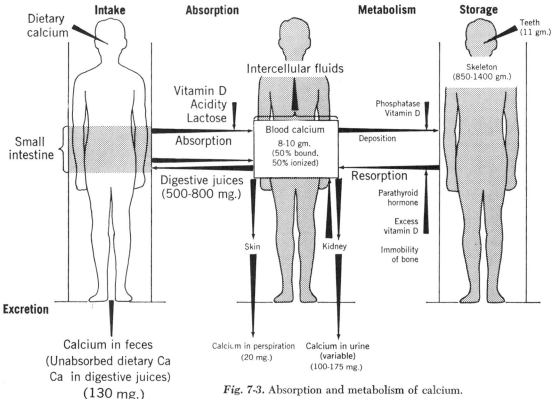

Fig. 7-3. Absorption and metabolism of calcium.

tion of the bone and an increased absorption of calcium from the gastrointestinal tract, with the resultant hypercalcemia.

The paths of the absorption and metabolism of calcium are shown schematically in Fig. 7-3.

Requirements

Controversy. In attempting to establish a recommended level for calcium intake, nutritionists have become involved in an intense controversy. Proponents of a lower allowance maintain that we have no evidence of adverse effects from low intakes, that there is no evidence that low calcium is a deterrent to growth, and that no clinical condition can be classified as a calcium deficiency. They maintain that conditions that have been classified as calcium deficiency diseases are in reality the result of inadequate vitamin D. Those who believe

that the present standard should be maintained are convinced that persons who have been on a restricted intake in their early years are more susceptible to osteoporosis as they grow older, that there is no evidence of harm from moderate intakes up to 2 gm., that not all people are able to adapt to low intakes, and that the larger amounts are readily available in the food supply to provide these levels for the American population. Where less calcium is available in the food supply and the population has adapted to lower intakes, a lower dietary standard is justified.

Calcium balance studies. Estimates of calcium needs have been based on the results of calcium balance studies in which the calcium content of the diet is compared to the amount of calcium excreted in the urine and feces. Urinary calcium represents that not resorbed by the kidney and fecal calcium, the endogenous calcium of the digestive secretions, plus any unabsorbed dietary calcium. This can range from 10% to 60% of the dietary intake. It has been assumed that when calcium intake exceeds calcium excretion, the body is in positive calcium balance and is storing calcium. When intake equals excretion, the body is in calcium equilibrium and is neither accumulating calcium nor losing it. When excretion exceeds intake, the body is in negative calcium balance and is releasing more body calcium than it is replacing, resulting in a net loss from the body that reflects decalcification of bone tissue in most cases.

Limitations. There are several limitations to the use of calcium balance data. Measurement of intake seldom involves a determination of the calcium in water, which in tropical areas with a hard water supply is an appreciable amount. Nor does it take into account the nonfood sources of calcium such as lime ingested by betel chewers and by persons eating Mexican tortillas made from lime-treated corn. An appreciable amount of calcium may be lost in perspiration and tears, which are seldom analyzed because we have not developed techniques to do so. Although under normal circumstances the loss of calcium in the sweat amounts to only 20 mg., for people living in the tropics this may amount to as much as 140 mg. and for those working hard at very high temperatures, as much as 1000 mg. This is sufficient to make a difference between positive and negative balance in many studies. Since some people adapt to a low calcium intake by conserving calcium either through a higher rate of absorption, a lower rate of excretion, or lessened secretions in the digestive juices, calcium balance data are meaningful only if there is information about dietary history. A person accustomed to an intake of 500 mg. could maintain calcium balance on 400 mg. more easily than could a person whose customary diet provided 1000 mg. The length of time required for adaptation

varies. Some persons adapt within two months to a lower intake, others much more slowly, and some, never. In addition, Ohlson observed that a positive or negative balance that had prevailed for weeks could be reversed without any dietary change in adult women. Calcium balances have been reported to reflect the emotional state of the individual, becoming negative under stressful circumstances and positive again as stress passes. Some evidence suggests that calcium balance data are useful only if considered in the light of phosphorus balance data, and one study has shown that the level of sodium in the diet also has a marked influence on calcium utilization.

Dietary allowances

In spite of the reservations that many scientists have expressed about the validity of calcium balance studies, they remain a widely used criterion for establishing a standard for calcium intake. These data must be critically appraised, taking into account previous calcium intake, adaptation, and physiological stress.

Recently the use of Ca^{47} with a relatively short half-life has proved useful in studying calcium metabolism as a basis for estimating requirements.

The recommended allowances proposed by the Food and Nutrition Board of the National Research Council in 1968 have been set at a level the Council believes will meet the needs of essentially all healthy individuals and one that can be readily achieved from the national food supply.

The Food and Agricultural Organization has released suggested practical calcium allowances. They believe these lower values represent a level that can more readily be achieved by a larger segment of the world's population, many of whom consume low amounts of calcium because of its limited availability in their national food supplies. The wide variation in the calcium available in the diets of various countries is evident from Fig. 7-4. The determination

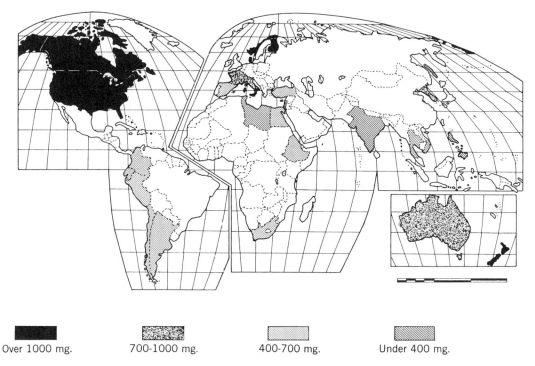

Over 1000 mg.　　700-1000 mg.　　400-700 mg.　　Under 400 mg.

Fig. 7-4. Amounts of calcium per capita available in food supply in different parts of the world. (Based on data from Calcium requirements, Report of Joint FAO/WHO Expert Committee, WHO Techn. Rep. Ser. No. 230, Geneva, 1962.)

Table 7-1. Comparison of standards for calcium intake for selected age and sex groups

	Age	Canadian dietary standard (1968)* (mg./day)	British† (mg./day)	NRC recommended dietary allowances (1968)‡ (mg./day)	FAO/WHO suggested practical allowances§ (mg./day)
Children	7-12 months	500	600	600	500- 600
	10-12 years	1200	700	1200	600- 700
Males	16-19 years	900	500	1400	500- 600
	Adult	500	500	800	400- 500
Females	16-19 years	900	600	1300	500- 600
	Adult	500	500	800	400- 500
	Pregnancy	1200	1200	1200	1000-1200
	Lactation	1200	1200	1300	1000-1200

*Dietary standards for Canada, Canadian Bulletin on Nutrition, vol. 6, No. 1, March, 1964; revised, 1968.
†Department of Health and Social Security: Recommended intakes of nutrients for the United Kingdom, Reports on Public Health and Medical Subjects, No. 120, London, 1969, Her Majesty's Stationery Office.
‡Food and Nutrition Board: Recommended dietary allowances, ed. 7, Publication No. 1694, Washington, D. C., 1968, National Academy of Sciences–National Research Council.
§Calcium requirements, Report of Joint FAO/WHO Expert Committee, WHO Techn. Rep. Ser. No. 230, 1962.

of these figures is complicated by the fact that there is little relationship between values obtained by calculations from tables of food composition and those obtained by actual analysis. A comparison of American, Canadian, British, and FAO recommendations listed in Table 7-1 shows that there is no general agreement regarding the optimal level of calcium intake. The FAO group, after evaluating all available data, suggests that there is no evidence that when vitamin D is adequate, there are any harmful effects from diets containing below 300 mg. or more than 1000 mg. of calcium per day.

Infants. There is relatively little data available on calcium needs of infants. It is assumed that the breast-fed infant who receives about 60 mg. per kilogram of body weight and retains two thirds of it receives adequate calcium. For the artificially fed infant who retains 35% to 50% of the 160 mg. per kilogram from cow's milk formula, an intake of 400 to 600 mg. is recommended. If undiluted whole milk with a relatively high fat content is fed, the amount of calcium absorbed is greatly reduced.

Children. The daily retention of 75 to 150 mg. of calcium per day requires a daily intake of 800 mg. of calcium for children 1 to 8 years of age. The rapidly growing skeleton of adolescents requires as much as 400 mg. of calcium per day, calling for an intake of 1400 mg. for boys and 1300 mg. for girls.

Adults. In establishing the recommended dietary allowances for the adult, it is assumed that the mandatory endogeneous calcium losses plus exogeneous calcium losses and losses in sweat and in the urine total 320 mg. per day. Assuming that 40% of dietary calcium is absorbed, it is suggested that an intake of 800 mg. per day will meet the needs of essentially all healthy adults. Balance studies show that the average person achieves calcium equilibrium on an intake of 10 mg. per kilogram

of body weight; however, the wide individual variations indicate that 18 mg. per kilogram would be needed to meet the needs of 95% of the population and 22 mg. if one were to be assured of meeting the needs of 99% of the population.

Pregnancy and lactation. Although the child is born with poorly calcified bones, the full-term fetus contains approximately 28 gm. of calcium, which must be provided from the mother's reserves. There is need for an increased maternal intake, not only for the calcification of the fetal teeth and bones that occurs during pregnancy but also to build the storage reserves of the mother to meet the high demands during lactation. Calcium is deposited in the fetal tissue at the rate of 25, 50, 85, 125, 175, 235, and 300 mg. per day during the last 7 months of pregnancy. Two thirds of fetal calcium is transferred from the mother to the fetus between the thirtieth and the fortieth week of pregnancy, when fetal calcium increases from 10 to 28 gm. Studies using radioactive isotopes of calcium in mothers' diets show that 85% to 90% of the calcium in the fetal skeleton and in human milk came from the mother's diet, and 10% to 15% was withdrawn from maternal reserves. Indications are that the ability to absorb calcium increases with need and that the pregnant woman may absorb up to 40% of dietary calcium. Even so, the National Research Council has recommended an additional 400 mg. per day over normal requirements to meet both fetal and maternal demands. A retention by the mother of two to five times fetal needs has been reported in the sixth and seventh months, indicating that maternal reserves are being built up at this time. Research also suggests a sharp reduction in muscular cramps frequently encountered in pregnancy upon administration of both vitamin D and calcium.

The transfer of calcium from mother to infant is greater during lactation than during pregnancy, about 50 gm. being secreted in milk during a six-month lactation period.

Human milk contains about 30 mg. calcium per 100 ml. To meet this demand for 200 to 300 mg. per day for the production of 850 ml. of milk without causing a severe depletion of the mother's reserves or a decrease in milk production, a maternal intake of 1300 mg. has been advised. At a 40% utilization rate, 750 mg. would be needed for milk production alone. This requires the use of large amounts of dairy products (a minimum of 1½ quarts of milk or its equivalent), plus generous use of other calcium-rich foods. Very few women maintain calcium equilibrium during lactation but draw on the calcium reserves built up during pregnancy to help provide the calcium transferred to milk. The ability of some women to maintain a successful level of lactation on very low calcium intakes is unexplained.

Old age. There is no basis on which to suggest an increase in calcium need with age, but all evidence points to the need for maintaining the adult intake of 800 mg. per day throughout the later years to reduce the likelihood of demineralization of the skeleton frequently observed, especially in women over 65 years of age.

Adequacy of calcium in the American diet. If the NRC recommended allowances are used as a criterion for adequacy, it is apparent from various studies of dietary intake that many persons in the United States fail to meet this standard. The extent to which the diets of Americans meet the National Research Council standards is shown in Fig. 7-5. This shows that men and boys are much more likely to consume adequate amounts than are women and girls. Milk was a major source of calcium in all diets, providing about three fourths of the calcium in most of the diets evaluated. Persons who do not drink milk, especially those who also restrict their use of other dairy products, find it virtually impossible to consume a diet reaching NRC standards. The inadequate intake in calcium in the diets of older women is of special concern because of the increased likelihood of osteoporosis in this group.

Food sources

Calcium is present in significant amounts in a very limited number of foods. Fig. 7-6 shows the contribution of various food groups to the total calcium available in the

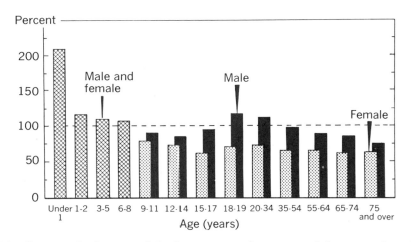

Fig. 7-5. Adequacy of calcium in daily diet as reported in survey of dietary intakes of households 1 day in spring, 1965. Calcium from 1 day's diet, as a percent of the recommended allowances (NAS-NRC, 1968). (From Food intake and nutritive value of diets of men, women and children in the United States—spring, 1965, Agricultural Research Service, Publication ARS 62-18, 1969.)

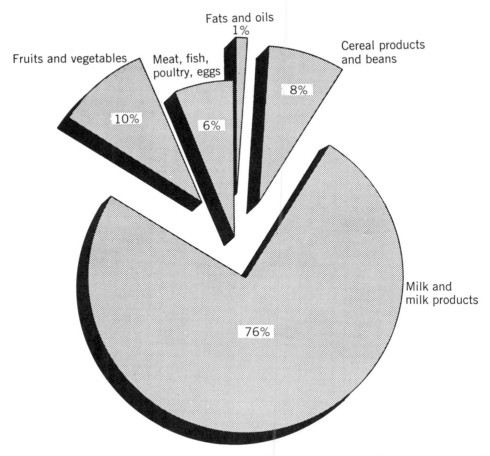

Fig. 7-6. Contribution of various food groups to the calcium content of the American food supply. (Based on Contribution of major food groups to nutrient supplies available for civilian consumption, National Food Situation No. 130, 1969.)

American diet, which has increased steadily from 0.86 gm. in 1906 to 1.16 gm. per capita per day in 1962. Milk and dairy products are the most dependable sources because of the many ways in which they can be consumed, their availability, and their relatively low cost. In addition, the calcium in milk is in complexes from which it is readily released. It becomes obvious from Fig. 7-7, showing the relative amounts of calcium from various food sources on the basis of 100 gm. and 100 kcal. of food, that should dairy products be excluded from the diet, the bulk of other foods needed to supply comparable amounts of calcium would make their use as a major source of calcium difficult. As sources of calcium they are also expensive.

Fish flour made from whole fish, including bones, has an extremely high calcium value both per 100 gm. portion and per 100 kcal. Although it may assume major importance as a source of both calcium and protein in countries where milk is not available, the possibility of its widespread use in the American diet is remote. Only a limited amount could reasonably be incorporated into a day's diet, and technically there are still many problems relative to flavor and keeping qualities to be solved.

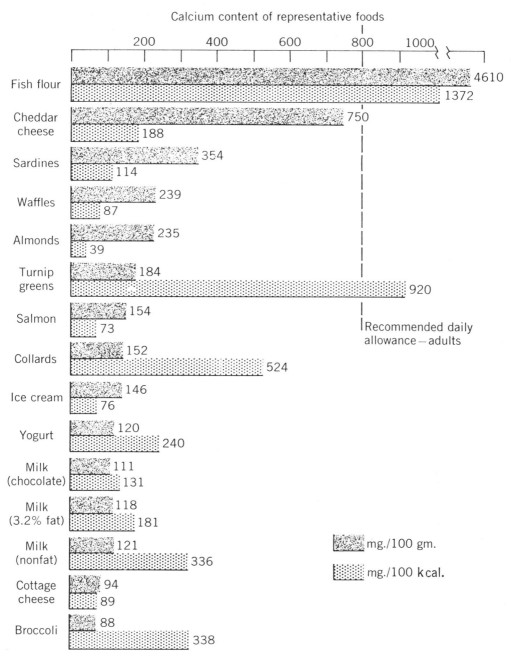

Fig. 7-7. Calcium content of some representative foods. (Based on Watt, B. K., and **Merrill**, A. L.: Composition of foods—raw, processed and prepared, U. S. Department of Agriculture Handbook No. 8, Washington, D. C., 1963, U. S. Department of Agriculture.)

Foods of low water content, such as sardines and almonds, have an appreciable amount of calcium in terms of 100 gm. portions, but their value to the diet is limited when one considers their contribution relative to calories—an especially important consideration for people on diets restricted in calories.

The most useful sources of calcium then become milk and milk products. The ultra-high temperature sterilization of milk does not affect the availability of milk calcium, nor do the more common practices of pasteurization or homogenization. The adding of chocolate to milk does not reduce significantly the availability of calcium. It is seen that nonfat milk and buttermilk are slightly better than whole milk as sources of calcium. This may be explained by the fact that when the fat portion, which is almost devoid of calcium, is removed, it is replaced by the calcium-containing portion of milk. Where cost is a prime consideration, nonfat products will provide calcium at one fourth to one third the price of whole milk. One ounce of cheddar cheese provides as much calcium as a cup of milk and often finds greater acceptance than milk as a source of calcium for adults. Cottage cheese is a variable source of calcium, depending on the method of processing used. Rennin coagulation retains more calcium in the curd than either a combination of acid and rennin coagulation or acid coagulation alone. All methods are used commercially. Cream cheese is a poor source, being made from the fat portion of milk that is low in calcium. Ice cream, a popular form of milk product, can be substituted at a level of one cup of ice cream for one half cup of milk as a source of available calcium.

The amount of calcium in milk from a particular species varies with the rate of growth of the offspring. It ranges from 0.02% in the milk of human beings, whose babies double their birth weight in 180 days, to 0.12% in the milk of cows, whose calves double their birth weight in 47 days, and 0.32% in the milk of dogs, who achieve the same proportionate increase in weight in 7 days.

Goat's milk contains slightly more calcium than cow's milk and often is substituted when an infant is allergic to cow's milk. Where cow's and goat's milk are not available or are not tolerated by young infants, calcium-enriched soybean milk preparations in either powdered or liquid form may be substituted as a satisfactory source of calcium. Evidence that many adults of Oriental extraction lack the enzyme lactase necessary for the digestion of lactose explains the aversion to milk often reported by this group. To promote the use of milk as a source of calcium cannot be justified under these conditions.

Next to milk products, broccoli and green leafy vegetables such as turnip greens and kale, which do not contain oxalic acid, have the most appreciable amounts of available calcium. The utilization of vegetable calcium is not as high because the increased gastrointestinal motility caused by the bulk of the vegetable increases rate of passage through the intestinal tract. In the case of the green leafy vegetables the fact that calcium is contained within the cell whose cellulose wall is digested with difficulty often limits the availability of this calcium. Considerable calcium may be lost in preparation of vegetables if thick skins are removed or the dark green leaves discarded.

Soybeans become a significant calcium source when consumed in large amounts. In Indonesia, for instance, a fermented soybean product, tempeh, and a dried soybean milk powder, saridele, are being advocated as potential sources of calcium and protein. In Oriental countries soy sauce may represent a significant source of calcium.

Although bread has not been traditionally considered a source of calcium, the current trend toward use of dried milk solids and calcium-containing mold inhibitors raises its available calcium to the point at which many adults receive as much as one seventh of their day's requirement from bread. Similarly, the calcium value of baked products such as muffins, waffles, and cakes should not be overlooked. There is also the potential for increasing their calcium value by adding additional milk solids up to the point at which the product remains palatable. The optional enrichment of flour with 500 to 1500 mg. of calcium per pound makes it a significant source. Data from food consumption studies in 1965 show that cereal products and beans contributed 21% of the calcium.

In tropical areas where milk products are produced and consumed by only a small segment of the population, other less traditional sources of calcium may assume much greater importance, although we have virtually no information regarding the extent to which they are utilized by the body. Where water consumption is high (as is common in the tropics) and its mineral content high (50 mg. or more per liter), water may provide up to 200 mg. or more per day. Small whole fish or fermented fish pastes are high in calcium. The mill powder used in grinding rice may adhere to the kernel in sufficient quantities to con-

tribute to the overall calcium intake. Lime used in making tortillas adds a significant amount of calicum to diets of Mexicans. Similarly, lime used by betel chewers adds to the calcium intake of these individuals, as does the ground rock, cal, used in porridges by the Peruvians. Even sweet potatoes, when they are a staple item in the diet as in the Papuan highlands of New Guinea, provide sufficient calcium to meet minimum dietary needs. In China, eggs may contribute a substantial proportion of the limited total calcium consumed, and in Malaya pregnant women eat a small shellfish, which is ground up whole and eaten. These represent but a few of the ways in which various populations perhaps acquire sufficient calcium, although they consume practically no dairy products.

Many diet supplements contain calcium salts, such as calcium carbonate, calcium gluconate, calcium lactate, and calcium citrate. These seem to be well utilized and may be of value during times of very high need such as pregnancy and lactation. However, the user is cautioned to read the label carefully, since multivitamin mineral pills seldom contain significant amounts of calcium. They should be considered a supplement to a calcium-rich diet but not a re-

Table 7-2. Relative costs of one third the adult daily calcium allowance from various food sources

Food	Amount required (oz.)	Cost*
Dried nonfat milk	0.67	$ .02
Cheddar cheese	1	$ .05
Fresh whole milk	8	$ .08
Chocolate milk	8	$ .08
Ice cream	6	$ .09
Sardines	2.5	$ .13
Cottage cheese	9	$ .19
Broccoli	10	$ .25
Almonds	3.5	$ .36

*Based on prices prevailing in northeastern United States, spring, 1970.

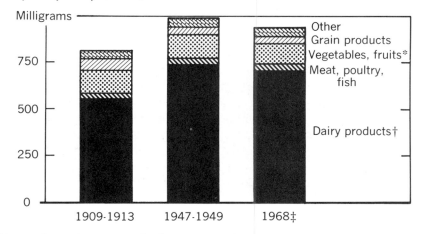

Fig. 7-8. Trends in consumption of calcium sources from 1909 to 1968. Sources of calcium, per capita per day. *Includes melons, potatoes, sweet potatoes, dry beans, peas, and nuts; †excludes butter; and ‡preliminary. (From Agricultural Research Service, U. S. Department of Agriculture, 1969.)

placement for dietary calcium. Purveyors of special food-blending devices are constantly promoting the consumption of pulverized eggshell as a feasible method of obtaining an adequate calcium intake. An eggshell does contain 2 gm. of calcium, but since we have no data on the utilization of calcium from this source, one can question the reliance on such a source, especially where adequate calcium is available from more conventional sources.

For people who have a restricted food budget, knowledge of the cost of a nutrient from various sources may be helpful in planning an adequate intake at minimum cost. Table 7-2 gives such information for some representative sources of calcium. Trends in sources of dietary calcium are shown in Fig. 7-8.

High calcium intake

Although we have no evidence of deleterious effects from excessive intakes of calcium per se, popular literature is suggesting with increasing frequency that a high intake of calcium is undesirable. In the several studies to assess the effect of high oral calcium intakes, (2 gm.) it was found that they had no effect on the level of

calcium in the urine of normal subjects, although they would result in high urinary calcium levels (hypercalcuria) in numerous disease states. In addition, there is no evidence that high dietary calcium levels have any effect on kidney stone formation or lead to deposition of calcium in other soft tissues in the absence of metabolic abnormalities.

Calcification of soft tissues does not occur in normal, healthy individuals solely as a result of high intakes of calcium. If, however, blood calcium levels become high because of increased bone resorption, it may be helpful to reduce dietary calcium in an effort to reduce the amount available for calcification of soft tissues such as the kidney. The abnormal deposition of calcium in soft tissues is more likely a result of low magnesium than of high calcium.

Work on animals has suggested that excessively high intakes of calcium have a depressing effect on the utilization of other nutrients, such as phosphorus, fat, iodine, zinc, magnesium, and iron, when the latter are present at minimal levels. However, the ratios at which this can occur are far beyond those calcium intakes that may be encountered in a normal diet. In adults high intakes of calcium lead to increased total absorption of calcium, although the efficiency of absorption is decreased. In children, however, an intake of 2300 mg. of calcium and 2400 mg. of phosphorus resulted in a depressed retention of calcium. This was accompanied by a marked increase in fat excretion in feces and may be caused by an inhibition of the fat-splitting enzyme pancreatic lipase in the presence of high calcium concentration in the intestine.

Once high urinary calcium levels occur as the result of some metabolic abnormality such as hypothyroidism, which stimulates calcium absorption, the restriction of dietary calcium to the levels considered adequate but not in excess of those required to meet body needs is likely a rational therapeutic approach.

Thus, although we have no evidence of additional benefits to be derived from calcium intakes in excess of recommended levels, neither can we point to any evidence of detrimental effects except for individuals with a tendency to deposit calcium in soft tissues.

Assessment of body calcium reserves

The major problem in assessing body nutriture in respect to calcium is the lack of a feasible method that is sensitive to changes in body calcium. Blood calcium levels are readily determined, but the action of the parathyroid gland in mobilizing bone calcium to maintain blood calcium at a level of at least 7 mg. per 100 ml. means that a drop in blood calcium is a more sensitive measure of the efficiency of the parathyroid than of calcium status. The hazards and cost involved in the use of radioactive isotopes of calcium restrict its usefulness to controlled studies on small numbers of subjects. Considerable work has been done to develop an x-ray measurement of bone density that will reflect the degree of mineralization of bone. Bones of the heel and finger, which have been investigated, do not show sufficient variation in mineralization within the normal range of human calcium intake to be of any use in assessing calcium nutriture. From 10% to 40% demineralization of bone may have occurred before the change will be reflected in x-ray measurements. The problem is further complicated by the fact that so far no deficiency symptoms can be attributed to a lack of dietary calcium.

Abnormalities of calcium metabolism

Osteoporosities. Osteoporosis is a condition found primarily among middle-aged women in which the absolute amount of bone in the skeleton has been diminished but the remaining bone mass is of normal composition. This is reflected in a shortening of stature and symptoms of low backache. It affects a minimum of 10% of the population over 50 years of age, and several studies have reported incidence as high as 50%. It is estimated that in 1963 there were over 4 million cases of severe osteoporosis in the United States, 80% of which were in women. Women lose 8% of their bone mass per decade after 40 compared to 3% in men.

Osteoporosis is now regarded as a condition of multiple origins. This has led to the proposal that it be referred to as the *osteoporosities*. The concept of multiple causation may help explain why high dietary calcium levels are not necessarily protective and low levels not necessarily associated with bone loss. The osteoporosities, then, have been attributed to decrease in bone mass as the result of long-standing dietary inadequacy of calcium, the action of the parathyroid in stimulating bone resorption, the failure to synthesize matrix collagen, the effect of immobility, and a loss of the stimulus to bone formation provided by the estrogens. It is now believed that in osteoporosis the rate of bone formation is normal but bone resorption occurs at an accelerated rate. The increased rate of bone resorption may occur to maintain normal blood levels of calcium when dietary intake is low or when dietary needs are abnormally high because of poor absorption. People with osteoporosis have usually been found to have had a lower than normal intake of calcium over a long period of time. Older people have been shown to absorb less calcium than do younger people, and those with osteoporosis less than do those free of the disease; in some cases people with osteoporosis also excrete more, but in all cases the gain in body calcium has failed to compensate for the losses, which has led to a resorption of bone tissue to maintain normal blood levels. Those with osteoporosis do not have the ability of normal people to reduce urinary calcium excretion when dietary intake is low. Thus it appears that the people who develop osteoporosis are those who cannot adapt to a low level of dietary intake, have impaired absorptive mechanisms, or persistently lose body calcium.

Treatment of osteoporosis with a diet high in calcium (15.5 mg. per kilogram of body weight) and with adequate vitamin D has been shown to arrest the resorption of the bone and has led to the observation that the prevention of osteoporosis with lifelong adequate calcium intakes is the best treatment. An accumulating body of evidence demonstrates that fluoride may protect against bone loss by substituting for the hydroxyl portion of the bone mineral, rendering it less susceptible to degradation. The high incidence of bone fracture among osteoporotic patients may be due to spontaneous fractures in which the break precedes the fall rather than being caused by falls. Osteoporotic bone breaks at loads 40% less than normal, and the healing period for fractures is considerably longer than normal.

Osteomalacia. Osteomalacia, on the other hand, is a condition in which there is a reduction in the mineral content of the bone but not in the total amount of bone. It is most likely to occur among women liv-ing in areas of low sunshine, those whose clothing prevents exposure to sunlight, those whose diets are low in calcium, and those for whom the demands of successive pregnancies and prolonged lactation have depleted their mineral resources.

Hypercalcemia. Hypercalcemia has been reported in infants as the result of high intakes of vitamin D or a diet in which the ratio of phosphorus to calcium is very high. These cases have been observed in connection with widespread supplementation of infant foods with vitamin D and the use of whole milk formulas in which the fat interferes with calcium absorption but not with phosphorus absorption. It is best corrected by reducing the vitamin D rather than the calcium in the diet.

Tetany and calcium rigor. When the level of calcium in the blood and hence in the extracellular fluids drops below a critical level, there is a change in the stimulation of nerve cells, resulting in increased excitability of the nerve and spasmodic and uncontrolled contractions of muscle tissue, a condition described as tetany. When calcium levels rise above normal, the muscle fibers enter a state of tonic contraction known as *calcium rigor*. Neither of these conditions is the result of abnormal dietary levels of calcium but rather both reflect an abnormality in parathyroid functioning.

PHOSPHORUS
Distribution

Since phosphorus constitutes 22% of the mineral ash in an adult body or 1% of body weight, it is classified as a *macronutrient* element. Its role as a major constituent of bones and teeth is recognized by even the casual student of nutrition. The fact that it is often discussed in connection with calcium has further emphasized its role in the formation of hard tissues, with the result that its other equally vital roles are often overlook or underestimated.

It is estimated that the adult body contains 12 gm. of phosphorus per kilogram of fat-free tissue. This amounts to about 670 gm. of phosphorus in the male and 630 gm. in the female. Of this phosphorus 85% to 90% is in the form of the insoluble calcium phosphate (apatite) crystals with a calcium to phosphorus ratio of 2:1, that give rigidity and strength to bones and teeth. The remaining 10% to 15% is distributed throughout all living cells of the body, with about half present in striated muscle. Specifically it is a part of the nucleus and the cytoplasm of every living cell, where it plays an essential role in many body processes and as a structural component. In fact, practically all biological reactions involve phosphorus to some extent, since it is vital to any reaction that involves the uptake or release of energy.

Functions

Regulates the release of energy. It is a phosphorus-containing substance, phosphate, that is responsible for the controlled release of energy resulting from the combustion or oxidation of carbohydrate, fat, and protein. A third phosphate molecule is attached to the compound ADP, (adenosine diphosphate) to form ATP (adenosine triphosphate) in a bond, or linkage, that stores energy. This linkage is referred to as a high-energy phosphate bond. As energy is needed, the ATP is changed to ADP, and a phosphate molecule and the energy that held it to ADP is released to supply energy slowly for many body reactions. If the cells were unable to convert energy into these high-energy bonds for storage, they would be incapable of regulating the rate at which it is available. Phosphate, and hence phosphorus, appears many times in the chemical reactions that occur in metabolism within the cell.

Facilitates absorption and transportation of nutrients. Phosphate is attached to many substances, such as monosaccharides, in a process known as phosphorylation, to facilitate their passage through cell membranes.

This occurs in absorption from the intestine, release from the bloodstream to the intercellular fluids, uptake into the cell, and uptake by the organelles of the cell. Fats that are insoluble in water are transported in the bloodstream as phospholipids, a combination of phosphate with the fat molecule that renders the fat more soluble. When glycogen is released from the liver or muscle storage sites to be used as a source of energy, it appears as a phosphorylated glucose compound, another manifestation of the essential nature of phosphorus.

Part of essential body compounds. The active form of some vitamins is one containing phosphorus—thiamin pyrophosphate (B_1) is an example. Since all enzymes are proteins and many proteins contain phosphorus, the essentiality of this mineral is obvious. Even more crucial is the role of phosphate as an integral part of the nucleic acids, DNA and RNA, both of which are essential, for cell reproduction through their vital roles in protein synthesis.

Calcification of bones and teeth. The use of the term *calcification* to describe the process in which calcium and phosphorus precipitate from the fluids bathing the bone cell matrix and crystallize as apatite in the organic framework of the bone to give it strength and rigidity has led to the erroneous belief that a lack of calcium is a major cause of failure of the process. Although bones contain half as much phosphorus as calcium, failure of bone calcification is as often the result of unavailability of phosphorus as of calcium. In cases of poor calcification of bone there is an increase in the enzyme phosphatase that facilitates the release of phosphorus from organic tissue compounds into the blood to create the proper calcium to phosphorus ratio for bone growth. The initiation of the calcification process involves the fixation of phosphate to the matrix, indicating a primary role of phosphorus in bone formation. The low phosphorus levels in the body are more likely a reflection of excessive excretion of phosphorus in the urine than of inadequate dietary phosphorus. It is well beyond the scope of this presentation to attempt to enumerate all the biological reactions in which phosphorus plays a key role. Those mentioned merely illustrate the diversity of reactions in which phosphorus participates.

Absorption and metabolism

Since practically all phosphorus must be absorbed as free phosphorus, that present in food as inorganic esters must be hydrolyzed, or split, in the intestinal tract by phosphorus-splitting enzymes, known as phosphorylases. The amount of phosphorus absorbed varies inversely with the amount of calcium, iron, strontium, and other elements that form insoluble complexes excreted in the feces. Fecal phosphorus also includes that which is part of substances secreted into the gastrointestinal tract. Unabsorbed phosphorus amounts to about 30% of dietary phosphorus. The control of the amount in the body is maintained through excretion in the urine rather than by absorption. Urinary phosphorus increases in catabolism of body tissue, representing the release of phosphorus from the tissues. It temporarily decreases after the ingestion of carbohydrates that require phosphorus for metabolism.

In addition to being associated in bone and tooth structure, both calcium and phosphorus metabolism are influenced by the same factors. The parathyroid, which regulates the level of calcium in the blood, affects the level of phosphorus in the blood and its rate of resorption from the kidney. Vitamin D, which facilitates the absorption of calcium from the gastrointestinal tract, also increases the rate of resorption of phosphorus from the kidney. In this way the levels of both calcium and phosphorus needed for calcification of bone are raised simultaneously. Blood levels of phosphorus range from 35 to 45 mg. per 100 ml., of which 3 to 5 mg. is in the form of inorganic phosphorus. Like calcium, phosphorus is constantly being released and rebuilt into bone tissue in the remodeling processes typical of bone. Evidence now indicates that the phosphorus of tooth enamel is exchanged with that in the saliva and the phosphorus in the dentin with that of the blood supply.

Food sources

Foods rich in protein are also rich in phosphorus content. Thus we find meat, fish, poultry, eggs, and cereal products are the primary sources of phosphorus in the average diet.

Whole-grain cereals contain phytic acid, a phosphorus-containing organic acid that is not available to the body. This phytic acid may combine with calcium in an insoluble complex from which neither nutrient can be absorbed. The amount of phosphorus in some representative foods is given in Table 7-3.

*Table 7-3. Phosphorus content of representative foods**

Food	Phosphorus (mg./100 gm.)
Cheddar cheese	478
Peanuts	401
Cod, broiled	274
Beef, lean round	250
Pork, lean	249
Halibut, broiled	248
Bread, whole-wheat	228
Eggs	205
Cottage cheese	152
Peas, fresh	116
Milk, whole	93
Bread, white enriched	90
Lima beans	67
Oatmeal	57
Rice, cooked	28

*Based on Watt, B. K., and Merrill, A. L.: Composition of foods—raw, processed and prepared, U. S. Department of Agriculture Handbook No. 8, Washington, D. C., 1963, U. S. Department of Agriculture.

Requirements

The NRC recommended allowances suggest a phosphorus intake of at least 800 mg., equal to the calcium allowance indicated for the growth period. Diets adequate in protein invariably provide an adequate amount of phosphorus. Experimental diets with a very low P/Ca ratio have been used to produce rickets, but an upset phosphorus to calcium ratio in human diets rarely occurs. About 70% of dietary phosphorus is absorbed.

For infants under 6 months the recommended intake of phosphorus is half that of calcium.

POTASSIUM
Distribution

Potassium is a monovalent cation with chemical properties similar to those of sodium, but physiologically unlike sodium in that potassium is concentrated inside the cell rather than in the extracellular fluid. A sodium to potassium ratio of 1:10 is maintained within the cell, compared to 28:1 in the extracellular fluids. Thus most of the 250 gm. of potassium normally present in the body is within the cells.

The amount of potassium in the blood plasma reflects the nature of cellular metabolism rather than body reserves. Plasma potassium rises when there is a breakdown of body tissue (catabolism) and also in acidosis as an indication that potassium is leaving the cell. It decreases when the rate of protein synthesis or glycogen deposition within the cell increases or in alkalosis, indicating that potassium is entering the cell. If the level of potassium in the blood and hence in the extracellular fluids increases too much, muscular coordination is disturbed, and in severe cases cardiac arrest occurs. This is usually the result of failure of the kidney to excrete potassium, since potassium is excreted primarily through the kidney. The body is less efficient in conserving or resorbing potassium than many other constituents so that there is normally a loss of about 7% of blood potassium in the urine. The presence of chlorine aids in the conservation of potassium.

Functions

Within the cell, potassium acts as a catalyst in many biological reactions, especially those involved in the release of energy and in glycogen and protein synthesis. If the sodium level increases in the intracellular material, it may counteract the catalytic effect of potassium and may interfere with cellular metabolism, especially protein synthesis. Potassium is a major factor in maintaining the osmotic pressure of the cell. Its presence within the cell is important in the maintenance of acid-base balance, although it is not as readily mobilized as sodium as a reserve base to offset excess of acid-forming elements. It also plays a role in the transmission of nerve impulses. Potassium acts along with magnesium as a muscular relaxant in opposition to calcium, which stimulates muscular contraction.

Potassium levels in the body have been found to reflect body composition, the levels increasing with an increase in lean body mass. This relationship has become the basis of a fairly simple and promising method of determining lean body mass, the *whole body counter.* In this method an estimate of the amount of radioactive potassium 40 in the body is made by a special Geiger-counting device. Since potassium 40 represents a constant percentage of the total dietary potassium, it is assumed that the same ratio holds in the body. By determining the amount of radioactive potassium in the body and from this the total amount of potassium, it is possible to estimate the amount of lean body mass. The difference between this value and total body weight provides information on total body fat. A drop in body weight without a concurrent drop in total body potassium indicates a loss of adipose tissue rather than lean body mass.

Deficiency

Potassium-deficiency symptoms are fairly well documented but seldom occur as a result of suboptimal dietary intakes. A deficiency state may occur in infants suffering from diarrhea when the passage of the intestinal contents is so rapid that there is a decreased absorption of dietary potassium and an increased loss of the potassium that is not resorbed from digestive secretions. Vomiting, the use of diuretics, and severe protein-caloric malnutrition may also lead to potassium depletion. Overall muscle weakness, poor intestinal tonus, heart abnormalities, and weakness of respiratory muscles are characteristic. Infants suffering from the protein-deficiency disease, kwashiorkor, respond to treatment only when potassium therapy is given along with an increased protein intake.

Because of the antagonistic relationship between sodium and potassium, an excessive intake of sodium may have the same effect as a suboptimal level of potassium.

A magnesium deficiency also leads to a decreased retention of potassium.

Requirements

The amount of potassium in the American diet has been estimated at 2 to 6 gm. per day or 0.8 to 1.5 gm. per 1000 kcal. Since potassium is distributed in a great many foods, its presence in the diet tends to parallel the caloric value of the diet. Although it has been established that potassium is a dietary essential, there is little information on minimal needs, which are estimated to be between 0.8 and 1.3 gm. There is no evidence that the amount generally found in the diet is suboptimal. The potassium content of some representative foods is shown in Table 7-4. Potassium in food occurs in very soluble form, increasing the possibility that a considerable amount may leach into the cooking water.

Plants are rich in potassium, and it is sometimes necessary to provide salt licks for herbivorous animals, such as cattle and

Table 7-4. Potassium content of some representative foods

Food	mg./100 gm.
Halibut	525
Baked potato	503
Lima beans	422
Pork, cooked	390
Beef, cooked	370
Lamb, cooked	290
Cabbage, raw	233
Asparagus, cooked	183
Waffles	145
Milk, whole	144
Egg, cooked	140
Grapefruit	135
Apples	110
White bread	85
Cheddar cheese	82

sheep, to provide sodium in the diet to prevent a sodium-potassium imbalance.

SULFUR

Sulfur, which represents 0.25% of body weight, is present in every cell of the body. It is concentrated in the cytoplasm. The highest concentration of sulfur is found in the hair, skin, and nails, as evidenced by the characteristic odor of sulfur dioxide given off when these keratin-containing tissues are burned. The sulfur-containing amino acids, cystine and methionine, are in high concentration in these tissues and are characteristic of keratin.

Sulfur in combination with hydrogen (SH) plays an important role in metabolism, since it is readily oxidized—a reaction essential for the formation of a blood clot. It is also able to form high-energy compounds that make it important in the transfer of energy. It is part of at least four vitamins—thiamin, pantothenic acid, biotin, and lipoic acid—which act as coenzymes necessary to activate the action of several enzymes. Compounds containing sulfur act as detoxifying substances by combining with toxic substances to convert them into harmless compounds that are excreted. Sulfur appears necessary for collagen synthesis and the formation of many mucopolysaccharides.

Sulfur is available to the body primarily as the organic sulfur in the amino acids, methionine and cystine. Inorganic sulfur or the sulfur as sulfate can contribute to the pool of sulfur in the body, but its availability depends on the ratio of organic to inorganic sulfur. Any excess of the element is excreted in the urine.

SODIUM

The necessity of salt, a major source of sodium, has been recognized for centuries, and many of the major conquests of the world revolved around a search for a salt supply. Trading in salt has had many social, political, and economic consequences. In spite of a long history, not until 1937 was the role of sodium as a dietary essential established. Salt is practically the only food not prepared in the home, although in many countries the only source of salt is the evaporation of seawater, frequently carried out on a small scale.

Distribution

Sodium is a monovalent cation present in the body primarily in the extracellular fluids—the vascular fluids within the blood vessels, arteries, veins, capillaries, and the intercellular fluids surrounding the cells. About 2 ounces or 50% of the total body sodium is found in these fluids, where it represents an important part of the cell's environment. Under normal conditions as little as 10% of body sodium is present within the cell, although the body has to work constantly to pump sodium out of the cell. The remaining 40% of body sodium is found in the skeleton bound in the surface of bone crystals, where about half of it acts as a reserve of exchangeable sodium available to the extracellular fluids when less dietary sodium is available or when losses from the body are high. In infants the bone cartilage can act as a reservoir of sodium. Except when low intakes occur in conjunction with increased demand, it takes a long period of sodium restriction to use up all the body reserves.

Absorption and metabolism

Normally from 3 to 7 gm. of sodium or 7.5 to 18 gm. salt are ingested daily, although the amount varies greatly with the extent to which table salt (sodium chloride) is added during cooking and at the table. Two teaspoons of table salt will provide 4 gm. of sodium. The body has an ability to handle considerably larger amounts. Although sodium can be toxic if consumed in excessive amounts, levels sufficiently high to become toxic are extremely unpalatable and unlikely to be consumed voluntarily.

A small portion of sodium is absorbed in the stomach, but most of it is absorbed rapidly from the small intestine. The absorption of sodium is an active (energy-requiring) process. Absorbed sodium is carried through the bloodstream to the kidney, where sodium is filtered out and returned to the bloodstream in amounts to maintain the blood levels within the narrow range required by the body. Any excess, which amounts to 90% to 95% of ingested sodium, is excreted in the urine. This regulation of sodium metabolism is controlled by aldosterone, a hormone secreted by the adrenal gland.

When the need for sodium increases, the secretion of the hormone aldosterone increases. This stimulates the absorption of sodium from the gastrointestinal tract and the resorption of sodium by the kidney. Conversely, when sodium intakes are high, the secretion of aldosterone diminishes and less sodium is retained. The level of sodium in the urine reflects dietary intake—being high when intake is high, and low when intake is low. Some sodium is also deposited in bone to become a reservoir available in time of need.

Since there is a limit to the amount of sodium that can be excreted in a certain volume of urine, blood levels and extracellular fluid levels will rise if dietary intake exceeds the kidney's ability to excrete it. When blood sodium levels rise, the thirst receptors in the hypothalamus of the brain react by stimulating the thirst sensation. This leads to greater fluid consumption, which in turn allows the kidney to excrete more urine and more sodium. Sodium blood levels drop, followed by a diminution of thirst.

Sodium is also lost from the body through perspiration. Normally these losses are minimal, but under environmental conditions that lead to excessive perspiration the loss of sodium by this route may be appreciable, one investigator reporting losses of 5 to 6 gm. of sodium chloride per day in the summer in the tropics. If losses through the skin become great, aldosterone secretion again stimulates the kidney to retain more sodium and to help minimize the effects from this sodium loss.

An additional intake of 1 gm. of salt for every liter of fluid lost in excess of 4 liters is recommended to help replace the lost sodium, although the acclimated person may need less and the unacclimated two to three times as much. Excessive vomiting may also result in appreciable loss of sodium.

The loss of body sodium leads to low levels in the extracellular fluids. In an attempt to equalize the osmotic pressure from electrolytes on either side of the cell membrane, potassium and water leave the cell. It is this cellular dehydration and loss of potassium that causes the feeling of fatigue that accompanies sodium depletion.

In contrast to potassium, sodium is an integral part of digestive secretions, such as bile and pancreatic and intestinal juices, which contain approximately 3 gm. per liter. A large amount (20 gm. per day) is secreted into the gastrointestinal tract by this route, but most of this is reabsorbed. Only under abnormal conditions, such as diarrhea, in which the digestive mass passes through the digestive tract very rapidly, is there a major loss of sodium through fecal excretions.

Functions

Sodium plays a vital role in performing the general functions of minerals discussed in Chapter 6.

As a cation in the extracellular fluids it helps maintain osmotic pressure on the outside of the cell membrane to counteract the similar effect of potassium within the cell and to maintain normal water balance. If the sodium concentration within the cell rises when the cell cannot pump it out quickly enough, water will be taken in to dilute the sodium to normal concentrations; the resulting waterlogged cells are described as edematous. If very marked uptake of water occurs, the condition is described as water intoxication.

As a base-forming element, sodium, accounting for 90% of the basic ions in the extracellular fluids, helps to maintain body neutrality by counteracting the acid-forming elements. When an excess of acid-forming elements appears in the body fluids, sodium can be released from the sodium reserves in the bone to offset the acid. One of the major causes of alkalosis is the ingestion of excess sodium-containing antacid preparations.

In the transmission of nerve impulses a change in the permeability of the nerve cell membrane allows sodium to enter and for a temporary period this changes the electrical charge on the membrane. This electrical charge travels down the nerve fiber as a nerve impulse or message. If the balance between sodium outside and inside the cell were not normal, this transmission of nerve impulses could not occur.

Sodium is also essential for the absorption of glucose and in the transport of other nutrients across membranes.

Requirement

The dietary requirement for sodium has not yet been determined, but it is generally observed that the usual intake far exceeds needs. The requirement for sodium is determined by the needs for growth, estimated at 1.8 gm. per kilogram of new tissue, the losses in sweat and other secretions, and the amount of potassium in the diet. The obligatory losses of sodium, which represent the minimum amount that would have to be replaced, have been estimated at 40 to 185 mg. per day. This includes 5 to 35 mg. lost in the urine, 10 to 125 mg. lost in the stools, 25 mg. through nonsweat losses from the skin, and 25 mg. in sweat. The usual intake of 3 to 7 gm. then represents many times the minimum requirement. Since a diet that provides only 100 to 150 mg. would be extremely unpalatable to most people, the likelihood of an insufficient intake is remote. The suggested requirement of 5 gm. represents as much as ten times the amount on which adequate sodium balance can be maintained.

Food sources

Dietary sources of sodium fall into two main categories: that present in food naturally and that added primarily as salt during processing and preparation.

Sodium is present in food in widely varying amounts, more generally being found in foods of animal origin than in those of plant origin. The sodium content of some representative foods is shown in Table 7-5. The amount found in a diet is as much a function of the amount of salt added in processing as of the amount present in the food. For instance, raw potatoes have only 0.001 mg. per 100 gm., but the same weight of potato chips has 0.34 mg. Cured ham has twenty times as much sodium as raw pork.

In some areas the sodium content of the water supply may be sufficiently high to make water a major source of sodium, perhaps exceeding that supplied by food. Many of the ion exchange units used as water softeners also produce water with a high sodium content. There is some evidence associating high sodium levels in the water with the incidence of atherosclerosis.

Sodium restriction

Under certain conditions, such as hypertension and kidney disorders, it has been considered important to restrict dietary

*Table 7-5. Sodium content of representative foods**

Low sodium	mg./100 gm.	Moderate sodium	mg./100 gm.	High sodium	mg./100 gm.
Apples	1	Milk	50	Graham crackers	670
Asparagus, cooked	1	Chicken		Cheddar cheese	700
		Light meat	64		
		Dark meat	86		
Grapefruit	1	Celery	100	Sauerkraut	750
Pineapple	1	Egg	122	Cornflakes	1000
Egg noodles	5	Tomato juice, canned	200	Processed cheese	1100
Sweet potato	10	Cottage cheese	290	Cured ham	1100
Broccoli, frozen	15	Sardines, canned	510	Olives, green	2400
Raisins	25				
Carrots	50				

*Based on Watt, B. K., and Merrill, A. L.: Composition of foods—raw, processed and prepared, U.S. Department of Agriculture Handbook No. 8, Washington, D. C., 1963, U. S. Department of Agriculture.

sodium intake. The degree of restriction varies with the severity of the condition. Mild restriction, with intake limited to 500 to 700 mg., can often be accomplished by limiting the use of salt at the table. For very strict restriction to 200 mg., it is necessary to choose foods naturally low in sodium, to eliminate all foods in which sodium is used in processing, and to use sodium-free salt substitutes and low-salt milk from which much of the sodium has been removed by a process in which there is an exchange of ions. Spices, except celery salt, parsley flakes, and vegetable salts, may be used, since they contain virtually no sodium.

The long-standing use of low-sodium diets to treat toxemia of pregnancy is now being challenged. Clinical studies on humans indicate that high-sodium rather than low-sodium diets are effective in preventing or relieving the symptoms of toxemia—high blood pressure, edema, proteinuria, and blurred vision. Extensive studies in rats have indicated an increased need for sodium during pregnancy, as evidenced by a decreased excretion of the element. The animals were better able to maintain normal bone and muscle sodium levels and gave birth to more and healthier young on elevated rather than reduced sodium intakes. Those on restricted intakes showed signs of sodium deficiency—general lethargy, debility, and a reduced amount of sodium in the blood and tissues.

With the current trend toward the early introduction of solid food into an infant's diet and the extensive use of commercially processed baby foods, to which have been added both salt and monosodium glutamate, there has been some concern that such a diet may predispose to hypertension when fed to young infants whose ability to concentrate urine is much less well developed than it is in an older child. Some manufacturers have responded to this concern by producing low-sodium infant foods.

CHLORINE

Chlorine, present as 0.15% of body weight, is widely distributed throughout the body, but is found in highest concentration as chloride in the cerebrospinal fluid and in the secretions into the gastrointestinal tract. Muscle and nerve tissue are relatively low in chlorine.

As a part of hydrochloric acid, chlorine is necessary to maintain the normal acidity of the stomach contents necessary for the action of gastric enzymes. It is an acid-forming element, and along with the other acid-forming elements phosphorus and sulfur, helps to maintain acid-base balance in the body fluids. Chloride ions are able to pass out of the red blood cell into the blood plasma easily. They contribute to the ability of the blood to carry large amounts of carbon dioxide to the lungs and to release it without changing its own reaction by moving in and out to balance the levels of carbon dioxide as carbonate in either the plasma or erythrocytes. This ready transfer of chloride in and out of the red blood cell is called a chloride shift.

Chlorine in the diet is provided almost exclusively by sodium chloride so that when salt intake is restricted, the chlorine level, first in urine and then in the tissue, drops. Whenever there are excessive losses of sodium, as in diarrhea, sweating, or vomiting, concurrent losses of chloride ions occur.

MAGNESIUM

The presence of magnesium in living organisms has been known since 1859. Although, it had long been used as an anesthetic and anticonvulsant, practically all the information on its biological functions has been gathered since 1950. By 1926 it had been identified as a dietary essential for mice and by 1932 as an essential for rats, but its role in human nutrition was much more difficult to establish. The sizeable reserve of magnesium in bone, some of which can be liberated to help meet the demands of the soft tissues, and the capacity of the kidney to resorb magnesium when needed have increased the difficulty of depleting magnesium levels in human beings sufficiently to study the effects of a deficiency.

In plant life it is an essential part of the green pigment chlorophyll, which differs from the hemoglobin of blood only in that magnesium replaces iron as the mineral in its structure.

Distribution and metabolism

The magnesium content of the infant's body at birth is approximately 0.5 gm. However, since magnesium crosses the placental barrier freely, the amount will vary with the amount available from maternal tissue. In the adult the magnesuim content of the body reaches 21 to 28 gm., of which 50% to 60% is concentrated in bone, where it represents 0.5% to 0.7% of the bone ash. About one third of the magnesium is closely bound with phosphate, and the remainder is absorbed on the bone surface, from which it can be mobilized to maintain normal blood and tissue levels.

In the soft tissues, magnesium is concentrated within the cell, and in the blood it occurs primarily in the red blood cells rather than in the serum. Serum levels are maintained from 1 to 3 mg. per 100 ml. In a deficiency the level in the red blood cells drops; in an excess the serum level rises.

Magnesium is absorbed primarily in the small intestine. Forty-three percent of an average intake is absorbed. When intakes are low, as much as 75% will be absorbed, and when intakes are high, the rate of absorption falls to 25%. The amount absorbed decreases as the amount of fat in the feces (steatorrhea) increases and as the dietary intake of calcium, protein, and vitamin D increases. Magnesium excretion is regulated through the kidney by the hormone aldosterone secreted by the adrenal gland. Urinary losses increase with the use of diuretics and with the consumption of alcohol.

Little endogenous magnesium appears in the feces. The amount lost in perspiration amounts to only 15 mg. per day. Since the gastric juice is relatively high in magnesium, vomiting may lead to large losses.

Functions

Within the cell, magnesium plays a very important role as catalyst to several hundred biological reactions, a major portion of which take place in the mitochondrion. It activates the production of ATP and all changes of ATP to ADP. This change is necessary in all reactions involving the expenditure or release of energy, such as synthesis of body compounds, absorption and transportation of nutrients, and any physical activity. The importance of magnesium in cellular metabolism is evidenced by the fact that the level of intracellular magnesium in metabolically active muscle tissue and liver is seven times that in the blood. Magnesium is crucial in cellular respiration, although in some reactions it may be replaced by other divalent elements such as manganese. Magnesium also influences protein synthesis by affecting the arrangement of the protein-synthesizing organelles of the cell, the ribosomes, and by facilitating the attachment of RNA to the ribosome. It is also necessary for the activation of amino acids so that they can be incorporated into protein molecules and for the synthesis, degradation, and stability of the genetic material DNA.

Magnesium is one of the minerals involved in providing the proper environment in the extracellular fluid of nerve cells to promote the conduction of nerve impulses and to allow normal muscular contraction. In this situation, magnesium and calcium play antagonistic roles, calcium acting as a stimulator and magnesium as a relaxor substance. The relaxing effect of magnesium is evident from the fact that with increasing levels of the element in the blood, there is an increasing anesthetic effect. At extremely high serum levels, coma and eventually heart failure will result. These levels may be reached in kidney failure in which the excretion of magnesium is depressed. On the other hand, low serum magnesium levels are associated with irritability, nervousness, and convulsions as the result of increased transmission of nerve impulses and increased muscular contraction. The competitive nature of the calcium-magnesium interrelationship is further evident during absorption and excretion. When a large amount of one is being absorbed or excreted, there is usually a reduction in the amount of the other.

Adequate magnesium may increase the stability of calcium in tooth enamel. It also influences the secretion of thyroxin and the maintenance of normal basal metabolic rate and facilitates adaptation to cold.

Deficiency

A recognized form of magnesium deficiency is a low magnesium tetany similar to that produced when the blood calcium level drops. The body's control over the contractions and relaxations of muscles is lost. The individual suffers from an uncontrolled neuromuscular activity diagnosed early as tremors but becoming increasingly involved until convulsive seizures occur in the more severe deprivation. These symptoms most often arise when a low dietary intake is superimposed on conditions that reduce the absorption and increase the excretion of magnesium. Alcohol increases the rate of magnesium excretion and may partially explain the loss of neuromuscular control diagnosed as magnesium tetany in alcoholics. Others who experience magnesium deficiency symptoms are infants suffering from kwashiorkor, persons maintained for long periods on magnesium-free fluids, as may occur postoperatively, or persons suffering prolonged losses because of nausea or diarrhea. High intakes of calcium aggravate the symptoms of low magnesium levels by favoring its excretion.

In the absence of adequate magnesium

the cardiovascular system and the renal system are also affected, with symptoms such as vasodilation and skin changes being frequent. Intramuscular injections of magnesium sulfate relieve these symptoms.

Assessment of reserves

Serum levels of magnesium do not provide a sensitive indication of the level in cells, since about 35% of the blood magnesium is bound to a protein and is not measured with current analytical techniques. Tissues may be depleted of magnesium while serum levels remain normal.

Bone formed when there is adequate magnesium available contains about 16% of its magnesium as a reserve that can be released to maintain blood levels when dietary magnesium drops. However, bone formed when little magnesium is available will have little or no magnesium and will tend to take up magnesium when the mineral becomes available from the diet, thus keeping blood levels low for a longer time.

The high levels of magnesium found in the red blood cells of mentally retarded children suggest that their ability to regulate magnesium metabolism is impaired.

Requirements

The Food and Nutrition Board of the National Research Council recommends an intake of 300 mg. per day for women and 350 mg. for men. These figures were arrived at after considering data from balance studies. They estimate that a typical American diet provides 120 mg. per 1000 kcal.—a level that will barely provide the recommended intake. When intakes were increased to 10 mg. per kilogram in an experimental situation, there was a period of large retention of magnesium, which later dropped, apparently after body stores were replenished.

The absence of magnesium deficiency symptoms in the American population, which apparently consumes too little to meet its needs, may be explained by the

Table 7-6. Recommended dietary
allowances for magnesium

Age	Magnesium (mg.)
1 to 10 years	70-250
10 to 12 years	250-300
12 to 19 years	350-400
Adult men	350
Adult women	300
Pregnancy	450
Lactation	450

fact that it experiences a very slight deficit that becomes significant only when a condition of stress is superimposed. Such situations may be the increased excretion that occurs with alcohol consumption, the impaired absorption accompanying the increased use of diuretics, or the decreased intake of magnesium of patients on fluid feedings.

Recommended allowances are presented in Table 7-6.

Food sources

Only recently have analytical methods provided satisfactory analyses of the magnesium content of foods. Table 7-7 classifies some common foods on the basis of their magnesium content. Precise figures are not given, since in several instances only single determinations have been made. The high chlorophyll content of green leafy vegetables accounts for their value in providing 30% of dietary magnesium. Absorption is reduced in diets high in phytic acid, normally found in the outer husks of cereal grains such as rice or oats. The magnesium in foods high in oxalic acid may be found in an insoluble complex.

Although milk is a relatively poor source of magnesium, it appears adequate to meet the needs of either breast- or bottle-fed infants.

Oriental diets with appreciable amounts of magnesium from rice, soybeans, and fish provide sufficient amounts to maintain magnesium balance. This observation is interesting in the light of findings that show that those persons with high magnesium intakes are less susceptible to cardiovascular disease than those on low intakes. Orientals are less susceptible than Westerners to cardiovascular disease and the adverse effects of cholesterogenic diets.

The increase in the undesirable calcification of soft tissues in magnesium deficiency may reflect the increase in calcium absorption that occurs when less magnesium competes with calcium for the com-

Table 7-7. Classification of some representative foods as sources of magnesium

Rich sources (> 100 mg.%)	Good sources (50-100 mg.%)	Fair sources (25-50 mg.%)	Poor sources (< 25 mg.%)
Cocoa	Clams	Oysters	Lobster
Nuts	Cornmeal	Crab	Pork
Soybeans	Spinach	Fresh peas	Lamb
Whole grains		Liver	Milk
			Eggs
			Veal
			Cod
			Most fruits and vegetables
			Fowl

mon carrier that transports them across the intestinal wall. This is often acompanied by an increase in the amount of calcium mobilized from the bone, which also increases the calcium available for deposi-

tion in soft tissues. High-calcium and low-magnesium diets also lead to an increase in magnesium excretion, further aggravating the antagonistic effects of these two elements.

SELECTED REFERENCES

Calcium

American Institute of Nutrition: Symposium on effects of high calcium intakes, Fed. Proc. **18:** 1075, 1959.

Calcium requirements, Report of Joint FAO/WHO Expert Committee, WHO Techn. Rep. Ser. No. 230, 1962.

Copp, D. H.: Endocrine control of calcium metabolism, Physiol. Rev. **32:**61, 1970.

Council on Foods and Nutrition: Symposium on human calcium requirements, J.A.M.A. **185:**588, 1963.

DeLuca, H. F.: Recent advances in the metabolism and function of vitamin D, Fed. Proc. **28:**1678, 1969.

Hegsted, D. M.: Nutrition, bone, and calcified tissue, J. Amer. Diet. Ass. **50:**105, 1967.

Hegsted, D. M.: Present knowledge of calcium, phosphorus, and magnesium, Nutr. Rev. **26:**65, 1968.

Leitch, I., and Aitken, F. C.: An estimation of calcium requirement; a re-examination, Nutr. Abst. Rev. **29:**394, 1959.

Lutwak, L.: Tracer studies in intestinal calcium absorption in man, Amer. J. Clin. Nutr. **22:**771, 1969.

Lutwak, L., and Whedon, G. D.: Osteoporosis—a mineral deficiency disease? J. Amer. Diet. Ass. **44:**173, 1964.

Rassmussen, H., and Pecht, M. M.: Calcitonin, **223:**4, 1970.

Roy, C. C., and O'Brien, D.: Calcium and phos-phorus: current concepts of metabolism, Clin. Pediat. **6:**19, 1967.

Potassium

Darrow, D. C.: Physiological basis of potassium therapy, J.A.M.A. **162:**1310, 1956.

Sodium

Bloch, M. R.: Social influence of salt, Sci. Amer. **209:**88, July, 1963.

Earley, L. E., and Daugharty, T. M.: Sodium metabolism, New Eng. J. Med. **281:**72, 1969.

Pike, R. L.: Sodium intake during pregnancy, J. Amer. Diet. Ass. **44:**176, 1964.

Magnesium

Caddell, J. L.: Magnesium deficiency in extremis, Nutr. Today **2**(3):14, 1967.

Hathaway, M. L.: Magnesium in human nutrition, Home Economics Research Report No. 19, Agricultural Research Service, Washington, D. C., 1962, U. S. Department of Agriculture.

Krehl, W. A.: Mg, Nutr. Today **2**(3):16, 1967.

Seelig, M. S.: The requirement of magnesium by the normal adult, Amer. J. Clin. Nutr. **14:**342, 1964.

Shils, M.: Experimental human magnesium depletion. I. Clinical observations and blood chemistry alterations, Amer. J. Clin. Nutr. **15:**133, 1964.

Wacker, E. C., and Parasie, A. F.: Magnesium metabolism, New Eng. J. Med. **278:**658, 712, 772, 1968.

IRON

The element iron was first recognized as a constituent of body tissue in 1713. Since that time it has been determined that iron represents about 0.004% of the body weight—an amount that varies from 3 to 5 gm., depending on age, sex, size, nutritional status, general health, and size of iron stores. Virtually all iron exists in combination with protein, and in almost all cases these essential compounds function because of the ability of iron to accept and release oxygen and carbon dioxide readily. Such reactions are essential to life.

Distribution

Iron is concentrated in the blood, but some is present in every living cell. The distribution of iron in various body tissues is shown in Table 8-1. About 70% of iron in the body is considered functional iron. The majority of this is present in the hemoglobin molecule of the blood. A small portion exists as iron in myoglobin in muscle, another iron complex that differs from hemoglobin only in the nature of the protein. The rest of the functional iron exists in the tissue enzymes, notably cytochrome oxidase and catalase, which are present in every living cell and are essential for cellular respiration. Functional iron amounts to about 35 mg. per kilogram of body weight. The remaining 30% of body iron is designated as storage, or nonessential, iron. It is stored in the liver, the spleen, and the bone marrow and amounts to 0.2 to 1.5 gm., with the lower values found characteristically in women. Storage iron is present in the liver as a soluble iron complex, ferritin, with a 20% iron content or as hemosiderin, an insoluble iron-protein complex, containing 35% iron.

In addition to the hemoglobin iron, the blood contains about 4 mg. of iron that is being transported from the site of absorption or the liver to the cells, bound to the protein transferrin. This transport iron is turned over so rapidly that as much as 35 to 40 mg. is exchanged each day.

Since the body has no mechanism for excreting iron, the level of both functional and storage iron is regulated through absorption. The body is extremely efficient in conserving iron and will avidly retain or salvage any iron that results from the catabolism, or breakdown, of iron-containing substances. Iron is absorbed in response to a need.

Functions
Carrier of oxygen and carbon dioxide

As a constituent of both hemoglobin and myoglobin, in which it represents 3.4% of the molecule, iron is responsible for the ability of these substances to act as a carrier for oxygen to make it available as needed for cellular respiration. Iron is also responsible for the capacity of these substances to carry carbon dioxide away from the cells to the lungs, where it is released as more oxygen is picked up.

Blood formation

Hemoglobin is a major component of the red blood cells, or erythrocytes. These cells are formed in the bone marrow in response

Table 8-1. Distribution of iron throughout the body

	Percent	Approximate amount (gm.)
Hemoglobin	60-75	2.0-3.0
Myoglobin	3	0.1
Storage iron (liver, spleen, and bone marrow)	20	0.2-1.5
Tissue iron	5-15	0.300
Transport iron		0.004

to the presence of the hormone erythro-poietin, produced in the kidney. The level of erythropoietin increases as the oxygen-carrying capacity of the blood decreases, with a decrease in the number of red blood cells. Erythrocytes begin as nucleated immature cells, known as erythroblasts. As these cells mature in the bone marrow, heme, an iron-containing compound, is synthesized in the presence of vitamin B_6, or pyridoxine, from the amino acid glycine and iron. The protein heme unites with another protein, globin, synthesized simultaneously from other amino acids. These hemoglobin-containing immature red blood cells, known as reticulocytes, are released into the bloodstream, where they lose their nuclei to become mature nonnucleated red blood cells capable of functioning as carriers of carbon dioxide and oxygen. Without a nucleus the red blood cells cannot synthesize the enzymes essential for their life. As a result, they live only as long as the enzymes present at maturity remain functional—usually about four months. As the red blood cells die, they are removed from the bloodstream by the cells of the reticuloendothelial system—the liver, bone marrow, and spleen.

In the spleen the iron and the amino acids of the hemoglobin molecule are removed. The iron is returned to the iron stores or to the bone marrow, where it is incorporated into new hemoglobin molecules. The amino acids are returned to the amino acid pool in the blood, making them available for the synthesis of new protein, or for deamination before being used as a source of energy. The remaining portion of the erythrocytes is excreted in the bile. By this mechanism, iron is carefully conserved and reused. The rate of destruction of red blood cells is accelerated in dietary deficiencies of ascorbic acid, vitamin E, and vitamin B_{12} (cobalamin).

Since the blood of the adult male contains 15 gm. of hemoglobin per 100 ml. (and that of the female 13.6 gm.), the total hemoglobin content of the 5 liters, or 5000 ml., of blood found in the adult male contains 750 gm. of hemoglobin. This amount of hemoglobin in turn contains 2500 mg. of iron. Since erythrocytes live only 120 days on the average, 1/120 of these cells are replaced every day. This means that 1/120 of the total iron, or approximately 20 mg., is released each day from old cells and is incorporated into the hemoglobin in the cells that replace them. As will be discussed later, it would be impossible to provide this amount of iron from dietary sources so that the process of conserving iron is essential to the survival of the organism.

A small amount of the total body iron is incorporated into tissue enzymes. The mechanism for this is not as well established as is that for hemoglobin synthesis. There is some evidence that in a dietary deficiency the level of iron-containing tissue enzymes may drop before the hemoglobin level of the blood drops.

Need for iron

Replacement of losses of body iron. Although iron is avidly conserved once it has been absorbed and there is no mechanism for excreting iron, there is some loss each day, which must be replaced. Since iron is present in every cell of the body, any loss of cells will represent a loss of iron. Thus the desquamation, or sloughing, of surface cells, the loss of cells lining the gastrointestinal tract, and the loss of hair or nails all contribute to the loss of body iron. A small number of red blood cells containing less than 0.1 mg. of iron appear in the urine. Perspiration is also believed to contain some iron. Daily fecal losses are estimated at up to 0.5 mg. per day, and those in the urine, perspiration, and desquamated cells vary from 0.2 to 0.5 mg. These small losses of 0.7 to 1 mg. per day are the only ones that the adult male must replace. Women, however, must in addition replace the iron lost in menstruation. Although this amount varies greatly among women, it is fairly consistent from month to month in the same woman, amounting to 16 to 32 mg. per month, or 0.5 to 1 mg. per day calculated

over the month. Ninety-five percent of women have a menstrual loss of less than 1.4 mg. per day. When these needs are added to those of the adult male, it becomes apparent that women must absorb from 1.2 to 2 mg. of iron daily to replace their losses (almost twice that for men).

Growth. Need for iron during growth is the result of an increase in blood volume with a concurrent increase in hemoglobin and in tissue mass, calling for more iron-containing enzymes. The increase in body iron from 0.5 gm. at birth to 5 gm. in the adult represents an increase of 4.5 gm. during the twenty-year growth period. Assuming a uniform rate of growth, this would amount to 225 mg. per year, or 0.6 mg. per day. This is in line with observations that infants retain from 0.2 to 1 mg. per day and adolescents, about 0.5 mg. Others have estimated growth needs at 60 mg. per kilogram increase in body weight.

It is recognized that the physiological iron needs for growth, menstrual losses, and other losses are great. Table 8-2 summarizes our knowledge about iron needs.

Blood donation. The gift of 1 pint of blood represents a loss of 250 mg. of iron that must be replaced before hemoglobin levels will return to normal. The blood volume and the cell number will return to normal quickly, but the return of hemoglobin levels can occur only at the

Table 8-2. Summary of iron requirements (mg./day)

Age group	Losses in feces	Losses in urine, perspiration, and desquamation	Needs for menstruation	Needs for growth	Needs for pregnancy	Total needs
Adult men	0.5	0.2-0.5				0.7-1.0
Adult women	0.5	0.2-0.5	0.5-1.0			1.2-2.0
Pregnant women	0.5	0.2-0.5			1.0-2.0	1.7-3.0
Children	0.5	0.2-0.5		0.6		1.3-1.6
Adolescent girls	0.5	0.2-0.5	0.5-1.0	0.6		1.8-2.6

expense of storage iron. To replace the amount of iron lost would require the absorption of an additional 0.7 mg. iron per day.

Absorption

Mechanism. Iron occurs in food, primarily in the oxidized form, ferric iron (Fe^{+++}), although some ferrous iron (Fe^{++}) has been found. Both occur attached to organic compounds, from which they must be released before being absorbed. The body can utilize either form, but evidence indicates that naturally occurring ferrous iron is used more efficiently than is ferric iron and that most iron is reduced to ferrous iron before being absorbed. The absorption of iron occurs in regulated amounts in the upper part of the small intestine, usually in the duodenum. Some is taken up in the stomach. The rapid rate of absorption has been indicated by studies with radioactive iron, which showed that significant amounts were absorbed within 4 hours after ingestion and appeared in the erythroblasts within 24 hours. From 2% to 10% of the iron content of food is absorbed. The many factors that influence this will be discussed later.

Since the body has no mechanism for excreting iron, the iron content of the body is regulated through a controlled absorption. The exact nature of the mechanism is not fully clear, but it now appears that dietary iron from the gastrointestinal tract passes into the epithelial or mucosal cells lining this area attached to a carrier substance, such as the carbohydrates fructose and sorbitol or some amino acids. These substances are usually called chelating agents, and the combination with iron, iron chelates. Within the epithelial cell the iron may remain attached to the carrier substance or may be transferred to a larger molecule, apoferritin, as long as there is free apoferritin present within the epithelial cells. The combination of iron and apoferritin is known as ferritin, the form

in which much iron is temporarily stored in the epithelial cells. The rate at which iron is released from the epithelial cell to the general circulation depends on the amount of a protein-carrier substance transferrin (beta-globulin), in the blood. This substance, capable of binding 2 atoms of iron per molecule, is able to carry iron to the tissues, bone marrow, and storage sites. When transferrin is saturated up to about one third of its total iron-binding capacity (TIBC), no more iron is absorbed from the mucosal cells except under conditions of excessive intakes. However, whenever there is more unbound transferrin, the iron in the epithelial cell recombines with a carbohydrate or amino acid carrier to again form an iron chelate. This iron-containing complex passes from the epithelial cell into the blood plasma, where it releases its iron to transferrin. The uptake of iron from the intestinal tract apparently depends on the presence of a suitable carrier, and its release into the bloodstream is believed to be regulated by the amount of transferrin present. The total transferrin in the blood is usually capable of transporting 4 mg. at once. If the iron is needed, it passes quickly into the bloodstream. If not needed, it remains in the epithelial cells and will be lost from the body through fecal excretion when these cells die and slough from the wall of the intestinal tract, as they do at a rate of 50 to 80 gm. per day, with complete renewal of the lining of the gastrointestinal tract occurring in less than two days.

Factors affecting absorption

Body's need for iron. The need for iron is reflected in the unbound transferrin level of the blood. When this rises, indicating that iron has been removed from the blood to the tissues or storage sites, more iron is absorbed to maintain a constant level in the blood. When the transferrin is saturated with iron, representing a decreased demand for iron on the part of the body cells, less is absorbed. Thus the iron absorption mechanism responds to the body's need for iron. A person with normal hemoglobin levels absorbs from 2% to 10% of dietary iron. A person with low hemoglobin levels and probably high demands for iron may absorb as much as 60% of dietary iron, although some reports set the figure as low as 10%. One study using the whole body counter for radioactive iron showed that iron-deficient subjects absorbed 29% of ingested iron, whereas normal subjects absorbed 10%. Increased iron absorption is noted in the latter half of pregnancy, when the demands of the fetus on maternal iron are great. Children may also absorb iron at a rate up to twice that of adults.

Form of iron. Although the body can absorb both the reduced ferrous (Fe^{++}) and the oxidized ferric (Fe^{+++}) iron, absorption is greater when iron is available in the reduced ferrous form. The ferric iron that predominates in food is usually reduced to the ferrous form prior to absorption, although during absorption it may be oxidized and reduced several times. The presence of any reducing substance, such as acid, is believed to enhance iron absorption. The hydrochloric acid secreted in the stomach keeps iron in the more readily available reduced form. Decreased iron utilization is sometimes noted in persons with a decreased secretion of hydrochloric acid in the stomach, known as achlorhydria. This is often associated with increasing age or with the consumption of alkaline powders in large amounts, as by ulcer patients. The addition of hydrochloric acid to the diets of people suffering from achlorhydria had no beneficial effect on iron absorption, suggesting that the decreased hydrochloric acid secretion may well be a result of and not a cause of poor iron absorption. Organic acids in food, such as ascorbic acid (vitamin C) found in citrus fruits, enhance iron absorption by helping reduce ferric to ferrous iron. It may play

an important role in diets of older people, in whom it may compensate for the reduced hydrochloric acid level. Since studies have shown that an increase in dietary vitamin C without an increase in iron is beneficial in iron-deficiency conditions, vitamin C is often included with iron supplements.

Bulk in diet. High bulk in the diet depresses the utilization of iron, which may account for the reports of poor absorption often noted from green leafy vegetables such as spinach. On the basis of this it has been suggested that iron supplements should be taken before meals to minimize the interference that the bulk of the diet may exert on iron absorption.

Size of dose. The percentage of iron absorbed varies inversely with the size of the dose. An intake of iron at a level of 0.25 mg. per kilogram of body weight resulted in 32% utilization, whereas at 4 mg. per kilogram only 4.1% was utilized. The administration of supplemental iron in smaller divided doses three or four times a day at a level commensurate with the body's ability to absorb it results in much better utilization than does a single large dose.

Other factors. Phytic acid is an organic acid found in some whole-grain cereal products, such as oatmeal. It combines with iron to form an insoluble iron complex that the body cannot utilize. The presence of phytic acid is not a cause for concern in a normal mixed diet, but should oatmeal or other foods high in phytic acid become staple items in the diet, then the adverse effects of phytic acid on iron absorption may become significant. Excess phosphorus may also have an inhibitory effect on iron absorption.

Steatorrhea, an abnormal condition in which higher than normal amounts of fat appear in the feces, is associated with a decreased rate of iron absorption.

The altitude at which a person lives also influences the extent of iron absorption. An increase occurs at high altitudes, whereas less is absorbed at lower altitudes.

Transportation and metabolism

Once iron has been absorbed from the epithelial cells into the blood, it is carried throughout the body bound to the protein carrier transferrin. From the blood it may be removed by several pathways. In response to the demands of all body cells it will be released for use in the synthesis of respiratory enzymes and other vital cellular constituents that require iron. Much of the iron in transit in the blood plasma, which may come either from dietary sources, from the breakdown of body cells, and/or from the storage depots, will be removed by the bone marrow to be used in the manufacture of hemoglobin for red blood cells. About 20 mg. of iron is used in the 7 to 8 gm. of hemoglobin liberated daily from the bone marrow in the newly formed red blood cells. Iron in excess of immediate needs of cells and bone marrow will be deposited in the iron storage depots of the body. Of approximately 1000 mg. (1 gm.) of iron stored in the body at any one time, 30% is in the liver, 30% in bone marrow, and the rest in the spleen and muscles.

On the other hand, if the dietary iron absorbed from the intestinal tract coupled with that obtained from the breakdown of red blood cells is not adequate to meet the needs of the bone marrow for hemoglobin synthesis and of other body cells for respiratory enzymes or cell growth, iron will be mobilized from the reserves in the liver, will be bound to transferrin in the blood, and will be recirculated throughout the body. If necessary, up to 50 mg. per day can be mobilized from storage iron. Only when the body's reserves of iron have been depleted will there be any evidence of iron deficiency symptoms. In infants the liver stores are adequate to last three to six months. A reserve of 1000 mg. in the adult lasts a male 1000 days and a woman over

500 days. The absorption and metabolism of iron are summarized diagrammatically in Fig. 8-1.

Recommended dietary allowances

Adults. The National Research Council recommended allowances for iron for adults are based on the assumption that an adult male must obtain approximately 0.7 to 1 mg. of iron a day to replace body losses and the adult female, 1.2 to 2 mg. per day. Since the average rate of iron absorption is 2% to 10% of ingested iron, it has been recommended that men obtain 10 mg. and women 18 mg. from dietary sources. For women whose needs range from 1.2 to 2 mg. per day, this represents a narrow margin of safety and may actually fail to meet the needs of some women.

Pregnancy. During pregnancy the recommended intake remains unchanged because the elimination of menstrual losses counterbalances the demands of the fetus, which amount to approximately 300 mg. for a full-term infant. Iron is stored rapidly in fetal tissue during the latter half of pregnancy, when the fetus is parasitic on the mother for iron. Iron will be transferred to fetal blood in an irreversible fashion even if the mother's hemoglobin level drops. The apparent drop in hemoglobin levels of the mother during pregnancy often reflects an increase in blood volume rather than an absolute drop in the amount of hemoglobin. Twins who must share a maternal iron supply and premature infants who have been deprived of part of the period in utero of maximum transfer of iron to the fetus are usually born with hemoglobin levels below the normally high infant levels of 18 to 22 gm. per 100 ml. of blood. Since their reserve of iron is usually lower also, it may be necessary to supplement their diets with iron at an earlier age than for a full-term infant.

Lactation. Milk contains relatively little iron; thus the demands for iron during lactation are not increased above needs

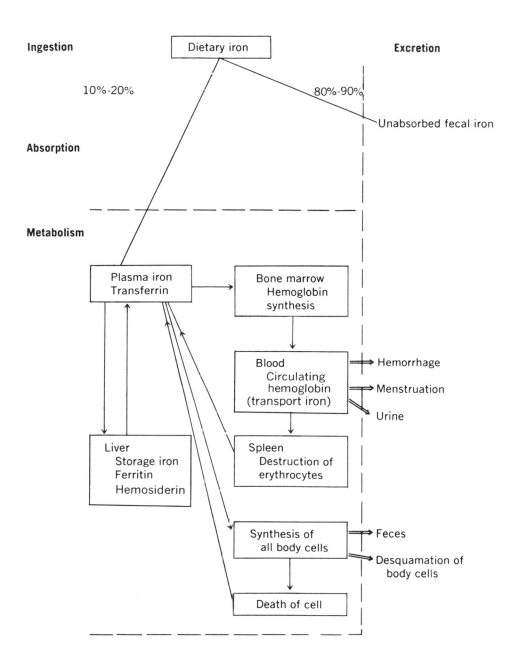

Fig. 8-1. Schematic representation of absorption and metabolism of iron.

for pregnancy. Human milk contains about 50% more iron than cow's milk. The addition of iron to the maternal diet has been ineffective in raising the amount transferred during lactation.

Infants and children. The reserve of iron in the liver of a full-term infant is sufficient to last from three to six months, during which time the infant doubles its birth weight. Thus the National Research Council sees no need to recommend a dietary source of iron other than milk until at least 3 months of age. The very high hemoglobin values in newborn infants drop rapidly to 12 gm. at 4 to 6 months of age and are maintained close to this level throughout childhood before rising in late adolescence to adult levels.

No advantage apparently results from maintaining the high birth levels. In fact, attempts to supplement the infant diet to prevent this drop have been unsuccessful, since little iron is absorbed in early infancy unless there is a physiological need for it. The current trend of adding iron to prepared infant formula is of limited usefulness until the infant has a need for a dietary source at about 3 months of age.

For infants over 3 months of age, dietary iron should be provided in adequate amounts to take care of the synthesis of hemoglobin required by the increasing blood volume and the demands of newly formed cells for iron. Needs of infants for dietary iron are greater per unit of body weight than adult needs and remain relatively high during childhood. Recommended iron intakes then increase in proportion to the increase in body size up to physical maturity, after which iron is needed only for replacement of iron lost from the body.

Evaluation of iron deficiency

Measurement of hemoglobin content of the blood has been the traditional method of assessing the adequacy of dietary iron. Its use has several limitations. First, little

agreement exists among hematologists regarding what level of hemoglobin is characteristic of iron deficiency. Second, hemoglobin levels fluctuate over the 24-hour period, and a single determination may give erroneous information. Third, hemoglobin levels drop only after iron stores have been depleted so that low hemoglobin values represent an advanced stage of iron deficiency. Last, anemia may be due to a deficiency of other nutrients.

Iron stores can be determined by an analysis of a bone marrow aspirate usually obtained from the sternum. This is a rather delicate procedure that does not lend itself to screening of a population. Perhaps the most sensitive method of identifying iron deficiency is to determine the percent saturation of transferrin in the blood. Saturation of less than 15% is indicative of iron deficiency.

Recently interest has centered on the possibility of determining the level of iron-containing enzymes as an indicator of iron adequacy. There is some evidence that the level of cytochrome C is reduced early in an iron deficiency and that the lack of this enzyme in the gastric mucosa may be a major factor responsible for a decreased absorption of iron.

Food sources

A diet adequate in most other nutrients will provide only 6 mg. of iron per 1000 kcal. Because of this it is difficult to obtain the recommended 18 mg. of iron for the adult woman, especially one whose caloric intake is below 3000 kcal.

The iron content of some representative foods in the American diet is given in Fig. 8-2. Liver is the only very rich source of iron, and as noted from Table 8-3 a sizeable difference exists, depending on the type of liver used. In any species the amount found in the liver will reflect the recent dietary intake of iron by the animal.

Since nutritionists have been singularly unsuccessful in increasing the popularity

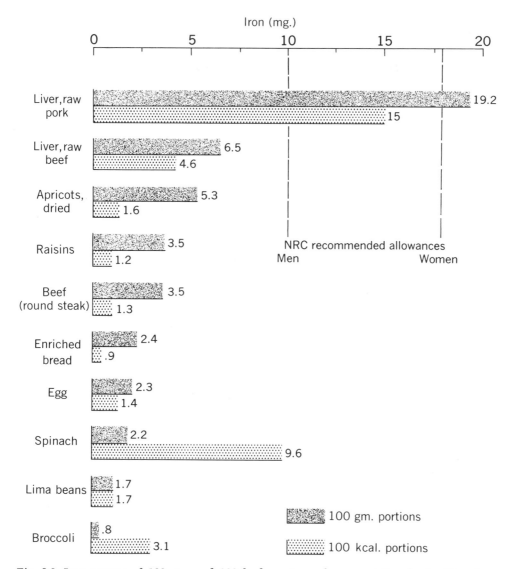

Fig. 8-2. Iron content of 100 gm. and 100 kcal. portions of representative foods. (Based on Watt, B. K., and Merrill, A. L.: Composition of foods—raw, processed and prepared, U. S. Department of Agriculture Handbook No. 8, Washington, D. C., 1963, U. S. Department of Agriculture.)

of liver in the American diet, most people depend on other sources. As there are virtually no other very rich sources, a variety of moderately good sources must be combined to meet needs.

From Fig. 8-3, showing the contribution of various food groups to the iron in the nation's food supply, it is clear that no one group is responsible for a large share of the iron in the diet, but that the meat, cereal, and fruit and vegetable groups make comparable contributions.

Because of wide differences in the degree to which iron from various sources is absorbed, knowledge of the iron content of foods does not always give a true picture of its availability. Difficulties inherent in the determination of the utilization of iron make it difficult to get agreement in data on iron absorption even with the use of radioactive isotopes of iron and even when balance studies are done with meticulous care. In all cases, absorption by iron-deficient subjects averaged 20%, whereas that from subjects with normal hemoglobin

Table 8-3. Iron content of different types of cooked liver°

Liver	mg./100 gm.
Chicken	8.5
Beef	8.8
Calf	14.2
Lamb	17.9
Pork	29.1

*From Watt, B. K., and Merrill, A. L.: Composition of foods—raw, processed and prepared, U. S. Department of Agriculture Handbook No. 8, Washington, D. C., 1963, U. S. Department of Agriculture.

levels averaged 2% to 10%, but a wide range of values is reported for each food tested.

The iron found in meat reflects the iron in both blood and muscle hemoglobin and is well absorbed. In eggs the iron is concentrated almost entirely in the yolk, but only about 4% is absorbed. The iron in chicken is well absorbed, with values up to 30% reported.

Fruits and vegetables are fairly good sources of iron, but often the bulk of the cellulose they also contain results in relatively poor utilization. The iron content of vegetables is influenced by soil and climatic conditions so that there is a wide range of values reported for the same product. Vegetables provide about three times as much iron in the American diet as fruits. Fruits and juices are rated as poor iron sources, potatoes and green stalks and leaves as good sources, and leguminous plants as excellent sources. Studies to determine the utilization of iron from various vegetable sources have not given

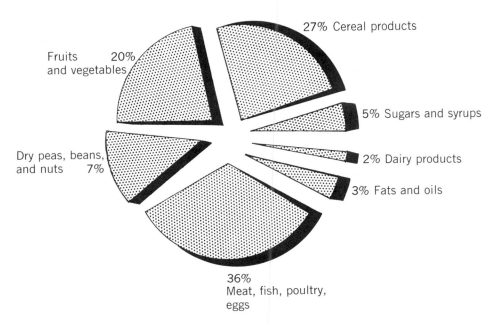

Fig. 8-3. Relative contribution of various food groups to total iron intake in American food supply. (Based on Contribution of major food groups to nutrition supplies available for civilian consumption, National Food Situation No. 130, 1969.)

consistent results. The pulp of fruits such as tomatoes and oranges contains twice as much iron as the juice. Occasionally canned fruits and vegetables or acid foods cooked in an iron container will pick up additional iron, which is equally as available as naturally occurring iron. Legumes such as peas and beans are relatively good sources, especially when the dry mature seed, which has had a prolonged growing period during which to accumulate iron, is used.

Raisins and other dried fruits are often recommended for their iron content. They will have no more iron than the original fruit from which they were derived. It should be remembered that the amount of dried fruit needed to make a significant contribution of iron also makes a significant contribution of calories. For instance, one-fourth cup of raisins, which provides 1.4 mg. of iron, also provides 115 calories.

About 28% of the dietary iron is available as the result of the fortification of foods with iron. Although only thirty states have laws requiring the enrichment of flour, about 90% of the flour and bread sold in the United States has been enriched with iron salts at a level that makes it comparable in iron content to the unrefined cereal. Evidence on the effectiveness of absorption of these added salts is fragmentary, but there is increasing evidence that some of the forms used may be poorly utilized and that the enrichment of dietary staples with iron will be of questionable value in preventing iron deficiency. This question is being actively investigated at the present time. The amount of iron added to enriched flour varies greatly from one country to another, ranging from 3 mg. per pound in England, to 6 mg. in Chile, to 12 to 16 mg. in Canada and Denmark. The Food and Drug Administration (FDA) proposed in 1970 that the amount of iron added to enrich flour be increased from 13 mg. to 50 to 60 mg. per pound and that in bread and rolls from 11 mg. to 32 to 38 mg. per pound.

Cereals, either enriched or whole grain, provide small amounts of iron per unit of weight, but because of the extent to which they may be consumed by certain groups, such as adolescent boys and families on restricted food budgets, they often make a significant contribution to the day's iron intake. Enriched bread, macaroni, and corn grits, for which enrichment standards have been set to provide a maximum as well as a minimum amount that can be added, contain slightly less iron than the whole-grain cereal from which they were derived. It is estimated that the use of enriched bread and cereals in place of refined cereals has increased the iron content of the diet by 14%. For other cereal products, however, iron can be added at any level within safe limits as long as the amount is declared on the label. Processors of such products as infant cereals and some prepared dried cereals have chosen to enrich their products at an extremely high level. This likely represents excessive enrichment to promote the sale of the product, but the consumer may be able to utilize only a small fraction of the added amount.

The only food group characterized as a poor source of iron is milk and milk products. The small amount of iron in milk is well utilized but still makes an insignificant contribution to the total dietary intake.

Some food sources that are relatively rich in iron but do not make a major contribution to the diet because of the infrequency with which they are consumed are oysters (6.3 mg. per serving), clams (6.1 mg.), and cocoa (1 mg. per tablespoon).

In some areas, iron in the drinking water may be a significant source to the body, especially when iron values of water exceed 5 mg. per liter.

Blackstrap molasses, a by-product of the sugar-refining process and widely extolled by food faddists, contains about 2.5 mg. per tablespoon. Because of the bitter flavor of the product, whether it can be considered a significant dietary item is questionable.

In 1959 the average per capita consumption of iron was placed at 16.3 mg. per day. Of all families 90% reported an intake of over 12 mg. per person per day, and 42% reported over 20 mg. per day, indicating intakes capable of meeting the needs for most adults.

Effect of cooking. Loss of iron in cooking arises from loss by solution into cooking water, which is discarded, and the removal of peelings, with the loss of the iron concentrated near the skin. Any cooking method that minimizes the possibility of iron dissolving in the cooking water, such as the use of relatively large pieces of food, cooking with skins on, and the use of simmering rather than boiling water, will increase the amount of iron available in the diet. Steamed vegetables have more iron than boiled vegetables; those cooked for a short time in a small amount of water have more than those cooked for a longer period and in a large amount of water; and those cooked in their skins have more iron than peeled ones. The use of vegetable stock in soups or gravies also helps minimize iron losses.

Deficiencies

Since the body is extremely efficient in conserving iron supplies, simple iron deficiencies occur only during the growth period or when intake fails to meet needs after loss of blood from the body or in women who have experienced frequent pregnancies in rapid succession. *Anemia,* a condition in which a deficiency occurs in the quantity and/or quality of the red blood cells, is the most common manifestation of iron deficiency.

Diagnosis. Anemia can be diagnosed by comparing to established standards blood hemoglobin levels measured as grams of hemoglobin per 100 ml. of blood and red blood cell counts measured as the number of red blood cells per cubic millimeter of blood. Standards for hemoglobin are 15 gm. of hemoglobin per 100 ml. of blood for men and 13.6 gm. for women. Clinical laboratories frequently report hemoglobin levels as a percentage of the standard. Thus a hemoglobin level of 90 means that the blood contained 90% of the standard, or in the case of men, 90% of 15 gm., or 13.5 gm. Red blood cell standards are 5 million per cubic milliliter of blood for men and 4.5 million for women. The total number of red blood cells in the body is so large that it defies comprehension—over 25 trillion. The number replaced every second is 2.5 million.

A third measurement, the color index, is useful in diagnosing the type of anemia. It involves the ratio of hemoglobin value expressed as a percentage of the standard to the red blood cell count expressed as a percentage of that standard, as follows:

$$\text{Color index} = \frac{\text{Percent normal hemoglobin}}{\text{Percent normal red cell count}}$$

Under normal conditions the color index is approximately 1. A value of more than 1 indicates a deficiency in the number of red blood cells with normal amounts of hemoglobin; a value of less than 1 indicates a lack of hemoglobin in the presence of an adequate number of cells.

Anemia can be classified into two categories based on the underlying cause—nutritional and hemorrhagic.

Nutritional anemia. Nutritional anemia is caused by the absence of any dietary essential involved in hemoglobin formation or by poor absorption of these dietary components. The most likely causes are lack of dietary iron or high-quality protein. But anemias have been reported associated with a lack of pyridoxine (vitamin B_6), which catalyzes the synthesis of the heme portion of the hemoglobin molecule; of ascorbic acid, which influences the rate of iron absorption and the release of iron from transferrin to the tissues; and of vitamin E, which effects the stability of the red blood cell membrane. Experimentally the omission of copper from the diet causes low hemoglobin values. Copper is not part of the hemoglobin molecule but apparently facilitates its formation by influencing either the absorption of iron, its release from the liver, or its incorporation into a hemoglobin molecule.

Nutritional anemia is usually characterized as hypochromic and microcytic. This broad classification suggests a lack of the pigment hemoglobin and the presence of small cells. Failure of the cell to grow in the absence of hemoglobin synthesis produces the small cells. As a result, nutritional anemia can be identified by a low color index and occurs primarily during the growth period when demands of growing cells and increased blood volume are not met by dietary intake of nutrients needed for hemoglobin synthesis. It is most pronounced in adolescent girls when the growth demands superimposed on the menstrual losses are difficult to meet by dietary means. This condition is sometimes described as *chlorosis* because of the greenish cast it gives the skin. A cursory diagnosis of hemoglobin status can often be made by a visual examination of the mucous membranes, especially on the underside of the eyelid or in the mouth, where the blood vessels are close to the epithelial surface. Pale membranes usually signify low hemoglobin values.

In adult men nutritional anemia is not likely to develop once normal levels have been reached because of the minimal need for iron and the relatively large liver reserves. Even on a diet devoid of iron it would take over six years to deplete the liver reserves and to cause a sufficiently large drop in hemoglobin values to lead to a diagnosis of anemia. In adult women a comparable situation could arise in four years.

Nutritional anemia does occur frequently in young infants who are maintained on a diet consisting solely of milk for a period of time exceeding the three- to six-month period during which fetal liver reserves are adequate. Infants utilize little dietary iron during the first three months of life, but after that the addition of enriched cereal, egg yolk, and meat to the infant's diet all provide good sources of iron. One study reported an incidence of anemia in 42% of breast-fed infants and 70% of bottle-fed infants at 1 year of age. Another study of nutritional intake of infants showed that unless the diet contained enriched cereals, it would fail to meet the recommended allowances for iron. Meat, fruits, and vegetables in the amounts consumed by these infants was not sufficient to meet the iron need without the use of cereal products.

Pernicious anemia. Pernicious anemia, a form of nutritional anemia in which the number of red blood cells and not the hemoglobin level is low, as shown by a high color index, is caused primarily by failure in the absorption of vitamin B_{12}, or cobalamin, rather than lack of a nutrient. It will be discussed in Chapter 12.

Hemorrhagic anemia. Hemorrhagic anemia is caused by an excessive loss of blood. This may occur after surgery, bleeding of wounds, internal hemorrhaging, excessive menstrual losses, blood donations, or in the presence of intestinal parasites. After a blood loss the blood volume is restored almost immediately, followed by an increase in the number of red blood cells and finally by the restoration of hemoglobin levels. A low color index also prevails in hemorrhagic anemia.

The loss of 1 pint of blood represents a loss of 250 mg. of iron. Even with the increased rate of iron absorption that occurs after blood loss, it takes at least 50 days to restore normal hemoglobin levels. This period may be reduced to 35 days if iron supplements and ascorbic acid are given. The wisdom of limiting blood donations to 4 to 6 pints per year, especially for women, is obvious.

Treatment. When iron-deficiency anemia with its symptoms of pallor, easy fatigue, decreased resistance to infection, soreness in the mouth, and palpitation after exercise is diagnosed, the use of a diet high in iron-rich foods with a concurrent intake of appreciable amounts of ascorbic acid is indicated. The use of iron salts in therapeutic doses is likely justified to speed the restoration of hemoglobin levels to normal, and in many cases it is the only way in which hemoglobin synthesis is adequately stimulated. Many iron salts, both organic and inorganic, such as ferrous gluconate, ferrous sulfate, ferrous citrate, ferric ammonium citrate, and ferrous fumarate, have been promoted by pharmaceutical firms. So far no preparation has been shown to be superior to ferrous sulfate, which contains 36% iron and is the least expensive of all these forms, costing from 1 to 15 cents per daily dosage. Therapeutic doses may contain as much as 250 mg. of iron, which may be absorbed at the rate of 150 mg. per day to bring about a maximum rate of increase in hemoglobin levels of 0.3 gm. per day. To provide this level of iron requires 0.8 gm. of ferrous sulfate or 1.2 gm. of ferrous gluconate. It is wise to build up therapeutic dosages slowly to develop a gradual tolerance to the iron and to prevent gastrointestinal upsets. Once normal hemoglobin levels are reached, the continued use of iron salts is not justified from either a nutritional or an economic point of view.

Excess

The theory that the absorption of iron was regulated in the intestinal mucosa suggested that the uptake of excess iron was impossible. This theory was questioned when it was reported that an African tribe, the Bantu, suffered from siderosis or hemochromatosis, a disease in which the iron reserves were found to be up to thirty times the normal 1 gm. reserve. The source of their iron, which amounted to 200 mg. per day, is thought to be the kettles in which the large amounts of beer they consume are fermented. An excess absorption as small as 3 mg. per day will result in 1 mg. of storage iron per day, which can accumulate to a sizeable amount over a period of years. A similar iron toxicity has been reported among persons who are overzealous in their use of therapeutic iron readily available on the open shelves in drugstores. There are many reports of ferrous sulfate toxicity in infants who have been given 3 to 10 gm. daily.

In siderosis, iron increased in the mitochondria of cells, reflecting increased tissue iron; serum iron increased, and the bone marrow became hyperplastic. The failure of the absorption mechanism to regulate iron absorption occurs at very high levels of iron intake. Under these circumstances the transferrin of blood is saturated at three times its normal level and is incapable of binding all the absorbed iron in a harmless complex.

Some evidence of iron overload has been noted in persons who have had successive blood transfusions. Even though the transfused blood is providing iron, they continue to absorb iron in a manner characteristic of an iron-deficient individual.

IODINE
Distribution

The essential trace mineral element iodine is present in the body in minute amounts, about 0.00004% of body weight, or 15 to 23 mg., in a healthy human adult. Like iron, iodine is present in every living cell of the body, with 70% to 80%, or about 10 mg., concentrated in a single tissue, the thyroid gland, where the level of iodine is twenty times that of the blood supplying it. The thyroid gland is a tissue consisting of two lobes or parts located in the neck area on either side of the trachea just below the larynx and weighing about 25 gm., or 0.2% of body weight. The two sides of the thyroid gland are joined by a thin strip of tissue, sometimes called the thyroid isthmus. Bile, hair, ovaries, and skeletal muscle rank next on the basis of concentration of iodine.

Our knowledge of iodine metabolism has been advanced with the use of radioactive isotopes of iodine, especially I^{131}, and the development of analytical methods sufficiently sensitive to determine the minute amounts of this element found in biological material.

Absorption

Iodine occurs in food primarily in the reduced iodide form but also as inorganic iodine or as an organically bound iodine complex. The latter is freed from its organic component, and the free iodine is reduced to iodide before absorption. Inorganic iodide is absorbed in all parts of the gastrointestinal tract but primarily in the small intestine. Some organically bound iodine is not absorbed and may be excreted in the feces, but it represents a maximum of 2% of ingested iodine. Even smaller amounts are excreted by the sweat glands. Iodine may also be absorbed through epithelial cells of the skin.

Once absorbed, the iodine appears immediately in the bloodstream, where it constitutes the major part of the "iodide pool"— all extracellular iodide. About 30% of the iodide in the blood plasma is absorbed by the thyroid gland, and the rest is taken up by the kidney to be excreted in the urine. The excretion of iodine not used by the thyroid gland provides a protection against the accumulation of toxic levels in other tissues.

Metabolism

The iodide picked up, or "trapped," by the thyroid gland is immediately oxidized to iodine within the thyroid gland. In this form one or two molecules unite with the amino acid tyrosine, which is attached to thyroglobulin, a mucoprotein rich in this amino acid, and with leucine, which is present in the center cells of the thyroid gland.

The iodated tyrosine molecules unite to form either thyroxin (T_4), with 4 atoms of iodine, or thyronine (T_3), with 3 atoms of iodine. These active hormones are released from storage in thyroglobulin by a protein-splitting enzyme, itself released under the stimulus of another hormone, and enter the circulation. Thyronine is a much more active form of the hormone than thyroxin but is present in relatively small amounts in the blood. There is some evidence that once thyroxin enters the individual cell, it becomes deiodated by the removal of 1 atom of iodine to form the more active thyronine with 3 atoms of iodine.

Function

Part of thyroxin. As part of the thyroid hormone thyroxin secreted into the circulating plasma, iodine plays a major role in regulating the growth and development of the organism and its rate of metabolism. The stimulating effect of thyroxin on metabolism can be appreciable, with the effects of a single dose persisting for six days or more. When the rate of metabolism increases, more oxygen is used up by the cells, indicating that more energy is being released from glucose and fatty acids to take care of the needs of the more active cells.

Although most attention has been focused on the role of thyroxin in energy metabolism, an increasing number of direct and indirect effects of thyroxin in metabolic functions are becoming apparent. The conversion of carotene, the precursor of vitamin A, to the active form of the vitamin, the synthesis of protein by ribosomes, and the absorption of carbohydrate from the intestine are more efficient when thyroxin production is normal. The synthesis of cholesterol is influenced by thyroxin levels, with above-normal cholesterol levels occurring in hypothyroidism and below-normal levels in hyperthyroidism.

Secondary to the effect of thyroxin in stimulating metabolism is its effect on nitrogen excretion. When energy needs increase, more of the calories from protein must be used as a source of energy rather than for growth or maintenance of tissue, leading to increased loss of nitrogen from the body. The rapid breakdown of body tissue occurring with protein catabolism leads to extreme body weakness that can be attributed to the loss of potassium that accompanies protein loss. If food intake is not increased to balance increased energy expenditure, body reserves of protein and fat will be depleted to meet the need, with a resultant loss of weight. Before the Food and Drug Administration ruled that thyroxin preparations would be available through prescriptions only, unscrupulous peddlers of weight-reducing aids were incorporating thyroid extract on the theory that these aids facilitated weight loss. They do indeed, but the undesirable side effects that accompany their uncontrolled use make such a practice potentially hazardous.

Since the only known function of iodine is in thyroxin formation, much of the discussion of iodine metabolism and needs centers around the activity of thyroxin and the thyroid gland.

Requirements

The Food and Nutrition Board of the National Research Council has suggested that an intake of 1 μg. of iodine per kilogram of body weight is adequate for most adults. To assure a margin of safety to take care of individual variations they recommend a daily intake of 100 μg. for women and 150 μg. for men. For pregnant and lactating women the need is 25 and 50 μg. higher. If, as is often recommended, the salt intake is restricted during pregnancy, eliminating a major source of iodine in the diet, precautions should be taken to see that sufficient iodine is available from other sources.

The needs for growing children, especially girls, may exceed the suggested level of 1 μg. per kilogram of body weight.

Food sources

Both food and water provide iodine in the human diet. The amount present in the water varies from one area to another and tends to parallel the iodine content of the soil. Iodine content of less than 2 μg. per liter is associated with iodine-deficiency conditions and that of 2 to 15 μg. with the absence of iodine deficiency. In the United States the iodine content of the water varies from 0.01 to 73 ppm.

Seafoods, such as lobster, shrimp, and oysters, are among the richest dietary sources, but because of the relatively minor role they play in the diet (except among people living in coastal regions), they do not make a major contribution to the iodine content of many diets. Saltwater fish contain 300 to 3000 μg. of iodine per kilogram of flesh compared to 20 to 40 μg. in freshwater fish. Fresh river water contains 0.5 to 2 μg. per liter; seawater contains 17 to 50 μg. Saltwater fish have an amazing capacity to concentrate this relatively small amount of iodine within their tissue.

The amount of iodine in dairy products and eggs is extremely variable and reflects the iodine content of the soil on which the rations of the animals were grown and the season of the year. The iodine content of milk rapidly reflects addition of iodine to the cow's diet. Most cereal grains, legumes, fruits, and vegetables are low in iodine content but, again, fluctuate with the iodine content of the soil in which they were grown. In general the leaves of plants have higher iodine concentrations than the roots. Spinach leaves are especially concentrated and have the highest iodine content of all plants. Corn is extremely low in iodine, which may make corn-eating people more susceptible to iodine deficiency conditions.

The variation in iodine content of vegetables from various sources can be illustrated by values of 240, 407, and 1283 μg. per kilogram of dry weight of carrots grown in Florida, Oklahoma, and Louisiana, respectively. Modern marketing practices in which the food supply of any one community comes from widely separated geographical areas have done much to assure a more uniform and more nearly adequate level of iodine for the average American.

The use of iodized salt in cooking has proved the most effective method of assuring sufficient iodine in the diet. It is added to salt as potassium iodide at a level of 100 mg. per kilogram, or 1 part per 10,000 parts salt, a level established to be completely safe and yet valuable in combatting goiter. This provides the person who consumes 6 gm. of table salt with 500 μg. per day. Some countries, such as Canada, Guatemala, and Colombia, have passed legislation to require the iodization of salt at 1 part iodine to 10,000 parts salt. In Europe 1 part iodine to 100,000 parts salt is used. Mandatory iodization has been recommended by the Food and Nutrition Board in the United States, but currently it is a voluntary measure on the part of the salt producers, who must comply only with the labelling requirements of the Food and Drug Administration. Currently less than half the salt sold in the United States is iodized, although 75% of all families report using it and only 4% say they never use it. The evidence of iodine deficiency uncovered in the *National Nutrition Survey* indicates that we have failed in our efforts to promote the use of iodized salt. A more stable iodate may replace potassium iodide as the enrichment agent, especially in countries where salt is moist, making iodide unstable.

Other methods of increasing the iodine intake of population groups in low-iodine areas have met with varying degrees of success. The addition of iodine to water supplies has been abandoned because of its failure to benefit people in rural areas and others with private water supplies. Iodized tablets or candies are rarely satisfactory even though they provide measured amounts of iodine because they depend on complete cooperation of a number of people. Where little baking of bread at home is done and where bread is a staple in the diet, the use of iodized salt in bread has been fairly effective. Failure of food processors to use iodized salt in packaged food products may be partially responsible for the suboptimal intake of many people.

In countries such as Japan where seaweed, which has a capacity to concentrate iodine from seawater, is consumed as a regular dietary item, it is a major source of iodine, containing 0.4% to 0.6% iodine on a dry weight basis. The value of recommending seaweed for consumption in a culture unaccustomed to its use is doubtful.

One of the few studies based on the chemical analysis of iodine content of American diets showed intakes varying from 65 to 529 μg. per day, the principal contribution being from vegetables and dairy products.

Evaluation of nutritional status

Since the dietary intake of iodine includes that in water as well as in food, the difficulties of conducting iodine balance studies to assess iodine nutriture are greater than those for other nutrients that are provided only by food. To obtain some assessment of the adequacy of iodine nutriture, use has been made of the determination of the iodine excretion in a single sample of urine in relation to the amount of creatinine excreted. In areas of low available iodine an excretion of about 25 μg. of iodine per gram of creatinine occurs, whereas in areas of high available iodine the excretion is at least 50 μg. Some excretion rates are as high as 1000 μg. per gram of creatinine.

Thyroxin

Since most of the iodine in the body is used in thyroxin synthesis, a convenient way to study iodine metabolism is to study thyroxin metabolism.

Measurement. The rate of thyroxin production can be measured in several ways.

The basal metabolic rate as determined by indirect calorimetry (described in Chapter 5) is closely related to the level of thyroxin production. A basal metabolic rate elevated at least 15% above the level predicted on the basis of body surface area or metabolic body size indicates a state of hyperthyroidism, an excess production of thyroxin. On the other hand, a depressed basal metabolic rate reflects a state of hypothyroidism, a decreased rate of thyroxin production.

A simpler, less costly method of assessing thyroxin level, the protein-bound iodine (PBI) test on less than 1 ml. of blood, has been developed. This method has an advantage over basal metabolism in that it is not influenced by previous meals or activity and is less costly. A positive relationship exists between the amount of iodine bound to protein circulating in the blood and the level of thyroxin produced, since 90% of the protein-bound iodine is in thyroxin, which is 65% iodine by weight. Normally PBI levels are 4 to 8 μg. per 100 ml. of blood. PBI blood levels above 11 μg. per 100 ml. are indicative of hyperthyroidism and levels below 3 μg., of hypothyroidism. It is not possible to calculate the exact extent of the change in energy expenditure using this method, but the relative level of basal metabolism can be determined.

Radioactive isotopes have proved useful in assessing the state of thyroxin production. Radioactive iodine is administered orally. The amount taken up by the thyroid gland is determined by measuring the radioactivity in the neck region and that taken up by other tissues, by a radioactivity reading in the thigh area. In hyperthyroidism a very rapid uptake of iodine by the thyroid occurs, followed by a gradual drop after 24 hours. Under conditions of normal thyroid function the uptake of radioactive iodine is gradual. In hypothyroidism the rate of uptake is rapid, and the iodine remains in the thyroid gland for much longer periods.

Regulation. The functioning of the thyroid gland is controlled by a thyroid-stimulating hormone (TSH) secreted by the pituitary gland in response to the level of thyroxin in the blood. This, in turn, reflects the availability of iodine for thyroxin synthesis. Many factors may influence the amount of TSH produced and hence the activity of the thyroid gland. When dietary iodine falls below 20 μg., which is inadequate for sufficient thyroxin synthesis, more TSH is produced. This results in an increase in size of the thyroid gland, known as simple goiter, in which both the size and number of thyroid cells increase. In addition, several antithyroid drugs have much the same effect in stimulating TSH production by inhibiting thyroxin formation. They may either interfere with the ability of the thyroid gland to trap iodine, block the oxidation of iodide to iodine, or block the organic binding of iodine. In any case, drugs such as thiourea or thiouracil stimulate the pituitary gland to secrete more TSH. Thiocyanates used in the treatment of hypertension inhibit the ability of the thyroid gland to concentrate iodine and so increase the work involved in producing thyroxin.

Certain foods contain substances called goitrogens because their presence predisposes a person to the iodine-deficiency disease goiter. They act in much the same way as the antithyroid drugs blocking the absorption or utilization of iodine. Foods of the cabbage family, such as rutabagas, turnips, and cabbage, contain a heat-stable substance, *pregoitren,* and a heat-labile activator that converts pregoitren to *goitren.* In raw foods the goitren that interferes with iodine utilization is formed; in cooked foods, however, the conversion cannot take place unless an activator is formed by bacterial synthesis. Evidence of the presence of such an enzyme in the gastrointestinal tract is increasing, which means that the pregoitren in cooked foods may also be converted to a goitren.

Ground nuts contain a substance, *arachi-*

doside, that also interferes with iodine utilization. The presence of this substance is one of the drawbacks to the use of nuts to improve the protein quality of the diet in areas where the diet consists of low-quality protein.

Sulfonamides, widely used antibiotics that reduce the conversion of iodide to iodine, are potentially goitrogenic but at the levels used in treating infection have little effect on thyroid activity. The extensive use of the vitamin-like substance para-amino-benzoic acid (PABA) has a similar effect. Some evidence also exists to support the theory that both high-calcium and high-fat diets may be goitrogenic. A diet very high in iodine may also be goitrogenic by limiting iodine absorption.

The salivary gland may play a role in regulating the level of thyroxin in the blood. It has the capacity to remove iodine (deiodate) from thyroxin, thus inactivating it. The iodine is secreted in the saliva and can be reabsorbed in the gastrointestinal tract.

Goiter

In 1920 iodine was recognized as an effective agent in the treatment of simple goiter, a condition in which the thyroid gland enlarges and causes a swelling in the throat, an effect evident from a profile view. A deficiency of iodine is the primary but not the only cause of simple goiter. Goiter may also be caused by factors that interfere with the availability of dietary iodine, impose abnormal demands on the thyroid gland, or interfere with the utilization of iodine by the thyroid. These interfering substances include chemicals naturally present in some foods or purposely introduced for therapeutic reasons or defects in an enzyme system necessary for the synthesis and release of thyroxin. In all these cases the thyroid gland enlarges to compensate for the lack of iodine needed for its normal functioning. Of the estimated 200 million cases of simple goiter in the world today, the majority are caused by a dietary lack of iodine and tend to occur in definite geographical regions.

Incidence. It has been established that the incidence of goiter is regional, occurring primarily in areas where the soil is of glacial origin or where flooding or tropical rains have leached the iodine from the soil. It is nonexistent in areas where iodine-laden vapors from the sea condense and deposit iodine on the soil. As shown in Fig. 8-4, in the United States areas of highest incidence are those bordering the Great Lakes—Michigan, Wisconsin, and Ohio—and the Rocky Mountain states. Coastal areas are relatively free of the condition, as are the southern states. Studies of the iodine content of the soils and water supplies of goitrous areas showed a very low concentration. Since simple goiter is not an incapacitating disease and in its early stages is a problem merely from an aesthetic point of view, people suffering from the condition were not motivated to seek medical help. Consequently little attention was paid to the disease. The increasing incidence reported by 1915 led to the first large-scale study on the control of goiter in human beings in Ohio from 1916 to 1920. There the addition of iodine tablets to the water supply twice a year effectively reduced the incidence of goiter in adolescent girls, the group most susceptible to the disease. Other methods have been tried, such as feeding iodized salt to cows to increase the iodine content of their diet in an effort to increase the amount appearing in the milk, the iodization of the water supply, and the iodization of salt. Of these, only the iodization of salt proved an effective method for reaching the majority of the population. The cost of adding iodine to the salt supply is so small that in most cases the manufacturers absorbed the cost.

In Michigan, where goiter among 47% of school children in 1921 constituted a major public health problem, an intensive educational campaign to promote the use of io-

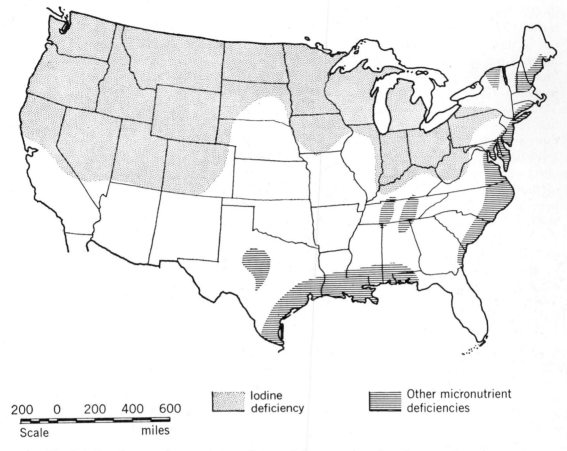

200   0   200   400   600
Scale   miles

Iodine deficiency

Other micronutrient deficiencies

Fig. 8-4. Distribution of micronutrient element deficiencies in soil in the United States. Some other micronutrient deficiencies also occur in scattered parts of goitrous areas. (Adapted from Beesom, K. C.: In Lamb, C. A., Bentley, O. G., and Blathic, J. M.: Trace elements, New York, 1958, Academic Press, Inc.)

dized salt was launched. The results were encouraging. By 1925 the incidence had dropped to 32%, and by 1951 only 1% of the population had simple goiter. Michigan's experience, however, has shown that it is necessary to maintain the educational program to keep the condition under control, since a letup in their educational efforts in 1951 resulted in a temporary increase. In 1970 a nutritional status survey in ten states revealed a shocking incidence of goiter, a condition that public health authorities believed was no longer cause for concern. In some areas as many as 5% of the population were afflicted—an incidence considered endemic.

The incidence of goiter is about six times as high in females as in males, and the most susceptible groups are adolescent girls and pregnant women. The practice of limiting the use of iodized salt in an effort to control adolescent acne, especially among girls, may be questioned because of the risk of stimulating the growth of the thyroid gland.

The distribution of goiter areas in the world is shown in Fig. 8-5 and a typical case of goiter in Fig. 8-6.

Treatment. Most goiters respond to iodine therapy, and it is now obvious that the effective agent in the successful use of sponges in treating goiter, reported as early as 1280, was iodine. The use of iodine

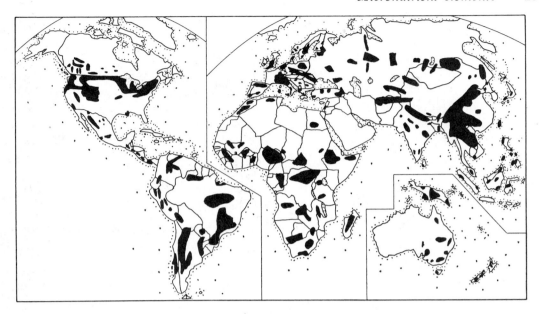

Fig. 8-5. Goitrous areas of the world.

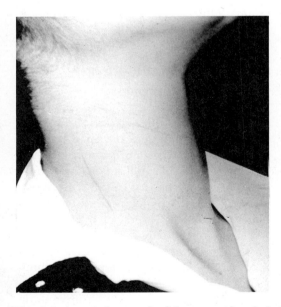

Fig. 8-6. A typical case of adult goiter identified in the 1970 *National Nutrition Survey.* (Courtesy Dr. W. J. McGanity, University of Texas, Galveston, Texas.)

salts in the treatment of goiter was recognized as early as 1820, although not until ten years later was it suggested that a lack of iodine in the diet may be a cause of simple goiter. Thirty years later the lack of iodine was associated with low iodine levels in the soil and water, but the suggestion of the French botanist Chatin that iodine be added to water in areas where goiter occurred was not then accepted. However, toward the turn of the century, when it was shown that iodine was a normal constituent of the thyroid gland and that the normal levels of 10 to 15 mg. dropped as low as 1 mg. in endemic goiter, a renewed interest came about in the use of iodine therapy in the treatment of goiter. Several investigations confirmed that endemic goiter was primarily the result of an iodine deficiency and could be controlled by raising dietary iodine intakes.

The most effective method of control is one of prevention, and the use of iodized salt has proved most useful. Simple goiter is a painless condition that has some undesirable effects on physical appearance, since once a simple goiter is formed in an adult, it cannot be reduced in size with iodine therapy. If the simple goiter continues to grow, the hazards increase until danger of blocking off the trachea occurs due to pressure from the growth of thyroid tissue on either side. Under these circumstances, treatment involves thyroidectomy, the surgical removal of part of the thyroid gland, an operation complicated by the fact that the parathyroid gland vital in the control of calcium metabolism is embedded in the surface of the thyroid gland. Ligating (or tying off of an artery leading to the thyroid) has occasionally been effective in controlling the growth of the gland.

Other abnormalities

Among children born to mothers who have had a limited iodine intake during adolescence and pregnancy and who live in areas where iodine deficiency has prevailed for years and where goiter is endemic, the condition cretinism is frequently encountered. Cretins who suffer from hypothyroidism are physically dwarfed, mentally retarded, and have enlarged protruding abdomens. If treatment is started soon after birth, many of the symptoms of cretinism are reversible, but if the conditions persist beyond early childhood, permanent mental and physical retardation cannot be prevented.

Adults who have had symptoms of hypothyroidism throughout their developmental period suffer from myxedema. These people have coarse sparse hair, dry yellowish skin, poor tolerance for cold, and a low husky voice. This can be due to a defect in the thyroid gland or in the pituitary, which produces the thyroid-stimulating hormone.

Both cretinism and myxedema are still found, but the use of iodized salt has greatly reduced the incidence in countries such as Switzerland where the soil and water is extremely low in iodine. A similar program in the Andes would undoubtedly lower the incidence in this mountainous low-iodine area.

Hyperthyroidism in which the basal metabolic rate may be elevated as much as 100% above normal is also known as Graves' disease and exophthalmic goiter. Persons suffering from overactivity of the thyroid gland experience nervousness, weight loss, increased appetite, intolerance to heat, tremors when the hand is outstretched, and protruding eyeballs. The increased rate of metabolism that accompanies increased thyroxin production puts an increased load on the cardiovascular system.

OTHER MICRONUTRIENT ELEMENTS
Essentiality

In addition to the seven macronutrient elements discussed in the previous chapter and the micronutrient elements iron and iodine discussed in this chapter, eight other mineral elements present in the body in small and variable amounts have been shown to play an essential role in metabolism in human beings.

A trace element is considered essential when the following are repeatedly demonstrated: a significant growth response to dietary supplements of this element alone, the development of a deficiency state on diets otherwise adequate, and a correlation of the deficiency state with the occurrence of suboptimal levels of the element in the blood or tissues of animals.

Seven others whose essential nature has not yet been established on the basis of these criteria may perform some functions similar to those deemed essential. Because some aspects of metabolism are common to many of them, they will be discussed as a group, followed by a brief discussion of unique aspects of several of them.

The use of the term *trace elements* to describe this group is unfortunate, since it may imply a lack of nutritional importance. Its use stems from the era when analytical techniques were sufficiently sensitive to detect their presence but not to measure the minute amounts needed. The extremely small concentrations at which these elements are functional is illustrated by the fact that 1 part in 10 million is active. The occurrence of micronutrient element deficiencies in the soil in the United States is shown in Fig. 8-4.

Role in the body

The small amounts needed bear no relationship to importance; a lack of one of these micronutrients can be equally as serious as a lack of one needed at a level many hundred times higher. Some may be catalysts to biological reactions, acting as a link between the enzyme and its substrate; others are part of essential body compounds, such as hormones and enzymes; and others are involved in the growth of tissue.

Because of the varied geographical sources of food in the average diet and the fact that the amount of these micronutrient elements present in food is a function of the soil on which they are grown, there is little evidence of naturally occurring dietary deficiencies of these nutrients. In fact, it has been difficult to purify experimental diets to the point at which an inadequate level of one nutrient and an adequate amount of all others are present. As a result, most of our evidence of the biological role of trace elements has been established by animal studies in which the source of food has been from a geographically restricted area where a deficiency of the element in the soil is reflected in a limited amount in the crops grown on these soils. Once the role of the nutrient has been elucidated in animals, it has often been possible to demonstrate a similar function in human nutrition. Frequently it is necessary to interfere with the absorption of or stimulate the excretion of an element as well as to eliminate it from the diet for long periods to demonstrate a deficiency.

Interrelationships

One of the major difficulties in acquiring precise information on the function of many mineral elements has been the extent to which the presence or absence of one element may influence the role of a second and modify the requirement of another.

The interactions between minerals may occur in the diet, in the intestine, at the sites of excretion in the kidney, intestine, or lungs, and at specific sites within the body cells.

As an example of interrelationships, it may be noted that an increase in the molybdenum content of the diet without a simultaneous increase in the copper or sulfur content results in depressed growth and restricted hemoglobin production. The copper-molybdenum antagonism is apparently reciprocal. As further examples, increased copper interferes with iron and zinc metabolism, high manganese affects iron metabolism, and excess cobalt interferes with the synthesis of the iodine-containing hormone thyroxin. Zinc-deficiency symptoms can be precipitated by diets high in calcium relative to zinc and can be relieved by correcting the imbalance. The fact that abnormally high levels of some elements can displace other elements that are essential parts of enzymes can lead to failure to produce a biologically active enzyme. In addition, it may also interfere with the use of the effective enzyme. The utilization of one mineral element can be evaluated only in the light of the availability and utilization of other nutrients with which it may have a close dietary and metabolic interrelationship.

The ability of one element to replace another in key compounds is one of the hazards of some of the multimineral supplements on the commercial market. Too often the basis of the formula is maximum profit to the promoter rather than any consideration of the nutritional needs of the individual. Unbalanced mineral supplements are potentially harmful. The Food and Drug Administration suggests that calcium, iron, and iodine are the only mineral elements that can be justified in dietary supplements and is promoting legislation to restrict the amounts that can be included.

Because of the complexities of the inter-relationships among trace mineral elements, it is necessary to assess the whole pattern of nutrient intake in studies of deficiency, toxicity, or requirements. Simple and uncomplicated deficiencies of single micronutrient elements seldom occur under normal conditions.

Toxicity

Some trace mineral elements essential in small amounts may be toxic when present at high levels. Most of the cases of toxicity from trace minerals have been the result of exposure to an environment saturated with the element, since minerals can enter the body through the respiratory tract and the skin as well as through the gastrointestinal tract. The manganese and selenium toxicity found among miners is believed to be caused by aspiration of air containing above-normal concentrations of the elements. Fluorine toxicity, which takes the form of a dental fluorosis, or mottled enamel, is the result of ingesting large quantities of water containing over 2.5 ppm of naturally occurring fluorine.

Selenium poisoning in animals is common in areas where the selenium content of the soil is high. High urinary levels are found in humans in the same area, although no definite evidence exists of selenium poisoning in man.

Deficiencies

Deficiencies of most trace mineral elements become evident only after prolonged dietary inadequacies and then usually only when associated with some defect in absorption and a change in other dietary components that leads to increased need. Usually the first evidence of an inadequacy appears in a reduction of enzymes of which the mineral is an essential part or a reduction in the activity of enzymes catalyzed by the element. Changes in blood levels of trace elements usually reflect the level of body stores rather than dietary intake, as body stores will be mobilized to maintain blood and tissue levels in the event of a dietary deficiency. Only when these are depleted and intake is inadequate will blood levels drop.

Requirements

The human requirements for most of the trace mineral elements have not been established. Their widespread presence in foods, the minute amounts involved, the absence of any deficiency states that can be attributed directly to lack of the nutrient, and the interrelationships among trace elements have made the assessment of dietary needs impossible with the techniques currently available. In addition, modification of the level of other nutrients of the diet, such as protein, may influence the amount of the element needed.

Food sources

The amount of trace elements present in vegetable foods is primarily a function of the amount present in the soils in which the crops were grown. In the case of animal foods the amount of some elements reflects the diet of the animal, whereas for others—especially those essential for the particular species—the animal may be able to regulate the amount present in its tissue by regulation of excretion. In any case, the ultimate source of the mineral content of food is the soil. The possibility of a trace mineral element deficiency is greatly reduced with modern marketing techniques that lead to the consumption of a diet from widely scattered areas rather than from a restricted geographical region. Some mineral elements are also introduced into foods through contamination during processing.

Milk is a relatively poor source of most micronutrient elements. This may be one reason to suggest the introduction of a wider variety of foods into the infant's diet after three or four months.

ZINC

Zinc has been recognized as an essential for fungi growth for almost a hundred years and for rat growth since 1934. It has only been since 1961, however, that evidence has existed to associate a dietary zinc deficiency with retarded growth, delayed sexual maturity, and delayed wound healing in humans. In Iran and Egypt, where zinc deficiency has been studied most extensively, it has been associated with a diet of wheat flour and little animal protein. In the United States some cases of retarded physical development have been attributed to a low dietary intake of zinc or to a defect in its absorption or utilization.

In animals a very rapid decline in growth rate and appetite occurs after the removal of zinc from the diet and an equally rapid restoration of these functions after its addition. This suggests that zinc in the body is not easily mobilized, that zinc plays some role in appetite regulation, and that the site of action of zinc is one where the metal is freely exchangeable.

Biological roles

Zinc is a stably bound constituent of at least twenty-five enzymes involved in digestion and metabolism. Among these is carbonic anhydrase, which functions in the maintenance of acid-base balance by facilitating the catabolism of carbonic acid. This is necessary for the transport and elimination of carbon dioxide, an essential aspect of respiration. As part of a protein-splitting enzyme of the pancreatic juice it plays a role in digestion, and as part of alkaline phosphatase it is involved in bone metabolism.

In addition to being an integral part of enzymes known to catalyze at least fifteen biological changes, many of which are involved in protein metabolism, zinc is required for the action of insulin.

Distribution

The 2 gm. of zinc found in the body is widely distributed. The high concentration found in the hair, skin, eyes, nails, and testes suggests a special function for zinc in these tissues.

In the blood 85% of the zinc occurs in the red blood cells, 4% in the leukocytes and platelets, and the remainder in the serum, where it is tightly bound to protein. Serum levels are maintained within a narrow range of 70-125 μg. per 100 ml. of serum, but they do decrease in many conditions, such as infection, pernicious anemia, hyperthyroidism, cirrhosis of the liver, pregnancy, and in women using oral contraceptives.

Requirement

The body's need for zinc appears to be met by intakes of 0.3 to 0.6 mg. per kilogram of body weight, the requirements increasing with an increase in dietary protein. High calcium levels depress utilization of zinc, necessitating higher dietary levels.

Table 8-4. Dietary sources of zinc

Rich sources (> 3 mg./100 gm.)	Moderate sources (1-3 mg./100 gm.)	Poor sources (< 1 mg./100 gm.)
Maple syrup	Beef	Lettuce
Oysters	Clams	Butter
Peas	Corn	Oranges
Whole-wheat cereals	Peanut butter	
Liver	Milk	
Oatmeal	Egg yolk	

Food sources

The zinc content of the diet varies but most provide 10 to 15 mg. per day. Diets high in protein and whole-grain products are usually higher in zinc. The zinc content of some representative foods is shown in Table 8-4. The zinc content of plant protein, such as soybean or sesame oil meal, is less available than that in animal protein. Phytic acid found in cereals depresses the absorption of zinc, as shown by an increased excretion in the feces.

The zinc concentration of human milk is 20 mg. per liter but drops to 0.65 mg. per liter at 6 months. This is less than the level in cow's milk.

Toxicity

Toxicity from excessive intakes of zinc may take place when galvanized utensils are used in processing acid foods or when carbonated beverages are sold in metal containers. Among the metabolic changes are a loss of iron from the liver, which may amount to 50% in three days, followed by a loss of copper much later. Both of these changes may result in anemia.

SELENIUM

Selenium is unique among mineral elements in that it is possible to consume natural foods containing either so little selenium that a deficiency results or so much that the food is toxic. The amount in food is a function of the amount of selenium in the soil on which it was grown. Areas of the United States with a high selenium content are in the Great Plains and the Rocky Mountains.

Biological role

Interest in selenium stems from the recognition in 1957 of its ability to replace vitamin E in some metabolic reactions, primarily those dependent on its antioxidant properties. In addition, selenium acts in conjunction with vitamin E in preventing certain conditions and under some circumstances, such as promoting normal growth and fertility, has specific functions of its own. Within the body the liver and kidney contain four to five times as much selenium as do muscles and other tissues. Once absorbed, selenium is excreted in the urine. Fecal selenium reflects unabsorbed mineral.

Selenium appears to be a complicating factor in kwashiorkor, in which treatment with adequate protein may be ineffective until sufficient selenium is provided.

In a study of dental caries in children it was observed that the total number of decayed, missing, and filled permanent teeth (DMF index) increased with an increase in the urinary excretion of selenium, although as yet we have no theory to explain this observation.

Food sources

Since cereals have a greater ability to concentrate selenium than do vegetables, they generally have a higher concentration, and within the cereal the bran and germ have the highest amounts.

Toxicity

At high levels of intake (5 to 10 ppm) selenium is toxic, apparently because of its capacity to replace sulfur in biological compounds and to inhibit the action of some enzymes. Likelihood of selenium poisoning in human beings is confined to persons exposed to industrial dusts containing the element. Toxicity is reduced by diets high in protein and is prevented completely in animals by arsenic. However, because it, too, is toxic, arsenic can be used only in limited amounts in humans.

Selenium found in cereal products is more toxic than selenium salts, which are only slightly soluble and are poorly absorbed.

MANGANESE

Although no deficiency of manganese has been demonstrated in man, it is considered an essential nutrient on the basis of our knowledge of its biochemical role in many essential biochemical reactions within the body. It is necessary for normal skeletal development, especially of the long bone. Manganese acts as a catalyst or as part of the essential enzymes involved in the synthesis of fatty acids and cholesterol; in the formation of urea, by which nitrogen is excreted; and in changes in the mitochondrion of the cell, essential for the release of energy.

Absorption and metabolism

Manganese is believed to be absorbed by a mechanism similar to that involved in iron absorption. A specific protein carrier, transmanganin, is available to transport manganese in the blood. Of the 10 mg. stored in the body, most is concentrated in the pancreas, bone, liver, and kidney. Little of the element is excreted in the urine. The major path of excretion is the bile, from which a significant amount is reabsorbed. Large intakes of calcium depress manganese absorption.

Requirement and food sources

Although the requirement for manganese has not been established, the 4 mg. per day found in a typical Western diet is considered adequate.

Whole-grain cereals and green vegetables are among the better sources of manganese, but the amount present de-

pends on the part of the plant and the geographical source. Tea (150 to 900 ppm) is an extremely rich source and in English diets is estimated to provide 3.3 mg. of manganese. Relative manganese values of common foodstuffs are given in Table 8-5.

Toxicity

Although the accumulation of excessive amounts of manganese is toxic, it is usually the result of inhalation as the result of industrial contamination rather than a high dietary intake. Weakness and psychological and motor difficulties are manifestations of high tissue levels. Iron metabolism is also adversely effected.

COPPER

Copper was first recognized as a dietary essential in 1928 when it was observed that anemia could be prevented only if copper as well as iron was available. Since that time many metabolic functions of copper have been identified but often have been difficult to assess because of the interaction of copper with other trace elements, such as zinc, molybdenum, and sulfur.

Functions

The role of copper in preventing anemia has been attributed variously to its effectiveness in facilitating iron absorption, in stimulating the synthesis of heme or globin fractions of the hemoglobin molecule, or in releasing stored iron from the liver. The

Table 8-5. Dietary sources of manganese

Rich sources (> 20 ppm)	Moderate sources (1-5 ppm)	Poor sources (< 1 ppm)
Nuts	Green leafy vegetables	Animal tissues
Whole-grain cereals	Dried fruits	Poultry
Dried legumes	Fresh fruits	Dairy products
Tea	Nonleafy vegetables	Seafood

evidence is conflicting, but most research supports the latter theory. There is some suggestion that copper is involved in the maturation of red blood cells or in their survival time in the blood.

In addition to its role in preventing anemia, copper is required for the synthesis of the phospholipids essential in the formation of the myelin sheath surrounding nerve fibers. It is part of the respiratory enzymes cytochrome oxidase, necessary for the release of energy in the cell, and catalase. Copper is part of the enzyme tyrosinase, needed for the conversion of the amino acid tyrosine to melanin, the dark pigment of hair and skin. The absence of this enzyme is associated with albinism. In conjunction with ascorbic acid (vitamin C), copper maintains the activity of the enzymes involved in the synthesis of the protein elastin in the wall of the aorta and is possibly necessary for collagen metabolism.

Absorption and metabolism

Typical diets provide from 2 to 5 mg. of copper, about 30% of which is absorbed. Copper is taken up rapidly from the stomach and upper intestine, where the contents are still acid. Absorbed copper appears in the bloodstream in as little as 15 minutes after ingestion. Initially it appears loosely bound to the protein albumin or to some amino acids. Both these chelates represent the transport form of copper, and the amino acid chelate appears to have the special function of facilitating the transport of copper across membranes into the cells. Transport copper represents only 7% of the serum copper. It remains in equilibrium with the copper in tissues and can enter the glomerulus of the kidney, from which it is excreted in the urine or resorbed. Copper is removed from the serum by the liver. There copper is either excreted into the bile stored in a protein complex containing 2% copper or used in the synthesis of ceruloplasmin, another protein-copper complex that is released

again into the blood, where it accounts for 93% of serum copper. Some serum copper enters the bone marrow, where it is used in the synthesis of erythrocuprein, which constitutes 60% of the copper within the red blood cells. Another nonerythrocuprein copper compound that accounts for the rest of the copper in the red blood cells may also be produced in the bone marrow or may arise from the serum copper directly. Copper is excreted by two pathways. Fecal copper represents unabsorbed, dietary copper and copper released in the bile and that lost through the intestinal wall in the albumin-copper complex of the serum. Urinary copper accounts for a mere 4% of copper loss.

Distribution

The total copper content of the body is estimated at 75 to 150 mg. Seventy-five percent of this is concentrated in the bones and muscles, but on a weight basis the brain is the most concentrated site of copper, followed by the liver, heart, and kidney. The newborn infant has liver stores five to ten times those of the adult, but they drop to adult levels as early as 3 months of age.

Requirement

A dietary intake of 2 mg. of copper per day appears to maintain copper balance in the adult. It is recommended that copper intake be 0.08 mg. per kilogram of body weight. Infants with large prenatal stores require considerably less.

Food sources

Copper is widely distributed in foods in widely varying concentrations. The amount is to a certain extent a reflection of the copper content of the soil on which the plant or animal was raised. Copper content of representative foods is given in Table 8-6. The use of copper pipes in water systems may be a source of some ingested copper.

Table 8-6. Dietary sources of copper

Rich sources (> 8 ppm)	Intermediate sources (2-8 ppm)	Poor sources (< 2 ppm)
Organ meats	Leafy vegetables	Milk
Shellfish (especially oysters)	Eggs	Butter
	Muscle meat	Cheese
Nuts	Fish	Sugar
Cocoa	Poultry	Fresh fruits
Cherries	Peas	and vegetables
Mushrooms	Beans	
Whole-grain cereals	Fresh fruit	
	Refined cereals	

Deficiency

Although low blood levels of copper have been reported, no specific deficiency symptoms have been associated with them. Hypocupremia seldom occurs as a result of low dietary intakes alone but is more often found in association with hypoproteinemia, which may reflect a loss of copper-protein from the body into the feces, and with anemia.

Toxicity

Copper is toxic to man when it exists as unbound copper ion. In this way it acts as an inhibitor to many enzyme systems. There is no evidence of toxicity as the result of environmental contamination. The ingestion of copper salts at levels ten times that found in a normal diet leads to nausea and vomiting, possibly as a result of a disturbance of the balance between absorption and excretion. Chronic copper toxicity occurs in the hereditary condition Wilson's disease, in which the level of ceruloplasmin is greatly reduced in the presence of a positive copper balance. This results in an accumulation of copper in the liver, brain, kidney, and cornea of the eyes, where it is identified visually by brown or green rings. Successful control involves the reduction of dietary copper to the point where its accumulation in these tissues is inhibited. More recently a penicillin derivative, penicillamine, that promotes the excretion of copper has been used to help reduce these stores to normal levels.

MOLYBDENUM
Biological role

It has been clearly established that molybdenum is an essential part of two enzymes—xanthine oxidase, which is involved in the formation of uric acid from the purine xanthine and also aids in mobilizing iron from liver reserves, and aldehyde oxidase, which is necessary for the oxidation of aldehydes. It is unconfirmed, however, that the human cannot perform these changes by other means. On this basis there has been a reluctance to classify molybdenum unequivocally as an essential nutrient. Evidence of molybdenum toxicity at high levels includes diarrhea, anemia, and a depressed growth rate.

Interrelationships

Most of the interest in molybdenum nutriture has centered around its metabolic interrelationships with copper and sulfate. The toxicity manifest in animals as depressed growth and hemoglobin production from high levels of molybdenum obtained by ingesting foods grown in soils high in the element can be overcome by the addition of copper to the ration. Similarly, a high molybdenum intake simulates a copper deficiency. High intakes of molybdenum alter the activity of alkaline phosphatase and produce certain bone abnormalities.

Absorption

Molybdenum is readily absorbed from the gastrointestinal tract and is excreted mainly in the urine, but the amount absorbed and excreted is influenced to a large extent by the amount of sulfate in the diet. High-sulfate diets increase urinary but not fecal excretion levels.

Food sources

Peas and beans are relatively rich sources (3 to 9 ppm); whole-grain cereals and dark green leafy vegetables, good (0.2 to 0.6 ppm); and fruits and vegetables, poor (less than 0.1 ppm). A dietary deficiency is almost impossible.

CHROMIUM

Chromium, an element found in concentrations as low as 20 to 50 parts per billion (ppb) in food, has important functions in both animal and human nutrition. Although it has been impossible to produce an experimental diet completely devoid of chromium, substantial evidence exists that a low dietary intake is associated with a reduced tolerance for glucose, decreased glycogen reserves, retarded growth, disturbances of amino acid metabolism, and increase in aortic lesions. The addition of chromium to the diet has been effective in increasing glucose tolerance and reducing the increase in blood cholesterol levels associated with an increased intake of refined carbohydrates.

Chromium is poorly absorbed, only about 3% of dietary chromium being retained in the body. It is excreted in both the urine and the feces. In the blood it competes with iron for a protein carrier.

Unlike other trace elements, the amount of chromium in tissues is reduced with age. Chromium is also associated with the decrease in glucose tolerance. The level of chromium in the American diet is lower than that in many other countries. This is attributed to the extensive use of refined cereals and sugar, which contain a much smaller amount of the element than do the less highly refined products. A suboptimal intake over a period of years may be one factor associated with the increase in diabetes that occurs with increasing age in the United States. It is thought the chromium acts to bind insulin, which favors the uptake of glucose to the receptor site on the cell. The high concentration of chromium found closely bound in the RNA molecule also suggests a role in protein synthesis.

In animals, chromium protects against the toxic effects of lead.

The concentration of chromium in foods varies with species, soil, and season, but vegetables have been found to provide 30 to 50 ppb; grains and cereals, 40 ppb; and fruit, 20 ppb.

The fact that chromium is present in high concentrations in the new organism and especially in proliferating tissues, that it accumulates in high concentration in the brain and nucleic acids, and that the level in the plasma changes with the need to metabolize glucose all suggest a biological role.

The most promising method of assessing chromium nutriture is to determine the content in the hair.

COBALT
Biological role

In human nutrition the major role of cobalt is as an essential part of vitamin B_{12}, or cobalamin, which is necessary to prevent pernicious anemia. The human being does not have the ability to synthesize the vitamin and must thus depend on animal sources of the nutrient. These have been synthesized by microorganisms in the intestine of animals that can incorporate the cobalt obtained from the plants they eat. Thus cobalt is a direct dietary essential for animals and an indirect one for humans. The cobalt content of plants reflects the cobalt content of the soil in which they are grown.

Food sources

The 5 to 8 μg. of cobalt in the adult diet appears to be about ten times the cobalt present in the cobalamin required, and since human tissues cannot synthesize vitamin B_{12}, little cobalt is retained from other than animal sources. Cobalt content of some representative foods is given in Table 8-7, but it must be remembered that the amount present is dependent on the cobalt in the soil in which plants are grown. Approximately half of ingested cobalt is absorbed.

Toxicity

There is some evidence that high intakes of cobalt may have toxic effects. One that has been observed is the goitrogenic effect after the prolonged ingestion of cobaltous chloride. The enlarged thyroid gland returns to normal after the cessation of cobalt administration. High intakes in animals have been observed to cause polycythemia (increase in the number of red blood cells) and hyperplasia (increase in quantity) of bone marrow, which are believed to be related to the production of erythropoietin, the hormone that stimulates red blood cell formation in the bone marrow.

VANADIUM

The role of vanadium in human nutrition has been studied only recently, and as yet evidence is insufficient to consider it a dietary essential.

Vanadium may be necessary in prenatal life for calcification of bones and teeth, but a relationship between dietary vanadium and dental caries rate has not been identified. It is possible that vanadium replaces phosphorus in apatite crystals and increases the hardness of the tooth enamel.

Vanadium in the diet of humans at a level of 100 to 125 mg. per day may inhibit the synthesis of cholesterol by counteracting the stimulating effect that manganese exerts on cholesterol synthesis.

So far we have no reason to attribute any toxic effects to vanadium, although there have been extensive investigations of its role in bone marrow, liver, kidney, or adrenal tissue.

FLUORINE

Fluorine has recently but not unanimously been considered an essential nutrient. Because of the widespread interest and frequent controversy regarding the nutrient in the popular press, its role in the human nutrition should be clarified.

Historical background

Interest in the possible nutritional role of fluorine dates back to 1931 when it was established that in communities where people had a remarkable freedom from tooth decay but suffered from an undesirable brownish appearance on the tooth surface, the water contained considerably more of the mineral element fluorine than did most communal water supplies. The efforts to identify the factor had started in 1902 when a dentist in Colorado Springs became curious about the brown stain known as *Colo-*

Table 8-7. Dietary sources of cobalt listed according to micrograms per grams dry weight

Excellent (> 5)	Good (1.5-5)	Poor (< 0.05)
Liver	Lean beef	Cereal grains
Kidney	Lamb	Leguminous seeds
Oysters	Veal	Green leafy vegetables
Clams	Poultry	tables
	Saltwater fish	Yeast
	Milk	

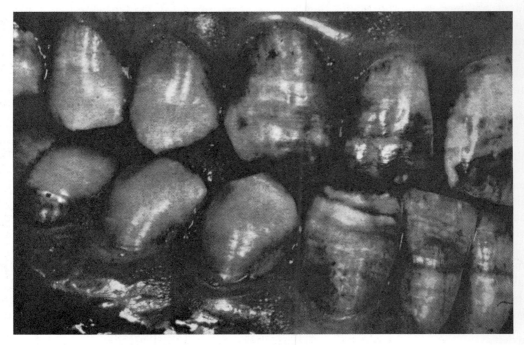

Fig. 8-7. Appearance of teeth in dental fluorosis. (From Duckworth, R.: Proc. Nutr. Soc. 22:79, 1963.)

rado brown stain on the teeth of many of his patients.

Once fluorine had been identified as the substance in the water supply responsible for the brown staining and the absence of dental caries, other studies soon showed that somewhat lower levels of fluorine in the water were responsible for a markedly lower incidence of tooth decay without the undesirable mottling of tooth enamel (dental fluorosis) illustrated in Fig. 8-7. The relationship between the fluorine content of the water and the rate of tooth decay was established in 1942. A water supply containing 1 ppm of fluorine accounted for a 50% to 60% lower incidence of tooth decay without any opacity or chalkiness in the tooth enamel. Only when the fluorine content of the water rose above 2.5 ppm did evidence of dental fluorosis occur.

Recognizing dental caries as a major public health problem and seeking some effective means of controlling it, the United States Public Health Service in 1945 initiated a study to determine if the addition of sufficient fluorine to the water supply to raise the natural fluorine content to 1 ppm would afford the same degree of protection against tooth decay as would a natural fluoride level of 1 ppm. Newburgh, on the Hudson River in New York, was chosen as the experimental city, with Kingston, across the river with a population of similar economic, racial, and cultural background and a low-fluorine water supply, serving as a control city. Careful records were kept of the incidence of tooth decay in both cities, and at the end of a ten-year period a report was made available. It showed that children under 10 years of age had received the greatest protection, having a DMF index 60% to 65% below those of their counterparts in Kingston. Children 12 to 14 years old who had consumed fluoridated water from early childhood but not since birth had a 48% reduc-

*Table 8-8. Reductions in decayed, missing, and filled permanent teeth (DMF index) reported among children in communities after ten years of fluoridation**

Community	Age studied	Percentage reduction
Grand Junction, Colo.	6	94.0
New Britain, Conn.	6-16	44.6
District of Columbia	6	59.1
Evanston, Ill.	6-7-8	91.3-64.6-62.6
Fort Wayne, Ind.	6-10	>50.0
Hopkinsville, Ky.	? (Children)	56.0
Louisville, Ky.	First 3 grades	62.1
Hagerstown, Md.	7, 9, 11, and 13	57.0
Grand Rapids, Mich.	6-7-8	75.0-63.0-57.0
Grand Rapids, Mich.	9-10	50.0-52.0
Newburgh, N. Y.	6-9	58.0
Newburgh, N. Y.	10-12	57.0
Newburgh, N. Y.	13-14	48.0
Newburgh, N. Y.	16	41.0
Charlotte, N. C.	6-11	60.0
Chattanooga, Tenn.	6-14	70.8
Marshall, Texas	7-15	54.0
Brantford, Ont.	6-7-8	60.0-67.0-54.0
Brantford, Ont.	9-10	46.0-41.0
Brantford, Ont.	11-13	44.0
Brantford, Ont.	14-16	35.0

*From Dunning, J. M.: Current status of fluoridation, New Eng. J. Med. **272:**30, 1965.

tion in tooth decay, and 16-year-olds who had been on it for an even shorter time had only a 40% reduction. A fifteen-year report on the same communities showed a similar degree of protection with no detectable adverse effects. A comparison of 6-year-olds in the two communities in 1962 showed that 33.9% of those in Newburgh were caries free compared to 16.4% in Kingston. In addition, comparable DMF rates were 0.09 and 0.65 per child respectively. These findings, showing that the earlier a child has an available source of fluorine the greater the protection it will provide, have since been confirmed and reconfirmed in fluoridation studies in many other communities. The child whose mother is drinking fluoridated water during pregnancy appears to receive maximum protection, although evidence shows that fluorine passes the placental barrier with difficulty.

However, evidence on this point is contradictory.

The effect of the fluoridation of the water supply on the dental health of children in various communities is shown in Table 8-8. The observed reduction of 50% to 60% approaches that observed in communities whose natural fluorine content is similar.

Several reports have been released showing an increase in tooth decay when a community dropped a fluoridation program that had been in effect for several years. Such reports indicating beneficial effects from the addition of fluorine and a reversal of these in its withdrawal help establish the fact that the benefits are caused by fluorine rather than other unidentified factors.

Aside from whatever benefits a pregnant woman *may* pass on to her child by drinking fluoridated water, there is little advantage as far as dental health is concerned from the consumption of fluoridated water by adults. However, there may be other benefits that accrue to the adult from the ingestion of fluorine-containing water. For instance, fluorine, by increasing the stability of the skeleton, may protect it against losses of calcium that often occur at menopause, under conditions of immobility, and, as recently observed, in space flight. The incidence of osteoporosis, an abnormality of bone metabolism that affects older people, is lower among persons using fluoridated water supplies than among those using low-fluorine water supplies.

Metabolism

Soluble fluoride is absorbed readily from the intestine, although some may be taken up by the stomach. About 90% of that ingested appears in the bloodstream. Of this, about 50% is excreted in the urine, and the other half is taken up readily by teeth and bones, where it apparently becomes an integral and important part of the tooth and bone structure. Regardless of the amount ingested, blood levels remain amazingly constant. Failure of blood plasma levels of fluorine to increase with an increase in dietary fluorine reflects the ability of the kidney to control the levels in body tissues by excreting amounts in excess of the body's needs. None appears in the soft tissues. The amount of fluorine appearing in other tissues, such as saliva, milk, and fetal blood, parallels that in the blood but at a slightly lower level.

Insoluble calcium and aluminum salts of fluorine retard the absorption of fluorine.

The affinity of bone for fluorine has given rise to concern over possible skeletal toxicity from the deposition of excess fluorine in the skeleton after ingestion of water with a high fluorine content. The homeostatic mechanism that maintains blood levels at a constant value undoubtedly prevents such a situation. Efforts to identify such an effect have shown that a lifelong ingestion of water containing 4 ppm of fluorine has no detrimental effects on bone formation. With continued exposure to high fluorine intakes, the bone ceases to take up more fluorine. Some evidence exists that fluorine delays the excretion of calcium, a factor that is advantageous in maintaining calcium balances. In fact, a dose of 50 mg. of fluorine per day has proved effective in improving calcium balance and preventing osteoporosis without any toxic effects.

Mode of action

The mechanisms by which fluorine imparts greater resistance to tooth decay have been studied extensively. It appears that where fluorine is available, some crystals of fluoroapatite replace the crystals of hydroxyapatite that are normally deposited during tooth formation. Fluorine at high concentrations may also replace some of the carbonate usually found in bone. These substances are apparently less soluble in acid and more resistant to the cariogenic action of acids in the oral environment. Fluorine is known to stimulate the action of some enzymes and to inhibit that of others. Consequently it may act in this way to reduce the formation of acid by the action of bacteria on carbohydrate in the mouth, thus reducing the likelihood of the solution of tooth enamel. It is known that both the dentin and enamel of teeth that have formed when fluorine is available do contain more fluorine than otherwise, indicating that fluorine does become an integral part of the tooth structure.

The enamel surface is still capable of taking up fluorine shortly after eruption during the final stages of tooth calcification. Fluorine available in the saliva is presumably preferentially absorbed on the tooth surface, adding strength and rigidity. In addition, some evidence exists that fluorine promotes the precipitation of calcium phosphate from saliva, which may facilitate the remineralization of teeth after decalcification in the oral environment during the initial stages of tooth decay. Larger, more nearly perfect crystals in bone have been observed as fluorine concentration of human bone increases. As much as 5000 to 6000 ppm in bone does not constitute a physiological hazard.

Sources

In addition to water, from which an adult usually ingests 1.5 mg. fluorine per day, another 1.3 to 1.8 mg. comes from tea and solid food high in fluorine content. The determination of the fluorine content of food is tedious. Results of some efforts are shown in Table 8-9.

Fluoridation of public water supplies

As soon as communities began to consider the fluoridation of their water supplies, groups of people began to oppose it for a wide variety of reasons, most of which revolved around its hazards, its ineffectiveness, and ethical considerations of so-called compulsory medication. Social issues assumed more importance than health issues. The opponents claimed that fluorine was toxic, that fluoridation of water supplies was a violation of the rights of the individual, and through a variety of highly emotional attacks on the program created doubt regarding the motives of the pro-

ponents of the measure. Any possibility of fluorine toxicity has been thoroughly investigated by the United States Public Health Service, which has been unable to find any evidence of detrimental effects from the addition of 1 ppm of fluorine to the drinking water no matter how large the water consumption. Based on the health records of 2 million people in artificially fluoridated areas, no evidence exists of increased deposition of fluorine in soft tissues, such as the kidney or heart, no increase in mortality and morbidity rates, no growth depression or abnormalities, no increase in cancer or nephritis, and no increase in birth rate of mongoloids, all of which have been claimed by the antifluoridation forces. Claims that fluorine interfered with cell growth and protein synthesis have been discredited by studies showing that cellular reproduction continues in the presence of an amount of fluorine far in excess of the amount that can be brought into the circulating fluids by oral intakes of fluorine. On the contrary, in addition to a reduction in tooth decay, a reduction in the amount of periodontal disease, a 30% reduction in the incidence of malocclusion, and among older people a decreased incidence of the bone abnormality osteoporosis was found.

Fluorine is toxic but only at levels well beyond that at which it is added to communal water supplies. Mottled enamel, or dental fluorosis, which presents only aesthetic problems, may occur at concentrations of 2 to 8 ppm, osteosclerosis at 8 to 20 ppm, growth depression at 50 ppm or more, and fatal poisoning at 2500 times recommended levels. Extreme precautions and constant surveillance of the level of fluorine in the water assure the public that the level in their water could not approach toxic levels. As an added precaution, it is suggested that in tropical areas where water consumption may be higher, the level of fluoridation should be reduced to 0.7 ppm.

Table 8-9. Fluorine content of some representative foods*

Food	mg./100 gm.
Tea	0.475
Coffee	0.250
Rice	0.07
Buckwheat	0.17
Soybeans	0.40-0.67
Spinach	0.02
Onions	0.05
Lettuce	0.01

*From Gordenoff, T., and Mender, W.: Fluorine, World Rev. Nutr. Diet. **2:**213, 1962.

In spite of the evidence that the addition of fluorine to the water supply to provide a total fluorine content of 1 ppm has no adverse effects at this level, and in spite of the endorsement of fluoridation by every medical and dental group in the United States, the United States Public Health Service, and many Asian and European countries, fluoridation remains a controversial issue. The antifluoridation groups have become so vocal that in many cases where fluoridation has come up for a public referendum, it has been defeated. In 1966 only 40.6% of the people on public water systems were receiving fluoridated water. Another 6% were consuming naturally fluoridated water. Of 1899 communities that have considered fluoridation up to 1966, 1126 rejected it. In most cases where it has been rejected, the decision was made at public referendum, and where it has been accepted, the decision was generally an administrative or legislative one.

In 1965 Connecticut become the first state to require fluoridation of the water supply in all cities over 50,000 population. By 1967 this had been extended to cities of 20,000 or more. Minnesota, Illinois, and Kéntucky have passed similar legislation. In a few cases, fluoridation has been terminated after a period of successful use. In spite of the efforts of the antifluoridation forces, 62 million people in over 2800 communities in 1968 were consuming water to which fluorine had been added, and another 10 million were drinking water in which the natural fluorine content was at a protective level. With the decision to fluoridate the water supply of New York City in 1965, another 8.5 million persons (for a total of 80 million) are receiving the benefits of a fluoridation program. In all cases where it has been introduced, a significant reduction occurred in tooth decay among children, a protection that carries over into adulthood.

Different forms of fluoride—sodium fluoride, sodium silicofluoride, and fluorosilicic acid—have all been used effectively to provide the fluoride ions as active agents in the water supply. None of these appear to influence the odor, taste, color, or hardness of the water, and all can be readily introduced into the community water system without causing a depreciation in plumbing equipment. The cost of fluoridation varies, depending on the chemical chosen and the engineering complexity of the water system, but most cities report a cost of from 10 cents to $1.15 per person per year. In the light of the fact that over 95% of the population without fluorine experience tooth decay and will stand to benefit financially as well as through a reduction in physical discomfort accompanying tooth decay, the cost seems small. In Philadelphia it was estimated that fluoridation had saved 360,000 teeth valued at over $2 million in dental bills during a thirteen-year period. In Newburgh the cost of the initial dental care of 5- to 8-year-old children who had been on fluoridated water all their lives was less than half and annual dental costs slightly more than half that of their counterparts in Kingston. Defluoridation, or the removal of natural fluorine from the water, has been undertaken in some communities where fluorine is naturally present at a level that causes mottling of tooth enamel. It has cost $1.00 per person per year.

Other methods of acquiring fluorine

Fluoridation of the water supply has proved the most feasible means of providing protection against tooth decay, but for persons who either do not have access to a community water supply or who live in communities that have not introduced it, other methods of obtaining the benefits of fluorine have been tried. The most frequent method is the use of sodium fluoride tablets. A year's supply of 2 mg. tablets to be taken daily that will release 1 mg. of fluorine costs only 15 cents per person, but distribution costs add another $3.50 per year. A major deterrent to the success of tablets is the failure of parents to continue to provide them throughout the whole growth period or at least for the first ten years. In Hawaii, where tablets were distributed free, 90% of the parents provided them for their children at the beginning of the program, but four years later only 12% were still using them. In Switzerland the use of tablets proved more successful, with only a 20% to 35% reduction reported. For infants the tablets must be dissolved in the formula or fruit juice, and care must be taken to see that they do not inadvertently get an overdose. Many of the commonly used infant vitamin supplements have fluorine added, but in areas where the water supply is fluoridated, their sale is restricted to prescription distribution.

Two studies on the feasibility of adding fluorine to the water supply in the schools in communities that did not have a community fluoridation program showed that a reduction in dental caries incidence of 33% could be achieved in an eight-year period by the addition of either 3 or 5 ppm of fluorine. This higher level was used to compensate for the fact that the children had access to the water supply for only part of the day, five days a week. There was no incidence of dental fluorosis.

A proposal that fluorine can be injected into the gum area just prior to the time that the teeth erupt, when they are most receptive to the uptake of fluorine ions, has received some scientific backing.

Topical applications of 8% stannous fluoride solution to the dry surface of teeth shortly after they erupt has been relatively successful, providing about 40% protection against caries, but the professional time involved makes the yearly treatment rela-

tively expensive and hence unavailable to many who would benefit most. The application of a phosphate fluoride every two years has resulted in a 70% reduction in caries. Although successful, these methods have limited value because of a shortage of dentists needed to carry out the process.

In Switzerland an attempt to add fluorine to salt was unsuccessful, especially since infants who need fluorine are seldom given salt. Attempts to add fluorine to the milk supply were also of limited usefulness.

The value of fluoridated dentifrices that contain about 0.1% fluorine is still being evaluated, and at the present time the evidence seems controversial. One problem revolves around the observation that fluorine content decreases with storage. It is possible that fluorine inhibits the action of enzymes or bacteria involved in the formation of acid in the mouth. It has been shown that the plaques that form on teeth, on which it is believed that bacteria act to produce the acid that initiates the solution of enamel and tooth decay, contain almost twice as much fluorine where there is a 2 ppm in the water supply compared to a fluorine-free area. Apparently the enamel surface is capable of taking in some fluorine ions from the fluids to which it is exposed in the mouth.

With concern over the waste that occurs when only 1% of the fluoridated water is used for human consumption, the possibility of adding flourine to a staple food item such as salt, flour, bread, milk, or sugar has been investigated. Of these, flour and salt seem to be utilized most effectively, although some limitations in their usefulness have been indicated.

SELECTED REFERENCES
General

Mills, C. F.: Metabolic interrelationships in the utilization of trace elements, Proc. Nutr. Soc. 23:38, 1964.

Underwood, E. J.: Trace elements in human and animal nutrition, ed. 3, New York, 1968, Academic Press, Inc.

Iron

Beaton, G. H., Thein, M., Milne, H., and Veen, M. J.: Iron requirements of menstruating women, Amer. J. Clin. Nutr. **23:**275, 1970.

Brown, E. B.: The absorption of iron, Amer. J. Clin. Nutr. **12:**205, 1963.

Brown, E. B.: The utilization of iron in erythropoiesis, Amer. J. Clin. Nutr. **12:**77, 1963.

Charley, P. J., Still, C., Shore, E., and Soltman, P.: Studies in the regulation of intestinal iron absorption, J. Lab. Clin. Med. **61:**397, 1963.

Council on Foods and Nutrition: Iron deficiency in the United States, J.A.M.A. **203:**119, 1968.

Crosby, W. H.: Intestinal response to the body's requirement for iron, J.A.M.A. **208:**347, 1969.

Editorial: Iron overload, J.A.M.A. **191:**668, 1965.

Finch, C. A.: The role of iron in hemoglobin synthesis, Conference on Hemoglobin, Publication No. 557, Washington, D. C., 1957, National Academy of Sciences.

Finch, C. A.: Iron-deficiency anemia, Amer. J. Clin. Nutr. **22:**512, 1969.

Hallberg, L., and Solvell, L.: Absorption of hemoglobin iron in man, Amer. J. Dig. Dis. **9:**787, 1964.

Jacobs, A., and Greenman, D. A.: Availability of food iron, Brit. Med. J. **1:**673, 1969.

Kasper, C. K., Whissell, V. E., and Wallerstein, R. O.: Clinical aspects of iron deficiency, J.A.M.A. **191:**359, 1965.

Linman, J. W.: Physiologic and pathophysiologic effects of anemia, New Eng. J. Med. **279:**812, 1968.

Man, Y. K., and Wadsworth, G. R.: Dietary intake and urinary loss of iron, Proc. Nutr. Soc. **27:**12A, 1968.

Peden, J.: Present knowledge of iron and copper, Nutr. Rev. **25:**321, 1967.

Schade, S. G., Cohen, R. J., and Conrad, M. E.: Effect of hydrochloric acid on iron absorption, New Eng. J. Med. **279:**672, 1968.

Scheffer, L. M., Price, D. C., and Cronkite, E. P.: Iron absorption and anemia, J. Lab. Clin. Med. **65:**316, 1965.

White, W. H.: Iron deficiency in young women, Amer. J. Public Health **60:**659, 1970.

Iodine

Matovinovic, J.: Endemic goiter, J. Amer. Med. Wom. Ass. **17:**427, 495, 571, 646, 1962.

Review: Endemic goiter, Nutr. Rev. **21:**73, 1963.

Vought, R. L., and London, W. T.: Dietary sources of iodine, Amer. J. Clin. Nutr. **14:**186, 1964.

Vought, R. L., and London, W. T.: Iodine intake and excretion in healthy nonhospitalized subjects, Amer. J. Clin. Nutr. **15:**124, 1964.

Zinc

Luecke, R. V.: Significance of zinc in nutrition, Borden Rev. Nutr. Res. **26:**45, 1965.

Mayer, J.: Zinc deficiency, a cause of growth retardation, Postgrad. Med. **35:**206, 1964.

Prasad, A. S.: Importance of zinc in human nutrition, Amer. J. Clin. Nutr. **20:**648, 1967.

Prasad, A. S.: A century of research on the metabolic role of zinc, Amer. J. Clin. Nutr. **22:**1215, 1969.

Sullivan, J. F., and Lankford, H. G.: Zinc metabolism and chronic alcoholism, Amer. J. Clin. Nutr. **17:**57, 1965.

Vallee, B. L.: The metabolic role of zinc, J.A.M.A. **162:**1053, 1956.

Selenium

Hadjimarkos, D. M., and Bonhorst, C. W.: The selenium content of eggs, milk and water in relation to dental caries in children, J. Pediat. **59:**256, 1961.

Copper

Cartwright, G. E., and Wintrobe, M. M.: Copper metabolism in normal subjects, Amer. J. Clin. Nutr. **14:**224, 1964.

Dowdy, R. P.: Copper metabolism, Amer. J. Clin. Nutr. **21:**887, 1969.

Gubler, C. J.: Copper metabolism in man, J.A.M.A. **161:**530, 1956.

Review: Copper deficiency in malnourished infants, Nutr. Rev. **23:**164, 1960.

Sturgeon, P., and Brubaker, C.: Copper deficiency in infants, Amer. J. Dis. Child. **92:**254, 1956.

Chromium

Mertz, R.: Chromium occurrence and function in biological systems, Physiol. Rev. **49:**163, 1969.

Schroeder, H. A.: The role of chromium in mammalian nutrition, Amer. J. Clin. Nutr. **21:**230, 1968.

Vanadium

Dimond, E. G., Caravaca, J., and Benchumol, A.: Vanadium excretion, toxicity and lipid effect in man, Amer. J. Clin. Nutr. **12:**49, 1963.

Fluorine

Ast, D. B., Cons, N. C., Carlos, J. P., and Polans, A.: Time and cost factors to provide regular, periodic dental care for children in a fluoridated and nonfluoridated area, Amer. J. Public Health **57:**1635, 1969.

Ast, D. B., and Fitzgerald, B.: Effectiveness of water fluoridation, J. Amer. Dent. Ass. **65:**581, 1962.

Blomquist, C. H., Singer, L., Pollock, M. E., McLaren, L. C., and Armstrong, W. D.: Sodium fluoride and cell growth, Brit. Med. J. 1:486, 1965.

Bonner, F.: Fluoridation—issue or obscession? Amer. J. Clin. Nutr. 22:1346, 1969.

Bransby, E. R., Forrest, J. R., and Mansbridge, J. N.: Dental effects of fluoridation of water with particular reference to a study in the United Kingdom, Proc. Nutr. Soc. 22:84, 1963.

Duckworth, R.: Fluoridation, Proc. Nutr. Soc. 22:79, 1963.

Dunning, J. M.: Current status of fluoridation, New Eng. J. Med. 272:30, 84, 1965.

Foster, R. D.: Self-application of topically applied stannous fluoride, J. Amer. Dent. Ass. 70:329, 1965.

Hodge, H. C.: Safety factors in water fluoridation based on toxicology of fluoride, Proc. Nutr. Soc. 22:111, 1963.

Korns, R. F.: Relationship of water fluoridation to bone density in two New York towns, Public Health Rep. 84:815, 1969.

Latham, M., and Grech, P.: The effect of excessive fluoride intake, Amer. J. Public Health 57: 651, 1967.

Review: Attitudes toward fluoridation, Nutr. Rev. 22:291, 1964.

Sapolsky, H. M.: Social science views a controversy in science and politics, Amer. J. Clin. Nutr. 22:1397, 1969.

Schlesinger, E. R.: Dietary fluorides and caries prevention, Amer. J. Public Health 55:1123, 1965.

Sognnaes, R. F.: Fluoride protection of bones and teeth, Science 150:989, 1965.

Weech, A. A.: Fluoridation, Amer. J. Dis. Child. 108:571, 1964.

9 | *Water*

If it is possible to say that one essential nutrient is more essential than another, we would have to concede that it is water. And yet it is the nutrient most often taken for granted to the point that it is sometimes omitted from a list of essential nutrients. The human being can live for weeks and even years without an intake of some essential vitamins and minerals but will survive only a few days in the absence of water, even though the body possesses rather involved mechanisms for conserving water when the supply is short. The longest time man has survived without water is seventeen days, but two or three days is the usual limit.

With 6% of the water in the adult body and 15% of that in the infant's body turned over each day, the exchange of water far exceeds that of any other nutrient. Although up to 8 pounds, or 4 quarts, of water may be taken in and another 4 quarts may be lost each day from the body, homeostatic mechanisms are so sensitive that a variation in body weight seldom occurs beyond ⅓ pound per day due to change in body fluids.

Distribution

Water constitutes 60% of the total body weight and 70% of the lean body mass. This proportion will vary from 50% to 75%, depending on age and the amount of body fat. Water is a constituent of every cell of the body. It is present in widely varying concentrations in different tissues, constituting 72% of muscle, 20% to 35% of adipose tissue, and 10% of bone and cartilage.

The distribution of fluids in the body is described in terms of an intracellular compartment representing the water within the cells, which accounts for two thirds of the total body water, and an extracellular compartment, comprising the other third. The compartments were shown in Fig. 6-2. The intracellular fluid is enclosed inside the cell membrane of each individual cell. The extracellular component is usually further subdivided into two compartments: the intravascular and the intercellular. The intravascular fluid includes the water in the blood vessels, arteries, veins, and capillaries and accounts for 4.5% of body weight and 7.5% of total body water. The intercellular (extravascular, or interstitial) fluid includes that which has left the blood vessels and is present in the spaces surrounding each cell. Exchange of fluids between the intracellular and intercellular compartments and between the intercellular and intravascular compartment, all of which are separated by a semipermeable membrane, occurs freely and is regulated by many factors, including the relative concentrations of protein and of electrolytes, such as sodium and potassium. The direction and the rate of exchange are determined by osmotic pressure due to the presence of electrolytes, oncotic pressure due to the presence of nonelectrolytes, such as protein, and hydrostatic pressure due to the force exerted by the pumping action of the heart on the fluid in the blood vessels. As much as 50 quarts of fluid cross membranes each day.

There are two other fluid compartments that do not participate as extensively in the dynamic exchange of fluid. Transcellular water is that which is present in such fluids as the spinal fluid, the ocular fluid in the eyeballs, the synovial fluid that lubricates joints, and the fluids in the mucous secretions of the linings of the respiratory tract, the gastrointestinal tract, and the genitourinary tract. It comprises 2.5% of total body water. The water in dense connective tissue, cartilage, and bone is part of its structural material and accounts for 15% of total body water.

Functions

Three to 5 liters of fluid are present in the arteries, veins, and capillaries, where the fluid acts as a solvent for the nutrients —monosaccharides, amino acids, fats (as phospholipids), vitamins, and minerals— and for the hormones secreted by the glands, all of which must be transported to all parts of the body if the individual cells are to be adequately nourished. This intravascular fluid also acts as a solvent and transporter of the waste products of metabolism, such as carbon dioxide, ammonia, and electrolytes, which must be carried from the cells to the lungs, skin, or kidney to be excreted.

Twelve liters of fluid in the extravascular, or interstitial, compartment carry nutrients that have left the blood vessels into close proximity to the membrane of the cell. It also collects waste products and hormones or other substances that may be secreted by the cell. Much of this fluid reenters the circulatory system, being pulled back when the oncotic pressures built up by the blood proteins that do not leave the bloodstream exceed the hydrostatic pressure that forced the fluid out of the intervascular compartment. Any remaining intercellular fluid in excess of normal amounts is accumulated by the lymphatic system and is eventually returned to the bloodstream. The amount of water in the extravascular, or intercellular, compartment fluctuates more than that in other compartments, since it can tolerate greater variations than other compartments. The blood volume is usually maintained at a fairly constant level at the expense of the intercellular fluid. Similarly, the intracellular fluid, which must also be maintained at a constant level to prevent the swelling or shrinking of cells, draws on the intercellular fluid. The intercellular fluid may thus be thought of as a buffer zone.

Within the cell intracellular water is used as a body builder, being incorporated in the synthesis of a new material. Glycogen, the form in which carbohydrate is stored, accumulates only in the presence of water. The deposition of fat involves the accumulation of an additional 20% water. Water also acts as a catalyst in many biological reactions within the cell and as a solvent for nutrients that must be transported from one organelle to another within the cell as well as for the waste products that must be eliminated.

In the transcellular fluids, such as saliva, water acts as a lubricant, facilitating the passage of food down the esophagus. In the stomach and small intestine, where digestion of food occurs, the water is necessary for the hydrolytic reactions required to break the complex nutrients into their simpler component parts, since most of these reactions are hydrolytic, or water requiring. Some of this water is derived from food and beverages, but a great deal of it comes from the digestive juices secreted into the gastrointestinal tract. This may amount to 8 to 10 quarts a day. In the synovial fluid of joints the prime function of water is to act as a lubricant.

In addition to the well-established roles of water in the body that we have already discussed, it is becoming increasingly evident that the amount of water in the diet exerts a definite influence on the metabolism of other nutrients. When 20% water was added to diets containing 6%, 9%, or 12% protein, a significant gain occurred in the protein efficiency ratio (PER), the weight gain per gram of protein. Some work has indicated that the intake of food is a response to the intake of fluid. Under circumstances such that thirst is depressed, food intake may also be reduced.

Studies to determine limiting factors in the work output of an individual suggest that a lack of water has a much more profound effect on work production than a lack of food.

Another important role of water, beyond acting as a solvent and transporter for nutrients and metabolic waste products and as a lubricant, is in the regulation of body temperature. Although some heat is lost by radiation and conduction from the skin, especially at low environmental temperatures, the evaporation of water from the surface of the body is the most effective method of ridding the body of extra heat produced in the metabolism of carbohydrate, fat, and protein. Some of this heat is required to maintain body temperature at 98.6° F., the temperature at which all enzymes crucial to metabolic processes operate most effectively. Because of its ability to conduct heat, water assists in the even distribution of heat throughout the body. But the metabolism of energy-yielding nutrients to provide energy for chemical, muscular, and osmotic work in the body yields as a by-product more heat than is necessary to maintain normal body temperature. If this is not released promptly, the body temperature increases to a point where all cellular enzymes will be inactivated. The evaporation of fluid from the skin requires energy in the form of heat, and the body is constantly cooling itself by causing water to be lost through evaporation. The loss of heat through the skin represents about 25% of the total caloric expenditure. This water loss, which amounts to 350 to 700 ml. per day under normal conditions of temperature and humidity, is referred to as "insensible perspiration loss." The greater the body surface area, the greater the amount of heat that can be lost

through the skin. A layer of subcutaneous fat that acts as an insulating material, reducing the speed with which heat is lost from the body, is an advantage in the winter and a disadvantage in the summer. Heat loss may also be affected by the proximity of the circulating fluids to the surface of the skin.

Water balance

Sources of body water. In contrast to all other nutrients, which must be provided in food, water is available to the body from several sources.

The major source is the fluids consumed as beverages. The amount of fluids will vary from one individual to another. Infants consume more per unit of body weight than do adults. Persons living in the tropics, where there is greater evaporation from the skin, consume more than those in temperate climates, and persons engaged in strenuous physical activity consume more than sedentary individuals. The amount consumed by adults as fluids varies from 900

Table 9-1. Water content of representative foods*

Food	Water (%)
Lettuce	96
Asparagus	92
Milk	87
Oranges	86
Potatoes	80
Cottage cheese	79
Veal	66
Chicken	63
Beef	47
Cheddar cheese	37
Bread	36
Butter	15
Gelatin	13
White sugar	0.5

*From Watt, B. K., and Merrill, A. L.: Composition of foods—raw, processed and prepared, U. S. Department of Agriculture Handbook No. 8, Washington, D. C., 1963, U. S. Department of Agriculture.

to 1500 ml., with an average of 1100 ml. under normal circumstances.

So-called solid foods vary in their water content from none to 96% water. The water content of some representative foods is given in Table 9-1, from which it is evident that many foods considered solid foods contain over 70% water. A 2000 kcal. diet chosen according to a typical food plan provides from 500 to 800 ml. of water.

The end products of combustion of carbohydrate, fat, and protein include water, in addition to carbon dioxide and energy. A constant amount of water is released during the oxidation or burning of each of these—1 gm. of carbohydrate yielding 0.6 gm. of water; 1 gm. of protein, 0.42 gm.; and 1 gm. of fat, 1 gm. This amounts to 15, 10.5, and 11.1 gm., respectively, from the ingestion of 100 kcal. from carbohydrate, protein, and fat. Thus, for an individual utilizing 2000 kcal. a day, 50% of which came from carbohydrate, 35% from fat, and 15% from protein, the water of metabolism would amount to 264 ml. per day, as shown in the calculation in Table 9-2. This amounts to 13.2 gm. per 100 kcal.

Loss of body water. Counterbalancing the intake of water, water is lost by several pathways—urinary losses, respiratory losses through the lungs, and evaporation losses through the skin.

Most of the ingested water is absorbed very rapidly through the walls of the intestinal tract—so rapidly that we find little relationship between the amount of water ingested and the amount found in the stomach.

Once absorbed, water is taken up by the bloodstream, which is 80% water, carried to the kidney, where it is used as a solvent for waste products from the body, and excreted as urine, which is 97% water. The fluid is filtered through the kidney tubule at the rate of 125 ml. per minute, which amounts to 120 to 190 liters per day. Here sufficient water is resorbed to retain normal blood volumes, and the rest, 1 ml. per minute, is excreted. If the fluid intake is high, urine volume is increased above the normal level of 1 to 2 liters, and the concentration of excretory products in the urine will be low. Such a urine has a low specific gravity. When fluid intake is low, more must be resorbed to maintain blood volume, and a much smaller amount will be used in the urine as a solvent for the excretory products. Since there is a limit to the extent to which the kidney can concentrate urine, there is a minimum urine volume necessary to rid the body of waste products. This minimum has been estimated at somewhere between 300 and 500 ml. but depends on the solute load to be excreted. If less than this amount of fluid is available for urine formation, waste products of metabolism will be retained in the tissue, where they may concentrate up to toxic levels. Under circumstances such as disasters and manned space flights when

Table 9-2. Calculation of water of metabolism produced on a 2000 kcal. diet

Source of kcal.	Percent of kcal. provided	Distribution of kcal. in 2000 kcal. diet	Weight of nutrient (gm.)	Water of metabolism per gram	Total water of metabolism
Carbohydrate	50	1000	250	0.6	150
Fat	35	700	77	1.07	82
Protein	15	300	75	0.42	32
					264

the fluid available is very limited and must be conserved, the mandatory excretion through the kidney can be reduced by limiting the intake of foods that normally give rise to metabolites, which must be excreted in the urine. Restricting protein and salt intake are the easiest, most effective methods of reducing the necessary urine volume. The provision of sufficient carbohydrate (100 gm.) to prevent ketosis will help reduce the solute load of ketones and electrolytes. Very young infants with poorly developed kidney function can excrete very small amounts of electrolytes.

Loss of water through the skin, as already discussed, amounts to 350 to 700 ml. per day. It has been reported as high as 2500 ml. per hour, and 500 ml. per hour is not uncommon at high environmental temperature and low humidity. Infants experience a high rate of evaporation from the skin, which compensates for small urinary losses.

Water along with carbon dioxide is constantly being lost through the lungs. The amount released this way is 300 ml. but will increase at high altitudes, which lead to increased respiration rates. Where the atmosphere is unusually dry, the total lost through the lungs and skin equals urinary losses.

During a 24-hour period as much as 8 to 10 liters of water (with 3700 ml. considered a minimum) may be secreted into the digestive tract as digestive juices. Practically all of this is reabsorbed as it passes down the gastrointestinal tract so that as little as 200 ml. will be excreted in the feces. These secretions include saliva, gastric juices, intestinal and pancreatic juices, bile, and secretion of lymph glands. The volume of digestive juices secreted is determined to a certain extent by the moisture content of the food. When food is dry, the secretion of saliva is increased to exert a maximum lubricating effect on the food, facilitating swallowing and the action of digestive enzymes. Secretion of bile is stimu-

Table 9-3. Water exchange in gastrointestinal tract

Source	ml.	
Gastric secretions		8200
Saliva	1500	
Gastric juice	2500	
Bile	500	
Pancreatic juices	700	
Intestinal juices	3000	
Water intake		2000
Total intake		10,200
Absorbed	10,000	
Fecal	200	

Table 9-4. Typical water balance in adult

Sources and loss	ml.
Sources of water	
Liquid food	1100
Solid food	500-1000
Water of oxidation	300- 400
Total	1900-2500
Loss of water	
Urine	1000-1400
Insensible perspiration	500
Perspiration and evaporation from lungs	300- 500
Feces	100
Total	1900-2500

lated by ingestion of large amounts of fat, and the volume of the gastric, pancreatic, and intestinal juices may fluctuate in response to the variation in moisture content of the food.

The sources of water in the gastrointestinal tract in a 24-hour period for a normal adult are shown in Table 9-3. These figures indicate that 10 quarts of fluid cross the intestinal wall in each direction each day.

• • •

In summary, it becomes obvious that to compensate for water losses in the urine

Table 9-5. Fluid requirement per kilogram of body weight	
Classifications	*ml./kg.*
Infants	110
10-year-old children	40
Adults	
72° F.	22
100° F.	38

and feces and through the skin and lungs, fluid intake must be at least 2 liters from food and beverages. Even under the most favorable conditions of low solute load, minimal physical activity, and absence of sweating, the total water from food, drink, and metabolic water should be at least 1.5 liters per day. About 40% of the liquid comes from tap water; the rest comes from milk and other beverages. Table 9-4 summarizes water balance within the body.

Requirements

The need for fluid in relation to body weight varies with age; the younger the person, the greater is the fluid requirement per unit of body weight. Fluid requirements under various conditions of age and environmental temperatures are shown in Table 9-5.

As a guide it is suggested that adults should consume 1000 ml. of water for every 1000 kcal. in the diet and infants, 1500 ml. Usually about two thirds of this comes from beverages and the remainder from solid food. Since this is considerably less than the 4700 to 17,000 ml. of water that may be turned over in the body each day, the body must have extensive mechanisms for conserving water.

Regulation of body fluid. The regulation of body fluid content is a function of the kidney, which resorbs a sufficient amount to maintain blood volume at a normal level. When the sodium concentration of the blood rises by as little as 1%, as it will when the volume diminishes, the thirst-regulating center of the brain is stimulated and the individual consumes more water. At the same time, the secretion of the antidiuretic hormone (ADH) will stimulate the kidney to resorb more fluid and to excrete a more concentrated urine when the blood volume drops.

Disturbances in water metabolism. Water is an essential part of cell cytoplasm, and the functioning of the cell is dependent on a certain concentration of nutrients in the internal environment of the cell. Any loss or accumulation of fluid in cells can lead to acute metabolic difficulties. This may result from abnormal loss, such as in diarrhea, nausea, or fever; abnormal retention; a defect in intestinal absorption; or an altered distribution of fluids within the body. When body fluids are reduced as much as 10%, symptoms of severe dehydration appear, whereas a 20% reduction is fatal. An increase to levels 10% above normal represents edema.

Under conditions of high environmental temperature the body loses large amounts of water through perspiration. Along with the water loss an appreciable loss of sodium occurs. The loss of water will stimulate the thirst center in the hypothalamus of the brain, leading to an increased consumption of water to replace that lost in perspiration. If this water intake is not accompanied by a source of sodium to replace that lost in perspiration along with the water, the individual suffers from a condition known as *water intoxication,* in which the sodium concentration in the fluids becomes very diluted. To protect against this, industries in which men work at high temperatures frequently require that their employees take salt tablets when they drink water. Travellers in tropical areas who are unaccustomed to high heat may find it necessary to use salt tablets to avoid the weakness that accompanies a loss of sodium from the body. A similar precaution may be necessary for persons who engage in strenuous physical exercise even in a temperate climate. Severe muscle cramps may result from the loss of electrolytes during sweating.

Another form of water intoxication, in which the intake of water exceeds the maximum rate of urine flow of 16 ml. per minute, is caused by an uptake of the extra water by the cells, again causing a dilution of the cellular constituents, in addition to the swelling of cells. When this occurs in brain cells, convulsions, coma, and death can result.

SELECTED REFERENCES

Brooke, C. E., and Anast, C. S.: Oral fluid and electrolytes, J.A.M.A. **179:**792, 1962.

Johnson, R. E.: Water and osmotic economy, J. Amer. Diet. Ass. **45:**124, 1964.

Robinson, J. R.: Water, the indispensible nutrient, Nutr. Today **5:**16, 1970.

Walker, J. S., Margolis, F. J., Teate, H. L., Weil, M. L., and Wilson, H. L.: Water intake of normal children, Science **140:**890, 1963.

10 | *Vitamins*

DISCOVERY

Vitamins were the last group of dietary essentials to be recognized. This is easy to understand, since they are needed in such very small amounts. Their presence in food is correspondingly low and hence was easily overlooked in the early analysis of foods. The minimum need for vitamins varies from a low of a few micrograms to a high of 30 mg., those needed in the smallest amounts being equally as important as those needed at a hundred or a thousand times that level.

Vitamins are now defined as organic substances, needed in very small amounts, that perform a specific metabolic function and must be provided in the diet of the animal. Those substances considered vitamins for one species that cannot synthesize them may not be vitamins for another species that has the ability to synthesize its own. For instance, vitamin C must be provided in the diet of man, monkeys, and guinea pigs but is synthesized by rats, rabbits, dogs, and other animals. The latter do not need to have them provided in the diet. Plants can manufacture vitamins from the elements available to them from the soil. In general, the more complex the animal, the more vitamins it must obtain from food.

The term *vitamine* was coined by Casimir Funk in 1912. Searching for the elusive substance in rice bran that had great power to cure the condition beriberi, he confirmed Eijkman's hypothesis that disease could be caused by a lack of a dietary constituent. This substance he correctly believed to be necessary for life (vita) and, in the case of the antiberiberi factor, nitrogen containing (amine); hence the term *vitamine*. He suggested, again correctly, that it was likely vitamins existed to protect against pellagra, scurvy, and rickets. Subsequent work showed that many "vitamines" existed, but only a few were "amine" in nature, and so the final e was dropped to give us the familiar term *vitamin*.

Shortly after Funk postulated his vitamin hypothesis, Osborne and Mendel and McCollum and Davis, two teams working independently, reported an elusive, unidentified substance in fat that was necessary for growth and reproduction in animals. This they designated fat-soluble A to differentiate it from the water-soluble B, believed to be responsible for preventing and curing beriberi.

From this simple classification of vitamins has grown a list of four completely different fat-soluble vitamins and eleven water-soluble substances that have been grouped together as the vitamin B complex and vitamin C. As our knowledge of the chemical and physical properties and the physiological roles of vitamins has grown, and the unique features of each member of the B complex has been clarified, an effort has been made to drop such designations as vitamin B_1, B_2, B_6, which imply a common functional or biochemical relationship. Since virtually no direct relationship exists except that they are all water soluble and most operate as coenzymes in metabolic reactions, terms that more adequately designate their composi-

Table 10-1. Discovery, isolation, synthesis, and nomenclature of vitamins

	Discovery	Isolation	Synthesis	Other names
Water-soluble vitamins				
Ascorbic acid (C)		1932	1933	Antiscorbutic factor Cevitamic acid
Thiamin (B$_1$)	1921	1926	1936	Aneurine Antineuritic factor Antiberiberi factor
Riboflavin (B$_2$)	1932	1933	1935	Yellow enzyme Vitamin G Lactoflavin Hepatoflavin Ovoflavin
Niacin	1936	1936		Nicotinic acid Nicotinamide or niacinamide Pellagra-preventive factor
Pyridoxine (B$_6$)	1934	1938	1939	Pyridoxic acid Pyridoxal Pyridoxol Pyridoxamine
Folacin	1945	1945	1945	Adermin Folic acid Citrovorum factor Pteroylglutamic acid *Lactobacillus casei* factor Vitamin M Vitamin B$_c$ Factor U
Cobalamin (B$_{12}$)	1948	1948	1955	Antipernicious anemia factor Cyanocobalamin Hydroxycobalamin Erythrocyte maturation factor
Panthothenic acid	1933	1938	1940	Animal protein factor (APF) Pantotheine Pantothenol Antichromomotriclia factor
Biotin		1935	1942	Antiegg white injury factor Bios II Vitamin H
Choline	1930	1962		
Inositol	1928	1928		Muscle sugar
Fat-soluble vitamins				
Vitamin A	1915	1937	1946	Axerophthol Retinoic acid Retinal Retinol Dehydroretinol
Vitamin D	1918	1930	1936	Antirachitic factor Cholecalciferol Ergocalciferol

Table 10-1. Discovery, isolation, synthesis, and nomenclature of vitamins—cont'd

	Discovery	Isolation	Synthesis	Other names
Fat-soluble vitamins—cont'd				
Vitamin E	1922	1936	1937	Tocopherol Antisterility factor
Vitamin K	1934	1939	1939	Phylloquinone Phytoquinone Farnoquinone Antihemorrhagic factor Menadione (synthetic) Synkayvite (synthetic) Hykinone (synthetic)

tion or structure, such as thiamin, riboflavin, pyridoxine, folacin, and cobalamin, are being used now. It will undoubtedly be some time before the old terminology disappears from the literature, but by pointing out the various systems of nomenclature, we hope to minimize the confusion.

Table 10-1 presents in historical sequence the discovery of vitamins. Gaps in the alphabetical and numerical designations can be explained by the fact that scientists, thinking they had discovered a new nutritional principle, would label it as a vitamin, only to discover later that either it did not have vitamin activity or was identical with another factor. It is clear no new vitamins have been elucidated in the last twenty-three years, and biochemists, physiologists, and nutritionists believe they can establish normal growth, reproductive capacity, and a high level of health by feeding a synthetic diet of the now known nutritional principles in which the balance of nutrients approximates that in natural foods. However, one can never dismiss the possibility that other factors will be discovered. This is especially true as biochemical technique and instruments become more refined and sensitive.

In spite of the fact that individual members of the fat-soluble group (vitamins A, D, E, and K) and the water-soluble group (all others) have unique functions, a few characteristics generally differentiate the

Table 10-2. General properties of fat-soluble and water-soluble vitamins

Fat-soluble vitamins	*Water-soluble vitamins*
Soluble in fat and fat solvents (water-miscible derivatives available)	Soluble in water
Intake in excess of daily need stored in the body	Minimal storage of dietary excesses
Not excreted	Excreted in urine
Deficiency symptoms slow to develop	Deficiency symptoms often develop rapidly
Not absolutely necessary in diet every day	Must be supplied in diet every day
Have precursors	Generally do not have precursors
Contain only the elements carbon, hydrogen, and oxygen	Contain the elements carbon, hydrogen, oxygen, and nitrogen and in some cases others, such as cobalt or sulfur

two groups. These are summarized in Table 10-2.

Related substances

Two groups of compounds chemically related to vitamins are of nutritional importance—vitamin precursors or provitamins, and antagonists or antivitamins.

Provitamins or precursors are substances that are chemically related to the biologically active form of the vitamin but have no vitamin activity until the body converts it into the active form. The conversion of the precursor to the active form takes place in different parts of the body with different degrees of efficiency, depending on the vitamin, the form of the precursor, and the complexity of the reactions required to convert it to the active form. For instance, carotenes are converted to vitamin A in the intestinal wall; 7-dehydrocholesterol to vitamin D in the skin, catalyzed by the ultraviolet rays from the sun; and tryptophan to niacin in the liver. Folic acid, or folacin, as it occurs in food, is actually the precursor of the biologically active citrovorum factor. In this case the conversion, which likely occurs in the cell, requires two other vitamins—ascorbic acid and niacin.

Antivitamins, vitamin antagonists, or pseudovitamins are usually but not always chemically related to the biologically active vitamin. In this case the body does not discriminate between the useful form of the vitamin and the antagonist and so incorporates either into essential body compounds. The active vitamin, as part of enzymes or coenzymes, allows biochemical reactions to occur normally. The antagonist not only does not function in the enzyme system but also stubbornly refuses to be replaced by the proper substance, which would allow the reaction to proceed. The situation is analogous to putting the key in a lock only to find that it does not work and cannot be removed so that the proper key can be used. Vitamin antagonists have been used to produce experimental vitamin deficiencies, especially of nutrients so widespread in nature that it is difficult to produce a diet sufficiently low in them to establish deficiency symptoms or to determine their metabolic role. Medically these are also proving useful in retarding the undesirable growth of tissues. A folacin antagonist, for instance, has shown some promise in retarding the growth of the rapidly growing leukocytes in leukemia but must be used with caution, since it also inhibits the growth of desirable cells.

Functions

In spite of our knowledge of the chemical structure of the vitamins and observations on the effects of their absence on body biochemistry, scientists still have been unable to determine the exact biochemical role of many of the vitamins. Those whose functions have been determined serve primarily as coenzymes needed to facilitate the action of enzymes. The chemical changes that occur in the products of digestion of food after it has been absorbed, which lead either to its incorporation into body structure or to the release of its energy, take place in individual cells. Each cell contains at least 500 enzymes that catalyze these changes. Some enzymes work alone to bring about the required changes; others require the help of coenzymes, most of which are vitamins attached to a protein, called an apoenzyme. The vitamin portion of the coenzyme is usually responsible for the attachment of the enzyme to the substrate. If the vitamins are not available to form the coenzymes, the sequence of chemical changes cannot proceed; the product whose change is blocked accumulates in the tissues or blood, or metabolism is diverted in another direction. In many cases the accumulated intermediary product of the biochemical changes that occur in a normal pattern is responsible for many of the symptoms associated with lack of a specific vitamin. Although the biochemical defect resulting from a vitamin deficiency is similar for all species, the clinical symptoms may vary considerably.

Deficiencies

Vitamin deficiencies may arise from one or several causes. Most common is the lack of the nutrient in the diet. Individuals show wide variation in normal needs; an amount adequate for one person may be insufficient for another. For instance, some adults can function with 0.2 mg. of thiamin, whereas others require as much as 0.8 mg. It is to take care of the needs of the latter that the National Research Council allows such a wide margin of safety over average needs in establishing its recommended dietary allowances.

Failure of the body to absorb the nutrient provided in food makes it unavailable to perform its function in the cell. For instance, persons whose secretion of bile is limited or absent usually absorb lower amounts of the fat-soluble vitamins than those who have an adequate amount of bile to facilitate fat absorption. A defect of gastric mucosa acid secretion precludes the absorption of cobalamin. Rapid passage of food through the gastrointestinal tract also inhibits absorption.

Increased need for a vitamin may precipitate symptoms on an intake that would normally be adequate. For instance, alcoholics experience an increased need for thiamin, persons with tuberculosis need more vitamin C, and now evidence is suggesting that an infant can be conditioned to need an abnormally high amount of pyridoxine or vitamin C if maternal tissues were saturated during fetal development.

Unusually high losses from poor methods of harvesting, storage, or preparation of the food reduce the actual content of the diet below expected levels.

Supplements

Knowledge of the beneficial effects of an adequate intake and the detrimental effects associated with an inadequate intake have resulted in an undue concern over the vitamin content of the diet. Many purveyors of vitamin supplements have capitalized on this concern and have created doubts on the part of the American public regarding the possibility of obtaining sufficient amounts of vitamins from food. In addition, they market supplements that contain vitamins at levels well beyond any conceivable need. As a result, many persons are buying and consuming vitamins in excess of their daily needs. Aside from the economic waste involved, little harm results from excess amounts of the water-soluble vitamins. However, as will be discussed later, excessive intakes of fat-soluble vitamins may have definite harmful effects, and indiscriminate use of such supplements should be discouraged. It is interesting and perhaps appalling to find that the United States produced 1200 pounds of ascorbic acid in 1962, enough to provide 20 mg. per person per day for a year for everyone in the world. Some was used in food preservation to preserve and maintain food quality eventually to end up in the diet, but an undue amount went into vitamin pills to be consumed by an overzealous public.

SELECTED REFERENCE

Report of the Committee on Nomenclature, American Institute of Nutrition: J. Nutr. **99**:244, 1969.

11 | *Fat-soluble vitamins*

VITAMIN A

Shortly after Casimir Funk designated the then-unknown accessory substances in food as "vitamines," two groups of scientists working independently recognized a fat-soluble substance in food necessary for growth in animals. This "vitamine," the first to be identified, was designated as fat-soluble A. It is still known as vitamin A, but it has since been established that there is a complex of chemically related substances, rather than one single active compound, with varying degrees of vitamin A activity. The term *axerophthol,* reflecting the role of one form of the vitamin in treating a condition known as xerophthalmia, has been applied occasionally to this same substance.

In 1912 Osborne and Mendel, working at Yale, reported that animals grew normally on diets containing milk fat but failed to grow when the milk fat was withdrawn. Growth failure was followed by an eye disease. Simultaneously, at the University of Wisconsin, McCollum and Davis were studying the growth of rats on a purified ration of carbohydrate, casein, minerals, and lard. They observed that after periods ranging from 70 to 120 days, growth ceased. They were able to restore growth and relieve the accompanying eye symptoms with an ether extract of butter, cod-liver oil, or egg yolk. Both groups concluded that a fat-soluble substance was necessary for normal growth in animals.

It was not until 1919 that Steenbock, also working in Wisconsin, recognized a similar growth-promoting property in diets containing a yellow vegetable pigment. He was stimulated in his work by Wisconsin dairy farmers' reports of better growth and improvement in fertility when cows were fed yellow corn rather than white corn. As a result of his observations, he was able to attach nutritional significance to the yellow coloring matter in plants such as corn, carrots, and sweet potatoes. By 1928 carotene, one of the yellow pigments of plants, was identified as a potent precursor of vitamin A.

The vitamin A activity of plant and animal foods is measured in terms of International Units (I.U.) or United States Pharmacopeia (U.S.P.) units. These are equal in potency and represent the amount of vitamin A or its precursor that will cause a specific growth response in rats whose reserves of vitamin A have been depleted. One International Unit is equivalent to 0.3 μg. of retinol or 0.6 μg. of β-carotene.

In spite of its early discovery, not until 1930 to 1932 did Swiss and British scientists identify the chemical structure of vitamin A. In 1937 it was crystallized from halibut-liver oil, which has a potency ranging from 2 million to 36 million I.U. per gram. By 1946 a method of synthesizing vitamin A had been developed. Synthetic vitamin A has a potency of 4.5 million I.U. per gram at a cost of about 20 cents. This amounts to 6 cents for a year's supply for an adult. It is now used in enrichment of many food products and in vitamin supplements. A water-miscible form is available for enrichment of nonfat products, such as dried

188

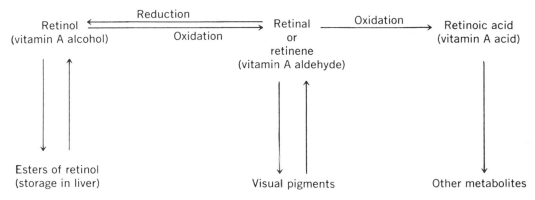

Fig. 11-1. Relationship of biological forms of vitamin A.

milk solids. Over 830 tons of synthetic vitamin A were produced in the United States in 1966.

Beta-carotene, a vitamin A precursor with a pronounced yellow color in its purified form, was produced synthetically in 1954. It is currently one of the few yellow pigments approved by the Food and Drug Administration for the artificial coloring of food. It is used extensively in gelatin, margarine, soft drinks, cake mixes, and cereal products. Ten tons were used in 1966.

Vitamin A is active in a variety of chemical forms, some of which are specific for certain physiological reactions. For instance, retinal has been associated with the visual process, but the forms active in other metabolic roles have not been identified. In an effort to simplify and standardize nomenclature, vitamin A alcohol has been designated as *retinol,* vitamin A aldehyde as *retinal,* and vitamin A acid as *retinoic acid.* Retinol and retinal can be reversibly oxidized and reduced, but as shown in Fig. 11-1, once retinoic acid has been formed, it cannot be converted back to retinal. Retinal has 90% and retinoic acid 60% of the potency of retinol. Vitamin A acid, which promotes growth but cannot prevent night blindness, cannot be stored and disappears rapidly, possibly by being converted into derivatives such as anhy-

droretinoic acid, which is excreted in the bile. Since vitamin A acid is capable of performing some but not all of the functions of vitamin A_1, it has been referred to as a partial vitamin.

With the exception of a small amount found in spinach, the biologically active form of vitamin A_1 is found only in foods of animal origin. A related form designated vitamin A_2, with a potency of 40% of A_1, is found only in livers of freshwater fish and is of little practical significance. Many plants, however, are rich in a group of compounds chemically related to vitamin A that are known as precursors or provitamins. Ten of these carotenoids have been identified in food. Of these, alpha-, beta-, and gamma-carotene and cryptoxanthine are the most important in human and animal nutrition. It is from these carotenoid compounds that animals are able to form vitamin A. The presence of the biologically active provitamins parallels the presence of green and yellow pigments in fruits and vegetables—a direct relationship existing between degree of pigmentation and potential vitamin A value. The green pigment chlorophyll is not itself a precursor but occurs universally in food in association with the yellow pigment that is. Since chlorophyll is darker, it masks the yellow pigment. Yellow pigments such as lycopene in tomatoes and xanthophyll in corn do not themselves have vitamin A potency, although both these foods do contain other vitamin A precursors.

Vitamin A is an almost colorless substance soluble in fat or fat solvents and stable under normal conditions of storage and food preparation.

Both carotene and vitamin A are relatively insoluble in water so that practically none is lost in cooking water. They are stable to heat, acid, and alkali but unstable to oxidation. Thus vitamin A is seldom lost in food preparation except when fat becomes rancid and is followed by the oxidation of vitamin A.

Functions

The metabolic roles of vitamin A appear to be numerous but are not well understood, in spite of the fact that it was the first vitamin to be discovered and has been chemically identified for almost forty years. The fact that we are only now gaining some information on it reflects the illusory nature of its biological role. It has been positively identified as participating in at least five distinct metabolic reactions. It is inferred that a common metabolic factor must exist in its effect on cartilage, bone, and epithelium, but so far no one has been able to identify the biochemical nature of this role. The clinical effects of vitamin A are many and seem to involve all human cells in one way or another, possibly through its effect on DNA synthesis.

Maintenance of visual purple for vision in dim light. The biochemistry of the action of vitamin A in dark adaptation is the only one of its functions that has been clearly defined. Vitamin A in the form of the aldehyde retinal or retinene combines with the protein opsin to form visual purple, or rhodopsin, the photoreceptor pigment in the special cells known as rods, in the retina of the eyes. These are responsible for vision in dim light. As light strikes the retina, the visual purple is bleached to

visual yellow, and retinene or retinal is separated from opsin. With this action a stimulus is transferred from the retina through the optic nerve fibers to the brain. During the process some vitamin A, which is split off from the protein, is reduced to retinol, most of which is reconverted to retinal, to recombine with opsin to regenerate visual purple, or rhodopsin. A small amount of retinol is lost, and vitamin A to replace it must come from the blood. The amount available in the blood determines the rate at which the rhodopsin is regenerated and is available to act again as a receptor substance in the retina. Until the cycle has been completed, vision in dim light is not possible. The mechanism involved is shown in Fig. 11-2.

Two good examples of this phenomenon are the visual reaction of persons on entering a dimly lit theater from a brightly lit street and the temporary blindness experienced by a driver at night after meeting a car with bright headlights. In both cases the bright light has caused excessive bleaching of rhodopsin, and vision in dim light, such as in the relatively dark theater or unlit road, will be possible only when a sufficient amount of visual purple has reformed to facilitate dark adaptation. This is illustrated in Fig. 11-3. The speed with which the eye adapts after exposure to bright light is believed to be directly related to the amount of vitamin A available to regenerate rhodopsin. The "dark adaptation" test, the speed of recovery of visual acuity in dim light as measured by an especially designed apparatus, was long considered the most sensitive measure of vitamin A status. It is now believed to be of limited usefulness.

Vitamin A is also part of another photoreceptor substance, iodopsin, in the cells in the retina known as cones, which are responsible for vision in bright light. The cones, however, are not as sensitive to changes in the amount of vitamin A available as are the rods.

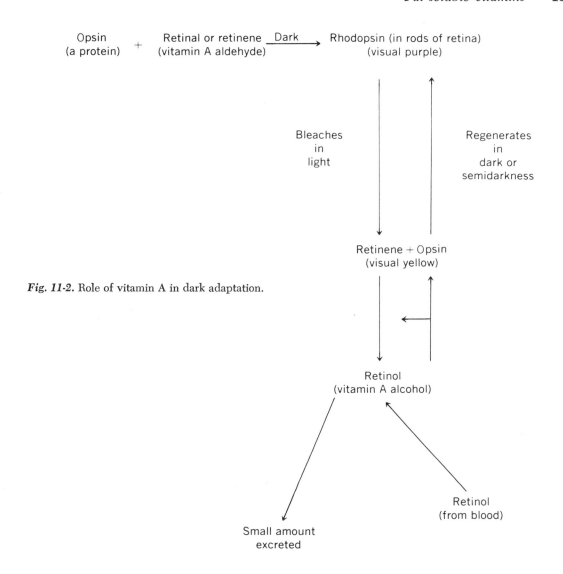

Opsin (a protein) + Retinal or retinene (vitamin A aldehyde) → Dark → Rhodopsin (in rods of retina) (visual purple)

Bleaches in light

Regenerates in dark or semidarkness

Retinene + Opsin (visual yellow)

Retinol (vitamin A alcohol)

Retinol (from blood)

Small amount excreted

Fig. 11-2. Role of vitamin A in dark adaptation.

Growth. The effect of vitamin A on growth is best illustrated by the fact that an animal deprived of vitamin A will cease to grow once vitamin A reserves have been depleted (Fig. 11-4). Growth failure shows up before any other symptoms. Bones fail to grow in length, and the remodelling process, an essential phase of bone growth, is poorly controlled. Since decrease in growth of nervous tissue is not concurrent, undue pressure may occur on the brain and other parts of nervous tissue whose growth is not depressed in vitamin A deficiency and that

are protected by a bony framework that fails to grow fast enough to accommodate them. Bone growth is stimulated when vitamin A is made available again.

A degeneration or defective formation of nervous tissue independent of the effect of a deficiency of vitamin A on bone growth may occur. One theory is that in the absence of vitamin A the protective layer of tissue surrounding nerve fibers does not form satisfactorily.

Reproduction. The role of vitamin A in promoting fertility in animals was one of

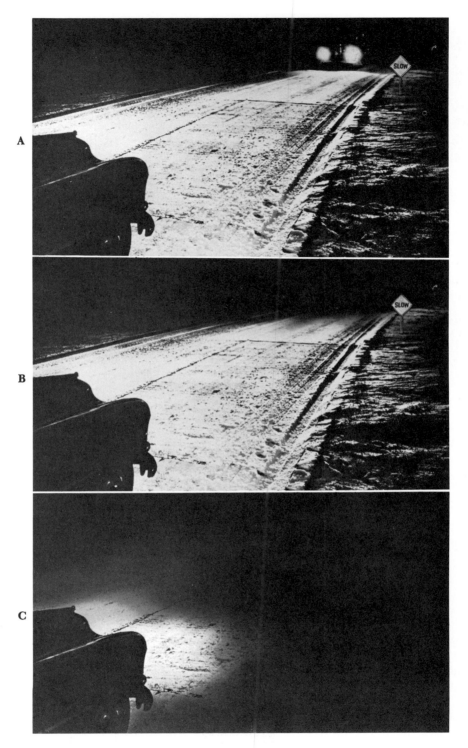

Fig. 11-3. Night blindness. Night blindness is a useful and early diagnostic sign of vitamin A deficiency. This loss of visual acuity in dim light after exposure to bright light is illustrated here. **A,** Both normal individual and vitamin A–deficient subject see headlights of an approaching car. **B,** After car has passed, normal individual sees a wide stretch of road. **C,** Vitamin A–deficient subject can barely see a few feet ahead and cannot see road sign at all. (Courtesy The Upjohn Co., Kalamazoo, Mich.)

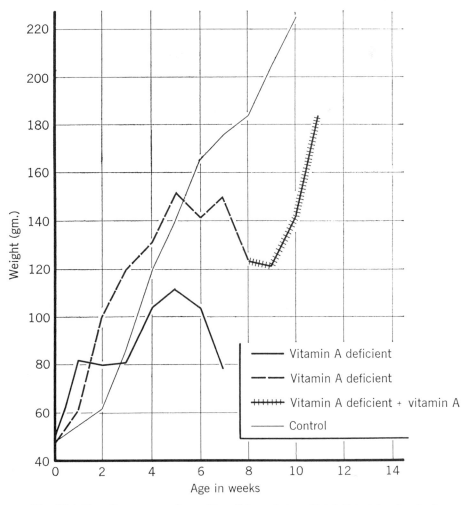

Fig. 11-4. Growth response of weanling albino rats to a diet deficient in vitamin A.

the first discovered. Either vitamin A alcohol (retinol) or its aldehyde derivative (retinal) is necessary for normal reproduction in rats. In its absence, failure of spermatogenesis occurs in the male, and fetal resorption in the female. The exact biochemical mechanism is unknown, but it has been shown that although the alcohol form of vitamin A is effective in stimulating normal reproduction, vitamin A acid will permit conception but will not prevent fetal resorption. A decrease in estrogen synthesis observed in vitamin A deficiency may be related to the abnormalities in reproduction.

Health of epithelial cells. Epithelial cells are found not only in the outer protective layer of skin but also the linings of all openings from the body, such as the respiratory tract, the gastrointestinal tract, and the genitourinary tract. In many cases these epithelial cells normally secrete mucus. The fact that certain sequences of degenerative changes occur when vitamin A is lacking supports the belief that vitamin A is essential to biochemical reactions necessary

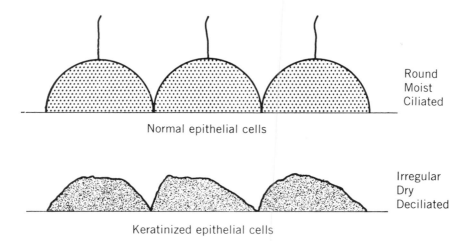

Round
Moist
Ciliated

Normal epithelial cells

Irregular
Dry
Deciliated

Keratinized epithelial cells

Fig. 11-5. Schematic representation of changes in epithelial cells in vitamin A deficiency.

to preserve health of epithelial cells. These cells are characterized by continuous replacement and progressive differentiation. They also tend to produce mucopolysaccharides as secretory products.

During a deficiency a drying or keratinization of the layer of cells occurs, followed by a loss of cilia or hairlike projections from the cell and the ability of the cells to secrete mucus. This depressed secretion of mucus is believed to be due to the fact that vitamin A is necessary for the synthesis of the carbohydrate mucopolysaccharide, a normal constituent of mucus. In addition, the ducts may become clogged by keratinized plugs. Finally, the outer layers pile up, leaving a layer of horny keratinized cells in place of the moist, rounded, ciliated cells of normal epithelium. The changes in epithelial cells are shown diagrammatically in Fig. 11-5. A large number of body processes are affected when vitamin A to promote the normal health of epithelial cells is inadequate. These effects will be discussed as results of deficiency of vitamin A.

Other functions. Studies have indicated that vitamin A (either as acid or alcohol) is necessary for the release of proteolytic, or protein-splitting, enzymes from particles in the cell known as lysosomes. These enzymes must be released to act on the cartilage of bone tissue during bone remodelling to cause a breakdown of the protein structure and the dissolution of the matrix itself. An excess of vitamin A may cause complete disintegration of the matrix by releasing too many enzymes too fast. An imbalance between the rate of breakdown of bone and bone formation is reflected in abnormal bone structure.

In addition to participating in reactions involving the stability of the membranes of subcellular particles, such as the lysosomes and mitochondria, vitamin A is involved in the stability of cell membranes. Some retinol is necessary to maintain a stable membrane, but excessive amounts make the membranes abnormally susceptible to rupture. This phenomenon is believed to be one factor in vitamin A toxicity.

Both vitamin A and vitamin A acid have been shown to be effective in the synthesis of the hormone corticosterone from cholesterol in the adrenal cortex. In the absence of vitamin A and with reduced corticosterone synthesis, the body loses the ability to synthesize glycogen, the storage form of carbohydrate.

The loss of appetite in a vitamin A deficiency has been attributed to changes in the taste buds. This may be due to a decrease in mucopolysaccharide synthesis.

Absorption and metabolism

From the time it is ingested until it is either used or excreted from the body, vitamin A changes form many times. Most of the vitamin A in food appears in combination with the fatty acid palmitic acid as vitamin A palmitate. Before it can be taken up from the intestine into the cells lining the intestine, it must be split by enzymes secreted in the pancreatic juice or produced in mucosal cells to form free retinol. These enzymes are dependent on the presence of bile before they can act. Once retinol is within the mucosal cell, it combines with fatty acid, usually palmitic, and is incorporated in the small particles of fat called chylomicrons. These are then released into the lymphatic circulation, which eventually enters the regular blood system to be carried to the liver. A small part of the retinol is oxidized first to retinal and then to retinoic acid. This form is converted into another chemical compound, a glucuronide, and is released into the portal circulation, which goes directly to the liver. Since vitamin A is fat soluble, factors that promote the absorption of fat enhance vitamin A absorption; conversely, factors that depress fat absorption depress vitamin A absorption. In addition, vitamin E enhances the absorption of vitamin A and the amount stored in the liver.

In the liver, retinol is again released from palmitic acid, and this time combines with a lipoprotein to be stored in the liver. Retinol is released from the lipoprotein with which it is stored in liver and attaches to a retinol-binding protein in the blood to be transported to the tissues in which it is used. Both retinoic acid and its derivative glucuronide can be excreted from the liver through the bile into the intestinal tract, from which as much as 80% of either may be reabsorbed. The rest is excreted in the

feces. Some retinol may be oxidized in the kidney to retinal and retinoic acid and excreted in the urine, but most of it is stored in the liver until needed. Retinoic acid, on the other hand, is excreted rather rapidly in the bile. The depressed utilization of vitamin A observed in protein deficiency can be explained by the number of proteins involved in its metabolism. Enzymes that are proteins are needed at many stages. Vitamin A is stored in a protein complex and is transported in the blood attached to a protein. In a protein deficiency the synthesis of all these proteins is depressed. Protein appears necessary for the mobilization of vitamin A reserves from the liver. This may explain low blood levels of vitamin A found in kwashiorkor that respond when protein and no additional vitamin A are given. Normal blood levels for vitamin A are approximately 130 I.U. per 100 ml. Any drop in plasma vitamin A levels reflects a depletion of liver reserves and a prolonged dietary deficiency rather than immediate dietary intake.

The four major vegetable precursors of vitamin A—alpha-, beta-, and gamma-carotene and cryptoxanthine—are absorbed in the presence of bile salts from the intestine after having been released from the plant cell during digestion. They are converted in the intestinal wall to vitamin A. The conversion of carotene to vitamin A is not complete, with some unchanged carotene being absorbed and entering the circulation, where normal carotene levels approximate 150 I.U. per 100 ml. of blood. Carotene levels reflect dietary carotene and do not reflect storage of vitamin A so that in decreased intakes a rather rapid drop in carotene values occurs. Unconverted carotene is stored in the fat depots rather than in the liver of human beings. Carotene levels have little significance as indicators of vitamin A status.

The amount of vitamin A formed from the precursor depends on the nature of the precursor. Beta-carotene is a symmetrical molecule made up of two vitamin A molecules. Although it could theoretically be changed into two molecules by breaking it in the center, evidence now shows that it is more likely to be broken down in a stepwise fashion from one end to give only one molecule of vitamin A. The other precursors can yield only one molecule of vitamin A, but usually yield less than beta-carotene. Approximately one third of the carotene in food is converted to vitamin A; carotenes in carrots and root vegetables undergo less than one-fourth conversion and those in leafy vegetables about one half. The conversion of carotene to vitamin A occurs primarily in the intestinal wall, although some may take place in liver and lungs. In any case the conversion is stimulated by thyroxin. Once converted into vitamin A, it is handled in the same way as is the preformed vitamin.

The absorption of vitamin A from foods is decreased in liver injury or in any condition in which the bile duct has an obstruction. Mineral oil has an affinity for both vitamin A and carotene, and since it is unaffected by digestive enzymes and passes through the digestive tract, it will carry with it much of the potential vitamin A in the diet. For this reason the practice of using mineral oil as a source of fat for low-calorie salad dressings on salad greens, one of the potentially good sources of vitamin A activity, is to be condemned. The intake of polyunsaturated fatty acids with carotene results in rapid destruction of carotene unless antioxidants are also present.

The concentration of vitamin A in human liver reflects long-term dietary intakes. The small number of studies reported have given values from 100 I.U. per gram in Great Britain, through 766 I.U. per gram for Americans, to a high of 1000 I.U. per gram among New Zealanders who live on a diet high in butter. It is estimated that a healthy person stores 500,000 I.U. in his liver, an amount that may last him several years. Autopsy data on livers of Canadians,

however, showed that 10% had no measurable reserves and 20% had no more than that normally found at birth.

Food sources

The vitamin A value of some representative foods is shown in Fig. 11-6.

Preformed vitamin A is available only in animal products in which the animal has metabolized the carotene of its food into vitamin A and has concentrated it in certain tissues. Liver, representing the storage site for vitamin A, reflects the dietary intake of the animal. It ranges from 2,000,000 I.U. per 100 gm. in polar bear liver to 45,000 I.U. in beef liver to 19,000 I.U. per 100 gm. in pork liver. Fish-liver oils are extremely rich, and until recently concentrates of these were the most widely used therapeutic sources of vitamin A.

Egg yolk with 2000 to 4000 I.U. per 100 gm. is a good source of vitamin A in the form of retinol and is the one usually introduced first into the diet to replenish the fetal reserves of a young infant. Since preformed vitamin A is colorless, the color of the yolk is no indication of its potency in the yolk. A deep yellow color may reflect unconverted carotene, but more often it is xanthophyll with no vitamin A activity. It is possible to increase the amount of vitamin A in an egg yolk by increasing the amount fed to the hen.

The vitamin A value of butter varies with the breed of animal and its diet and shows a definite seasonal variation. In winter, butter averages 9000 I.U. per pound, whereas in summer, values may exceed 15,000 I.U., the amount with which margarine in the United States is usually fortified. In neither case is color an indication of vitamin A value.

In milk the vitamin A is present in the fat portion; this is absent in nonfat milk. Average values for milk are 390 I.U. per cup, which is relatively low, and the loss of vitamin A when nonfat milk replaces whole milk becomes important only when

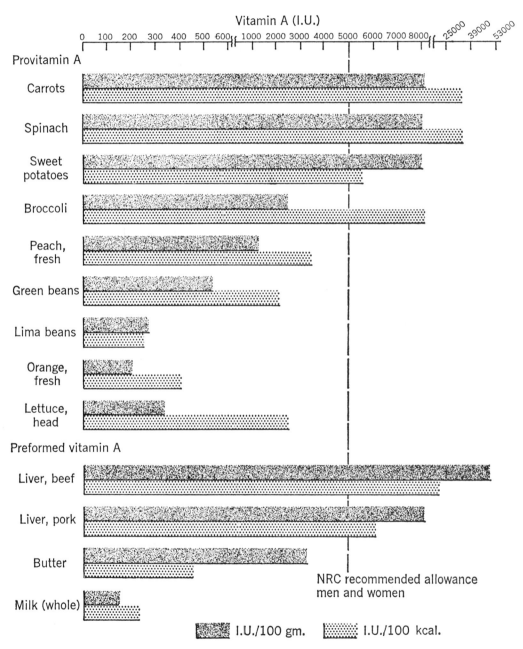

Fig. 11-6. Vitamin A value of 100 gm. and 100 kcal. portions of some representative foods. (Based on Watt, B. K., and Merrill, A. L.: Composition of foods—raw, processed and prepared, U. S. Department of Agriculture Handbook No. 8, Washington, D. C., 1963, U. S. Department of Agriculture.)

milk is the sole item in the diet, as it is for very young infants. Any yellow color in milk is due to presence of carotene, reflecting inefficient conversion to vitamin A by the cow. Fresh fluid nonfat milk and dried nonfat milk solids of homogenized whole milk are often enriched with vitamin A. The amount of vitamin A in cheese is the same as that in the milk from which it is made. Aside from milk products, eggs, and

Table 11-1. Vitamin A values of representative foods

Food	I.U. of vitamin A activity
Fruits and vegetables	
Spinach (½ cup)	10,600
Carrots, diced (½ cup)	9065
Broccoli (½ cup)	2550
Kale (½ cup)	4610
Asparagus (½ cup)	910
Peas (½ cup)	575
Brussels sprouts (½ cup)	260
Lima beans (½ cup)	230
Cabbage, cooked (½ cup)	75
Apricots, dried (½ cup)	8195
Apricots, canned (½ cup)	2260
Papaya (½ cup)	1595
Watermelon (2-pound wedge)	1265
Peaches, raw (½ cup)	1115
Orange (1 medium)	290
Banana (1 medium)	95
Pineapple, raw (½ cup)	90
Dairy products	
Milk, fresh whole (1 cup)	390
Milk, fresh nonfat (1 cup)	10
Cheese, cheddar (1 ounce)	378
Cheese, processed cheddar	
(1 ounce)	300
Butter (1 tablespoon)	230
Margarine (1 tablespoon)	230
Meat, fish, poultry, and eggs	
Egg, whole	590
Egg yolk	580
Liver (3 ounces)	
Beef	45,450
Lamb	43,000
Chicken	27,000
Calf	19,000
Pork	12,000

liver, animal products contain virtually no vitamin A. Muscle meats are devoid of vitamin A value.

Fruits and vegetables contain no preformed vitamin A but only precursors. Because of this, tables of food composition report vitamin A activity or vitamin A value of foods, reflecting the potential vitamin A available from the food based on ability of the body to make the conversion.

Generally, as seen from Table 11-1, the vitamin A value of fruits and vegetables is directly proportional to the amount of carotene or chlorophyll present in the food. Thus the deeper the orange, yellow, or green color of fruits and vegetables, the higher the vitamin A value. In addition, if one examines the vitamin A values of a food such as a head of lettuce, one finds a tenfold increase as one progresses from the inner bleached leaves to the outer leaves higher in chlorophyll and carotenoids. Unfortunately a high concentration of chlorophyll is often accompanied by an astringent bitter taste, as in very dark green endive leaves, so that a potentially rich source of vitamin A is unpalatable. Some fruits, such as mangoes, increase their carotene content with storage.

The yellow pigments lycopene, found in watermelon and tomatoes, and xanthophyll, found in corn and egg yolk, do not have vitamin A value. Another yellow pigment, cryptoxanthine in corn, does have vitamin A potential of about 3.5 I.U. per gram. In countries where red palm oil is used in cooking, its carotene content represents a major source of vitamin A activity, with 800 I.U. per gram.

The ability of the body to utilize carotene varies with the food and the form in which the food is ingested. For instance, grated carrots have greater value than carrot slices. Utilization varies from 30% to 70% of available vitamin A.

Vitamin A is stable to heat, light, acid, and alkali, and little is lost under normal conditions of food preparation. Excessive

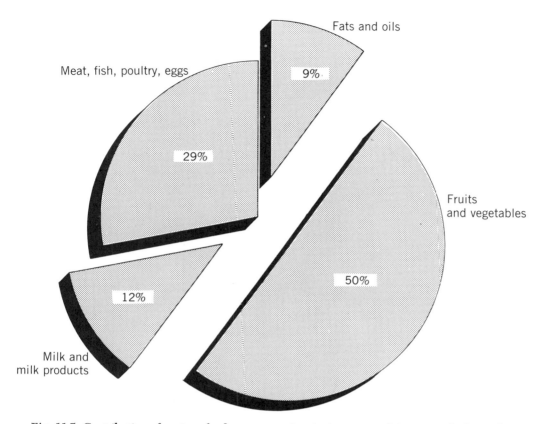

Fig. 11-7. Contribution of various food groups to vitamin A content of American food supply. (Based on Contribution of major food groups to nutrient supplies available for civilian consumption, National Food Situation No. 130, 1969.)

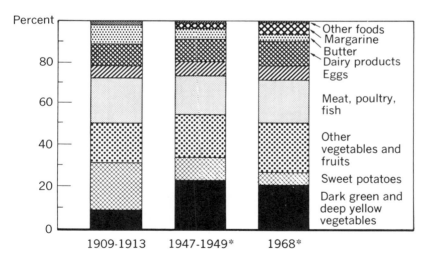

Fig. 11-8. Trends in consumption of dietary sources of vitamin A value from 1909 to 1968. *Includes fortification; †data preliminary. (From Agricultural Research Service, U. S. Department of Agriculture, 1969.)

temperatures in frying oils high in carotene, such as palm oil, that are used extensively in tropical countries, may cause its destruction, as will the oxidation that occurs in rancid fats. The small amount of green and yellow pigment that may appear in cooking water from fruits and vegetables represents an insignificant portion of that present in the food. Sun-drying of fruits may lead to some loss of vitamin A.

The contributions of various food groups to the vitamin A content of the American diet are shown in Fig. 11-7, and Fig. 11-8 depicts the change in the contribution of the various food groups to vitamin A value between 1909 and 1968. Preliminary results of the *National Nutrition Survey* show that vitamin A is the nutrient for which intakes are most often below recommended levels and that blood levels are correspondingly low.

In the United States average daily intake is 7500 I.U., 50% of which comes from vegetable sources, compared to about 4300 I.U. in Britain, two thirds of which is from animal sources. In Central and South America 93% of the vitamin A comes from the precursor and one third of this from yellow maize. India has an intake of less than 1000 I.U. per day, and the simultaneous low protein intake keeps the level of utilization low.

Recommended allowances

The National Research Council recommended allowances for vitamin A have been established assuming that one third of the vitamin A value of a mixed diet comes from animal sources and two thirds from vegetable sources. The recommended allowances have been set at 5000 I.U. for an adult per day. If preformed vitamin A from animals is the sole source, 3000 I.U. is considered sufficient. During pregnancy the recommendation is increased to 6000 I.U., and in lactation 8000 I.U. is deemed adequate. The recommended amounts for other age groups are shown in Appendix C.

The discrepancies in recommended levels of vitamin A intake in various standards result from assumptions of different proportions of vitamin A and carotene in diets and different interpretations of the efficiency with which carotene is converted into vitamin A.

The need for vitamin A varies under varying conditions. Tiring work, especially in hot weather, tends to raise needs. This may be a manifestation of the decreased ability to convert carotene into vitamin A at higher temperatures. Also, more vitamin A is needed after removal of the gallbladder, in hypothyroidism, and in conditions of impaired intestinal absorption.

Deficiency

Vitamin A deficiency symptoms will show up only after liver reserves have been depleted. This depends on the extent of the reserves, determined by previous dietary intake. In animals, growth ceases when the reserves of vitamin A have been used up. Most symptoms of a vitamin A deficiency as seen in human beings are a reflection of its role in maintaining the health of epithelial cells. They may result from low dietary intakes, interference with absorption and storage, interference with conversion of carotene to vitamin A, or rapid loss of vitamin A.

Night blindness. One of the earliest symptoms of vitamin A deficiency is night blindness. In low intakes the liver reserves drop, followed by a drop in blood levels and a subsequent drop in the level available in the retina of the eye, which eventually shows up in a slow dark adaptation time and finally night blindness.

Changes in the eye. The cornea of the eye is affected early. The lachrymal gland fails to secrete, possibly as a result of decreased ability to synthesize mucopolysaccharide or of a blocking of the lachrymal duct. This is followed by a keratinization, opacity, and sloughing of epithelial cells of the cornea, with eventual rupturing of the

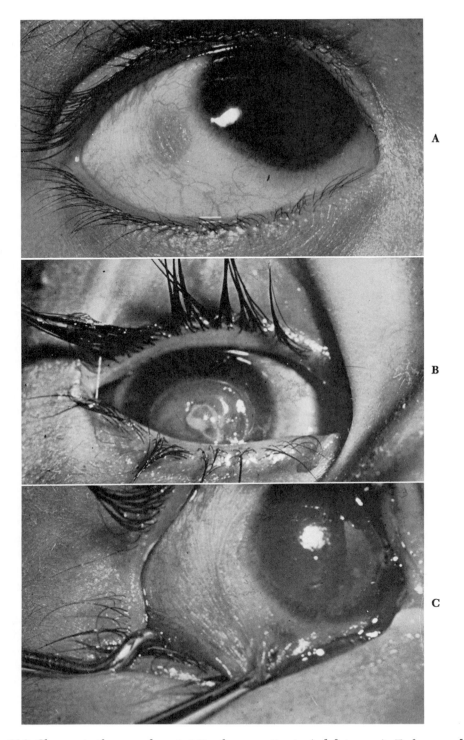

Fig. 11-9. Changes in the eyes characteristic of severe vitamin A deficiency. **A,** Early corneal xerosis, with infiltration in lower central cornea. **B,** Keratomalacia—softening and protrusion of whole central area of cornea. **C,** Generalized xerosis, with clearly demarcated Bitot's spots. (From McLaren, D. S., Shirajan, E., Tschalian, M., and Khoury, G.: Amer. J. Clin. Nutr. **17:**117, 1965.)

corneal tissue. Infection apparently sets in, pus is exudated, and the eye will hemorrhage. This condition is known as Bitot's spots in its mildest form, as xerosis conjunctivae in moderately severe form, and as xerophthalmia in advanced stages. These conditions were prevalent in children in Denmark during World War I when occupation troops deprived them of dairy products, their most dependable source of vitamin A. It is now reported frequently in Indonesia and other tropical countries where a low protein intake may also be a contributing factor. Typical eye symptoms of severe vitamin A deficiency are shown in Fig. 11-9. Total blindness is a frequent result and most frequently affects children. It is suggested that many children succumb to other forms of vitamin A deficiency before xerophthalmia develops.

Respiratory infections. Vitamin A has often been designated as the anti-infective vitamin because of the high incidence of respiratory ailments associated with a vitamin A deficiency. Since vitamin A does not directly attack the infective organism, the use of this term has been questioned. However, evidence exists that when the epithelium of the trachea and bronchi become keratinized, deciliated, and deprived of their mucous secretions and a break occurs in the integrity of the mucous membranes, they become a good harbor for microorganisms that would not normally penetrate a healthy epithelial layer. In animals the changes in epithelium during vitamin A deficiency usually lead to terminal bronchial pneumonia. Recovery among tuberculosis patients has been more rapid when the diet is high in vitamin A. Efforts to relate susceptibility to the common cold to vitamin A intake have shown no relationship, but those on diets high in vitamin A have had colds of shorter duration.

Changes in skin. A dry rough skin, especially in the area of the shoulders, may be an early sign of a vitamin A deficiency. This condition, known as folliculosis, in which there are simply eruptions near the base of the hair follicle that subsequently undergo a keratinization, is used as an indication of possible vitamin A deficiency in many nutritional status studies.

Changes in genitourinary tract. Keratinization of epithelial cells seems to favor calcium deposition and may well predispose to kidney stones.

Changes in gastrointestinal tract. Many disturbances in the gastrointestinal tract, such as diarrhea, have been linked by various investigations to the changes in epithelial tissue that takes place in the absence of vitamin A.

Failure of tooth enamel. The integrity of the enamel layer of teeth may reflect the adequacy of vitamin A in the first five years of life. In vitamin A deprivation in animals the enamel layer of teeth is absent.

Toxicity

The possibility that excessive amounts of vitamin A may produce detrimental rather than desirable results has been recognized only recently. Symptoms have appeared as a result of the use of polar bear liver, which has a very high vitamin A potency, the treatment of a skin disorder in adolescents with daily doses of vitamin A of 50,000 to 100,000 I.U., and the use of large doses of vitamin A supplements for infants by overzealous mothers. The symptoms of vitamin A toxicity are many, ranging from headache, drowsiness, nausea, loss of hair, and diarrhea in adults to a scaly dermatitis, weight loss, anorexia, and skeletal pain in infants to loss of hemoglobin and potassium from red blood cells, cessation of menstruation in young girls and women, and rapid resorption of bone in adults. The period between the initiation of high intakes and the onset of symptoms varies from six to fifteen months. Wide individual differences in sensitivity to high levels seem to exist, some persons showing symptoms after long-term dosages of 50,000 I.U. daily and others exhibiting a reaction only at levels of 150,-

000 to 200,000 I.U. daily. Recovery is rapid and complete on withdrawal of excess intake, with symptoms subsiding in 72 hours in many cases. Toxic reactions can occur only from overconsumption of the preformed vitamin but not of the precursor. Permanent effects of vitamin A toxicity are rare. Some workers are concerned that long-standing high intakes on the part of the mother, resulting in storage levels in the liver of 1000 I.U. or more per gram, may have harmful effects in the fetus even if the mother has not exhibited a toxic reaction herself. In animals single injections of vitamin A in the pregnant female have produced congenital skeletal abnormalities in her young. Even though vitamin A acid cannot be stored, it can contribute to toxic reactions, and thus it is suggested that toxicity is caused by oxidation of the acid.

The Food and Drug Administration has become sufficiently concerned to ask that a ceiling be placed on the amount of vitamin A that can be included in a multivitamin preparation available without a prescription. The availability of vitamin A supplements of high potency at a low price often leads people to oversupplement the diet. This, coupled with the widespread practice of enriching food products for trade advantages, increases the possibility of a person receiving a toxic dose. The possibility of this occurring in a normal mixed diet is remote.

VITAMIN D

Vitamin D is now officially designated cholecalciferol (vitamin D_3) or ergocalciferol (vitamin D_2), depending on whether it is derived from animal or vegetable sources. It had been known previously as the *sunshine vitamin* because sunshine is one of its sources to the body, and as the *antirachitic factor,* or *rickets-preventative factor* because of its effectiveness in curing rickets.

Since vitamin D_3 can be produced in the body, it is technically a hormone, but if insufficient amounts are produced in the body, either vitamin D_2 or vitamin D_3 must be supplied by the diet, in which case they are technically vitamins. Vitamin D is necessary for all animals with a bony skeleton, since it facilitates the absorption and utilization of calcium and phosphorus for normal bone formation. Like vitamin A, vitamin D is measured in terms of International Units defined in terms of a biological response to the administration of the vitamin to a depleted animal. One International Unit of vitamin D weighs 0.025 μg., and 1 mg. contains 40,000 I.U.

Rickets

Rickets is a condition that has plagued infants in the temperate zone for many years. It was so common in England that some writers referred to it as the *English disease.* Before a dietary factor was implicated as causative agent, many environmental factors had been investigated. The fact that it occurred more frequently among people living in the crowded, smoky, industrial areas of cities where standards of sanitation were often poor suggested that rickets was a disease of bacterial origin. Dark-skinned people moving from the tropics to the temperate zone were susceptible to rickets. Since they frequently lived in crowded housing, the environmental theory seemed to be supported. From time to time it was suggested that sunshine had a curative effect on rickets, but the relationship between sunshine and rickets was not established until the late 1920's, after the nature of vitamin D had been clarified.

Rickets is essentially a disease of defective bone formation that manifests itself in many ways. Basically it is due to an inadequate deposition of calcium and phosphorus in bone. The bones, normally poorly calcified at the time of birth, remain soft and pliable. Deformities develop when these poorly calcified bones are called upon to perform functions for which they are not sufficiently strong. Bowing of legs occurs when a child starts to walk before the bones have become sufficiently rigid to support the weight of the body. The ends of the long bones become enlarged, causing difficulties in movement. Knock-knees are a manifestation of this enlargement, which results from the flattening that occurs when the poorly calcified ends of the bones are subjected to the weight of the body. Deformities of the ribs result in a concave breast (pigeon breast) that causes crowding in the chest cavity. Ribs also develop irregularly spaced areas of swelling that take on the appearance of beading, which has led to the use of the term *rachitic rosary* to describe this syndrome. The failure of the fontanel of the skull to close

allows rapid enlargement of the head, sometimes interpreted as a sign of health in a child, as witnessed by the number of rachitic infants who have been judged "best baby in the show."

Teeth erupt later, are less well formed than is normal, and decay earlier. Growth is generally retarded, but the severity of the disease as measured by other symptoms is frequently greater in children who have undergone rapid growth.

Rickets is a condition that primarily affects children. The symptoms are very slowly reversible so that some symptoms produced during early childhood may remain throughout adulthood. The long-held belief that rickets does not develop in chil-

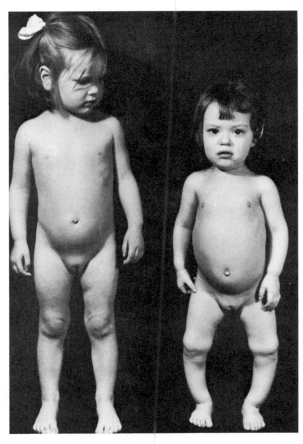

Fig. 11-10. Typical case of rickets. (From Arneil, G. C.: World Rev. Nutr. Diet. **10:**239, 1969.)

dren over 2 years of age is no longer tenable. Many of the cases that have been associated with a recurrence of rickets in the 1960's in both Great Britain and the United States have been identified in children between 2 and 4. They show a growth retardation and the typical bowed legs. A typical case of rickets is shown in Fig. 11-10.

The term *adult rickets* is sometimes applied to the disease osteomalacia, which reflects a defect in bone formation but not a vitamin D deficiency.

Discovery

The discovery of vitamin D followed by six years the identification of fat-soluble A. In 1918 a British nutritionist, Mellanby, presented the first evidence of a fat-soluble substance with antirachitic properties. By 1919 scientists had produced rickets experimentally by feeding animals diets in which vegetable or animal fats replaced cod-liver oil. By 1922 the recognition that the antirachitic properties of cod-liver oil, which had been used as a folk remedy since early in the nineteenth century, were not destroyed by oxidation that destroyed its vitamin A value led to the suggestion that a second fat-soluble vitamin existed. It was soon identified as vitamin D.

The existence of provitamin D, which could be activated by the short ultraviolet rays of the sun, was discovered in 1922. This antirachitic factor was isolated in a crystalline form in 1930, twelve years after the first report of the substance. By 1937 its chemical structure had been elucidated. Most vitamin D used in the enrichment of food products has been obtained from the irradiation with ultraviolet light of the precursors of vitamin D. Methods are now available for the synthesis of two derivatives of vitamin D that are even more active than the naturally occurring vitamin.

Functions

The role of vitamin D in promoting normal calcification of the bone has been known for some time, but scientists were at a loss to explain the basis of the biochemical and physiological changes that occurred in a vitamin D deficiency and that were prevented or reversed when adequate amounts of the vitamin were available. The most usual changes were the following:

1. Reduced intestinal absorption of calcium and phosphate
2. Reduced resorption of phosphate and amino acids by the kidney
3. Hypocalcemia (low blood calcium levels) and a failure to mobilize bone calcium
4. Reduced concentrations of citrate (an organic compound intermediary in cellular respiration) in body fluids and bones
5. Increase in level of the enzyme alkaline phosphatase in the blood

Since 1960 a surge of interest has taken place in attempts to determine the metabolically active form of the vitamin and the molecular basis for its action. It now appears that vitamin D does not operate in the calcification process per se but facilitates it by causing an elevation in calcium and phosphorus levels in the blood to the point where the blood is supersaturated and calcification can occur. Although some questions are still unanswered regarding the exact mode of action of vitamin D, at least some aspects of the mechanism have been elucidated. Vitamin D_3 or cholecalciferol, is absorbed from the intestinal tract and is carried attached to alpha-globulin$_2$, a protein in the blood to the liver. There some vitamin D is converted into a metabolite of cholecalciferol, 25-hydroxycholecalciferol, which is transported to the bone and small intestine. It enters the nucleus of the cells lining the gastrointestinal tract and stimulates the synthesis of a protein that acts as a carrier necessary for calcium absorption. In the presence of a source of energy the calcium in the intestinal lumen is picked up and transported into the mucosal cell. The carrier transports the calcium across the intestinal cell and releases it into the bloodstream in an exchange process involving sodium. At the same time that calcium is being taken up from the intestine, an increase occurs in an enzyme within the cell that in the presence of calcium leads to the release of inorganic phosphate into the blood. In this way the calcium and phosphate of the blood are increased simultaneously—a situation that favors calcification of the bone. It is believed that the same derivative of vitamin D_3 is carried to the bone, where it acts in a similar way to facilitate the uptake of calcium by the bone for deposition in the bone matrix. The fact that there is a delay from the time vitamin D is administered until calcium absorption is affected can be explained by the fact that the ingested vitamin must first be converted into an active form before it can stimulate the synthesis of the carrier that is necessary for calcium absorption. The drop in citrate level in vitamin D deficiency could be a manifestation of the increased need for energy for calcium uptake.

Failure of calcification of bone is more often caused by an inadequate supply of phosphate than of calcium, although the term *calcification* to describe the deposition of calcium phosphate crystals in the bone matrix implies that calcium is primarily involved. The addition of vitamin D to the diet increases the rate of absorption of phosphate, but likely of greater importance is the fact that it increases the resorption of phosphate from the tubules of the kidneys. In the absence of vitamin D much phosphate is lost in urinary excretions, and the blood levels of phosphate drop. Alkaline phosphatase, which is produced in large amounts in the growing surfaces of bone, helps release inorganic phosphate into the blood from organic compounds, another method of increasing phosphorus available for calcification.

Vitamin D also influences the rate of resorption of amino acids in the kidney tubules. Evidence indicates that the level of amino acids in the urine (amino-aciduria) is a fairly sensitive indication of vitamin D status, increasing in a deficiency and decreasing when vitamin D restores the normal rate of resorption.

The importance of maintaining blood calcium at a level of at least 7 mg. per 100 ml., is so great that calcium is mobilized from the old, or deep, bone matrix to hold this level even in a dietary calcium deficiency. In a vitamin D deficiency the mechanisms for mobilizing calcium fail to function, with a resultant drop in blood calcium levels (hypocalcemia).

A discussion of the role of vitamin D would be incomplete without mention of the antagonistic relationship between vitamin D and hydrocortisone, a hormone secreted by the adrenal gland and used therapeutically in the treatment of many conditions. Hydrocortisone can depress the high blood levels of calcium associated with excessive intakes of vitamin D. It can also decrease the permeability of the intestinal membrane and hence calcium absorption when administered along with normal levels of vitamin D.

As noted in the discussion on calcium, the parathyroid hormone augments the vitamin D—mediated mobilization of calcium from reserves of exchangeable calcium in bones. Vitamin D appears to permit or regulate the action of the parathyroid hormone. It is evident that three factors—vitamin D, hydrocortisone, and the parathyroid hormone—all operate to regulate calcium balances and bone metabolism. The nature of the interrelationship is not clear. In the case of the effect on resorption of phosphates, the action of vitamin D, which favors resorption, is antagonistic to the action of the parathyroid hormone, which inhibits the process in the kidney.

The rate of intestinal absorption of calcium is greatly increased in the presence of adequate dietary vitamin D; a rate of 10% absorption without vitamin D may be increased to 33% in the presence of the vitamin.

Absorption

Vitamin D is absorbed in the intestinal tract in the presence of bile. Absorption is complete regardless of the form of the vitamin—cholecalciferol or ergocalciferol—or of the medium in which it is presented—oil or aqueous. Conditions in which fat absorption is reduced, such as steatorrhea or obstructive jaundice, result in a decreased rate of absorption of vitamin D. Some vitamin D is converted in the liver to the active form, some remains unchanged and accumulates in the liver and kidney, some forms esters with long double-chain fatty acids, and some appears in an unidentified form. In contrast to vitamin A, vitamin D is stored in only limited amounts in mammals, with most of it being stored in the liver, kidney, adrenal glands, and bone. Rachitic bone has a greater affinity for it than nonrachitic bone. Vitamin D is excreted through the bile and the intestinal wall.

Requirements

Because of the two sources of vitamin D, the evaluation of minimum requirements is difficult. Indications are that between 100 and 400 I.U. of vitamin D will protect against rickets and will promote growth when adequate amounts of calcium and phosphorus have been ingested. Increased intake appears to provide no greater protection against rickets and at levels over 1800 I.U. may have detrimental effects, reversing the beneficial effects of lower levels. Both breast- and bottle-fed infants should receive a dietary supplement of vitamin D by 2 weeks of age to provide the NRC recommended intake of 400 I.U. per day. If fortified milk or commercial infant formulas are used, it is not only unnecessary but also possibly undesirable to add a supplement. Vitamin D in milk is up to ten times as potent as that in oil.

Premature infants whose calcium reserves are much lower than those of full-term infants, in whom half the calcium is deposited in the last six weeks of fetal life, have a need for vitamin D to facilitate the absorption of the high level of calcium needed to meet the demands of their rapid growth. Apparent ineffectiveness of dosages of 400 I.U. of vitamin D in breast-fed premature infants may be a function of the low calcium content of breast milk rather than of an increased need for vitamin D.

During pregnancy and lactation an intake of 400 I.U. is deemed desirable, although these recommendations are not well documented. Otherwise adults appear to obtain sufficient amounts if they are exposed to some degree of sunshine and have a varied diet. If occupational or clothing habits are such that exposure to sunlight is limited, a dietary source for adults is recommended.

In older children and adults who seldom develop rickets, who have a greater exposure to ultraviolet light and many other food sources, and whose growth rate is relatively slow, it is much more difficult to evaluate minimal needs, since no other criterion of adequacy of vitamin D has been established.

It is only when exposure to sunlight is inadequate, dietary intake of vitamin D is restricted, and needs are relatively high that deficiency symptoms develop.

Sources

Irradiation of precursor in skin. Vitamin D is available to the body by two separate pathways. The skin normally contains a fat-related substance, 7-dehydrocholesterol, which constitutes 0.15% to 0.42% of the sterols in the skin and which performs no biological function. However, when exposed to the short ultraviolet rays from 275 to 300 mμ in length from the sun or from mercury vapor sunlamps, it is converted into the biological active substance vitamin D_3, or cholecalciferol. This is then absorbed from the skin into the general circulation. It is still not clear whether the conversion takes place in the epithelial cells of the skin or on the surface of the skin, but evidence seems to favor the latter. The amount of vitamin D available through the irradiation of the precursor in the skin is influenced more by the amount of ultraviolet light to which the individual is exposed than by the amount of the precursor present. In the summer in the temperate zone ultraviolet rays may penetrate sufficiently far north for a maximum of four hours in the middle of the day. In winter this time may be reduced to less than an hour. Ultraviolet rays are incapable of penetrating fog, smog, clouds, smoke, ordinary window glass, window screening, clothing, or skin pigment. The presence of any or all of these reduces the potential vitamin D available through irradiation. The pigment in the skin, which acts as a protection against overproduction of vitamin D in dark-skinned people living in the tropics, reduces the benefits from the much smaller amount of irradiation available in the temperate zone. For this reason the incidence of rickets among dark-skinned infants in the temperate zone is much higher than among light-skinned infants and than among dark-skinned infants in the tropics. Some protection against overirradiation is necessary, since it can lead to the production of potentially toxic substances, such as tachysterol, toxisterol, and suprasterol.

A special window glass, mercury quartz, permits the transmission of ultraviolet rays. The benefits from its use in windows in hospital nurseries where patients are unable to be taken out-of-doors may justify the cost, which is over ten times that of regular glass.

Dietary intake. The other source of vitamin D, and in the temperate zone the major source, is ingested vitamin D. Some foods of animal origin, such as eggs, milk, butter, and fish-liver oils, constitute the major sources of the preformed vitamin, but they are characteristically poor and un-

reliable sources, the amount present varying with the diet and breed of the animal. Vegetables are poor sources. Even when all potential dietary sources are included, it is possible to obtain only about 125 I.U. per day. This would include egg yolk, with 2 to 5 I.U. per gram; butter, with 0.1 to 1.0 I.U. per gram; and milk, with 5 I.U. per cup. As a result it is now customary to rely on foods enriched with vitamin D or nutritional supplements during periods of maximum need for vitamin D. A study of the sources of vitamin D in diets of children showed that vitamin D in preparations and fortified milk were the major sources, with natural foods providing less than 25% and other fortified foods up to 50%. These other fortified foods provided vitamin D in excess of needs that were adequately met by natural foods, vitamin preparations, and fortified milk.

Milk, a carrier of both calcium and phosphorus needed for calcification of bones, is the food most commonly fortified with vitamin D. Evaporated milk, irradiated to provide 400 I.U. per quart of reconstituted milk, was the first food to be sold as an irradiated product. Now practically all homogenized milk and nonfat milk and much of the dried nonfat milk solids have vitamin D added. Regular milk, in which a cream layer rises to the top, is not fortified because the fat-soluble vitamin D would concentrate in the cream layer. About 85% of all milk sold in the United States is fortified with vitamin D at a level that will permit maximum utilization of its calcium and phosphorus. The cost of fortifying 100 gallons of milk is estimated at 4 cents.

Although milk is the only product that has been endorsed for fortification, vitamin D is being added to many other products, such as infant cereals, prepared breakfast cereals, milk flavorings, margarine, bread, and even some beverages. If a person consumed even one serving of each of these along with 1 quart of fortified milk a day, the intake could readily reach 1000 I.U. per day! However, since manufacturers are continually changing the amount they are adding to foods and the foods to which they are adding it, to assess the amount of vitamin D in the diet is difficult without access to the labels on the products. For instance, in the United States, millers have the option of adding from 250 to 1000 I.U. of vitamin D per pound of flour. Although the United States does not allow the addition of vitamin D to margarine, England requires 1300 to 1600 I.U. per pound and Germany 135 I.U.

In the temperate zone, where neither sunshine nor a diet of nonfortified products can be relied upon to provide enough vitamin D for protection from rickets, it has become standard pediatric practice to introduce a supplementary source of vitamin D in infant diets. The use of cod-liver oil, which had been traditional since the early 1920's, has been almost completely replaced by water-miscible preparations of vitamin D. This overcomes the problem of lipoid pneumonia in infants, caused by aspirating the oily cod-liver oil. The odor of the cod-liver oil was much more objectionable to mothers than to infants, as was the problem of oil-stained clothing. Water-miscible preparations traditionally contain vitamin A and also ascorbic acid. Most drug companies had voluntarily reduced the recommended dosage to provide only 400 I.U. of vitamin D per dose rather than the 800 I.U. previously suggested before the Food and Drug Administration made 400 I.U. mandatory in 1965.

Cod-liver oil preparations, which are still used, are standardized to provide 85 I.U. per gram, or 340 I.U. per teaspoon.

A solution of irradiated ergosterol (ergocalciferol) in a neutral oil is marketed as viosterol. The use of this very concentrated source of vitamin D increases the likelihood of an overdose.

The presence of calcium salts with vitamin D in therapeutic preparations may adversely effect the stability of vitamin D.

Distributors of mineral-vitamin preparations are being discouraged from combining vitamin D with mineral supplements, even though it may seem a logical combination.

In Europe, where the habit of using daily supplements of vitamin D or foods enriched with vitamin D has not been established, physicians have found that massive injections of 300,000 I.U. of vitamin D at intervals of six weeks to three months is an effective way to control rickets. Apparently no adverse effects result from such large doses, but in the United States smaller daily doses are preferred.

Toxicity

Since the demonstration over forty-five years ago that cod-liver oil was effective in preventing rickets, the disease has ceased to be a cause of concern to medical and public health authorities, although the *National Nutritional Survey* in 1970 revealed a 2% incidence of rickets. Now the cause for concern lies at the other end of the continuum, with attention being directed toward the problem of overuse of vitamin D. In one of the earliest studies to assess the need for vitamin D, Jeans and Stearns showed that no extra benefit was derived from levels above 400 I.U. per day, and that levels of 1800 I.U. per day actually retarded linear growth. More recently reports of hypercalcemia in infants, in which practically all tissues of the body are adversely affected, have focused attention on the possibility that high levels of vitamin D are causative. The withdrawal of all sources of vitamin D alleviated the high blood calcium levels with their rapid onset of symptoms of loss of appetite, nausea, weight loss, and failure to thrive. The level of vitamin D intake that precipitates hypercalcemia varies greatly from one individual to another. Adults receiving 100,000 I.U. of vitamin D for weeks or months will develop symptoms. An intake of 1000 to 3000 I.U. per kilogram of body weight in infants

(10,000 to 30,000 I.U. per day) is usually toxic. Apparently some infants experience a hypersensitivity to vitamin D and exhibit toxic symptoms on levels as low as 1000 I.U. per day, although the lower limit of toxicity is likely closer to 2000 to 3000 I.U. All forms of vitamin D are potentially dangerous, and the effects of an overdose resemble those of toxisterol or suprasterol.

The fact that benefits did not increase from vitamin D intakes in excess of 400 I.U. per day and a possibility that detrimental effects exist for sensitive individuals at levels above 2000 I.U. have led British authorities to persuade processors of vitamin D–enriched products to reduce the level of fortification so that a person consuming the recommended amount of the food would be protected against rickets and yet would not be in danger of excessive intake if he consumed all such fortified products. A report three years after the introduction of this policy, which reduced vitamin D intakes by one third to one half, indicated a decrease in the incidence of hypercalcemia and no increase in the incidence of rickets. It is generally recommended that the dose of vitamin D should not exceed that shown to be safe for children most reactive to vitamin D.

Large doses of vitamin A given concurrently with potentially toxic doses of vitamin D tend to reduce the incidence of toxic symptoms. Little is known about the mechanisms of the toxicity, but it is suggested that the liver may fail to inactivate the excessive amounts ingested.

VITAMIN E

Vitamin E, now known to be needed by twenty species, including man, was first recognized as a dietary essential in 1922. At that time it was found to be necessary for normal reproduction in animals. Since a deficiency was shown to produce permanent sterility in male animals and a decrease in the ability of female animals to conceive or to carry a fetus to term if conception did

occur, vitamin E became known as the antisterility factor. Although it is now understood that a failure in normal reproduction in animals is only one of the results of a vitamin E deficiency and that human reproduction is unlikely to be affected, the use of this term has persisted. Vitamin E deficiency states have been experimentally produced in many species, and some theories of its biochemical role have been advanced, but its role in human nutrition is still poorly understood. The understanding of vitamin E is complicated by the fact that a variety of other nutrients are capable of performing some but not all of the functions of this nutrient, and in some but not all species.

Chemical forms

The term *vitamin E* is applied to a group of chemical compounds known as the tocopherols (from Greek, *to bear child*). So far eight related tocopherols have been identified as having vitamin E activity. Chemically they differ only slightly, but biochemically more marked differences exist in their effectiveness. Alpha-tocopherol is considered the biologically active form.

Functions

Since vitamin E deficiencies have only recently been produced in human beings, most of our knowledge of vitamin E functions has come from experimentation on animals, such as chicks, rats, rabbits, and guinea pigs. From these it has become obvious that vitamin E affects different species in different ways. It has been possible, however, to postulate several functions for vitamin E.

Antioxidant in both animal and plant tissue. By being readily oxidized itself, tocopherol reduces the amount of oxygen available to other substances that may otherwise be destroyed or changed undesirably by the uptake of oxygen. Thus fats containing vitamin E are less susceptible to oxidation and the resulting rancidity than are those devoid of vitamin E. Vitamin A, unsaturated fatty acids, and vitamin C in foods are similarly protected against destruction when vitamin E is present. Tissue lipids are likewise less susceptible to excessive oxidation (peroxidation), which may modify structure of the tissue and hence its function.

Oxidation of the fat in the membrane and the stroma of the erythrocyte, or red blood cell, occurs when the protection against oxidation is lost as levels of tocopherol drop. The resulting weakness in the structure of the membrane results in hemolysis or breakdown of the cell. Other evidence of the antioxidative role of vitamin E has been established. In fact, some investigators believe that no other biochemical function can be attributed to vitamin E and that a loss of this antioxidant property and the resultant lipid oxidation can provide an explanation for all manifestations of a vitamin E deficiency. Others dispute this on the basis that other antioxidants can substitute for or can spare vitamin E in some but not all of its metabolic roles.

Cellular respiration. Vitamin E plays an essential role in the final biochemical changes by which energy from glucose and fatty acids is finally released and water is formed. This function has not been completely clarified. The fact that it seems to be involved primarily in respiration in heart and skeletal muscles may provide a rationale for earlier but unsuccessful attempts to treat human heart diseases and muscular dystrophy with vitamin E.

Synthesis of essential body compounds. In species capable of synthesizing vitamin C, tocopherol acts as a necessary cofactor. It also stimulates the synthesis of coenzyme Q, essential in the respiratory chain and plays a regulatory role in the incorporation of pyrimidines into the nucleic acid structure. This seems to be especially true in the bone marrow, where red blood cells are manufactured. In a vitamin E deficiency, abnormally large red blood cells (macro-

cytes) are formed when vitamin E fails to regulate the formation of nucleic acids.

Absorption and metabolism

As a fat-soluble substance, vitamin E requires the presence of bile for absorption, either from oil solutions or aqueous emulsions. It is apparently absorbed unchanged into the lymph and is transported in the bloodstream as tocopherol. Tocopherol is stored in various tissues, but adipose tissue, muscle, and liver are the major sites, with the uterus, testis, pituitary, and adrenals also containing high amounts.

A newborn infant has approximately 20 mg. of vitamin E stored in the body.

Requirements

In 1968 was the first time the Food and Nutrition Board of the National Research Council believed that sufficient information existed on which to base recommended dietary allowances. They determined the desirable intake was related to a unit of metabolic body size (weight in $kg.^{3/4}$) rather than to body weight or caloric intake and recommended that the diet provide 1.25 I.U. per unit of metabolic body size. The definition of 1 I.U. is 1 mg. of the acetate of alpha-tocopherol. They point out that the requirement will increase with an increase in the level of polyunsaturated fatty acids in the diet at the usual level of fat intake—40% of the calories coming from fat.

The requirements for pregnancy and lactation have not been determined, but it appears that vitamin E is transferred much more effectively through the milk than through the placenta to the infant.

Serum tocopherol levels are low at birth (0.25 mg. per 100 ml.), although the mother's level increases to a high of 1.5 to 2 mg. per 100 ml. at the end of pregnancy. These levels are associated with preparation for lactation. Human milk, which provides approximately 0.5 mg. per kilogram of body weight of the infant, is higher in vitamin

E than cow's milk and results in a faster increase in serum tocopherol levels of breast-fed babies. Infants with defective fat absorption may need supplementary vitamin E. Premature infants have low serum vitamin E values, which reflect the fact that most of the vitamin E is transferred to the fetus in the last two months of fetal life. After delivery these infants exhibit no other signs of vitamin E inadequacy regardless of dietary intake.

Food sources

Tocopherols occur in greatest concentration in vegetable oils, wheat germ oil being the source from which vitamin E was first obtained. The vitamin E value of this and other vegetable oils is given in Table 11-2. Generally speaking, amount of naturally occurring vitamin E in oils increases along with an increase in polyunsaturated fatty acids. Tocopherols are also present in a wide variety of other plant and animal tissues, as shown in Table 11-3.

A study of the vitamin E activity of typical meals showed that breakfasts ranged from 0.59 to 3.68 mg., lunches from 0.44 to 5.37 mg., and dinners from 1.61 to 6.38 mg. Only by choosing the meals highest in tocopherol from each group was it possible to obtain 15 mg. per day, which is believed to be an adequate level of intake. A range for three meals of 2.6 to 15.4 mg., with an average intake of 7.4 mg., was found. This was considered low in the light of the increased consumption of polyunsaturated fatty acids that increases the need for tocopherol.

These same investigators found a 63% to 74% decrease in the tocopherol content during freezer storage of foods fried in oil. Since an increasing number of foods are being stored frozen, this may be additional cause for concern when coupled with the low intake. The heating of cooking oils destroys virtually all the tocopherol present,

Table 11-2. Tocopherol content of 100 gm. of various oils°

Food	mg./100 gm.
Wheat germ oil	260
Corn oil	
Unhydrogenated	100
Hydrogenated	105
Cottonseed oil	
Unhydrogenated	91
Hydrogenated	80
Soybean oil	
Unhydrogenated	101
Hydrogenated	73
Safflower oil	
Stabilized	59
Unstabilized	36
Soybean oil	130
Coconut oil	8

*From Bunnell, R. H., Keating, T., Quaresimo, A., and Parmin, G. K.: Alpha-tocopherol content of foods, Amer. J. Clin. Nutr. **17:**1, 1965.

Table 11-3. Vitamin E content of 100 gm. of some representative foods°

Food	mg./100 gm.
Mayonnaise	50.0
Margarine (made with corn oil)	46.7
Yellow cornmeal	3.4
Whole-wheat bread	2.2
Beef liver, broiled	1.62
Egg	1.43
Fillet of haddock, broiled	1.20
Butter	1.0
Tomatoes, fresh	0.85
Green peas, frozen	0.65
Ground beef	0.63
Pork chops, pan-fried	0.60
Chicken breast	0.58
Cornflakes	0.43
Banana	0.42
White bread	0.23
Carrots	0.21
Orange juice, fresh	0.20
Potato, baked	0.055

*From Bunnell, R. H., Keating, J., Quaresimo, A., and Parmin, G. K.: Alpha-tocopherol content of foods, Amer. J. Clin. Nutr. **17:**1, 1965.

but esters of tocopherol such as tocopherol acetate are less than one fifth destroyed.

Fruits and vegetables are relatively poor sources of tocopherol, but fresh and frozen vegetables retain much more than canned products. Little is lost in normal cooking procedures.

Sixty-four percent of dietary tocopherol comes from oils, shortening, and margarine; 11%, from fruits and vegetables; and only 7% from grains.

Deficiency

In animals. A lack of vitamin E in animals is manifest in a wide variety of seemingly unrelated ways, with symptoms involving the muscles, nervous system, reproductive organs, vascular system, and glandular system. Chicks show characteristic changes in the central nervous system, known as *encephalomalacia.* Ubichromenol will delay the onset of symptoms. Rats show necrotic liver degeneration. These symptoms can be relieved or prevented by the amino acid cystine or the mineral element selenium, both of which can substitute for vitamin E in this instance. A condition known as *exudative diathesis,* in which large patches of fluid accumulation appear beneath the skin on the breast, legs, abdomen, and neck, also occurs in rats and chicks. This condition is also relieved by selenium. Reproductive failure in rats, mice, and guinea pigs has been well documented. Degeneration of the epithelium results in permanent sterility in males. Female rats that do conceive will resorb the fetus by the eighth day of the 22-day gestation period. Fetuses can be salvaged if vitamin E is given by the fifth day, but if it is delayed until after the sixth, many congenital abnormalities appear.

The accumulation of a brown pigment (ceroid) at resorption sites in the uterus and in the kidney of rats has been attributed to vitamin E or selenium deficiency and is likely related to oxidative changes in unsaturated fatty acids. A similar pigment that occurs in nerve cells in human senility shows up in nerve cells when stress factors are superimposed on a vitamin E–deficient diet. Ceroid is also associated with the fatty streaks in the arterial wall that precede the formation of the arterial plaque of atherosclerosis.

Muscular dystrophy, characterized by muscular weakness caused by fragmentation of muscle fibers, accumulation of fluid in interstitial spaces, and deterioration of hyaline membrane, occurs in vitamin E deficiency in guinea pigs, rabbits, and monkeys. The premature release of enzymes from the cell lysosome when the membrane becomes more susceptible to lipid peroxidation and accompanying breakdown has been suggested as a cause of muscular dystrophy. No relationship has been established between vitamin E nutrition and human muscular dystrophy, believed to be a hereditary condition causing extensive wasting of certain voluntary muscles, with an onset from birth to adulthood. Monkeys exhibit a characteristic megaloblastic anemic reaction to vitamin E inadequacy.

In human beings. Except experimentally, vitamin E deficiency is rarely seen in human beings. Certain biochemical changes have been associated with a low dietary intake coupled with either an increased need, as in a diet high in vegetable oils with a high polyunsaturated fatty acid content, or with conditions that interfere with fat absorption. Increased susceptibility of the membrane of the erythrocytes to hemolysis is the most easily detected evidence of vitamin E deficiency. Other indications of vitamin E inadequacy are a drop in the level of tocopherol in blood, an increase in urinary excretion of creatine, and a decrease in creatinine excretion.

Work done on induced vitamin E deficiencies in mental patients in Illinois indicates that with 3 mg. of tocopherol in the diet, plasma tocopherol levels drop below normal values of 1 mg. per 100 ml. of blood. This drop is accompanied by increased tendency to hemolysis in red blood cells, especially below 0.5 mg. tocopherol. When the lard in the diet (low in polyunsaturated fatty acids) was replaced by corn oil (high in polyunsaturated fatty acids), a further drop occurred in serum tocopherol levels. An already high rate of erythrocyte hemolysis was not increased further. Larger amounts of vitamin E were required to maintain normal blood tocopherol levels when corn oil was substituted for lard.

Low serum levels of vitamin E have been associated with a macrocytic anemia in which the life-span of the red blood cells is decreased and the synthesis of both DNA and RNA is increased. Children with kwashiorkor and the vitamin A deficiency disease xerophthalmia have much lower serum tocopherol levels and a greatly reduced chance of responding to therapy than do children with kwashiorkor without xerophthalmia. Some evidence suggests the muscular changes that occur in infants suffering from cystic fibrosis of the pancreas resemble those of vitamin E deficiency in animals. Some studies have also shown an accumulation of the ceroid pigment in muscles.

Substitutes

Much of the confusion over the role of vitamin E has arisen because of the ability of many other chemically unrelated substances to substitute for some or all of the many biochemical functions of the tocopherols. The mineral selenium either replaces vitamin E as an antioxidant or spares it so that several vitamin E deficiency symptoms do not develop. The distribution of selenium to certain tissues may be low, thereby offering an explanation of its failure to protect against all vitamin E deficiencies, such as encephalomalacia and muscular dystrophy. Selenium does not have the same effect that vitamin E does in maintaining coenzyme Q levels in tissues. The distribution of selenium in the diet is unrelated to vitamin E in diet.

Ubichromenol has been shown to have vitamin E activity, especially in delaying onset of symptoms. The effect of selenium may be to enhance the ubichromenol activity in various tissues, which in turn may control the release of proteolytic enzymes from lysosomes.

A chemical antioxidant, DPPD (*N,N'*-diphenyl-*p*-phenylene), can replace all functions of vitamin E, at least for a considerable period of time. It is effective in preventing fetal resorptions.

The presence of the sulfur-containing amino acid cystine is also involved in influencing the antioxidative effectiveness of vitamin E and its substitutes.

Clinical uses

Because of the seemingly unrelated pathological changes in tocopherol deficiencies in animals there has been a temptation to use vitamin E in the treatment of a large number of conditions, even though no relationship between vitamin E nutrition and these conditions has been confirmed. Some 2000 papers have appeared on the therapeutic uses of vitamin E. Contradictory reports on their effectiveness continue to appear, and in a few cases reasonable evidence of its therapeutic value exists. Perhaps most controversial is its use with women who have suffered repeated spontaneous abortions. Some evidence supports such therapy, but much gives negative results. Some forms of ulcers have responded well to the use of vitamin E, but evidence is insufficient to support claims for its effectiveness in heart disease, muscular dystrophy, male infertility, diabetes, complications of menopause or gangrene. Recent evidence has shown that vitamin E in tissues provides some protection against the detrimental effect of pollutants in the air.

Good evidence exists to support the therapeutic use of vitamin E when absorption of fat has been depressed, when the intake of polyunsaturated fatty acids has increased, or in severe protein deficiency.

VITAMIN K

Vitamin K was first discovered in 1934 by a Danish scientist who identified it as the fat-soluble factor necessary for the co-agulation of the blood. Since the Danish word for the process is spelled *koagulation* he designated this factor as vitamin K. The term *vitamin K* is used to designate a group of substances belonging to a chemical group known as quinones. These include naturally occurring fat-soluble vitamins K_1 and K_2 and the chemically related synthetic substance menadione, which is also known as vitamin K_3. Vitamin K_3 serves as an intermediary substance in the formation from both vitamin K_1 and K_2 of the biologically active form of the vitamin believed to be vitamin K_2-20. (The twenty designated the number of carbon atoms in a carbon chain that is part of the vitamin molecule.) Vitamin K_1 occurs primarily in green leafy plants. It was first isolated from alfalfa meal and is now known as phylloquinone or phytoquinone. Vitamin K_2, which has 35 carbons in its carbon chain as it occurs in nature, is produced by bacterial synthesis in the gastrointestinal tract. It has also been isolated from putrified fish meal and has been designated as farnoquinone. Vitamin K_1 either in its natural form or in a synthetic form is available for therapeutic purposes. Any one of these forms is usable, but they do differ in the extent to which they may cause side effects when used therapeutically.

In addition to the naturally occurring vitamin K and synthetic menadione, all of which are fat soluble, the following have been produced synthetically: Hykinone and Synkayvite, both of which are water solu-

Table 11-4. Interrelationship and properties of compounds with vitamin K activity

Naturally occurring	Synthetic		
Fat-soluble	Fat-soluble	Water-soluble	Water-miscible
Form			
Vitamin K_1		Synkayvite	Mephyton
Phylloquinone		Hykinone	Konakion
Green plants			Mono-Kay
Vitamin K_2	Vitamin K_3 menadione		
Farnoquinone	Biologically active		
Bacterial synthesis	K_2-20		
Mode of administration			
Orally (except for infants)	Subcutaneously		Orally
Intravenously	Intramuscularly		Intramuscularly
Subcutaneously			Subcutaneously
Intravenously			Intravenously
Uses			
Orally several days before	Obstructive jaundice		1 mg. to newborn
delivery	Woman in labor		
To counteract anticoagulants	Newborn		
Gastrointestinal surgery			
Special precautions			
No side effects	Small margin of safety		Wide margin
	Safe after first few weeks		of safety
	Large doses produce hemolytic		
	anemia, hyperbilirubinemia,		
	and kernicterus		

ble, and Mephyton, Konakion, and Mono-Kay, all of which are water miscible. These latter forms have properties that make them especially suited to the treatment of vitamin K deficiencies when fat absorption is impaired. The relationship among these various forms is somewhat confusing. Table 11-4 attempts to clarify these interrelationships and tabulates the special properties of each.

The naturally occurring fat-soluble forms of the vitamin may be stored in the body, primarily in the liver.

Vitamin K is stable to heat and reducing agents but is destroyed by light, acid, alkali, and oxidizing agents.

Functions

The ability of the blood to coagulate is dependent on the presence of many factors, among which are prothrombin and proconvertin. Vitamin K is necessary for the synthesis of prothrombin and proconvertin in the liver, although it is not a part of either substance. Prothrombin levels in the blood determine the rate at which the blood will clot, high levels indicating good coagulability, low levels a depressed rate of coagulation. Proconvertin, also known as factor VII, is also required for the coagulation of the blood. There is some reason to believe that vitamin K is required for the synthesis of other factors involved in blood-clotting. It has also been suggested that vitamin K takes part in an oxidation reduction system in which the SH group in fibrinogen is oxidized to the S-S group to form the clot, fibrin.

Vitamin K is involved in a process called phosphorylation in which phosphate is added to glucose to facilitate its passage through cell membranes and its conversion into glycogen.

Coenzyme Q, which is a link in the respiratory chain of reactions involved in the ultimate release of energy from fatty acids and glucose, is similar to vitamin K chemically. Vitamin K participates in cellular respiration in lower forms of animals.

Absorption

Since vitamin K is fat soluble, its absorption is regulated by the same factors that govern fat absorption. An obstruction of the bile duct limiting the secretion of fat-emulsifying bile salts, as occurs in obstructive jaundice, will reduce absorption, as will failure of the liver to secrete bile. The use of a nonutilizable oil such as mineral oil will cause the excretion of vitamin K in the feces.

Vitamin K is absorbed in the upper part of the gastrointestinal tract, as are other fat-related factors. This raises the question of how much of the vitamin K synthesized in the lower part of the gastrointestinal tract will be absorbed.

An anticoagulant, Dicumarol, which is similar chemically to vitamin K, apparently replaces vitamin K in the liver, where it not only is ineffective in promoting prothrombin synthesis but also blocks a normal synthesis. The widespread use of anticoagulant drugs in phlebitis or thrombosis has made the use of vitamin K therapy more important to control hemorrhaging.

Requirements

The National Research Council recognizes vitamin K as a dietary essential but has been unable to make any quantitative evaluation of needs because of its abundance in most diets. Only for newborn infants does any need for special attention to vitamin K appear, and for them an intake of 1 to 5 mg. should be adequate. One study of depleted adults showed a need for 0.03 mg. per kilogram.

Sources

For most individuals adequate levels of vitamin K are provided by green and yellow vegetables and from the synthesis of the vitamin by intestinal bacteria. The concentration of vitamin K in foods is highest in dark leafy green vegetables, with some being found in fruits, tubers, and seeds. It usually occurs in association with chlorophyll in the chloroplasts. Alfalfa is an especially rich source, but in spite of the efforts of food faddists, is not an accepted item in average diets. No evidence of adult dietary inadequacies exists to warrant suggestions that the diet be supplemented with such a rich source.

Since much of the bacterial synthesis occurs in the lower intestine, only a small portion of that synthesized may actually be absorbed. The amount synthesized will also be reduced when substances are taken that depress the growth of intestinal bacteria. Salicylic acid, an ingredient in most pain depressants of the aspirin type, and certain antibiotics and sulfonamides may act in this way. Young infants are the ones most likely to suffer from a subnormal level of intestinal synthesis, for during the first few days of life their relatively sterile intestinal tract does not contain the organisms that synthesize vitamin K. Little vitamin K passes the placental barrier from the maternal circulation to be stored in fetal tissue, although if vitamin K is given to the mother at delivery, a sufficient amount passes to stimulate prothrombin synthesis. Milk is low in vitamin K so that even those who receive nourishment in the first few days of life do not receive an appreciable amount of vitamin K. Breast-fed infants are at an even greater disadvantage than bottle-fed infants because mother's milk is often not produced in significant amounts for several days, it contains about one fourth the amount of vitamin K as does cow's milk, and there is less chance of vitamin K–synthesizing bacteria developing in the lower intestine.

Deficiency

Because vitamin K can be synthesized and also is provided in adequate amounts in practically all diets, a deficiency in adults is invariably caused by a failure in absorption. Low prothrombin levels can also be due to failure of the liver to synthesize it.

In infants, however, the lack of bacteria to synthesize vitamin K, the low stores of vitamin K in the infant at birth, and the small amount provided in milk characteristically lead to low prothrombin levels and a prolonged coagulation time. This occurs at a time when the incidence of hemorrhage is high. The association between vitamin K and blood coagulation times led to the routine administration of vitamin K to the mother just prior to delivery or to the infant in the first days of life to reduce neonatal deaths caused by hemorrhage. After its use had become routine, however, an increase in a hemolytic type of anemia, an accumulation of bilirubin in the blood, and a condition known as kernicterus, in which bile pigment accumulates in the gray matter of the central nervous system, were attributed to vitamin K toxicity from the uncontrolled use of synthetic vitamin K. An evaluation of vitamin K therapy in newborn infants has shown that it is desirable but that certain precautions should be observed to provide the greatest benefits and the greatest margin of safety. Several studies have shown that the normal incidence of hemorrhage of the newborn of 1 in 400 infants is markedly reduced with vitamin K therapy and especially in babies who may get less than adequate oxygen at birth. Natural vitamin K_1 is considered the most desirable form, as there have been no reports of toxicity from oral administration of 1 to 2 mg. Doses of 0.5 to 1 mg. of a water-miscible preparation provide protection when given intravenously or intramuscularly to the infant. Menadione, a synthetic vitamin K_1, cannot be given orally, as it causes vomiting. A dose of 2 to 5 mg. given to the mother usually transfers adequate protection to the infant, but larger doses that ensure adequate levels for the infant may be hazardous to some infants. It is recommended that protection be provided by administering natural vitamin K_1 to the infant after birth rather than to the mother, with larger doses recommended for an infant whose mother has been given anticoagulant therapy. It can be given orally, subcutaneously, intramuscularly, or intravenously. The Food and Drug Administration has prohibited the inclusion of menadione (vitamin K_3) in prenatal supplements.

SELECTED REFERENCES
Vitamin A

Ames, S. R.: Factors affecting absorption, transport and storage of vitamin A, Amer. J. Clin. Nutr. 22:934, 1969.

Chopra, J. G., and Kevany, J.: Hypovitaminosis A in the Americas, Amer. J. Clin. Nutr. 23:231, 1970.

Dowling, J. E., and Wald, G.: Role of vitamin A acid, Vitamins Hormones 18:515, 1960.

Editorial: Hypervitaminosis A.: its broadening spectrum, Amer. J. Clin. Nutr. 6:335, 1958.

Goodman, D. S., and Huang, H. S.: Biosynthesis of vitamin A with rat intestinal enzymes, Science 149:879, 1965.

Greaves, J. P., and Tan, J.: Vitamin A and carotene in British and American diets, Brit. J. Nutr. 20:819, 1966.

McLaren, D. S., Shirajan, E., Tchalian, M., and Khoury, G.: Xerophthalmia in Jordan, Amer. J. Clin. Nutr. 17:117, 1965.

McLaren, D. S., Tchalian, M., and Ajans, Z. A.: Biochemical and hematalogic changes in the vitamin A-deficient rat, Amer. J. Clin. Nutr. 17:131, 1965.

Olson, J. A.: The alpha and omega of vitamin A metabolism, Amer. J. Clin. Nutr. 22:953, 1969.

Olson, J. A.: Metabolism and function of vitamin A, Fed. Proc. 28:1670, 1969.

Owen, E. C.: Some aspects of the metabolism of vitamin A and carotene, World Rev. Nutr. Diet. 5:132, 1965.

Roels, O. A.: Present knowledge of vitamin A, Nutr. Rev. 24:129, 1966.

Underwood, B. A., Siegel, H., Weisell, R. C., and Dolinski, M.: Liver stores of vitamin A in a normal population dying suddenly or rapidly from unnatural causes in New York City, Amer. J. Clin. Nutr. 23:1037, 1970.

Wolf, G.: Some thoughts on the metabolic role of Vitamin A, Nutr. Rev. 20:161, 1962.

Wolf, G.: International symposium on metabolic function of vitamin A, Amer. J. Clin. Nutr. 22:903, 1969.

Vitamin D

Bransby, E. R., Berry, W. T. C., and Taylor, D. M.: Study of the vitamin D intake of infants in 1960, Brit. Med. J. 1:1661, 1964.

Committee on Nutrition: The prophylactic requirement and toxicity of vitamin D, Pediatrics 31:512, 1963.

Committee on Nutrition: Vitamin D intake and the hypercalcemic syndrome, Pediatrics 35:1022, 1965.

DeLuca, H. F.: Recent advances on the metabolism and function of vitamin D, Fed. Proc. 28:1678, 1969.

Ebel, J. G., Taylor, A. N., and Wasserman, R. H.: Vitamin D–induced calcium-binding protein of intestinal mucosa, Amer. J. Clin. Nutr. 22:431, 1969.

Harris, F., Hoffenberg, R., and Blach, E.: Calcium kinetics in vitamin D deficiency rickets, Metabolism 14:1101, 1965.

Harrison, H. E.: Vitamin D and permeability of intestinal mucosa to calcium, Amer. J. Physiol. 208:370, 1965.

Kimberg, D. V.: Effect of vitamin D and steroid hormones on the active transport of calcium by the intestine, New Eng. J. Med. 280:396, 1969.

Norman, A. W.: Actinomycin D and the response to vitamin D, Science 149:184, 1965.

Ponchon, G., and DeLuca, H. F.: Metabolites of vitamin D3 and biologic activity, J. Nutr. 99: 157, 1969.

Seelig, M. S.: Vitamin D and cardiovascular, renal, and brain damage in infancy and childhood, Ann. N. Y. Acad. Sci. 147:537, 1969.

Taylor, A. N., and Wasserman, R. H.: Correlations between vitamin D–induced calcium-binding protein and intestinal absorption of calcium, Fed. Proc. 28:1834, 1969.

Wasserman, R. H.: Vitamin D and the intestinal absorption of calcium, New York, J. Med. 64:1329, 1964.

Vitamin E

Booth, V. H., and Bradford, M. P.: Tocopherol content of fruits and vegetables, Brit. J. Nutr. 17:575, 1963.

Bunnell, R. H., Keating, J., Quaresimo, A., and Parman, G. K.: Alpha-tocopherol content of foods, Amer. J. Clin. Nutr. 17:1, 1965.

Century, B., and Horwitt, M. K.: Biological availability of various forms of vitamin E with respect to different indices of deficiency, Fed. Proc. 24:906, 1965.

Committee on Nutrition, American Academy of Pediatrics: Vitamin E in human nutrition, Pediatrics, 31:324, 1963.

Green J. and Bunyan, J.: Vitamin E and the biological antioxidant theory, Nutr. Abstr. Rev. 39:321, 1969.

Herting, D. C.: Perspectives on vitamin E, Amer. J. Clin. Nutr. 19:210, 1966.

Herting, D. C., and Drury, E. E.: Plasma tocopherol levels in man, Amer. J. Clin. Nutr. 17:351, 1965.

McMasters, V., Lewis, J. K., Kinsell, L. W., Van Der Veen, J., and Olcott, H. S.: Effect of supplementing the diet of man with tocopherol on the tocopherol levels of adipose tissue and plasma, Amer. J. Clin. Nutr. 17:357, 1965.

Roels, O. A.: Present knowledge of vitamin E, Nutr. Rev. 25:33, 1967.

Tappel, A. L.: Will antioxidant nutrients slow aging processes? Geriatrics **23**:97, 1968.

Vitamin K

Committee on Nutrition: Vitamin K compounds and the water-soluble analogues, Pediatrics **28**:501, 1961.

Goldman, H. I., and Amades, P.: Vitamin K deficiency after the newborn period, Pediatrics **44**:745, 1969.

Johnson, B. C.: Dietary factors and vitamin K, Nutr. Rev. **22**:225, 1964.

Olson, R.: Present knowledge of vitamin K: In Present knowledge of nutrition, ed. 3, New York, 1967, Nutrition Foundation, Inc.

Owen, G. M., Nelson, C. E., Baker, G. L., Connor, W. E., and Jacobs, J. P.: Use of vitamin K_1 in pregnancy, Amer. J. Obstet. Gynec. **99**:368, 1967.

Wefring, K. W.: Hemorrhage in the newborn and vitamin K prophylaxis, J. Pediat. **63**:663, 1963.

12 | *Water-soluble vitamins*

ASCORBIC ACID

Vitamin C, cevitamic acid, hexuronic acid, and ascorbic acid are names that have all at one time or another been applied to the antiscorbutic or scurvy-preventative substance discovered in 1932 by King and Waugh. They isolated it from lemon juice. Almost simultaneously, Szent-Györgyi found it in the suprarenal gland, located near the kidney, and in oranges and cabbage.

Descriptions of scurvy can be traced as far back as a papyrus from 500 B.C. found at Thebes, the writings of Hippocrates in 400 B.C., and other recurring references in early recorded history. It had been known for 250 years that scurvy could be controlled by dietary means and since 1906 that it was a deficiency disease, but the search for the effective agent ended only with the isolation of the relatively simple white crystals of vitamin C in 1932.

The conquest of scurvy is of special historic interest because it was in an effort to cure this "scourge of the Navy" that the first carefully conceived nutrition experiment was conducted with human beings. British seamen who embarked on long sea voyages without an opportunity to replenish supplies for long periods did so knowing that a large portion of the crew would die or be incapacitated by scurvy. For instance, Magellan lost many of the 196 men who started around Cape Horn with him in 1520, and in 1497 Vasco da Gama lost 100 of 150 men. In 1775 Captain Cook's crew was spared by his insistence that they eat a thick soup he called "sour krout." In 1747 Dr. James Lind, a British physician, hypoth-

esized that various "acidic principles" might have antiscorbutic properties. To test his theory he distributed twelve sailors suffering from scurvy into six groups of two each and fed them the ship's basic diet plus one of six potential cures—oil of vitriol, or sulfuric acid, in water three times a day, 2 teaspoonsful of vinegar three times a day, ½ pint of seawater per day, and 2 oranges or 1 lemon per day. The results of his experiment are now legend—both oranges and lemons had miraculous curative powers, the sailors assigned to this treatment being restored to active duty within six days, whereas those on other treatments showed no progress. Not only did he prove that scurvy could be cured, but he laid the foundation for the theory that lack of an essential food element could cause illness. Others had advanced similar theories even a century earlier, but their observations had gone virtually unnoticed.

It was fifty years later before the British Navy recognized Lind's work to the point of requiring that all ships leaving British ports carry sufficient lime juice to have it available for its crew throughout the whole voyage. The routine use of lime juice led to the use of the term "limey" to refer to a British seaman, a term that now has been extended to all British servicemen.

Although the British Navy was the first to take steps to prevent scurvy, many other groups had suffered from it and in some cases had found a cure. Crusaders believed that those who could survive the pain that attacked feet and legs and the changes in their gums until spring would usually be cured by warm temperatures. Cartier's expedition, which was forced to spend a winter near Montreal in 1535, was spared when the Indians taught his group to use the bark of a pine tree, the ameda, to cure scurvy. French and Spanish sailors were saved because of the quantities of onions and leeks they consumed. Sailors in the Mediterranean were seldom away long enough to deplete their tissue reserves of vitamin C. Scurvy had been known to occur in the late spring in European cities but not in rural areas. By this time, city dwellers had been reduced to a diet of meat and bread, whereas their counterparts in the country still had some cabbage, onions, and potatoes left in storage. After failure of the potato crop even rural populations experienced scurvy outbreaks. As late as 1846 Mormons making their way west to Utah were forced to winter in Nebraska on a diet of mush. Many of them succumbed to scurvy. Spaniards landing after long sea voyages in California in 1602, 1603, and again in 1769 lost many of their numbers, and their first task after landing was the search for an herb or plant to cure scurvy.

Medical authorities who have considered scurvy a disease of the past have been appalled by some reports of infantile scurvy in the 1960's. Infantile scurvy was first reported in the late nineteenth century and paralleled the change from the use of wet nurses to preserved milk. It increased again when pasteurization of milk became mandatory. Again, it seems to be occurring among bottle-fed infants whose formula has been subjected to prolonged heat treatment and who receive no fruit juice or vitamin C concentrate. Canadian authorities, faced with a rapid increase in scurvy among 6- to 12-month-old babies, have suggested the enrichment of commercial formula preparations with ascorbic acid, the use of supplements, and the encouragement of breast-feeding, since human milk contains about six times as much vitamin C as pasteurized

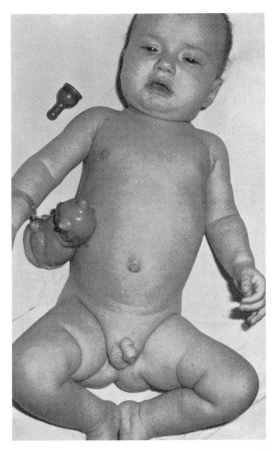

Fig. 12-1. Infant with scurvy. Note frog position of legs and apprehension of infant in anticipation of handling of tender limbs. (From Grewar, D.: Clin. Pediat. [Phila.] 4:82, 1965.)

cow's milk. American nutritionists believe that education in the early use of orange juice or a vitamin preparation is a more reasonable approach to the problem. Australia, with the highest rate of infantile scurvy, has considered providing free orange juice or multivitamins rather than enriching milk. A typical case of infantile scurvy is shown in Fig. 12-1.

Chemical properties

Chemically ascorbic acid is a simple 6-carbon compound closely related to the monosaccharides. The synthetic form of the vitamin, first produced in 1933, is derived

$$\text{Reduced ascorbic} \underset{1}{\overset{2}{\rightleftarrows}} \text{Dehydroascorbic} \xrightarrow{+H_2O} \text{Diketogulonic}$$
$$\text{acid} \qquad\qquad \text{acid} \qquad\qquad 1 \qquad \text{acid*}$$

1   Oxidation

2   Reduction

Fig. 12-2. Relationship of various chemical forms of ascorbic acid.

*   Biologically inactive

from the monsaccharides—glucose of sugar or galactose of milk sugar. The body cannot discriminate between natural and synthetic forms so that they can be used interchangeably.

Vitamin C, with the formula $C_6H_8O_6$, is known as reduced ascorbic acid and is susceptible to oxidation. It has now been established that the first product of the oxidation of this biologically active compound, dehydroascorbic acid ($C_6H_6O_6$), which has 2 less hydrogens, can be used equally as well by the body. It is apparently reduced again to the active form by the body before taking part in biological reactions. Further oxidation of dehydroascorbic acid produces a product, diketogulonic acid, with no antiscorbutic properties, and the oxidative process is irreversible. The changes are shown schematically in Fig. 12-2.

Some evidence exists that reduced ascorbic acid is changed in kidney cells to dehydroascorbic acid, a form in which it is more readily transported to the tissues. It also penetrates into the cell more easily in this oxidized form.

Most animals have the ability to synthesize ascorbic acid and therefore need no dietary supply of it. This synthesis takes place primarily in the microsomes of the cell, especially liver cells. So far only five species have been found that lack the enzyme necessary to complete the conversion of glucose or galactose to ascorbic acid. Man, monkey, the guinea pig, the Indian fruit bat, and the red-vented bulbul bird are the only species known to rely on a dietary source of ascorbic acid. Of these, the guinea pig is used most extensively in research.

In plants ascorbic acid is accumulated during the ripening process, presumably synthesized in the plant cells from the natural glucose in fruit.

d-Ascorbic acid, structurally related to the biologically active l-ascorbic acid, is not utilized by the human being unless it is given in small doses throughout the day. It is being used extensively as a preservative in processing meat. To avoid possible confusion and any implication that d-ascorbic acid is a vitamin, it has been recommended that the term *erythrobic acid* be applied to this compound.

Other reducing compounds have been found that can replace ascorbic acid in some of its biological roles, but none is effective in curing scurvy.

Functions

Although ascorbic acid is a relatively simple compound that has been available in a purified form at reasonable cost for over thirty-five years, biochemists, nutritionists, and physiologists have been unable to shed much light on the nature of its biochemical role. In contrast to most water-soluble vitamins, it has no clear-cut role as a catalyst, nor is it part of any enzyme or structure. Fragments of knowledge that will eventually form the total picture are suggesting some of its potential roles, but we still find the same general terms applied to ascorbic acid deficiency now as were used fifty years ago. The following are some of the more widely accepted roles.

Collagen formation. The primary defect in scurvy is the failure of collagen formation in the fibroblasts in connective tissue. Collagen, the protein substance that binds the cells together in much the same way that mortar binds bricks, is characterized by the amino acid, hydroxyproline. Hydroxyproline, which constitutes one third of the amino acid composition of collagen, is not available from food. It is formed by the hydroxylation of proline once it has been incorporated in the amino acid chain of the collagen molecule. This reaction is catalyzed by ascorbic acid. Thus in an ascorbic acid deficiency this change does not occur to provide the basic building material for collagen, and a collagen with a low hydroxyproline content is formed. A failure in collagen synthesis is observed primarily in tissues subjected to stress. Most collagen is inert metabolically and once laid down does not require vitamin C for maintenance, but certain fractions of collagen in some tissues are highly active and subject to rapid breakdown in ascorbic acid deficiency.

When the collagen is not formed or maintained in a scorbutic animal, the failure shows up in many ways. The need for ascorbic acid in healing of wounds is great. Here, new connective tissue, which is primarily collagen, must be formed. The high concentration of ascorbic acid found in scar tissue and the drops in blood level of the vitamin, which occur during healing, suggest that it is mobilized to the site of the healing. High levels are maintained after the scar tissue has been completely formed,

indicating a need for maintenance of scar tissue. There is some controversy regarding the need for increasing the dietary intake preoperatively and postoperatively for individuals whose tissues are apparently saturated with vitamin C. Some authorities recommend intakes of 100 to 300 mg. per day to ensure rapid and complete healing, whereas others believe this is unnecessary. However, since we have no evidence of adverse effects from higher levels, there is little reason to forego possible benefits from larger intakes.

Decrease in elasticity of the cell walls, which become fragile and frequently rupture to cause small pinpoint hemorrhages, is at least partially the result of failure of collagen in the muscle in which small blood vessels are embedded. These subcutaneous hemorrhages show up most often in areas subjected to mechanical stress, such as in the gums, which often become soft, spongy, and hemorrhage easily, and in the ends of the long bones. Such changes occur when tissue saturation falls below 60% to 90% of normal levels.

The matrix of the bone shaft, which is primarily collagen, may be defective when collagen formation fails. It is less capable of holding calcium and phosphorus during bone calcification, resulting in weakened bone structure. The intercellular spaces do calcify, however. Sometimes bones are displaced when supporting cartilage is weakened as a result of a lack of vitamin C for maintenance. Characteristic bone changes in scurvy are shown in Fig. 12-3 and gum changes in Fig. 12-4.

Dentin formation. Changes in tooth structure have been related to ascorbic acid status during a critical period in tooth formation. The dentin layer, arising from a group of cells known as odontoblasts, does not form normally in scorbutic animals, apparently because of the degeneration and death of the odontoblasts at the time calcification of the dentin layer should occur. This, of course, produces a tooth with a

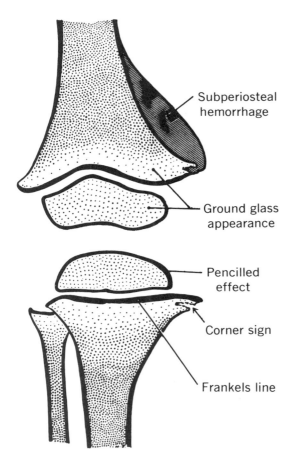

Subperiosteal hemorrhage

Ground glass appearance

Pencilled effect

Corner sign

Frankels line

Fig. 12-3. Radiographic signs of scurvy. (From Grewar, D.: Clin. Pediat: [Phila.] **4**:82, 1965.)

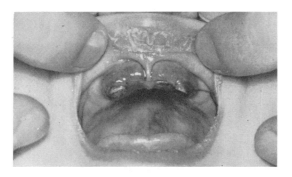

Fig. 12-4. Gum hemorrhage in scorbutic infant. Note occurrence only where teeth have erupted; it does not occur in edentulous gum. (From Grewar, D.: Clin. Pediat. [Phila.] **4**:82, 1965.)

structural weakness that is less able to resist mechanical injury or to resist decay once it is initiated.

Tyrosine metabolism. The role of ascorbic acid in the utilization of the amino acid tyrosine is the one most clearly established by biochemists. It is necessary only when large amounts of tyrosine are being used. Under these circumstances, vitamin C is needed to protect one of the enzymes involved in the oxidation of tyrosine from destruction by the substrate on which it acts. When the enzyme is destroyed, intermediate products of tyrosine metabolism appear in the urine, indicating abnormal use of the amino acid and a failure of the body to oxidize it. Premature infants on high-protein diets often show a similar defect.

Utilization of iron and calcium. The absorption of iron from the intestinal tract is facilitated by the presence of vitamin C, which is effective as a reducing agent to keep ferrous iron in the reduced form in which it is most readily absorbed. The interrelationship with iron is also evident in that vitamin C activates some iron-containing enzymes. The role of ascorbic acid in facilitating calcium absorption may involve preventing its precipitation as an insoluble complex.

Utilization of folic acid. The conversion of the inactive form of the vitamin folic acid to the active form, the citrovorum factor, is catalyzed by ascorbic acid. It may be in this way that vitamin C is effective in preventing the megaloblastic anemia of infancy.

Other functions. Many other functions have been attributed to ascorbic acid. In some cases the evidence is not clear cut. In others, when the evidence indicates a strong possibility of a relationship, no explanation of the biochemical mechanism involved has been found.

Ascorbic acid is believed to be involved in the production and secretion of hormones of the adrenal gland, but the mechanism is unclear, since scorbutic subjects are able to produce normal levels of these steroids and adrenal glands respond normally to usual stimulation.

Considerable evidence exists that cholesterol deposition in the ground substance in the arterial wall rises in an ascorbic acid deficiency and falls on the administration of the vitamin. This may indicate a role in lipid metabolism.

The conversion of the amino acid tryptophan to serotonin involved in regulating blood pressure levels is dependent on ascorbic acid, again because it stimulates hydroxylation. Although only 1% of the tryptophan is used this way, the production of serotonin is very essential.

Reports on the role of ascorbic acid in combatting infection have been contradictory. When it has been found beneficial, the role has been obscure. No beneficial effects from intakes of 200 mg. of vitamin C could be demonstrated on the incidence and cure of the common cold, but Pauling believes that 1 to 2 gm. are effective. The low blood levels of ascorbic acid reported in infections such as tuberculosis may be caused by a shift of the vitamin to the infected tissue. Much the same mechanism seems to operate during stress, with the mobilization of ascorbic acid from tissues of the body to be concentrated in traumatized areas.

In the case of burns, skin grafts heal more quickly when ascorbic acid is present.

Large doses of ascorbic acid (525 mg. per day) have been demonstrated as beneficial in exposure to low environmental temperatures. The subjects maintained skin temperature more readily and experienced fewer and less severe symptoms of frostbitten feet. It is postulated that vitamin C accelerates the metabolism of the amino acids tyrosine and phenylalanine, precursors of the hormones thyroxin and adrenaline, which may stimulate basal metabolic rate and hence heat production.

Massive doses of ascorbic acid have been reported effective in treatment of such conditions as poisoning, hay fever, arsenic sensitivity, and muscular pains.

Biochemically evidence exists that ascorbic acid has a sparing action in relation to several vitamins of the B complex group—thiamin, riboflavin, niacin, pantothenic acid, biotin, and folic acid. In some cases it appears to replace them; in others it prevents their destruction.

Absorption and metabolism

Ascorbic acid is absorbed in humans in the upper part of the intestine, possibly by simple diffusion, and is circulated in the blood. From the bloodstream it is picked up by the tissues, passing readily into the adrenal tissue with 66 mg. per 100 gm. of tissue, kidney with 12 mg.%, liver with 32.8 mg.%, and spleen with 41.9 mg.%, most of which appears to be in equilibrium with serum. The eye, muscles, testes, and brain also accumulate some, but the concentration is markedly different from that in the blood serum. In the kidney some reduced ascorbic acid is changed to dehydroascorbic acid, in which form it more readily penetrates the cell barriers of erythrocytes, brain, and placenta, which it enters by active transport, or an energy-requiring process. Although the body has no extensive storage areas for vitamin C, some tissues, such as the adrenal tissue (especially the cortex), retain relatively large amounts that act as a buffer for other body tissues when dietary intake is low. Early estimates placed body stores at 5 gm., but more recent work studying the excretion of ascorbic acid through the respiratory tract suggests a figure as low as 1 gm. That this reserve is called upon in times of dietary deficit is evidenced by the fact that it takes as long as seventeen weeks for the white blood cell level to drop to zero, which occurs before any detectable signs of scurvy are found in a diet devoid of vitamin C.

Isotopic studies with C^{14}-labelled ascorbic acid have provided a means of studying ascorbic acid catabolism in the body. Depending on the dose administered, between 20% and 66% of the dose has been exhaled as carbon dioxide within 24 hours. The larger the dose, the more is oxidized in this fashion. From 15% to 30% is excreted in the urine after a medium dose. This appears in the urine primarily as oxalic and threonic acids and some dehydroascorbic acid. A small amount, usually less than 1%, is found in the feces. The remaining portion, between 30% and 50% of the dose, is usually retained in the body. The higher the ascorbic acid intake of the previous diet, the less is retained in the body. Since the body's capacity to store ascorbic acid is limited by the saturation level of various tissues, any excess is excreted in the urine or is oxidized and is exhaled as carbon dioxide. No evidence has been found of toxic effects from high levels of ascorbic acid.

Requirements

In the case of ascorbic acid there has been considerable controversy as to what criteria should be used in establishing recommended allowances.

Adults. Current standards are based on the assumption that an intake leading to saturation of vitamin C reserves in the tissues is the most desirable. As a result, recommended levels are many times those known to prevent frank signs of scurvy. It has long been recognized that intakes as low as 6.5 mg. per day are sufficient to prevent scurvy. (Lind provided 20 to 30 mg. of ascorbic acid in the dose he prescribed for the British Navy.) Taking into account the exhalation of CO_2 from the catabolism of ascorbic acid (in addition to the urinary excretion rate), research suggests that minimum requirements may be even lower. In adults 10 mg. has been shown to prevent scurvy for a year and to cure it in ten to fourteen weeks. However, the level for maintenance of optimal health is undoubtedly higher.

Recommended allowances for adults are 60 mg. for men and 55 mg. for women, based on a level of 2.5 mg. per kg.[3/4] body weight. These should allow for maintenance of an optimal level of health, optimal re-

sistance to physiological and pathological stress, and maintenance of healthy gums. Saturation of adult tissues can be achieved at intakes of slightly over 80 mg. in five weeks. No increase in benefits occurs with a large dose of 340 to 400 mg. No evidence exists to indicate that needs increase with age, although high levels may improve iron absorption in older persons whose level of hydrochloric acid secretion may be low.

Pregnancy. American standards for ascorbic acid intake in pregnancy are 60 mg. This is based on studies indicating a drop in blood serum levels and a decreased urinary excretion during pregnancy. It has been established that the developing fetus is parasitic on the mother in respect to vitamin C. Plasma levels in the fetus remain high (two to four times as high as maternal levels), and a high concentration is also found in the placenta. The placenta may act as a barrier for the return of the vitamin to maternal circulation. Too high an intake by the mother during pregnancy may condition the infant to a rich supply so that he is much more susceptible to deficiency symptoms on restricted intakes.

Lactation. The ascorbic acid content of mother's milk reflects to a certain extent the dietary intake of the mother and usually varies from 4 to 8 mg. per 100 gm. of milk. An intake of 60 mg. per day by the mother should result in optimal levels in her milk.

The lack of agreement regarding what constitutes a desirable level of intake of ascorbic acid is evident from Table 12-1, which compares recommendations prevailing in various countries. Even when the different philosophies on which the standards are based are considered, some obvious discrepancies still remain.

Infants. Based on the amount of ascorbic acid found in mother's milk (average, 4 to 8 mg. per 100 ml.), it is believed that a breast-fed infant receives 15 to 50 mg. per day. This leads to plasma ascorbic acid levels of 0.5 to 1.5 mg.%. Cow's milk provides only 4 to 6 mg.% and maintains much

Table 12-1. Comparison of dietary standards for ascorbic acid for selected age groups (in milligrams) *

	NRC	U.S.S.R.	Canada	Japan	Great Britain	Australia	Norway
Children 1-2 years	40	40	20	30	15	—	30
4-6 years	40	50	20	40	20	30	30
Boys 12-14 years	55	70	30	80	25	30	50
Men	60	70	30	65	30	30	30
Women	55	70	30	60	30	30	30
Pregnancy	60	100	40	100	60	80	50
Lactation	60	120	50	150	60	100	75

*Adapted from Young, E. G.: Dietary standards: In Beaton, G., and McHenry, E. W.: Nutrition, II, New York, 1964, Academic Press, Inc.

lower blood levels. It is recommended that 25 mg. be a minimum level of supplementation and that premature infants receive double the dose. Ascorbic acid supplementation should be started within the first ten days of life. Orange juice diluted with water has been satisfactory for most children, but the fact that some developed allergic reactions when a portion of the oils from the rind were extracted along with the juice has resulted in more reliance on synthetic preparations, especially as provided in multivitamins for early feeding of vitamin C. Fruit juices other than citrus juices do not provide enough vitamin C to make them effective in the diet of infants. For children the National Research Council recommendations increase from 35 mg. for those 1 to 3 years of age to a high of 55 mg. for girls from 13 to 18 years and 60 mg. for boys 16 to 18 years. Research on which recommended allowances are based presents discrepant findings. Long-term studies show that children with an adequate supply of ascorbic acid have a better general condition in regard to growth and resistance to infection.

Food sources

Vitamin C is found almost exclusively in foods of plant origin. Aside from liver, no other animal food is considered a significant source. The amount present in a plant tissue depends on many factors.

Part and type of plant. The head of broccoli was shown to have 158 mg. of vitamin C per 100 gm. of vegetable compared to 115 mg. per 100 gm. of stem. But stems retained 82% during a 10-minute cooking period, whereas heads retained only 60%. Counteracting some of the difference, thin-stemmed vegetables contained more vitamin C than do thick-stemmed ones. Vegetables that wilt lose much more vitamin C than do those that do not wilt. Kale loses 1.5% of its total vitamin C per hour at room temperature, whereas cabbage loses much less. Roots lose vitamin C slowly, but the loss is accelerated at higher temperatures.

Stage of maturity. Since the vitamin accumulates throughout the ripening process from the setting of the fruit, the longer the fruit remains on the vine or tree before harvesting, the higher the ascorbic acid content.

In contrast, immature seeds, such as peas and beans, contain some ascorbic acid but lose it all at maturity. Sprouting of peas or beans results in a vegetable with an appreciable amount of vitamin C, however.

Conditions of storage. Storing of vegetables at refrigerator temperatures at high humidity with a minimum of air movement will reduce ascorbic acid losses. The amount present in fresh vegetables bought in the temperate zone in the winter months is a function of the storage conditions during harvesting, shipping, and display in stores previous to selling. Losses are minimized at low temperatures and minimum exposure to air.

Season of year. A study of the ascorbic acid content of broccoli showed wide fluctuations, with low values reported in May and peak values in December.

Method of processing. Any method of food processing that involves the application of heat is likely to result in a reduced ascorbic acid content. If processing is done in the absence of air, losses will be much lower. In frozen and canned foods that are picked at the peak of maturity and are processed immediately under optimal conditions, the resulting product may have a higher vitamin C value than does the fresh product, for which the period between harvesting and consumption may be long and characterized by poor storage facilities.

Blanching of vegetables prior to freezing is necessary to destroy certain enzymes that otherwise would catalyze the destruction of ascorbic acid. In home-frozen vegetables the vitamin C content is likely to be less than that in commercially frozen vegetables that have been picked at the peak of maturity and processed immediately.

Irradiation of potatoes results in no decrease in ascorbic acid values.

Method of cooking. Many of our best sources of ascorbic acid are normally consumed raw. For those characteristically cooked, however, the effect of cooking method assumes much importance.

In most cooking the greater part of the losses occur in the early stages of cooking. For instance, broccoli heads lose 40% of their ascorbic acid values in the first 10 minutes. In the case of broccoli most of the loss is represented by leaching into the cooking water. On the other hand, cabbage,

with a lower initial amount, loses more by heat destruction of ascorbic acid, than by leaching. The amount of water used has a greater effect on losses than does the total cooking time. Steaming was found to lead to higher retentions, 69% versus 45%, than did boiling when tested on five vegetables. Steaming had no advantage over pressure-cooking.

Electronic cooking caused less destruction of ascorbic acid than did either pressure-cooking or boiling. In the case of broccoli, retentions of 85%, 80% and 45%, respectively, were reported. For cabbage comparable values were 80%, 70%, and 38%.

Method of preparation. Any method that reduces the surface area exposed to air or water minimizes losses. Thus finely shredded cabbage loses more ascorbic acid than do cabbage wedges. In the case of cabbage, however, the practice of serving it in vinegar, as in coleslaw, helps counteract the losses from exposure on the surface. Potatoes peeled, cut into smaller pieces, and cooked lose more than those cooked whole in their skins. The use of a dull knife in cutting fruit and vegetables may mash the cell, resulting in increased losses. The practice of crisping vegetables in cold water is undesirable, since it results in the leaching of ascorbic acid into the water.

In Fig. 12-5, which shows the contribution of various food groups to the ascorbic acid in the American diet, it is seen that fruits and vegetables provide 94% of the ascorbic acid. The remaining 6% comes from meat, fish, poultry, and eggs and dairy products. Cereal products contribute none. Although one would have expected an increase in the total amount of vitamin C in the diet in recent years with the greater use of frozen vegetables and the increased availability of fresh produce the year round, dietary studies indicate that the ascorbic acid in the American diet was lower in 1959 than in either 1947 to 1949 or 1935 to 1939. A shift from rich toward poorer sources has

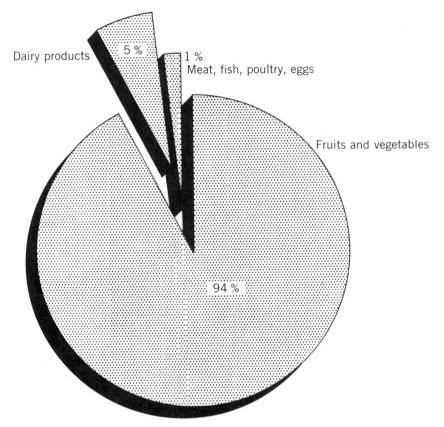

Fig. 12-5. Contribution of various food groups to ascorbic acid content of American food supply. (Based on Contribution of major food groups to nutrient supplies available for civilian consumption, National Food Situation No. 130, 1969.)

taken place in both vegetables and fruit juices.

The change in the sources of ascorbic acid in the American diet between 1909 and 1968 is depicted in Fig. 12-6. Fig. 12-7 shows the adequacy of the dietary intake as reported in the 1965 household consumption food study for different age groups.

Recent tables of food composition have continued to record only the reduced ascorbic acid content of fruits and vegetables, although considerable evidence exists that the body utilizes both reduced and dehydroascorbic acid. In spite of the fact that values representing total ascorbic acid would be more meaningful, the food composition table in Appendix F is based on reduced

ascorbic acid except for frozen fruits and vegetables, for which total values are provided. The ascorbic acid content of 100 gm. and 100 kcal. portions of some representative foods is presented graphically in Fig. 12-8. Table 12-2 gives both reduced, dehydroascorbic, and total ascorbic acid values for some representative foods for which data is available.

Aside from the more frequently used sources of vitamin C, such as citrus fruit and citrus juices, broccoli, spinach, strawberries, and melon in season, several other sources are rich. Parsley has a high content (per 100 gm.) but is consumed in such small quantities that it is not an important source. Many of the early concentrates of

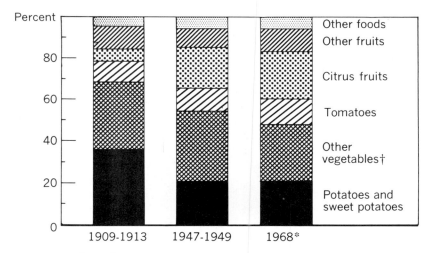

Fig. 12-6. Sources of ascorbic acid in food supply from 1909 to 1968. *Includes fortification, data preliminary; †excluding tomatoes, potatoes, and sweet potatoes. (From Agricultural Research Service, U. S. Department of Agriculture, 1969.)

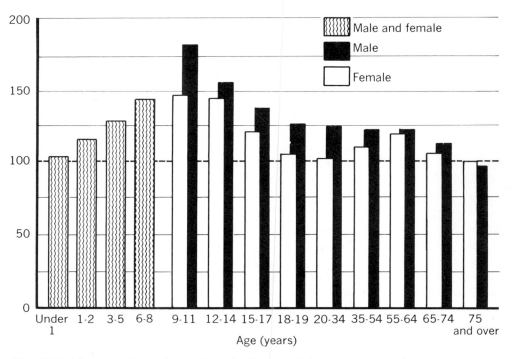

Fig. 12-7. Adequacy of ascorbic acid intake from 1 day's diet as reported in 1965 dietary survey of households in the United States. (From Food intake and nutritive value of diets of men, women and children in the United States—spring, 1965, Agricultural Research Service, Publication ARS 62-18, U. S. Department of Agriculture, 1969.)

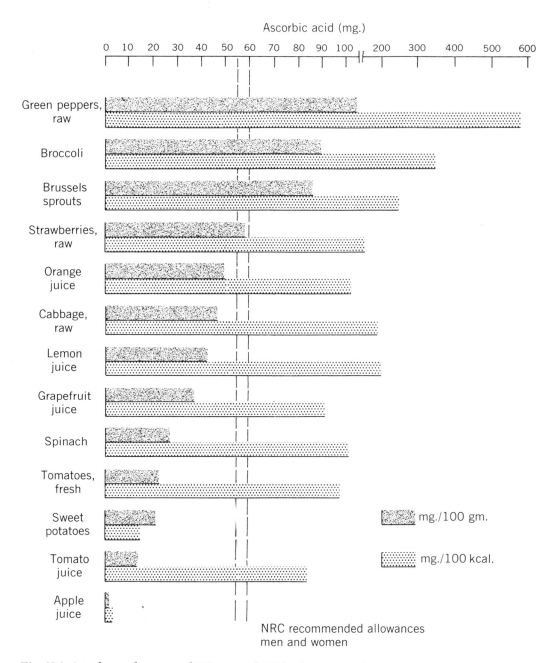

Fig. 12-8. Ascorbic acid content of 100 gm. and 100 kcal. portions of some representative foods. (Based on Watt, B. K., and Merrill, A. L.: Composition of foods—raw, processed and prepared, U. S. Department of Agriculture Handbook No. 8, Washington, D. C., 1963, U. S. Department of Agriculture.)

*Table 12-2. Reduced, dehydroascorbic, and total ascorbic acid in 100 gm. of some representative foods (in milligrams)**

Food	Reduced ascorbic acid	Dehydroascorbic acid	Total ascorbic acid
Asparagus	7.9	26.9	34.8
Broccoli	48.2	9.8	58.0
Brussels sprouts	60.9	4.4	65.3
Cabbage, raw	54.4	22.3	76.7
Cantaloupe	15.5	18.2	33.7
Green pepper	41.0	4.8	45.8
Strawberries	53.8	12.9	66.7
Sweet potatoes	18.8	8.1	26.9
Tomato juice	15.2	2.3	17.5

*From Davey, B. L., Dodds, M. L., Fisher, K. H., Schuck, C., and Shih, D. C.: Utilization of ascorbic acid in fruits and vegetables. 1. Plan of study and ascorbic acid content of 24 foods, J. Amer. Diet. Ass. **32:**1064, 1956.

vitamin C before synthetic vitamin C was readily available were made from rose hips gathered mostly by Indians in northern Alberta. Recently the acerola cherry, native to the tropics, has been identified as an extremely rich source (1500 mg. per 100 gm.), and although unpalatable alone, it is being used to fortify fruit juices less rich in ascorbic acid, especially for infant feeding. Camu-camu, a fruit native to South America, averages even more with 2000 mg. per 100 gm.

In the food industry, especially among processors of fruit juices and fruit juice mixtures, the trend is to add vitamin C at a level of about 30 mg. per 4-ounce serving to give them a better chance of competing with citrus juices. For consumption by persons who do not recognize the difference in ascorbic acid values of various juices, this is a commendable practice, although evidence exists that analyzed values many times vary considerably from value declared on the label, indicating a need for greater quality control. In keeping with the policy of recommending the enrichment of food products only when there is evidence of a lack of the particular nutrient in a sig-

nificant segment of the population, it is hard to rationalize such a practice. However, in Canada the enrichment of apple juice with ascorbic acid has the approval of government agencies, since it conceivably puts a native product in a better place competitively with an imported one. The addition of ascorbic acid to dehydrated potatoes is a questionable practice because of the likelihood of its being destroyed by heat and oxidation in preparation and service. The enrichment of milk or carbonated beverages with ascorbic acid has not been endorsed in the United States. In the processing of frozen fruits, such as peaches and apples, ascorbic acid is frequently added because of its reducing properties that help prevent discoloration of the fruit.

Evaluation of nutritional status

In spite of the fact that the biochemistry of ascorbic acid in the cell is less well understood than is that of other nutrients, the assessment of nutritional status in regard to ascorbic acid is more satisfactory.

Several methods have been used to assess nutritional status for vitamin C in the body. Since no one method alone is completely

Table 12-3. Comparison of biochemical data on ascorbic acid at different levels of saturation in the tissues

	Saturated	*Less saturated*	*50% saturation*	*25% saturation*
White blood cell levels of ascorbic acid	27-30 mg.%			20 mg.%
Serum levels of ascorbic acid	1 mg.%	0.4-1 mg.%	Too low to measure	
Urinary excretion; percent of test dose	60%-80%	20%-60%	Very low	
Dietary intake	> 100 mg.	40-100 mg.	10-15 mg.	5-7 mg.

satisfactory, a more accurate assessment is possible by a combination of several methods. By these methods it is possible to detect a difference between optimal and less than optimal nutrition.

Serum ascorbic acid levels have been widely used but do not bear a direct relationship to either dietary intake or white blood cell levels, which are believed to reflect state of tissue saturation. When serum values fall below 0.4 mg.%, they parallel white blood cell levels, but correlation for individuals is low. When tissues are less than 50% saturated, serum levels are too low to measure, making this determination virtually useless in discriminating between low and scorbutic levels of tissue saturation. When tissues are saturated, serum levels are close to 1 mg. per 100 gm. of blood.

The white blood cell, or leukocyte, level of ascorbic acid is a much more sensitive test of ascorbic acid nutrition. When tissues are completely saturated, leukocyte values are between 27 and 30 mg. per 100 gm. of blood. The fall in white blood cell level parallels the degree of saturation of the tissues so that a fall in these levels is indicative of depletion of body reserves. Scurvy does not develop until tissues are less than 20% saturated, indicated by a white blood cell level of less than 20 mg.%. This will not occur unless levels of intake fall below 10 mg. per day.

A measure of the amount of a test dose excreted in the urine within a short period after its administration has been the basis of the urinary excretion test for vitamin C status. The theory behind this test is that a depleted tissue will take up more of a test dose than will saturated tissues. Thus, when the intake has been adequate, the percentage of a test dose recovered in the urine will be high. When tissues are depleted, the amount appearing in the urine decreases, showing that more has been retained in the body. Table 12-3 shows the levels of these measurements under varying degrees of saturation.

Deficiency

Scurvy represents the most severe form of ascorbic acid deficiency but is relatively rare, especially in adults, now that its cause and cure are known. When it does develop, however, the early symptoms are relatively nonspecific, such as listlessness, fatigue, weakness, shortness of breath, muscle cramps, aching bones, joints, and muscles, and loss of appetite. These are followed by more specific symptoms, such as swollen, sensitive gums, hardening and roughness around hair follicles, and small pinpoint or petechial hemorrhages under the skin. The skin becomes dry, feverish, and rough and is covered by severe reddish blue spots. The hemorrhaging of the gums often predisposes to secondary infection. Five out of 9 prisoners subjected to experimental scurvy developed ocular lesions, mostly in the form of hemorrhages in the conjunctiva.

Infantile scurvy, illustrated in Figs. 12-1 and 12-4, is most likely to occur in the period of rapid growth between 5 and 24 months of age. Breast-fed infants never have scurvy, but bottle-fed infants whose diets are not varied by 6 months of age develop symptoms of irritability, anorexia, growth failure, tenderness of lips, and anemia. The onset is very rapid and unless treated promptly the condition may result in rather rapid death. If treated, the recovery is equally as dramatic.

Delayed or incomplete wound healing is a frequent manifestation of ascorbic acid deficiency, and anemia invariably occurs after two months of restricted intake. A drop in white blood cell levels is also frequent.

THIAMIN

The discovery of the chemical structure and the synthesis of thiamin by Williams in 1936 marked the end of a long and tedious search on the part of German, English, and American scientists to identify the substance in rice bran responsible for the cure of *beriberi*. As early as 1855 Takaki had cured beriberi in the Japanese Navy by using meat and milk to supplement the regular diet of the seamen, among whom over 30% were usually afflicted with the disease.

In 1890 Eijkman, a Dutch physician, was able to cure the paralytic polyneuritis that had developed in chickens fed scraps of polished rice from hospital wards by feeding unhusked rice or rice polishings. He also showed that he could cure human beriberi by similar treatment. His method of treatment worked, although his explanation that rice starch contained a toxin has since been shown to be erroneous. By 1910 Vedder in the Philippines had recognized that an active factor was present in a rice bran extract, *tikitiki*, capable of curing polyneuritis

in chicks and beriberi in humans. By 1926 Dutch scientists had produced thiamin crystals, but another ten years elapsed, however, before they were chemically identified and synthesized by Williams. By the following year, 1937, both Swiss and American firms were producing thiamin commercially at a cost of approximately $450 a pound, and Britain was formulating plans to use it to enrich bread. By 1961 thiamin production in the United States had risen to 200 tons, and the price had dropped to $9 a pound.

Beriberi

Beriberi is a disease that was virtually unknown until the middle of the nineteenth century, although it had been described by the Chinese as early as 2600 B.C. With the trend toward the use of more highly refined cereals having increased storage life, beriberi became a major health problem. This was especially true in countries where a staple food item such as rice provided as much as 80% of the calories in the diet. The cause of beriberi was not identified at first as a dietary deficiency resulting from the removal of the outer layers of cereal grains. Instead, various other theories were advanced, such as the presence of a toxic substance in the starch of rice for which there was an antidote in rice bran, the presence of a microbe, the absence of nitrogen in the diet, or the production of a toxic substance in the stomach from the use of rice. None of these theories withstood scrutiny, and eventually the search narrowed to one for the active substance in a rice bran extract that had almost magical curative properties in beriberi, especially infantile beriberi. It was identified as a water-soluble substance easily destroyed by heat and alkali.

In spite of our knowledge of food sources of thiamin and the ready production of synthetic thiamin at reasonable prices, beriberi is still a problem in many parts of the world. The Philippines still reports an incidence of infantile beriberi deaths of 75 per

100,000 births. There, beriberi is listed as the fourth leading cause of death and led to 15,200 infant deaths and 6,130 adult deaths in the period of 1954 to 1958. In addition, it is estimated that at least 1.5 million persons suffer from some manifestation of the disease, either clinically or subclinically. The incidence of beriberi can be attributed to the fact that the mills, which have taken over all but 5% of the rice milling, are producing a highly polished rice and with few exceptions are failing to comply with government regulations regarding enrichment even at a cost of less than one fifth of a cent per pound. The practice of repeatedly washing the milled rice to remove the dust that accumulates during marketing in open bins causes a further loss of thiamin. It is estimated that after milling, washing, and cooking losses are considered, the average consumption of slightly less than 1 pound of rice per day provides only 0.27 mg. of thiamin. On the basis of the Food and Agricultural Organization criterion of 0.27 mg. of thiamin per 1000 nonfat kcal. in the diet, this level of intake will not protect against beriberi.

Infantile beriberi occurs most frequently from 2 to 5 months of age, is very rapid in onset, and unless treated within a matter of hours often results in death. Beriberi occurs more often in breast-fed than bottle-fed infants, reflecting the failure on the part of the lactating mother whose dietary thiamin is too low to produce a milk with sufficient thiamin to protect her infant. Human milk normally contains less than half as much thiamin as cow's milk, but that of a woman on a thiamin-deficient diet is much lower. The situation may be complicated by the transfer of methyl glyoxal, a product of metabolism that accumulates in the body in thiamin deficiency, to the mother's milk. Milk from mothers suffering from beriberi has been found to contain about half as much thiamin as that from normal mothers. A baby with beriberi develops very rapidly such symptoms as cyanosis (too much car-

bon dioxide in blood, causing a bluish color), tachycardia (a very fast heartbeat), and a characteristic cry changing from a loud piercing one to a thin weak almost inaudible one, sometimes accompanied by vomiting and convulsions. Once thiamin is administered, symptoms are relieved within a matter of hours.

In adults, beriberi is a different condition and takes two distinct forms. In wet (edematous) beriberi the victim suffers from swelling of the limbs, usually starting at the feet and progressing upward throughout the body until the accumulation of fluid in heart muscle leads to eventual heart failure and death. Early signs of this edematous form are wristdrop and ankledrop.

In dry (wasting) beriberi a gradual loss of body tissue occurs, the patient becoming thin and emaciated. In both forms, symptoms are irritability, vague uneasiness, disorderly thinking, and nausea, all suggesting an involvement of the nervous system.

The disease continues to be a problem in areas of the world where polished rice is a staple in the diet and where the milling of rice has shifted from the home to the mill. In the United States, alcoholics are almost the only group in which the disease ever occurs. However, considerable evidence exists of subclinical thiamin deficiency, especially among persons who eliminate bread and cereal products, our most reliable source of thiamin, from their diets in an effort to lose weight.

Early work in the study of beriberi was facilitated by the observation that chickens fed the beriberi-producing diet developed polyneuritis (inflammation of many nerves). These animals showed loss of neuromuscular coordination, had a poor sense of balance, and died within a short time of onset of the symptoms.

Chemical properties

Thiamin, which is available as the biologically active but more stable thiamin hydrochloride, is a white crystalline substance, soluble in water, and easily destroyed by heat or oxidation, especially in the presence of alkali. The term *thiamin* indicates that it is a sulfur-containing substance (thio) and it is also amine- or nitrogen-containing. It has also been known as aneurin, indicative of its role in preventing symptoms involving nerves. It is also referred to as the antineuritic factor.

Functions

Vitamin B_1 is known to be a part of the coenzyme thiamin pyrophosphate (thiamin with two molecules of phosphate attached to it), or cocarboxylase, which is required in metabolism of carbohydrate. The metabolism of carbohydrates has three stages at which the absence of thiamin as part of a coenzyme leads to a slowing or complete blocking of the chemical changes. Although it has not been confirmed, it has been postulated that an accumulation of the intermediary products of metabolism blocked by the absence of the necessary thiamin-containing enzyme causes typical thiamin deficiency symptoms. Since thiamin is part of the cocarboxylase necessary for the decarboxylation (removal of carbon dioxide) from pyruvic acid as it is prepared to enter the citric acid cycle, pyruvic acid tends to accumulate when thiamin is lacking. A similar role for cocarboxylase in oxidative decarboxylation exists at the stage in the metabolic cycle at which another intermediary product of both fat and carbohydrate metabolism, alpha-ketoglutaric acid, is decarboxylated to succinic acid. A third enzymatic role of thiamin is in activating transketolase, an enzyme necessary in the direct oxidative pathway for metabolism of glucose that occurs in all cells except skeletal cells. Even though this pathway involves less than 10% of all glucose, it is essential, since it is the only way the body can produce both ribose, the sugar needed for the synthesis of RNA so essential in cell reproduction, and also an intermediary product needed for the synthesis of fatty acids. The level of transketolase found in the red blood cells has been shown to be a sensitive indicator of thiamin status. There, the level of transketolase falls before any other manifestations of thiamin deficiency occur. Since it reflects dietary intake, it can be used in detecting suboptimal nutritional status. In birds a decreased transketolase level reduces the ability of the red blood cells to oxidize glucose directly. This leads to the accumulation of methyl glyoxal, apparently due to a failure to oxidize it.

Absorption

The absorption of thiamin occurs primarily in the duodenum of the small intestine, reaching a maximum at intakes of 2.5 to 5 mg. per day. Large intakes such as 10 mg. are absorbed three times as well in four divided dosages as in one single dose. The use of sustained-release preparations of thiamin have yielded contradictory results.

Thiamin absorption is an active process requiring energy. Any thiamin synthesized in the lower gastrointestinal tract appears as cocarboxylase, which cannot be absorbed at this point, so that intestinal synthesis in humans appears to have no significance.

A substance in onion oil and garlic oil, alliin, combines with thiamin to form alliithiamin, a form in which the vitamin is more readily absorbed. The widespread use of onions and garlic in oriental diets with marginal amounts of thiamin may thus help to alleviate thiamin deficiencies. Another thiamin compound, thiamin bisulfide, is absorbed more freely than thiamin hydrochloride.

Since thiamin pyrophosphate (cocarboxylase) is too large a molecule to pass through the cell membrane, it becomes clear that this coenzyme is produced in the cell as needed and that the thiamin existing in either animal or plant foods as cocarboxylase must be split before being absorbed. With the aid of enzymes it is then rejoined to phosphates as needed in individual cells to produce cocarboxylase.

The decrease in gastric acidity that occurs in thiamin deficiency decreases the release of thiamin from thiamin complexes in the gastrointestinal tract, inhibiting its absorption and accentuating the deficiency symptoms.

Metabolism

The adult body contains from 30 to 70 mg. of thiamin. Although there is no storage site for the vitamin, it has been observed that normal levels of 2 to 3 μg. per gram of heart muscle, 1 μg. per gram of brain, liver, and kidney, and 0.5 μg. per gram of skeletal muscle double after thiamin therapy and rapidly drop to half these values in thiamin depletion.

It is known that thiamin in excess of body needs is excreted in the urine. A measure of urinary thiamin in relation to dietary thiamin has been the basis for balance studies to assess the adequacy of intake. When thiamin excretion is low, a larger portion of the test dose is retained, indicating a tissue need for thiamin. A high excretion, on the other hand, indicates tissue saturation. On low intakes excretion drops to zero. A radio-

active test dose of thiamin appears in the urine as thiamin, thiamin disulfide, and about sixteen other degradation products.

Requirements

Efforts to determine the minimum needs and optimal intakes for humans for thiamin have involved thiamin balance studies, in which the relationship between dietary intake and urinay excretion have been determined. A level of intake that leads to minimum but not zero excretion is believed to represent minimal needs but provides no protection against further reduction in thiamin intake.

Recommendations for all age groups assume a relationship between caloric intake and thiamin need. The assumption is based on the fact that thiamin is part of the coenzyme needed in at least three places in the metabolism of carbohydrate. As caloric intake varies with age, size, physical activity, environmental temperature, or physical state of the animal, carbohydrate intake changes, and an increased carbohydrate intake creates an increased need for thiamin. The current recommendations of the National Research Council based on a level of 0.5 mg. of thiamin per 1000 kcal. are pre-

Table 12-4. Recommended daily intake for thiamin (in milligrams)

		United States*	Great Britain†	Canada‡
Children	2- 3 years	0.6	0.6	0.4
	6- 9 years	1.0	0.8	0.7
Boys	12-15 years	1.4	1.1	0.9
Girls	12-15 years	1.4	0.9	0.8
Men	18-35 years	1.4	1.1	0.9
	35-55 years	1.3	1.0	0.9
Women	18-35 years	1.0	0.9	0.7
	35-55 years	1.0	0.8	0.7

*Food and Nutrition Board: Recommended dietary allowances, ed. 7, Washington, D. C., 1968, Publication No. 1694, National Academy of Sciences–National Research Council.
†Department of Health and Social Security: Recommended intakes of nutrients for the United Kingdom, Reports on Public Health and Medical Subjects, No. 120, London, 1969, Her Majesty's Stationery Office.
‡Dietary Standards for Canada, Canadian Bulletin on Nutrition 6, No. 1, 1964; Revised, 1968.

sented in Table 12-4. In keeping with their philosophy of setting recommendations at a level compatible with the potential of the nation's food supply to provide it and sufficiently high to provide a margin of safety to take into account practically all individual variations in need, efficiency of absorption, and normal losses in food preparation, these figures represent optimal intakes, for the most part about 100% above minimal requirements. These levels protect against deficiency symptoms and provide a buffer against zero intakes of thiamin. We have no evidence of benefits to be derived from intakes in excess of these levels. Since thiamin is water-soluble and the body has limited capacity to store it, excesses are ex-creted, and we have no indication of toxicity from its use.

Studies of older people show that their needs are relatively high, they excrete less at all levels of intake, they experience a faster reaction to moderate depletion, and they respond more slowly to the addition of thiamin to the diet.

The need for thiamin increases with an increased consumption of alcohol. This accounts for the reported incidence of beriberi among alcoholics in the United States. It appears that the vitamin is necessary for the metabolism of acetaldehyde, an intermediary product in alcohol metabolism.

The amount of fat in the diet, especially medium-chain fatty acids, influences the

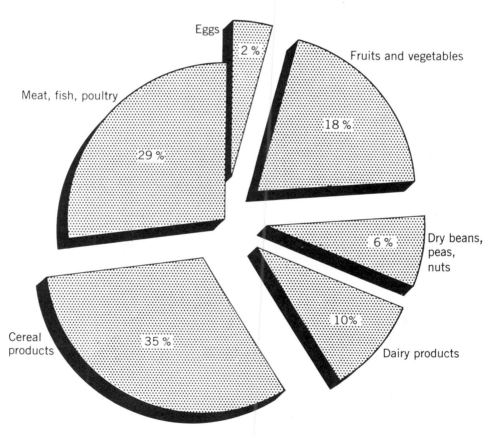

Fig. 12-9. Contribution of various food groups to the thiamin content of the American food supply. (Based on Contribution of major food groups to nutrient supplies available for civilian consumption, National Food Situation No. 130, 1969.)

need for thiamin, and fat has frequently been referred to as a "thiamin sparer." Since only one of the reactions for which thiamin is needed is involved in the metabolism of fatty acids, it follows that when fat calories replace carbohydrate calories, less thiamin will be required. Thus, thiamin intakes that are suboptimal in a high-carbohydrate diet prove adequate when fat replaces some of the carbohydrate. It is suggested that a toxic product, presumably methyl glyoxal, arises from carbohydrate metabolism but not from fat metabolism in the absence of thiamin. A third possibility is that fat protects thiamin from loss or destruction in the body.

Considerable evidence exists that the need for thiamin decreases when some sulfonamides and other antibiotics are given. Several theories have been suggested to explain this effect, but no clear-cut evidence has been established to support any one of them.

Food sources

As shown in Fig. 12-9, cereal products provide about one third of the available thiamin; meat, fish, and poultry, about one fourth; and dairy products, about one tenth of that available to the American public.

Fig. 12-10 shows the thiamin content of 100 gm. and 100 kcal. portions of some of the more dependable sources of thiamin in the average American diet. Thiamin in vegetables is in nonphosphorylated form, whereas that in meat occurs primarily as cocarboxylase or diphosphate, from which it must be released before it is absorbed.

The richest sources of the vitamin are pork products. For that segment of the population who eat pork frequently, it represents a dependable source of thiamin. Those whose religious beliefs prohibit consumptions of pork must and do obtain adequate amounts from other sources.

Peas and other legumes are good sources. As will be noted from a comparison of fresh

and dried peas, amount of thiamin increases with increasing maturity of the seed. The amount of the nutrient actually obtained from dried legumes will be reduced if they are soaked for a long period in water, which is discarded, or if baking soda is used to hasten the cooking time by softening the cellulose. The United States Department of Agriculture now suggests that the use of minute amounts of baking soda (1/16 teaspoon per cup of beans) is satisfactory, since reduced cooking time reduces thiamin losses sufficiently to compensate for increased losses resulting from the addition of an alkali.

Whole-grain cereals contain the greater part of their thiamin in their outer husks, the part that is removed in the milling process.

Enriched or whole-wheat bread may at first appear as an insignificant source, but in the amounts consumed, especially by low-income families, the use of bread products provides enough thiamin to ensure an adequate intake in diets that would otherwise be marginal. The use of enriched bread that has come with the mandatory enrichment laws in thirty states has been credited with decreasing the incidence of beriberi among alcoholics, many of whom eat bread or bread products—one of the cheaper sources of calories. Of bread and flour marketed in the United States 90% is now enriched at a cost of approximately 4 cents per 100 pounds. The effect of the enrichment program on the thiamin content of the American diet is evident from Fig. 12-11.

Dried brewer's yeast and wheat germ, both rich in thiamin, assume little importance in the American diet because of the infrequency of their use. Live yeast, found in compressed yeast cakes, is high in thiamin, but it has been established that these same yeast cells deprive the body of thiamin and may precipitate thiamin-deficiency symptoms. Cooking, of course, kills the yeast cells; thus it is only when live

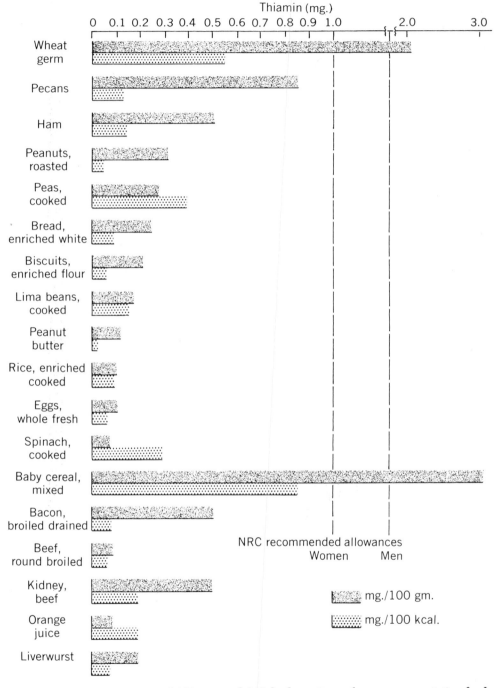

Fig. 12-10. Thiamin content of 100 gm. and 100 kcal. portions of some representative foods. (Based on Watt, B. K., and Merrill, A. L.: Composition of foods—raw, processed and prepared, U. S. Department of Agriculture Handbook No. 8, Washington, D. C., 1963, U. S. Department of Agriculture.)

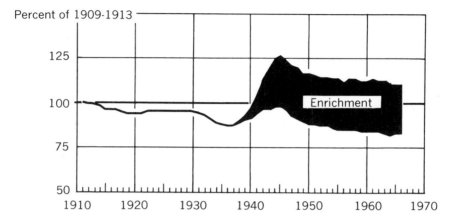

Fig. 12-11. Effect of enrichment program on thiamin content of American diet from 1910 to 1966. Thiamin per capita consumption, five-year moving average. (From Agricultural Research Service, U. S. Department of Agriculture, 1969.)

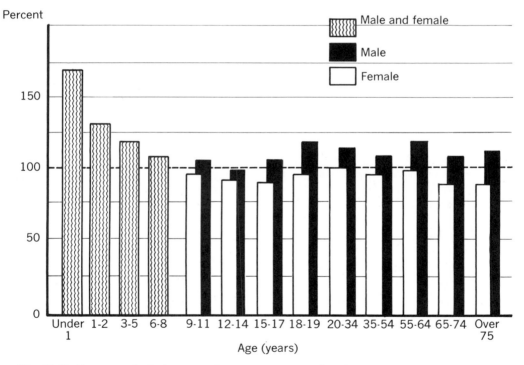

Fig. 12-12. Extent to which American diets meet recommended dietary allowances for thiamin. Thiamin from 1 day's diet as a percent of the recommended allowances. (From Food intake and nutritive value of diets of men, women and children in the United States—spring, 1965, Agricultural Research Service, Publication ARS 62-18, U. S. Department of Agriculture, 1969.)

yeast is taken, as was once recommended as a therapeutic agent in certain skin conditions, that a problem occurs.

The enrichment of other cereal products, such as rice, macaroni, corn grits, and flour, assumes practical importance, depending on the extent to which these items are a staple food item in a diet.

The United States Department of Agriculture reports that the American food supply provides about 1.8 mg. per person per day, which is not much above the daily adult requirement. The extent to which the American diet meets established dietary allowances for thiamin is shown in Fig. 12-12.

Certain freshwater fish, a few saltwater fish, bracken ferns, and some shellfish, such as clams, shrimp, and mussels, contain a thiamin-splitting enzyme, thiaminase. Fortunately this enzyme is heat-labile (its coenzyme is heat-stable) so that only in circumstances in which raw fish is regularly consumed is the presence of this enzyme detrimental in human nutrition.

Effect of cooking

The extent to which foods lose thiamin in preparation is determined by the physical and chemical properties of the vitamin.

Loss in solution. Since thiamin is water-soluble, it will leach out of a product in proportion to the amount of water available, the extent to which it is agitated, and the surface area of the food exposed to the water. Any method of preparation that minimizes the length of time a food is in contact with water and the amount of surface area will decrease thiamin losses. As much as 18% of the thiamin in rice is reportedly lost in the method used by Orientals of washing the rice several times before cooking. Modern marketing procedures, which protect the food from contamination from the air, eliminate the necessity for preliminary washing of rice. In fact, most packages warn the housewife not to wash rice and to cook it in a minimum of water to reduce cooking losses. This is especially important when the rice is enriched by coating it with an enrichment mixture.

Loss due to heat. Thiamin is destroyed by heat. The higher the temperature and more prolonged the exposure to heat, the greater the loss. Roasting pork at 325° F. allows a retention of 75% to 100% of the original thiamin, whereas higher temperatures give lower yields. Destruction appears no greater in cooking in electronic ovens than in conventional ones. Thiamin in food is less susceptible to heat destruction than is the free form of thiamin. Also, a difference is found in rate of heat destruction between various foods, that in spinach, heart, liver, and lamb being more susceptible than that in peas, beans, pork, and carrots.

Loss due to oxidation. Cooking procedures that increase the amount of oxygen in contact with the food, especially under conditions of moist heat, speed up the destruction of thiamin. The use of rapidly boiling water in cooking vegetables is an example of this.

Loss due to alkali. The destruction of thiamin is greatest in the presence of alkali. The addition of baking soda, an alkali, to cooking water, is sometimes suggested as a means of preserving the bright green color of fresh vegetables. Its use for such purposes cannot be recommended because of the destructive effect it has on both thiamin and vitamin C.

Loss due to irradiation. The thiamin content of pork is virtually destroyed by the irradiation procedures sometimes used in food preservation.

Evaluation of nutritional status

The most sensitive test available for the determination of thiamin status is the red blood cell transketolase activity. These values reflect changes in dietary intake before any other signs of thiamin inadequacy are detectable. In animals, growth response is considered a fairly sensitive indicator of thiamin intake but is not as specific to thiamin as is transketolase activity, which was shown to drop 30% at one week and 51% at two weeks in rats who continued to grow during this period of thiamin deficiency.

Another promising indicator of thiamin status of an individual is the carbohydrate index, which is a function of pyruvic acid, lactic acid, and glucose in the blood after the administration of glucose and a standard exercise test. It, of course, is useful only for persons able to exercise.

The urinary excretion test for thiamin involves measuring the amount of thiamin excreted in the urine following a test dose. Persons with low levels of saturation in the tissues will retain more and excrete less than will persons whose intake has been more adequate.

Deficiency

Thiamin deficiency may result under several sets of circumstances aside from a low dietary intake, which frequently occur when the diet is very low in calories or limited in variety. Failure of absorption, usually caused by some abnormality in the gastrointestinal tract, the inability of tissues to accumulate adequate stores of the vitamin, failure to utilize available thiamin, or an increased requirement such as occurs in a diet high in carbohydrate or alcohol may lead to deficiency symptoms. At the moment we have no clear-cut indication of the relationship between clinical symptoms and biochemical changes that occur in a thiamin deficiency. Several explanations have been considered—first, that a lack of thiamin causes a failure to provide energy for the cell; second, that in thiamin deficiency some product essential for metabolism in heart or muscle cells is not formed, and alternatively, that some toxic product accumulates.

Since thiamin deficiency in humans usually occurs along with symptoms of deficiencies of other vitamins of the B com-

plex, it is difficult to attribute symptoms specifically to thiamin. The condition is often complicated by symptoms brought on by concurrent infection and varies with degree of deficiency and presence of stress situations such as pregnancy. However, in cases where thiamin has been effective in relieving particular symptoms, it is customary to consider them specific to thiamin. The following have been associated with a lack of thiamin, although similar symptoms may occur as a result of other dietary inadequacies, especially those of B complex vitamins.

Loss of appetite. Loss of appetite, or anorexia, has been clearly demonstrated in experimental animals and has been related in many cases to thiamin inadequacy in humans. Anorexia accompanied by vomiting was the first sign of deficiency shown by a group of normal men subjected to an induced thiamin deficiency. Even at intakes of 0.2 mg. per 1000 kcal., which did not cause any other symptoms, loss of appetite, nausea, and constipation occurred. Although increased intake of thiamin will restore a depressed appetite to normal levels, it is ineffective in stimulating the appetite beyond a normal level.

Decreased muscle tonus. The tonus or elasticity of the wall of the lower gastrointestinal tract is decreased in thiamin deficiency to the point that normal gastric motility is decreased, the colon becomes distended, and constipation results. Thiamin has been used with varying degrees of success in treating constipation in older people in whom gastrointestinal motility is frequently subnormal.

Depression. Mental depression and confusion sometimes alleviated by the administration of thiamin has led to the somewhat misleading designation of thiamin as the "morale vitamin." Persons on low thiamin intakes show pronounced mood changes, vague feelings of uneasiness, fear, disorderly thinking, and other signs of mental depression. Mental changes associated with inadequate thiamin respond readily to thiamin supplements. This is well illustrated in a study of 10 older women (52 to 72 years of age) limited to 0.33 mg. of thiamin per day. They all showed increasing irritability, complained of fatigue and headache, and voluntarily restricted their social engagements. Urinary excretion of thiamin dropped progressively. Immediate improvement was observed when they were given 1.4 mg. for one day. Similarly, the restoration of thiamin to the diets of men who had been on a restricted thiamin intake led to the restoration of normal attitudes. Reports demonstrating that the use of thiamin supplements with children was effective in raising their I.Q. and intellec-

tual performance have subsequently been discredited. In beriberi the most acute symptom is mental confusion leading to coma.

Neurological changes. Nystagmus caused by a weakness in the sixth cranial nerve is known as Wernicke's syndrome. This symptom, a manifestation of changes occurring in the central nervous system, is easily reversed by thiamin administration. Levels of thiamin in the brain can be reduced by 50% without any noticeable clinical signs; further reduction to 30% of normal leads to slow and unsteady gait, and at 20% severe disturbance of posture and equilibrium occurs.

Peripheral neuritis, in which the nerves

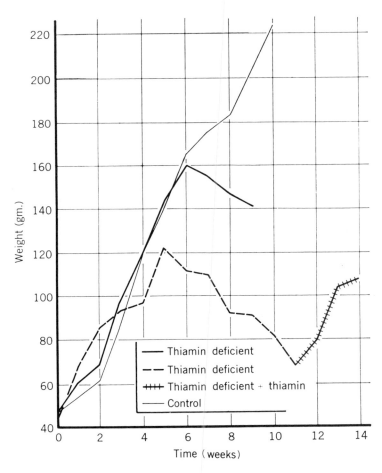

Fig. 12-13. Growth patterns of weanling albino rats with and without thiamin.

that control the extremities fail to function properly, shows up in a variety of ways in humans, usually affecting the legs first.

Neuromuscular coordination is affected in persons on low thiamin intake, resulting in decreased work output and mechanical efficiency. Motor speed, eye-hand coordination, and body and manual steadiness reactions that had deteriorated on an intake of 0.05 mg. of thiamin per 1000 kcal. were quickly restored with thiamin supplementation. Other signs of peripheral nervous system involvement are loss of ankle and knee jerk, painful calf muscles, and general atrophy of leg muscles manifest as difficulty in walking.

Beriberi. Beriberi, the final form of thiamin deficiency that manifests itself in either the wet or dry form, has been mentioned earlier.

Deficiencies in animals. In experimental thiamin deficiency in rats complete deprivation leads to death in three to six weeks, with no specific clinical symptoms, but when small amounts are provided, death is delayed to eight to twelve weeks. Rats develop spasticity of muscles and usually die in convulsive seizures complicated by heart lesions unless treated promptly.

Growth retardation accompanying a dietary lack of thiamin is readily demonstrated in animals. Typical growth patterns of rats with and without thiamin are shown in Fig. 12-13.

In birds a condition, polyneuritis (inflammation of many nerves), occurs upon thiamin deprivation. Birds lose their sense of balance and have depressed appetite and a chronic state of head retraction. All symptoms are relieved with thiamin intake.

Clinical uses

Thiamin has been used in the medical treatment of a wide variety of conditions other than beriberi. A survey of the literature showed that it had been tried in 230 different conditions. In the period from 1936 to 1945 these included neuritis, neuralgia, pains of various origins, diseases of the central nervous system, and cardiovascular symptoms. A renewed interest in thiamin therapy from 1951 to 1960 found it used in acidosis, diabetic coma, pyruvemia (accumulation of pyruvic acid in the blood), and toxemia of pregnancy. In addition, it is widely used as a supplement to stimulate a poor appetite. The possibility of observing beneficial results are greatest when malnutrition, nutritional imbalance, or impaired intestinal absorption have precipitated the symptoms.

RIBOFLAVIN

Riboflavin, which has also been known as vitamin B_2, vitamin G, and the yellow enzyme, was recognized in 1917 when it became clear that vitamin B retained some growth-promoting properties after its antiberiberi properties had been destroyed by heat. To differentiate the heat-labile component from this heat-stable fraction, the two components were designated vitamin B_1 and vitamin B_2, respectively.

At the time of the discovery of riboflavin, reports appeared almost simultaneously announcing the isolation of four substances necessary for growth—hepatoflavin, lactoflavin, ovoflavin, and verdoflavin. These investigators, obviously isolating their factors from liver, milk, eggs, and grass, respectively, had agreed that they were flavin compounds—substances that produce an intense yellow-green fluorescence in water. These substances had been concentrated from natural foods in 1925 and isolated in 1932, at which time it became evident that the active factor was composed to a protein plus a pigment, the flavin. With the synthesis of riboflavin in 1935 it soon became clear that the 5-carbon sugar ribose was common to all forms, which were then designated riboflavine. Shortly afterward the final *e* was dropped but has been recently (1961) added in the official spelling in Britain.

Chemical properties

Riboflavin is a relatively stable vitamin; it is resistant to the effects of acid, heat, or oxidation. It is unstable in the presence of alkali and light. Since it is slightly soluble in water, some losses occur when riboflavin-containing vegetables cut in small pieces are cooked in large amounts of water for long periods of time. The major loss of riboflavin in food is due to the action of either the ultraviolet or visible rays of sunlight on milk, a significant source of riboflavin in the American diet. Efforts of the dairy industry to reduce this loss have met with much popular resistance. The use of brown glass bottles that filter out the harmful rays of the sun are considered suitable only for less nutritional beverages! The flavor that housewives claim arises from the use of more opaque wax-lined cardboard or plastic containers has limited their acceptance, although advances in packaging are reducing the problem. The most successful efforts have been the provision of covered insulated boxes that protect the milk from exposure to sunlight after home deliveries.

Functions

Riboflavin is a part of several enzymes and coenzymes in which it contributes to their capacity to accept and transfer hydrogen atoms, or positive charges. These reactions are essential for the release of energy from glucose and fatty acids and within the cell mitochondrion. The two coenzymes, flavin mononucleotide (FMN), or riboflavin monophosphate, and flavin adenine dinucleotide (FAD), which is FMN with two phosphates and an additional ribose group, are attached to a variety of enzymes known as flavoproteins. Before riboflavin can function as a part of these enzymes, it must be phosphorylated (have a phosphate group attached to it). This addition usually occurs in the intestinal cells during absorption. Riboflavin is also an integral part of other enzymes specifically involved in the transfer of hydrogen atoms in protein meta-

bolism. Riboflavin is necessary before the amino acid tryptophan, a source of the vitamin niacin in the body, can be converted into the active form of the vitamin.

Some substances chemically related to riboflavin can replace riboflavin completely; others are effective for a short time, apparently replacing the reserves of riboflavin but leading to death as soon as the original reserves are depleted; and still others act as riboflavin antagonists. These antagonists replace riboflavin in enzyme systems in which they cannot function as riboflavin does and in so doing prevent any available vitamin from functioning. In human beings, riboflavin deficiencies have been produced experimentally by the use of the riboflavin antagonist galactoflavin, in which the 5-carbon ribose is replaced by a 6-carbon sugar, galactose.

Absorption

Although not equally available from all sources, riboflavin is absorbed through the walls of the intestine by passive diffusion; that is, it passes through the epithelial cells of the intestine without an expenditure of energy. The rate of absorption is proportional to the size of the dose. Within the intestinal cells it is phosphorylated (linked with a phosphate molecule), in which form it is carried to the tissues, where it may be attached to a protein as a flavoprotein. There is relatively little storage of riboflavin in the body although the liver, with 16 μg. per gram, and kidney, with 25 μg. per gram, contain slightly higher concentrations than do other tissues, such as muscle with 2 to 3 μg. per gram. Some unabsorbed riboflavin appears in the feces, which also contains riboflavin of bacterial origin. However, most excretion occurs through the kidney. The amount of riboflavin excreted after a test dose of the vitamin reflects the extent to which tissues are saturated with the vitamin. The smaller the amount excreted, the greater the amount retained—presumably to bring the levels in

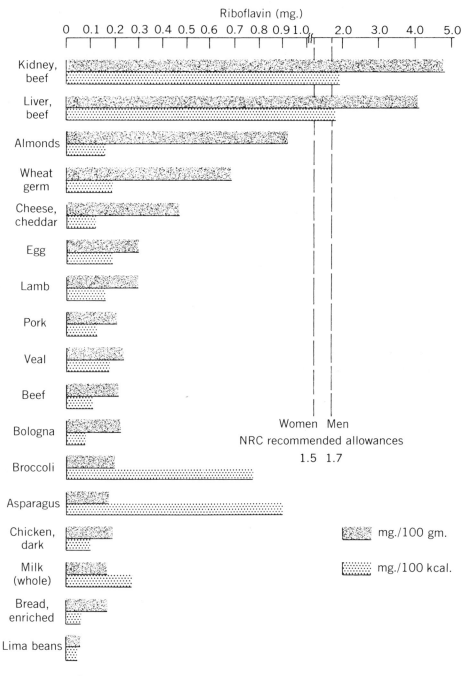

Fig. 12-14. Riboflavin content of 100 gm. and 100 kcal. portions of representative foods. (Based on Watt, B. K., and Merrill, A. L.: Composition of foods—raw, processed and prepared, U. S. Department of Agriculture Handbook No. 8, Washington, D. C., 1963, U. S. Department of Agriculture.)

the body tissues up to saturation levels. A loss of protein from the body is accompanied by a loss of riboflavin.

Requirements

Although in previous editions of *Recommended Dietary Allowances* by the Food and Nutrition Board of the National Research Council, riboflavin requirements had been based on caloric intake, the current edition uses metabolic body size (weight in kg.[3/4]) as a criterion. This takes into account body size and metabolic rate but does not consider rate of growth, which is also believed to influence riboflavin requirements. For the adult 0.07 mg. of riboflavin per kg.[3/4] is recommended to ensure tissue saturation with the vitamin. This estimate was based on data from studies of excretion relative to intake when intake was

above normal. Similar observations on infants led to a recommendation of an intake of 0.1 mg. per kg.[3/4]. Recommendations were arbitrarily decreased with an increase in age throughout childhood as needs for growth decrease.

The FAO/WHO committee has continued to base their recommendations on caloric intake and has set 0.55 mg. per 1000 kcal. as a practical goal. The needs for pregnancy call for a 0.3 mg. increase in intake and lactation, for a 0.5 mg. increase beyond the needs of an adult woman.

Food sources

Riboflavin is widely distributed in both animal and vegetable foods. The amount present in 100 gm. and 100 kcal. portions of representative foods is presented graphically in Fig. 12-14 and Fig. 12-15 shows

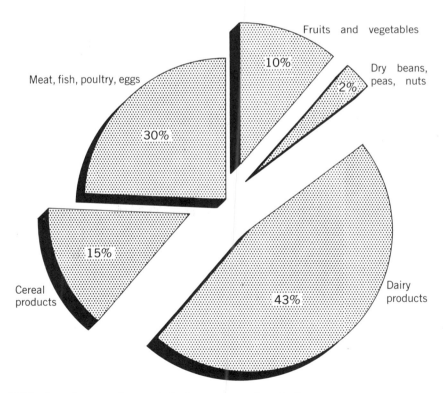

Fig. 12-15. Contribution of various food groups to the riboflavin content of American food supply. (Based on Contribution of major food groups to nutrition supplies available for civilian consumption, National Food Situation No. 130, 1969.)

the relative contributions of the major food groups.

Milk makes a significant contribution, with 1 quart providing all the recommended intake suggested for all ages and 2 cups providing a sufficient amount to take care of minimal needs. This assumes that adequate precautions are taken to minimize exposure to sunlight, which drastically reduces the amount of riboflavin available.

Cereals are low except after germination. Enriched cereals have about twice as much riboflavin as do whole-grain cereals, but still contribute only one seventh of the intake. Neera, a palm juice used in India, has been found to be high in riboflavin and accounts for a positive improvement in health during the time when it is in season. Evidence exists that riboflavin is synthesized by bacteria in the gastrointestinal tract, but there is little indication that a significant amount is absorbed in humans except when the diet is high in starch. A diet high in starch, cellulose, and lactose stimulates riboflavin synthesis in the intestines, whereas fat and protein have an inhibitory affect.

Deficiency

The lack of riboflavin manifests itself in a wide variety of ways.

In humans an early form of ariboflavinosis (a lack of riboflavin) is a condition known as *cheilosis,* in which cracks appear at the corners of the mouth and the lips become inflamed. The tongue becomes smooth and takes on a characteristic purplish red color in a condition described as glossitis. These two signs are the ones used most frequently in nutrition surveys as indicative of low riboflavin intakes, although the intake must be low for several months before these symptoms manifest themselves. Changes in the skin, causing dryness and scaliness, have been associated with low riboflavin intakes but are not specific to this vitamin.

As is true in a deficiency of all vitamins, growth retardation occurs with a lack of riboflavin. Reproductive capacity is also reduced when riboflavin is lacking, and if conception does take place, certain congenital malformations such as harelip and cataracts have been associated with a deficiency at a crucial stage in early (embryonic) development. This effect has been clearly demonstrated in animal experiments, but the relationship is much more difficult to establish in human pregnancy.

Other effects of a lack of riboflavin in the diet of animals for which no counterpart symptoms have been established in humans are loss of hair (alopecia) and infiltration of blood vessels into the cornea of the eye (corneal vascularization), which may eventually form cataracts.

Toxicity

No reports of riboflavin toxicity have appeared even though amounts as high as 10 gm. per kilogram have been given to animals. Neither is there evidence of human toxicity.

NIACIN (NICOTINIC ACID)

Niacin, another water-soluble vitamin identified with the B complex, has been known as nicotinic acid and as the pellagra preventative (P-P) factor. It is a white crystalline substance first isolated from yeast and rice bran in 1912. It was not associated with pellagra until many years later, however. The term *niacin* is now used to include nicotinamide, the amine form, as well.

History

The disease known as *pellagra* in Italy and *mal de la rosa* in Spain was first described in the eighteenth century when it occurred mainly among the poor, for whom corn was the dietary staple. Although there was evidence that the disease could be cured by changing the diet, not until 1917 was it associated with the absence of a dietary factor.

The association of pellagra with diets

monotonously high in highly refined maize, or corn, led to the theory that it was caused by a mold or a toxic or infectious substance in spoiled corn. A lack of nitrogen was implicated, and later the absence of lysine, tryptophan, or cysteine in conjuction with high leucine content in corn diets suggested an amino acid imbalance as a cause. The skin symptoms associated with pellagra were aggravated by exposure to sunlight, leading to the belief that the disease was the result of sun poisoning. Since the pellagragenic corn diets, in which molasses and salt pork were often the only other foods, were consumed by persons on limited incomes often living in crowded unsanitary surroundings, theories suggesting an infectious or parasitic nature for the disease received further support. The fact that several members of one family often developed pellagra seemed reason to look for a hereditary factor.

Only in 1917 when Goldberger, a physician working with the United States Public Health Service, confirmed his theory by producing pellagra by dietary restriction was progress made in controlling the disease. His experiment with a group of prisoners who were promised reprieve if they would switch from the prison diet to one typical of the villages in which pellagra was prevalent is now classical. Since this diet was in many cases the one most familiar to the prisoners, they were willing subjects. After about five months, however, these men began to develop the classical symptoms of pellagra—dermatitis, diarrhea, and depression—whereas those on regular prison fare remained healthy. This fairly well refuted the theory that pellagra was an infectious condition and established the theory that a dietary factor was involved. It took an additional twenty years to identify the nutritional factor.

Pellagra, first reported in the state of New York in 1875, is the only vitamin-deficiency disease that has ever been considered endemic to the United States and a major public health problem. Its incidence has been fairly well confined to the small mill villages of the southern states where the diet is predominately corn, molasses, and salt pork. In 1918 an estimated 10,000 deaths from pellagra and another 100,000 cases were reported, primarily in cotton-growing areas. At that time, when a dietary deficiency was suspected but the identity of the lacking nutrient had not been established, the most effective means of controlling the disease was to encourage the increased use of meat and milk products by promoting home production of food.

Efforts to isolate the dietary factor responsible for preventing or curing pellagra were complicated by the fact that many other deficiencies produced similar skin symptoms. Not until 1937 did Elvehjem, working at the University of Wisconsin, show that nicotinic acid was effective in curing blacktongue, a condition in dogs analogous to human pellagra. The use of nicotinic acid in treating human pellagra brought dramatic results and the census of pellagra victims in southern hospitals dropped precipitously.

Pellagra is still found in corn-eating countries such as Romania, Yugoslavia, and some parts of Egypt. The fact that it is not found in Central America, where corn provides 80% of the calories, can be attributed to the use of alkalis (usually soda lime) in its preparation. This helps liberate the niacin bound in the cereal.

Tryptophan-niacin relationship

A chemical analysis of some foods such as milk effective in curing or preventing pellagra indicated a low niacin content. Moreover, diets low in niacin were not always pellagragenic. This apparent discrepancy was explained in 1945 with the discovery that the amino acid tryptophan was also effective in curing pellagra. The role of tryptophan as a precursor of niacin has since been well established. Although for a while some investigators were convinced that tryptophan promoted the intestinal synthesis of niacin, only with the use of radioactive isotopes was it unequivocally proved that tryptophan was converted to niacin in the cells. It has now been shown that 60 mg. of tryptophan can yield 1 mg. of niacin. Although current food composition tables do not record the niacin equivalent values for foods, the sum of the preformed niacin and the niacin equivalent of the tryptophan more accurately reflects the pellagra-preventative value of the food. Dietary requirements are expressed as niacin equivalents. Tryptophan needed for synthesis of body protein will not be available for conversion to niacin, although it has not been clearly defined which need has priority. The conversion of the amino acid tryptophan to the vitamin niacin requires the presence of at least three other vitamins, thiamin, pyridoxine, and riboflavin and possibly biotin. Since vitamin B_6 is involved in the formation of niacin, it has not been surprising to find symptoms of pellagra appearing when isonicotinic acid hydrazide (INH, or isoniazid), a vitamin B_6 antagonist used in the treatment of tuberculosis, is administered in high doses. Only the L form of tryptophan can be converted; D-isomers are biologically inactive.

Chemical properties

Niacin is extremely stable to heat, light, acid, alkali, and oxidation. Because of its stability little of the nutrient is lost in normal procedures of food processing and preparation. It is active either as the acid or as the amide nicotinamide. The amide is preferred for therapeutic doses, since the use of large amounts of the acid, which acts as a vasodilator, may lead to flushing of the skin and tingling sensations.

Functions

Niacin is required by all living cells, where it plays a vital role in the release of energy from all three energy-building nu-

trients—carbohydrate, fat, and protein—and is involved in the synthesis of protein, fat, and pentoses. It is part of a coenzyme to which it contributes the ability to accept and release hydrogen atoms in at least forty of the places where these exchanges are involved in metabolism. The coenzymes of which niacin is an essential part are now identified as nicotinamide adenine dinucleotide (NAD) and nicotinamide adenine dinucleotide phosphate (NADP), both of which can accept or release hydrogen atoms readily. Because of this, they are effective in assisting a group of enzymes known as dehydrogenases in removing hydrogen in many biological reactions. They have previously been known as coenzymes I and II and as DPN and TPN (di- and triphosphopyridine, nucleotide), and the use of these terms still persists in some literature. No other biochemical role for niacin has been established yet, but the central role it plays as a part of these coenzymes means that without it the body is unable to utilize carbohydrate, fat, or protein.

Evidence exists that pharmacological doses of 1 to 2 gm. three times a day of niacin but not of nicotinamide may result in lowered blood cholesterol levels apparently because of its interference with cholesterol synthesis in the liver. It also leads to a reduction in levels of triglycerides and lipoproteins possible by inhibiting the mobilization of free fatty acids. Other mechanisms by which it could possibly act as a hypocholesterolemic agent have been investigated but have not proved fruitful. The side effects of niacin are overcome as the treatment continues.

Absorption and metabolism

Niacin is readily absorbed and is stored to a limited extent. Any excess niacin is methylated and excreted either as N-methyl nicotinamide or as the pyridone of N-methyl nicotinamide. The observation that animals excrete some radioactively labelled vitamin as carbon dioxide through the lungs has not been tested in human beings. About two thirds of the niacin metabolized by adults may come from tryptophan.

Requirements

In establishing the recommended dietary allowances, the National Research Council has defined a niacin equivalent as 1 mg. of niacin or 60 mg. of tryptophan.

Since niacin is intimately involved in the release of energy from food, it is not surprising to find that the recommended allowance for niacin is based on the caloric intake. The minimum need has been established at 4.4 niacin equivalents per 1000 kcal., to which a 50% margin of safety has been added in the recommended allowances of 6.6 niacin equivalents per 1000 kcal. It is also suggested that a minimum intake of 9 to 13 equivalents be maintained regardless of caloric intake, since this appears to be a level needed to prevent pellagra.

The amount required is influenced by factors other than caloric intake. In an amino acid imbalance the need for niacin increases. The type of carbohydrate may also have some effect, as data shows that carbohydrates containing fructose increase the need for niacin.

During the second and third trimesters of pregnancy an increase of 2 equivalents over normal needs is indicated. For lactation, when human milk contains 0.5 to 0.7 niacin equivalents per 100 ml., the maternal diet should provide 7 equivalents more than that needed under normal circumstances. This will provide the breast-fed infant with 4 to 5 equivalents per day, which apparently satisfies his needs. Bottle-fed infants almost always have a higher intake.

Most American diets that are adequate in protein tend to supply sufficient niacin. Animal protein contains 1.4% tryptophan and 1% vegetable protein. Thus a diet with 60 gm. of protein provides a minimum of 600

Table 12-5. Niacin, tryptophan, and niacin equivalents of some representative foods (milligrams per 100 gm. food)

Food	Niacin*	Tryptophan†	Niacin equivalent of trytophan‡	Total niacin
Beef liver	16.5	296	4.9	21.4
Peanut butter	15.7	330	5.5	21.2
Chicken, cooked	7.4	250	4.1	11.5
Beef, round	5.6	203	3.4	9.0
Bread, enriched	2.3	91	1.5	3.8
Orange juice	0.4	3	0.05	0.45
Spinach	0.3	37	0.6	0.9
Cottage cheese	0.2	179	2.9	3.1
Whole milk	0.1	49	0.8	0.9
Eggs	0.1	211	3.5	3.6

*From Watt, B. K., and Merrill, A. L.: Composition of foods—raw, processed and prepared, U. S. Department of Agriculture Handbook No. 8, Washington, D. C., 1963, U. S. Department of Agriculture.
†From Amino acid content of foods, Home Economics Research Report No. 4, Washington, D. C., 1957, U. S. Department of Agriculture.
‡Since 60 mg. of tryptophan can be converted into 1 mg. of niacin, niacin equivalent = $\frac{\text{mg. tryptophan}}{60}$.

mg. of tryptophan, which can be converted into 10 mg. of niacin. Any tryptophan needed for the synthesis of body protein would not be available for niacin formation. However, once the growth process is completed, much more tryptophan can be diverted for niacin synthesis.

Most diets contain a sufficient surplus of tryptophan to result in 8 to 14 mg. of niacin. An additional 8 to 17 mg. of preformed niacin makes a total of 16 to 33 mg., an amount sufficient for practically all adult needs. Only when the diet is low in protein and relatively high in a tryptophan-poor cereal is a deficiency likely to occur. Gelatin is one protein completely devoid of tryptophan. In general the niacin equivalent of American diets is considered to be 50% above the niacin content.

Food sources

The major sources of niacin are shown in Table 12-5. Liver, meat, poultry, peanut butter, and legumes are the richest sources. Milk and eggs, although low in preformed niacin, contain high amounts of tryptophan and as such have a high niacin equivalent. Fig. 12-16 shows the relative contribution of different food groups to dietary niacin. These values are based on niacin content and not niacin equivalents.

Evidence shows that much of the niacin in cereals such as rice and corn occurs as niacinogen or niacytin. In this form it is

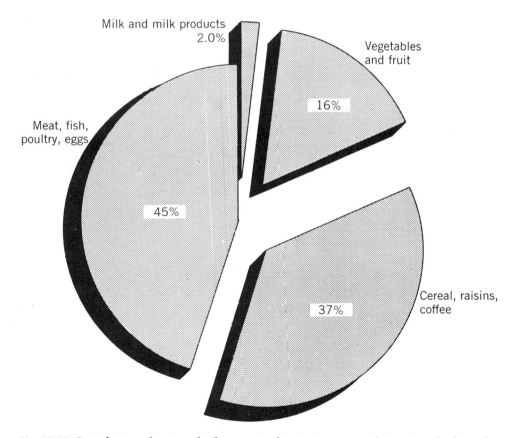

Fig. 12-16. Contribution of various food groups to the niacin content of American food supply. (Based on Contribution of major food groups to nutrient supplies available for civilian consumption, National Food Situation No. 130, 1969.)

closely bound to protein composed of at least seventeen different amino acids, from which it can be separated with great difficulty except by alkaline hydrolysis. For this reason the niacin in these foods has low biological value and does little to meet the body's requirement for the vitamin unless prepared with alkali, as is done in the preparation of corn tortillas.

As much as 80% to 90% of the niacin of cereals is in the outer husk and is removed in the milling process. The addition of niacin in enriched cereal products has done much to compensate for this loss.

Evaluation of nutritional status

Since there is little storage of this water-soluble vitamin in the body, we have learned much about it by studying the forms and the amounts in which it is excreted in the urine after a test dose. When the dietary intake is adequate, a large percentage of the test dose is excreted, and most is in the form of methylated end products of niacin metabolism. In diets low in niacin, the excretion of the pyridone drops long before any clinical symptoms of pellagra are observable. The combined excretion of N-methyl nicotinamide and its pyridone derivative drops to less than 2 mg. compared to normal excretion of 5 to 8 mg. of N-methyl nicotinamide and 7 to 10 mg. of the pyridone. When the dietary intake of both tryptophan and niacin has been low, less of the test dose is excreted, indicating that the body needs to retain more. Most of that excreted is in the form of N-methyl nicotinamide. Recently the use of a ratio of urinary excretion of pyridone to urinary excretion of N-methyl nicotinamide per gram of creatinine (indicative of muscle mass of the body) has provided a criterion on which to evaluate nutritional status of population groups with respect to niacin adequacy. A ratio of less than 1:1 is considered indicative of pellagra, whereas a ratio between 1:1 and 1.3:1 is considered borderline.

Deficiency

In pellagra the skin, the gastrointestinal tract, and the central nervous system are affected. The symptoms progress through *dermatitis, diarrhea,* and *depression* preceding *death* in what has been characterized as the four D's of pellagra. The dermatitis of pellagra is often complicated by symptoms of other B vitamin deficiencies, but when a niacin deficiency occurs, the character of the skin inflammation is specific. It occurs almost exclusively on areas of the skin exposed to sunlight and in a symmetrical pattern on both sides of the body. There is a clearly demarcated line between the afflicted and healthy areas of the skin. As the mucous linings of the gastrointestinal tract become involved, the patient suffers from diarrhea and other manifestations of infection. The hydrochloric acid secretion normally present in the gastric juice may be absent, and this may reduce the bactericidal function of the gastric juice and may allow the growth of infection-producing organisms. These changes in the gastrointestinal tract usually precede the degenerative changes that occur in the mental outlook of the patient. The irritability, headaches, and sleeplessness of early stages is soon followed by more severe mental symptoms, such as loss of memory, hallucinations, delusions of persecution, and finally a severe depression that almost inevitably precedes death.

PYRIDOXINE (PYRIDOXOL)

The terms *vitamin B₆* and *pyridoxine* are used to denote at least three chemically, metabolically, and functionally related substances—pyridoxol, pyridoxal, and pyridoxamine—all of which are biologically active for all animals studied so far. Pyridoxine was first identified in 1934 as vitamin B₆ or *adermin,* a substance capable of curing a characteristic dermatitis in rats that did not respond to any of the three factors then known in the B complex. This was followed by its isolation in 1938 and the elucidation of its structure and its synthesis one year later in 1939. The same year, Gyorgy suggested the name pyridoxine. Since then many scientists have attempted to elucidate its role in metabolism.

Pyridoxine is found widely distributed in nature. In plants it occurs as pyridoxol, the alcohol form bound to protein, a form in which it is not readily absorbed. Pyridoxamine and pyridoxal, the most prevalent forms in animal tissues, are readily available. Pyridoxine is relatively stable to heat but is destroyed by oxidation and ultraviolet light. Pyridoxal is labile to alkali, but all three forms are stable to acid. The broad distribution of pyridoxine in food coupled with a relatively small need for the vitamin makes it difficult to induce a human deficiency sufficiently severe to produce characteristic symptoms by the use of a diet low in the vitamin. However, certain undesirable biochemical changes do occur on a diet containing suboptimal amounts of pyridoxine, although no physical changes may be observed. The use of an antagonist, deoxypyridoxine, in conjunction with a diet low in vitamin B_6 has made it possible to produce deficiency states more rapidly in both animals and humans for experimental purposes.

Functions

Pyridoxine in the form of pyridoxal phosphate functions as a coenzyme for many biological reactions. Zinc or magnesium catalyzes the formation of this active coenzyme. In contrast to thiamin, riboflavin, and niacin, which act primarily as coenzymes for energy metabolism, pyridoxine plays no direct role in energy metabolism. Instead it is involved primarily with reactions occurring in protein metabolism, being necessary in the synthesis and catabolism of all amino acids. Pyridoxine is necessary for the process of transamination, in which the characteristic amino (NH_2) group from an amino acid is transferred to another substance to produce a different amino acid.

Deamination, the removal of the amino group from some amino acids, is dependent on enzymes containing vitamin B_6–deaminases. This process of deamination must take place before protein in excess of needs for growth can be used as a source of energy. In addition, the removal of the carboxyl (COOH) group from certain amino acids in a process called decarboxylation also requires pyridoxal phosphate. This decarboxylation is a necessary step in the synthesis of the vital body regulators serotonin from tryptophan, norepinephrine from tyrosine, and histamine from histidine. In a vitamin B_6 deficiency only histamine synthesis is retarded. The decarboxylation of glutamic acid in the brain is dependent on vitamin B_6 and is necessary for the regulation of neuronal activity. It also functions in the metabolism of sulfur-containing amino acids such as cysteine, from which it facilitates the removal of sulfur.

Pyridoxal phosphate plays a role in hemoglobin synthesis as a cofactor in the formation of a precursor of porphyrin, a substance that is an essential part of the hemoglobin molecule.

The most intensively studied role of vitamin B_6 in protein metabolism is in the conversion of the amino acid tryptophan into the vitamin niacin. This conversion involves several biochemical steps, in one of which an intermediary product is converted to kyneurenine in a reaction catalyzed by pyridoxal phosphate. Kynurenine in turn is changed to niacin. If large amounts of tryptophan are fed in what is known as a tryptophan load test, a person whose diet is low in pyridoxine does not produce enough pyridoxal phosphate to allow the conversion of all the kynurenine produced from tryptophan to niacin. Instead, xanthurenic acid, a substance that is not utilized by the body, is produced from kynurenine. It is excreted in the urine, and a determination of xanthurenic acid in the urine is used as an indication of the availability of pyridoxine. High urinary xanthurenic acid levels occur when available pyridoxine is limited, and low levels occur when available pyridoxine is sufficient to allow normal conversion of tryptophan to niacin. Efforts to confirm beliefs that the conversion of the essential fatty acid linoleic acid to arachidonic acid was dependent on pyridoxine have been unsuccessful. Vitamin B_6 may be involved in fat synthesis, however.

In carbohydrate metabolism, pyridoxine, as part of the enzyme glycogen phosphorylase, facilitates the release of glycogen from the liver and muscle as glucose-phosphate. This must occur before any stored carbohydrate can be available to the cells as glucose to be used as source of energy. One half of the pyridoxine stored in the body is in the form of this enzyme in the muscle. Evidence indicates that pyridoxine may be needed for the formation of other enzymes involved in carbohydrate metabolism. Low blood glucose levels, low glucose tolerance tests, and a sensitivity to insulin in a pyridoxine deficiency provide additional evidence of a relationship with carbohydrate metabolism.

The role of pyridoxine in the metabolism of the central nervous system is the concern of many workers. Changes in electroencephalograms used to evaluate the functioning of the nervous system occur in pyridoxine deficiency and in severe deficiency convulsive seizures take place. Pyridoxine may be necessary to present uncontrolled excitation of the central nervous system and eventual uncontrolled muscle seizures. The reduction in the enzymes, dependent on pyridoxal phosphate as well as in the pyridoxal content of the brain, suggests that pyridoxine may regulate the formation of these enzymes.

Vitamin B_6 is essential for the production of antibodies, as evidence by the reduced production as available pyridoxine drops. This is believed to be due to a reduced incorporation of amino acids into protein and a deficient production of messenger RNA necessary to direct protein synthesis in the cells that normally produce antibodies. Skin grafts take longer to heal in the absence of pyridoxine, apparently because of delayed hypersensitivity.

A possible role for pyridoxine in cholesterol metabolism has been suggested from studies on monkeys that showed that pyridoxine-deficient animals developed arteriosclerotic changes similar to those found in man. However, efforts to identify the relationship have been unsuccessful. These animals had four times as much dental caries as animals with adequate pyridoxine and also showed changes in the fat in their liver.

A further relationship between pyridoxine and protein metabolism is reflected in

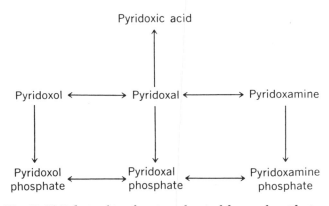

Fig. 12-17. Relationship of various chemical forms of pyridoxine.

the fact that when pyridoxine is increased, D-methionine, normally not available to the body, is equally as available as L-methionine; D-tryptophan, 50% as available as L-tryptophan; and D-valine, 33% as available as L-valine.

Metabolism

Vitamin B_6 is active as pyridoxal phosphate, which can be formed in the body from any one of the three forms found in food—pyridoxine, pyridoxal, and pyridoxamine. The pathways by which these substances can form pyridoxal phosphate are shown in Fig. 12-17. The maximum amount of pyridoxine that can be converted to the coenzyme form is 7 mg. per day.

Since pyridoxine is a water-soluble vitamin, virtually no storage of it occurs in the body. Any excess of the vitamin is oxidized to pyridoxic acid, which is metabolically inert and is excreted in the urine. Most persons excrete 0.3 to 0.4 mg. per day, but levels as high as 0.7 to 0.8 mg. have been reported. Some pyridoxine (about 0.7 to 0.9 mg. per day) is excreted in the feces, but it arises primarily from synthesis by intestinal microorganisms and does not indicate loss of ingested pyridoxine.

Requirements

Since pyridoxine is necessary for practically all aspects of protein metabolism, the requirement for the vitamin varies directly with the protein content of the diet, the requirement of which in turn is a function of body size.

Not until 1968 did the National Research Council believe adequate data existed on which to base recommendations for the dietary intake of pyridoxine. After evaluating evidence indicating that the need for vitamin B_6 was a function of the amount of protein in the diet and relatively independent of the caloric content of the diet, they recommended an intake of 2 mg. per day, which they postulated would be adequate to allow for the metabolism of 100 gm. of protein. For the pregnant woman, who transfers sufficient pyridoxine to the fetus to maintain a level of the vitamin in fetal blood five times that in the maternal blood, an additional intake of 0.5 mg. is recommended. This is based on evidence that the stress of pregnancy increases the need for pyridoxine, as the body is then less able to handle large amounts of tryptophan. Although supplemental vitamin B_6 should be given during the third trimester of pregnancy, large supplements should be avoided because of the danger of conditioning the infant to a higher requirement. A similar intake of 2.5 mg. is considered adequate to take care of the needs of lactation when 0.1 mg. per 100 ml. is transferred to human milk.

The recommended intake for infants is based on the observation that both human and cow's milk contain approximately 0.015 mg. per gram of protein, or 0.04 mg. per 100 kcal., levels which allow for adequate metabolism of protein. For the older infant and the child 0.5 to 1.2 mg. are suggested and for the adolescent 1.4 to 2 mg. appear desirable.

Older people may have increased needs for the vitamin. They have a lower level of the enzyme transaminase in the plasma, have less pyridoxal kinase in the brain, and excrete more xanthurenic acid after a tryptophan load test.

Food sources

Few foods can be considered poor sources of vitamin B_6. Among the richest, however, are muscle meats, liver, vegetables, whole-grain cereals, and egg yolks.

Since the pyridoxine in vegetable sources is more resistant to losses during processing and storage than is the pyridoxal and pyridoxamine found in animal sources, vegetable sources make a more significant contribution to the total dietary intake.

Although the vitamin B_6 content of foods is not listed in standard tables of food composition, the U. S. Department of Agricul-

Table 12-6. Pyridoxine content of average servings of some representative foods*

Food	μg. per serving
Beef liver	840
Bananas	510
Round steak	435
Ham	400
Egg yolk	300
Canned salmon	300
Cabbage	160
Lima beans, frozen	150
Spinach	150
Egg	110
Potatoes	91
Cheddar cheese	80
Strawberries	55
Milk, whole	40
Grapefruit	34
Orange juice, frozen	28

*From Orr, M. L.: Pantothenic acid, vitamin B_6 and vitamin B_{12} in foods, Home Economics Research Report No. 36, Agricultural Research Service, Washington, D. C., 1969, U. S. Department of Agriculture.

ture has prepared a separate table of food composition in which the pyridoxine content of food is given. The pyridoxine content of some representative foods is shown in Table 12-6.

Freezing of vegetables causes a 25% reduction in the amount present, and milling of cereals leads to losses as high as 80% to 90% of the original values. At the present time, pyridoxine is not added to enriched cereals, although adequate justification could be found for such a practice on the basis of data suggesting that the intake of pyridoxine is marginal in many American diets.

Evaluation of nutritional status

Although no specific nutritional deficiency disease can be attributed to a lack of the vitamin, evidence exists that certain biochemical changes do occur when the in-take is low or the needs of the individual are above normal.

A relative pyridoxine deficiency can be detected by measuring the amount of xanthurenic acid excreted after a test dose of 10 gm. of the amino acid tryptophan. In another test, requiring only one sample of blood, the amount of pyridoxal phosphate in the blood following an oral dose of 100 mg. of pyridoxine is determined. This indicates relative tissue saturation. Since pyridoxine is necessary for transaminase activity, the level of the enzyme transaminase in the blood is thought to reflect levels of vitamin B_6 available.

Since most pyridoxine is converted into pyridoxic acid before it is excreted in the urine, the determination of the level of this metabolite in the urine is a useful indicator of vitamin B_6 status. The excretion of 0.1 to 0.2 mg. of pyridoxic acid is considered indicative of a state of vitamin B_6 depletion, and excretion of less than 1 mg. in 24 hours suggests that the adequacy of the intake should be questioned. This is especially true if blood levels of the vitamin are low. In severe deprivation, pyridoxic acid disappears from the urine entirely.

Deficiency

In 1951 it was first observed that infants who were inadvertently given a formula providing less than 0.1 mg. of pyridoxine showed signs of hyperirritability and convulsions. These symptoms disappeared on the administration of the vitamin. It has been postulated that these symptoms were the result of a low dietary intake by infants who were fed a formula in which vitamin B_6 had been destroyed by heat and who had an increased need for the vitamin, possibly conditioned by high levels of supplementation of the maternal diet during pregnancy.

In adults the only symptom that has been attributed to lack of pyridoxine is a microcytic hypochromic anemia in association with high serum iron. Other less specific symptoms, such as weakness, nervousness, irritability, insomnia, and difficulty in walking, have been associated with inadequate intakes of vitamin B_6. Efforts to induce a deficiency state by dietary deficiency in humans produced only symptoms of irritability after fifty-four days. When the vitamin antagonist deoxypyridoxine was fed, skin changes (glossitis, cheilosis, and stomatitis), different from those of a riboflavin or niacin deficiency occurred.

Changes in urinary components occur in a pyridoxine deficiency. The amount of oxalate increases and the amount of urinary citrate decreases. Since citrate favors the solubility of oxalates, it is possible that the formation of urinary calculi, or kidney stones, which occurs in pyridoxine deficiencies, reflects decreased solubility of the oxalate. This may also be explained by the low levels of the transaminases necessary to convert oxalic acid to the nonessential amino acid glycine. However, when magnesium as well as pyridoxine is low, the appearance of urinary calculi is prevented.

Clinical uses

Vitamin B_6 has been used in the treatment of many conditions. When isoniazid (isonicotinic acid hydrazide), which is chemically related to pyridoxine, is used in the treatment of tuberculosis, patients develop many of the symptoms of a pyridoxine deficiency, including an increase in xanthurenic acid in the urine. These symptoms are readily counteracted with the use of higher than normal amounts of pyridoxine. Apparently isoniazid combines with pyridoxal phosphate and inactivates the enzyme involved in decarboxylation of amino acids.

Pyridoxine has been used in doses of 50 mg. per day in the treatment of the nausea of pregnancy with at least some success. Pyridoxine-containing lozenges sucked three times a day during pregnancy significantly reduce the incidence of new cavities, possibly because of an inhibitory effect on the growth of microorganisms that favor caries development. A similar reduction in tooth decay was observed in 10- to 15-year-old adolescents who were given lozenges with 3 mg. of B_6 three times a day.

Some types of anemia have responded to treatment with large (50 mg.) doses of pyridoxine, which may be necessary for the synthesis of the heme in iron-containing portions (protoporphyrin) of the hemoglobin molecule. The use of pyridoxine in treating acne, Parkinson's disease, and muscular dystrophy has met with no significant or consistent results.

PANTOTHENIC ACID
Discovery

Pantothenic acid, identified first as vitamin B_3, was so named to designate its widespread occurrence in foods (from the Greek word *pantos,* everywhere). As knowledge of its role in biological reactions has developed it may have been so named for its universal and central role in the metabolism of carbohydrate, fat, and protein.

Pantothenate had been recognized as a growth factor for yeast and as a cure or prevention for dermatitis in chicks and graying of hair in rats before it was finally isolated in 1938 and synthesized in 1940. A yellow viscous oil, pantothenic acid has never been crystallized, although its synthetic calcium salt, calcium pantothenate, has been available in crystalline form for some time. It is in this form that it is incorporated into most nutritional supplements. The alcohol form pantothenol is used in supplements and cosmetics.

Chemical properties

Pantothenic acid is a water-soluble vitamin that is stable in moist heat in neutral solution but is readily destroyed by dry heat. In acid or alkali it is relatively unstable. There is little loss in cooking at normal temperature.

Chemically, pantothenic acid is a relatively simple compound containing the

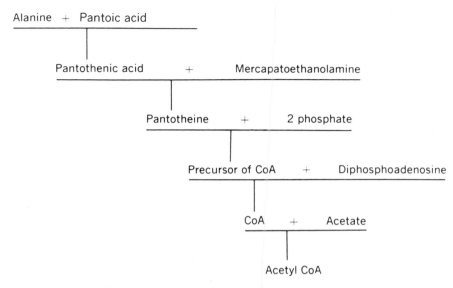

Alanine + Pantoic acid

Pantothenic acid   +   Mercapatoethanolamine

Pantotheine   +   2 phosphate

Precursor of CoA   +   Diphosphoadenosine

CoA   +   Acetate

Acetyl CoA

Fig. 12-18. Relationship between pantothenic acid and CoA.

amino acid alanine. Before it participates in biological reactions, it unites with a sulfur-containing compound to form pantotheine, which in turn adds phosphate and an adenine molecule to form coenzyme A (also called CoA). Coenzyme A is the form in which most pantothenic acid is found in microorganisms and in animal tissues and in which it participates in a central role in most biological reactions. The activation of CoA involves the addition of the 2-carbon acetate compound to form acetyl coenzyme A, or acetyl CoA. These acetate molecules are readily accepted and are transferred from the CoA molecule.

The relationship between pantothenic acid and activated CoA is shown in Fig. 12-18.

Since CoA appears within the cell but not in the blood, it must be synthesized within the cell and can pass the cell membrane with difficulty, if at all. CoA appears in highest concentration in the liver, adrenal gland, kidney, brain, and heart, all of which are tissues characterized by high metabolic activity.

Functions

As part of coenzyme A, pantothenic acid participates in the release of energy from all three energy-yielding nutrients—carbohydrate, fat, and protein. Products in the oxidation of each of these eventually react with CoA in the Krebs cycle before all their energy is released. In addition, CoA—and hence pantothenic acid—is necessary for the synthesis of fat. Besides functioning in the transfer of acetate groups to the Krebs cycle, CoA is involved as a source or acceptor of acetate groups for amino acids, vitamins, and sulfonamides. It provides acetyl groups for the formation of acetylcholine needed in the transmission of nerve impulses and for the detoxification of certain drugs. It is essential for the formation of porphyrin, a part of the hemoglobin molecule, and for the synthesis of cholesterol and some of the steriods produced by the adrenal glands. In essence, because of its central role in energy metabolism, it can be considered vital to all energy-requiring processes within the body.

Table 12-7. Food sources of pantothenic acid*

Food	mg./100 gm.
Beef liver	7.70
Egg yolk	4.40
Beef kidney	3.85
Wheat bran	2.90
Whole egg	1.60
Broccoli, frozen	1.45
Lima beans, frozen	1.24
Beef, round	0.62
Cornmeal	0.59
Cheddar cheese	0.50
Milk, nonfat	0.37
Milk, whole	0.34
Bananas	0.26
Almonds	0.25
Yellow corn, canned	0.22

*From Orr, M. L.: Pantothenic acid, vitamin B_6 and vitamin B_{12} in foods, Home Economics Research Report No. 36, Agricultural Research Service, Washington, D. C., 1969, U. S. Department of Agriculture.

Requirements

It is well established that human beings and practically all other animals and microorganisms have a need for pantothenic acid. The amount needed has not been estimated with any certainty but is generally believed to be about 10 mg., or ten times the thiamin requirement. A 3000 kcal. diet will usually provide from 13 to 19 mg. of total pantothenic acid, of which 5 to 10 mg. will occur as free pantothenic acid. From 7 to 10 mg. is excreted daily in the urine. The wide range of intakes, blood values, and urinary excretion levels that appear in individuals with no evidence of deficiency make it difficult to determine a minimum intake. Except for periods of stress, when needs may be relatively high, most diets will provide adequate amounts of pantothenic acid.

Food sources

The amount of pantothenic acid in foods representative of the main food groups is given in Table 12-7. Pantothenic acid is a component of all living matter. Although organ meats and whole-grain cereals are the richest sources, all food groups make a significant contribution to the dietary intake. The richest sources so far determined have been royal jelly from the queen bee and fish ovaries prior to spawning.

Foods processed in dry heat are relatively poor sources of pantothenic acid.

Deficiency

The wide variety of reactions for which pantothenic acid is necessary is paralleled by an equally wide variety of deficiency symptoms. Chicks show a characteristic dermatitis around the eyes, a degeneration of the spinal cord, changes in the thymus gland, and fatty degeneration of the liver. Ducks experience anemia; rats experience growth failure, the accumulation of the reddish pigment porphyrin in their whiskers, and hemorrhaging in the adrenal gland; and pigs experience changes in the sensory nerves. Biochemically an increase in copper in the skin has occurred in a pantothenic acid deficiency.

Although humans apparently do not experience pantothenic acid deficiencies of sufficient magnitude to precipitate deficiency symptoms in most mixed diets, the low intakes may slow down many metabolic processes, resulting in a wide variety of subclinical symptoms. When human volunteers were fed a pantothenic acid antagonist along with a diet low in pantothenic acid, the list of symptoms reportedly reversed by the vitamin was rather extensive. It included irritability, restlessness, burning feet, muscle cramps, impaired muscular coordination, sensitivity to insulin, decreased antibody formation, easy fatigue, mental depression, gastrointestinal disturbances, and upper respiratory infections. This list likely reflects impaired health of cells in many tissues. The site at which the symptoms first appear may be a function of some particular metabolic stress factors. High levels seem to improve the ability to withstand stress.

Pantothenic acid neither prevents nor cures graying of hair in humans in spite of any claims to the contrary by vendors of food supplements.

Clinical uses

Pantothenic acid has been used successfully in treating the paralysis of the gastrointestinal tract after surgery, which causes the accumulation of gas and severe abdominal pain. It appears to stimulate gastrointestinal motility.

FOLACIN
Discovery

Folacin was discovered in the course of the search for the factor in liver responsible for its effectiveness in curing pernicious anemia, a fatal condition characterized by large red blood cells and degeneration of nervous tissue. Although folacin (earlier known as folic acid) does not have the antipernicious anemia properties attributed to it in 1945, it has been established as a dietary essential for man, many animals, and microorganisms. It has been isolated from spinach, yeast, and liver, occurs in a wide variety of foods, and participates in many biological reactions.

The many names by which folacin has been known gives some indication of the various paths by which the substance was identified. As early as 1930 the Wills factor now believed to be folacin was identified in yeast and crude liver extracts and was found to be effective in curing a tropical macrocytic anemia. In 1938 the term *vitamin M* was applied to a growth factor for monkeys, in 1939 factor U and vitamin B_c were used to identify growth factors for chicks, and by 1940 the *Lactobacillus casei* factor or nor-eluate factor was found to be essential for the growth of that microorganism. As the chemical nature of all these substances became known, it was learned that the effectiveness of all these was due to the presence of pteroylglutamic acid (PGA). Since this substance could be extracted from green leafy vegetables such as spinach, it was designated in 1941 as folic acid (from the Latin, *folium*, leaf). The term has now been changed to *folacin* in keeping with current practices in nomenclature. Since many substances are now known to give rise to folacin in the body, the use of the term has been restricted to pteroylmonoglutamate, the form from which the active coenzymes are directly derived, and the term *folate* is applied to the broader group of substances that give rise to folacin in the body. Substances with folic acid activity are synthesized by plants, in animal tissues, and by microorganisms in the intestinal tract. By 1945 scientists knew the chemical structure of pteroylglutamic acid and had succeeded in isolating and synthesizing it. Folic acid has been established as a dietary essential for chicks, monkeys, and man, but it is not needed by rats, dogs, and rabbits.

Chemical composition

Folate as it occurs in food is a combination of the chemical compounds pterin and para-aminobenzoic acid (PABA), which together are termed pteroic acid and to which are attached either one, three, or seven molecules of the amino acid glutamic acid. It is interesting to note that earlier in the history of nutrition, para-aminobenzoic acid was itself considered a vitamin. Before these complexes can be used in the body as a vitamin, all but one of the glutamic acid molecules must be split off to form an unconjugated folic acid, or folacin, molecule, pteroylmonoglutamic acid (PGA). This release of the extra glutamic acid molecules is facilitated by specific enzymes and vitamin B_{12}. The folic acid is then reduced in the presence of ascorbic acid and the niacin-containing coenzyme NADPH to tetrahydrofolic acid (THFA). This unstable compound unites readily with a single carbon unit, which can be derived from

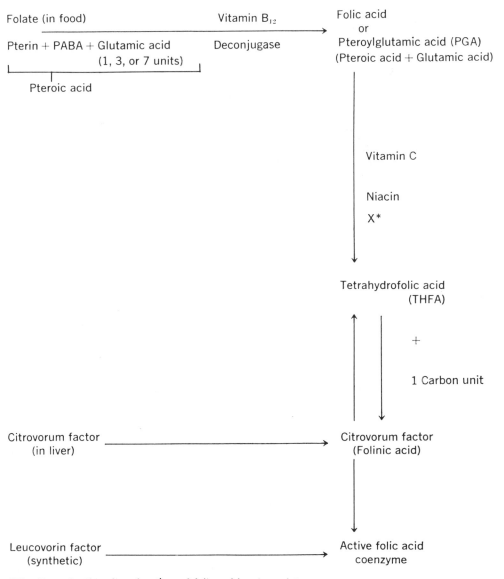

*The X marks the site of action of folic acid antagonist

Fig. 12-19. Relationship among various chemical forms of folacin. (PABA = para-amino-benzoic acid.)

many sources, to form a more stable substance known as the citrovorum factor, or folinic acid, considered the biologically active form of the vitamin. This conversion of folic acid to folinic acid must occur before it can perform its role as part of a coenzyme. Anything that blocks this conversion renders ingested folate unavailable. The citrovorum factor undergoes minor structural changes to become the coenzyme responsible for the many roles played by folacin. The synthetic form of the citrovorum factor is known as leucovorin. In addition, the citrovorum factor occurs preformed in liver, either in the active form or combined with extra glutamic acid molecules that need only be removed to give a biologically active substance. Apparently the body stores folacin as the citrovorum factor in the liver. The relationship among the various forms of the vitamin is shown in Fig. 12-19.

Folic acid antagonists such as aminopterin and amethopterin, which are chemically related to folic acid, block the action of folacin by interfering with its conversion to THFA. This explains why the citrovorum factor has been effective in overcoming the effect of the antagonist, whereas folate has not.

Absorption and metabolism

Folic acid is absorbed in the upper part of the intestine by both active transport and diffusion. Its absorption is facilitated by ascorbic acid and by some antibiotics. It is believed that some of the glutamic acid molecules of the conjugates or complexes of three or seven glutamic acid units with folacin, which constitute 80% of dietary folate, are split by enzymes in the pancreatic juice or in the intestinal mucosa and absorbed in both the upper and lower gastrointestinal tract. Absorbed folacin is removed rapidly from the serum into the tissues, which apparently have a protein that actively binds folacin. Little folic acid is excreted. The liver is the major storage site with reserves to last four to five months.

The absorption of folic acid is reduced in nontropical sprue, a condition in which structural and functional abnormalities occur as a result of the degenerative changes in the jejunum portion of the small intestine. Consequently, symptoms of folacin deficiency occur in nontropical sprue.

Functions

It was determined shortly after the discovery of folacin in 1945 that although it cured macrocytic anemia by stimulating the regeneration of both red blood cells and hemoglobin, folacin was not the antipernicious anemia factor for which scientists were searching, since it was ineffective in relieving the neurological symptoms. It did, however, play several essential roles in metabolism. Of the biochemical roles that have been clearly established, several are closely involved in blood formation.

Folacin functions in all biological reactions involving the transfer of single-carbon units, such as methyl (CH_3) groups, from one substance to another. In this role it appears to act as an intermediary, accepting the single-carbon group from one compound and passing it on to the next. Examples of this function are the formation of the amino acid methionine from one of its precursors, homocystine; the formation of the 2-carbon amino acid serine from the single-carbon amino acid glycine, the formation of the vitamin choline from its precursor ethanolamine, and the synthesis of the amino acid histidine. The conversion of nicotinic acid to N-methyl nicotinamide, the form in which it is excreted, depends on the addition of a methyl (single-carbon) unit obtained from folacin.

The synthesis of the purines adenine and guanine and the pyrimidine thymine, all part of the nucleic acids DNA and RNA, is dependent on folic acid coenzymes. Because of this role in nucleic acid synthesis, folic acid is especially important in conditions in which rapid cell division is occurring. The formation of each new cell requires the synthesis of DNA to carry the genetic information to it. Since nucleic acids control protein synthesis, folic acid exerts an indirect effect on the synthesis of enzymes and other essential protein compounds.

The conversion or oxidation of the essential amino acid phenylalanine to tyrosine also requires folacin, as does the oxidation and decarboxylation of tyrosine and the formation of part of the structure of hemoglobin—the porphyrin group.

Requirements

The need for folate has not been clearly established. It is believed that the minimum need for adults lies between 0.025 and 0.25 mg. The National Research Council has set the recommended dietary allowances for adults at 0.4 mg. Information on the minimum daily requirement indicates that 0.05 mg. is adequate. After a deficiency this level of folic acid will stimulate normal red cell production and normal bone marrow tissue but will not immediately cause an increase in serum folic acid levels or any storage of the vitamin. The minimum level may also be influenced by body size and metabolic rate. However, the amount of folic acid in food to provide this level is variable because of uncertainty about how much is destroyed in cooking and processing and the extent to which it is absorbed, which varies greatly with the source. The requirement for folic acid increases with the increased consumption of alcohol and in any condition having a marked increase in the metabolism of single-carbon units, such as pregnancy, hyperthyroidism, and hemolytic anemia. Synthetic folic acid is much more completely utilized, with 0.1 mg. protecting against folic acid deficiency. The need for infants is almost as high as that for adults because of the rapid rate of growth.

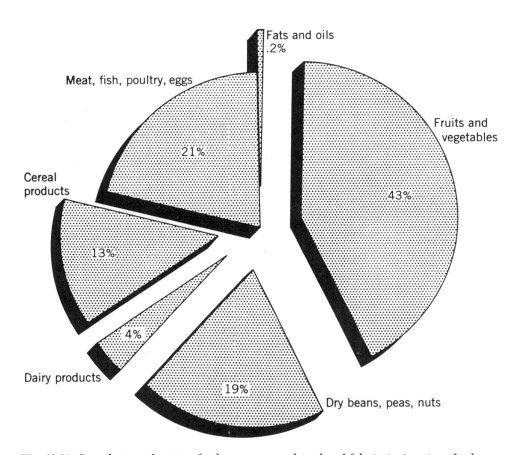

Fig. 12-20. Contribution of various food groups to total intake of folacin in American food supply. (Based on Contribution of major food groups to nutrient supplies available for civilian consumption, National Food Situation No. 130, 1969.)

Food sources

The usual dietary intake of folacin is unknown, although it is believed to be between 0.15 to 0.2 mg. per day. However, estimates vary greatly, depending on the method of analysis used. Although the content of the vitamin in many foods has not been established, data rate liver, kidney, yeast, and mushrooms as the best sources. Among vegetables, asparagus, broccoli, lima beans, and spinach rank highest, and lemons, bananas, strawberries, and cantaloupes are rich fruit sources. Milk contains little folacin. Fig. 12-20 shows the contribution of various food groups to the total intake in the American diet. Table 12-8 gives values for the folic acid content of various foods.

Losses of folic acid in processing and in cooking may range as high as 50% to 90%. Exposure to light also causes loss of folate. A high percentage of folacin in liver, yeast, and eggs is absorbed, but for other foods as little as 10% may be available.

The microbiological methods of assessing the folate activity of foods apparently do not give an accurate picture of the avail-

ability, since persons consuming diets that may contain 500 to 1000 μg. of folate do not respond as well as they do to 25 to 50 μg. of synthetic folic acid.

Evaluation of nutritional status

Since folacin is involved in normal blood formation, an analysis of the blood of humans or animals has proved the best method of detecting an inadequacy of the nutrient. A folic acid deficiency is diagnosed by low serum levels and a response to a physiological dose.

In human folacin deficiency abnormally large red blood cells, or erythrocytes, known as megaloblasts, form when the newly formed immature red blood cells, or reticulocytes, fail to mature and to lose their nuclei. Under these conditions the number of red blood cells decreases, but the amount of hemoglobin they contain does not decrease. These changes show up as high color index (>1), in which the percentage of normal hemoglobin level is compared to the percentage of normal red blood cell count. Normally the color index is approximately 1.

An analysis of the urine to determine the presence of the substance formiminoglutamic acid (FIGLU), which accumulates when folate is deficient, shows promise as a method of evaluating the folacin status of an individual. The metabolism of histidine involves its conversion to glutamic acid. If folic acid is lacking, the complete change does not occur, and an intermediary product, formiminoglutamic acid, accumulates because there is no way to remove the formyl (single-carbon group) from the molecule. If folinic acid is present, it removes the single carbon to form the active folic acid coenzyme. If folacin is inadequate, coenzymes are not formed, and the single-carbon unit (formimino) is not removed from the formiminoglutamic acid.

Deficiency

Folic acid–deficiency symptoms may result from inadequate intake, impaired ab-

Table 12-8. Folic acid content of average servings of representative foods

Food	μg.
Pork liver	126.0
Asparagus	109.0
Kidney beans (½ cup)	57.6
Carrots	22.0
Round steak	10.5
Potatoes	6.8
Cheddar cheese (1 ounce)	4.5
Peaches, canned	4.0
Bread (1 slice)	3.4
Chicken, light meat	2.8
Orange juice (½ cup)	2.6
Apple, medium	2.6
Egg, whole	2.5
Shrimp	1.8
Milk, whole	1.5

*From Hardinge, M. G., and Crooks, H.: Lesser known vitamins in foods, J. Amer. Diet. Ass. **38:**240, 1961.

sorption, excessive demands, and metabolic derangements.

With increasing knowledge of folate metabolism have come increasing numbers of reports of folate deficiency. A deficiency of the vitamin has been implicated in conditions ranging from toxemia of pregnancy (20% of pregnant women found to be deficient) to rheumatoid arthritis. In pregnant women and in women using contraceptive pills, absorption of folacin is decreased—probably the result of estrogens. It has been suggested that as the relationship between folate deficiency and biochemical disorders is clarified, it may be apparent that folate deficiency is the most prevalent of all vitamin deficiencies. Almost all symptoms can be attributed to a failure to metabolize single-carbon units.

In experimental deficiency conditions it took adults about five months to develop symptoms of megaloblastic anemia. Infants with low reserves and higher needs for growth developed symptoms in eight weeks. Inadequate folate may reduce the production of leukocytes or white blood cells and hence the ability of the body to produce antibodies.

Although no clear reason is known for the relationship, it has been found that 90% of all alcoholics suffer from a folacin deficiency.

In folic acid deficiencies the blood picture is affected differently in different animals. In monkeys a reduced number of white blood cells (leukopenia) occurs, with a reduced resistance to intestinal infection and an increase in enlarged red blood cells (macrocytes). Chicks also show macrocytic anemia, low hemoglobin and hematocrit, and slow growth.

Clinical uses

Folacin is effective in treating nutritional megaloblastic anemia caused by folate deficiency, the megaloblastic anemia of pregnancy and infancy, and some other anemias that fail to respond to vitamin B_{12}. In addition, it is effective in relieving some of the

symptoms that occur in tropical sprue, such as anemia, glossitis, and gastrointestinal disturbances.

Although folacin does relieve the anemia and glossitis associated with pernicious anemia, it not only fails to alleviate the degeneration of nervous tissue but also accentuates the changes. Thus, in addition to failing to provide a complete cure for pernicious anemia, the use of folic acid may be potentially dangerous in allowing the irreversible nervous system symptoms to develop.

Concern over the possibility that a dose of folacin, curing the megaloblastic anemia of pernicious anemia, may eliminate the most effective means of diagnosing the disease has led the Food and Drug Administration to set a limit of 0.1 mg. of folic acid as the amount that is permissible for use in vitamin supplements. This would be sufficient to protect against a folacin deficiency without curing megaloblastic symptoms of pernicious anemia. If the megaloblastic anemia has been primarily caused by vitamin B_{12} deficiency but has responded to folic acid therapy, the anemia is likely to recur.

The use of a folic acid antagonist such as aminopterin to interfere with the formation of the active coenzyme, which is necessary for the production of white blood cells (leukocytes), has been effective in decreasing the rate of leukocyte formation in leukemia, a fatal condition characterized by overproduction of white blood cells. Unfortunately, such a treatment also restricts the growth of other cells so that it can be used only intermittently and provides only temporary relief.

COBALAMIN
Discovery

Until 1926 pernicious anemia was a fatal disease of unknown origin with no known cure. In 1926 Castle established that the condition could be cured if the patient were fed large amounts of raw liver (at least three quarters of a pound per day). Noting that pernicious anemia patients had an abnormal gastric secretion, he postulated that the antipernicious anemia substance was formed by the combination of an *extrinsic factor* in food, especially liver, and an *intrinsic factor* in the normal gastric secretion. Both the extrinsic and intrinsic factors were considered necessary for the prevention or cure of the disease. Castle's theory was held during succeeding years while scientists attempted to isolate and identify the active substance in food. The story of this search is the story of the discovery of cobalamin, or vitamin B_{12}, now recognized as Castle's extrinsic factor.

The attempts to identify the active principle in liver were hampered by the fact that no animal other than man had exhibited a need for the substance. Thus all clinical evaluations of new liver concentrates had to be made on human subjects suffering from pernicious anemia. Since persons were frequently in widely separated locations, their availability as subjects was limited. Medical investigators were able to isolate progressively more concentrated extracts of liver that showed antipernicious anemia potency, but the progress was discouragingly slow in spite of the fact that with each advance pernicious anemia patients benefitted. Only with the discovery that the microorganism *Lactobacillus lactis* also needed the antipernicious anemia factor for growth could more extensive experimental work be attempted, and the final isolation of the effective principle became possible. Clinical tests, which showed that an injected dose of the liver extract was much more effective than the same amount ingested, began to cast doubt on Castle's theory and eventually led to the conclusion that Castle's extrinsic factor in food was indeed the antipernicious anemia factor and that the intrinsic factor secreted by the parietal cells of the gastric mucosa was responsible and necessary for the active absorption of the substance. The favorable results that had been obtained when large amounts of liver were fed by mouth were explained on the basis that such large amounts of cobalamin were absorbed by diffusion rather than by active transport across the intestinal membrane, which required the intrinsic factor.

Chemical composition

By 1948, two years after folic acid had been discovered and determined *not* to be the sought-after antipernicious anemia factor, workers in Britain and the United States almost simultaneously succeeded in isolating small red crystals with high antipernicious anemia potency from the liver extracts. This substance was soon identified chemically as one containing about 4% of its weight as the mineral cobalt, previously known to be essential only in the diets of sheep and cattle. The cobalt was present in the center of a chemical molecule resembling hemoglobin or chlorophyll, in which iron and magnesium are the characteristic mineral elements. In addition to containing cobalt, one active form of the vitamin was found to possess a cyano- group closely bound in the molecule. The antipernicious anemia factor was first identified as vitamin B_{12}, but the term cobalamin is now the accepted name. The synthesis of cobalamin has still not been accomplished.

Once cobalamin was isolated and chemically identified, its role in biological reactions was more easily studied. In contrast to other vitamins, a deficiency of cobalamin is primarily the result of a defect in the mechanism by which it is absorbed rather than a dietary deficit.

The term *cobalamin* is now used to designate all of the many forms in which the vitamin may appear in animal tissues as an active coenzyme. Hydroxycobalamin, cyanocobalamin, nitritocobalamin, and thiocyanate cobalamin are among the forms known to exhibit vitamin effects, although others have been identified. Of these forms, cyanocobalamin is the most active, although hydroxycobalamin appears to be retained longer by the body.

The animal protein factor (APF) known to stimulate growth in animals was found to be identical with vitamin B_{12}. It appears to promote the retention of nitrogen and hence to raise the biological value of the protein of the diet, leading to more rapid growth per unit of food. The apparent beneficial effects of the antibiotics aureomycin and penicillin in stimulating growth in animals is now attributed to the fact that they inhibit the growth of organisms that destroy vitamin B_{12}. Their use, then, essentially increases the vitamin B_{12} available and indirectly enhances growth. The usefulness of cobalamin as a growth factor for children has been investigated. Although results are inconclusive, they suggest that it is effective only in underweight children and only if the general nature of the diet improves.

Absorption

The absorption of vitamin B_{12} is governed by a heat-labile mucoprotein secreted from the parietal cells of the wall of the stomach and found in normal gastric juice. As it mixes with food in its passage through the digestive tract, this intrinsic factor, which is different in each species, releases vitamin B_{12} from the protein complex in which it occurs in food. It then helps attach the vitamin to a receptor in the intestinal mucosa of the ileum portion in a reaction catalyzed by the mineral calcium. Cobalamin is released to the mucosa or absorbing cells in the intestinal wall by the action of intestinal enzymes, which also are different in each species. A failure in any stage in the absorption can render dietary cobalamin unavailable.

The percentage of the intake that is absorbed decreases as the actual amount in the diet increases. On an average intake of 16 μg., from 3 to 5 μg. are absorbed. However, in minimal intakes of 0.5 μg. as much as 70% is absorbed.

If the gastric juice of a person lacks this intrinsic factor necessary for absorption of cobalamin, there is no uptake of the vitamin at all from the amounts normally provided in food. However, if amounts about a thousand times the normal dosage are given, as in oral doses of liver extract, sufficient amounts to meet the needs of an individual may pass through the intestinal wall by diffusion. Since the intrinsic factor in the hog's stomach is similar to that from the human gastric mucosa, it has been possible to administer a concentrate of hog's stomach to facilitate the absorption of cobalamin from either food or therapeutic preparations.

Experimentally it has been demonstrated that the vitamin may be taken in by inhalation. It is poorly absorbed, however, if administered rectally. It is most effective if injected intramuscularly to bypass the defective absorptive mechanism.

The efficiency of absorption appears to diminish with increase in age, with a pyridoxine deficiency, with an iron inadequacy, and in hypothyroidism but increases during pregnancy and when an intrinsic factor concentrate is fed along with it. The use of sorbitol, an alcohol derivative of carbohydrate, has also improved cobalamin absorption, especially among older people with depressed gastric secretions.

The administration of a radioactive dose of cobalamin and measurement of its excretion gives an indication of the effectiveness of absorption. In feces of normal subjects 30% is found, whereas pernicious anemia patients excrete 70%. About 50% to 70% is absorbed by normal subjects, with one third of this being excreted in the urine. Small amounts appear in the bile.

Metabolism

Once cobalamin is absorbed, it passes into the bloodstream, where it is bound again to a protein, the form in which it circulates to various tissues. Any vitamin absorbed in excess of the capacity of the blood to bind it is rapidly excreted in the urine, and evidence exists that in some cases a vitamin B_{12} deficiency may be caused by limitations in the cobalamin-binding capacity of the blood. The body holds on to any absorbed protein-bound vitamin tenaciously, storing any excess beyond immediate needs in the form of a cobamide enzyme in combination with protein, primarily in the liver, which has 1 to 2 μg. per gram. The uptake in the liver is facilitated by ascorbic acid. The average storage amounts to 2000 μg., an amount sufficient to last about six years.

Functions

Cobalamin is necessary for normal growth, for maintenance of healthy nervous tissue, and for normal blood formation. The exact biochemical role of the vitamin in maintaining all these functions has not been determined, but some aspects have been identified. In many respects a complex interrelationship exists between the roles of cobalamin and folacin.

The functional form of the vitamin is a coenzyme that has many forms but is generally referred to as a cobamide coenzyme. The conversion of the vitamin to this active form involves many nutrients, including niacin, riboflavin, and manganese.

In the bone marrow where erythroblasts, the forerunners of red blood cells, are formed, cobalamin coenzymes are necessary for the synthesis of thymine, which is an essential part of the genetic material DNA. If DNA is not produced, the cells cannot divide but instead continue to produce RNA and to synthesize protein, increasing in size to become the large cells called megaloblasts. The red blood cells produced by these megaloblasts are large and immature macrocytes that are characteristic of the blood of pernicious anemia patients and differ from the mature erythrocytes in normal blood. Once cobalamin is available, the megaloblasts are no longer formed, and the erythroblasts produce normal mature red blood cells, the erythro-cytes. The role of cobalamin in nucleic acid synthesis, which may include the formation of deoxyribose from ribose as well as thymine synthesis from methyl groups, is important in all body cells, but its effect is more pronounced in erythrocytes, which develop very rapidly at a rate of at least 200 million per minute.

The way in which cobalamin affects the nervous system is not clear. However, it is known that vitamin B_{12} keeps glutathione, an integral part of several enzymes involved in carbohydrate metabolism, in the reduced state in which it is biologically active. Since the nervous system relies entirely on carbohydrate as its source of fuel, anything that disrupts carbohydrate metabolism will deprive nervous tissue of its energy source and hence will interfere with its normal functioning. Since the nervous system has a limited range of pathways by which it can handle carbohydrate, it may be dependent on vitamin B_{12}. Levels of pyruvic acid and lactic acid, intermediary products in carbohydrate metabolism, increase from 50% to 100% in a cobalamin deficiency, suggesting a block in glucose metabolism.

Like folate, cobalamin is concerned with metabolism that involves single-carbon units such as methyl groups. Unlike folate, which aids the transfer of these single-carbon units from one substance to another, cobalamin is necessary for the synthesis or formation of these units, which in turn are vital in the formation of many essential body compounds.

In the metabolism of folic acid, vitamin B_{12} catalyzes the release of folic acid with one glutamic acid molecule from folic acid conjugates of three or seven glutamic acid molecules that occur in foods. In addition, it facilitates the formation of the folic acid coenzymes from the citrovorum factor, or folinic acid.

Besides its direct role in folic acid and nucleic acid metabolism and its more indirect role in carbohydrate metabolism, the vitamin appears to play a role in fat and protein metabolism, but the mechanisms have not been clarified.

Food sources

Vitamin B_{12} is found only in foods of animal origin. Animals absorb the vitamin after it has been synthesized by bacteria in their rumen from the plant foods they eat, provided sufficient cobalt is available. Microorganisms in the gastrointestinal tract of human beings are also able to synthesize the vitamin, but the site of synthesis is too far down in the colon to permit absorption.

The best sources of cobalamin are the animal foods—liver (which contains about 1 ppm), kidney, milk, and meat, in all of which it occurs in a protein complex. This is illustrated in Table 12-9. In diets of everyone except strict vegetarians, who make absolutely no use of animal products, the intake is always adequate. Deficiency symptoms result from failure in the absorptive mechanisms rather than any lack of the nutrient.

Commercially, cobalamin is produced by

specific organisms capable of synthesizing it. If it is obtained from liver, 1 ton of liver is required to yield 20 mg. of the vitamin. It is sometimes advertised as the red vitamin because of its bright red crystals.

Cyanocobalamin is stable to acid and oxidation but is destroyed by alkali. About 70% is normally retained in cooking.

Requirements

The need for cobalamin is extremely small and has been difficult to determine, but it is now recommended that a diet containing 3 to 5 μg. per day, from which 1 to 1.5 μg is absorbed, will satisfy the need of most adults. On the other hand, studies of the whole body turnover of the vitamin suggest a need ranging from 0.5 to 2.5 μg. Body stores normally range from 800 to 11,000 μg. Pernicious anemia patients will experience relief on as little as 0.1 μg. by intramuscular injection or 5 to 15 μg. taken orally with the intrinsic factor.

Deficiency

As indicated earlier, virtually no evidence is found of a deficiency state from a lack of dietary source of the nutrient except among strict vegetarians, who develop neurological symptoms but not changes in their blood pattern. Pernicious anemia, the major manifestation of an inadequate amount of the nutrient, results from a lack of the intrinsic factor secreted by the glands of the stomach, from partial or complete removal of the stomach, from a lack of the protein in the blood that binds absorbed cobalamin, or from a lack of the substance that releases it from the mucosal cells to the blood. Intestinal infestation with a fish tapeworm that avidly absorbs any available vitamin also produces an induced deficiency state. Diagnosis of vitamin B_{12} deficiency can be made on the basis of blood levels of the vitamin, which are determined by microbiological techniques. Normal levels of 100 to 1000 μg. per milliliter fall below 100 in pernicious anemia, and changes in

Table 12-9. Cobalamin content of some representative foods*

Food	μg./100 gm.
Beef liver	80.0
Oysters	18.0
Lamb	2.2
Egg, whole	2.0
Salami	1.4
Frankfurters	1.3
Haddock	1.3
Cheddar cheese	1.0
Shrimp	0.9
Pork	0.7
Chicken	0.5
Milk, whole	0.4

*From Orr, M. L.: Pantothenic acid, vitamin B_6 and vitamin B_{12} in foods, Home Economics Research Report No. 36, Agricultural Research Service, Washington, D. C., 1969, U. S. Department of Agriculture.

the nature of red blood cells from small nonnucleated cells to larger nucleated ones help confirm the diagnosis.

Pernicious anemia can now be readily controlled by injections of cobalamin. About 1000 μg. are given twice in the first week, followed by 250 μg. per week until the blood pattern has returned to normal. A dose of 250 μg. every three weeks is usually sufficient to protect against recurrence of the condition. The most crucial aspect of pernicious anemia therapy is a sufficiently early diagnosis that treatment can be begun before neural degeneration has become irreversible. In contrast to the victim of pernicious anemia prior to 1925, who faced almost certain death, or after 1926, who was forced to eat large amounts of liver daily, today's patient has at his disposal a relatively simple and inexpensive form of treatment.

BIOTIN
Discovery

Recognition of biotin as a dietary essential occurred in 1924 when it was identified as bios II, one of three factors necessary for the growth of microorganisms. Between this time and the time of its synthesis in 1943, various scientists had sought the nature of substances they had named vitamin H and coenzyme R. Once the chemical nature of this sulfur-containing nutrient was determined, it was clear, as had been the case in the study of many other nutrients, that all three were the same substance, now identified as biotin.

Symptoms of biotin deficiency occur in animals only after the ingestion of a diet low in biotin and high in raw egg white. Raw egg white includes a carbohydrate-containing protein, *avidin,* which binds biotin in a complex too big to be absorbed but which the body cannot break to release biotin. Experimentally it was found that in humans the diet had to provide 30% of its calories from raw egg white to induce a biotin deficiency. Since this represents ap-

proximately 27 egg whites in a 3000 kcal. diet it is obvious that the ingestion of the occasional raw egg white is not going to precipitate a deficiency state. Cooking denatures avidin so that it no longer has the ability to bind biotin.

Chemical properties

Biotin has been isolated in at least five active forms from food. One of these, biocytin, is a combination of biotin and the amino acid lysine. Other forms are biotin sulfone, which is a potent antagonist, and biotinal, which can be oxidized to an active form.

In animal tissues the protein-bound biotin is fat soluble, whereas the free biotin found in plants and excreted in the urine is water soluble.

Biotin is stable to heat but labile to alkali and oxidation. As a water-soluble vitamin some will be lost in cooking water.

Functions

Biotin is an active substance participating in many biological reactions. In animal cells it occurs bound to protein where it acts as an enzyme.

The best established role of biotin coenzymes is in the addition (carboxylation) or removal (decarboxylation) of carbon dioxide in various reactions. Since these reactions are common in nature, we find biotin involved in both the synthesis and oxidation of fatty acids and the oxidation of carbohydrate. Its role in deamination, which must occur before amino acids can be used as a source of energy, has been established for at least three amino acids—aspartic acid, threonine, and serine. It is necessary for the synthesis of nicotinic acid, but the mode of action is not clear. The synthesis of the digestive enzyme pancreatic amylase is another biotin-dependent reaction.

Failure of some of these functions shows up in an impaired utilization of glucose, a decrease in the incorporation of amino acids into protein, and up to 30% reduction in fat caused by failure in the synthesis of fatty acids.

Requirements

So far it has been impossible to establish whether or not humans need a dietary source of biotin and, if so, the magnitude of the need. It is thought that the body uses approximately 150 μg. per day, an amount adequately provided by the diet even without that provided by intestinal synthesis.

Food sources

Most of the biotin in food occurs bound to protein from which the body can readily liberate it. Liver, kidney, milk, egg yolk, and yeast have been shown by biological assay to be the richest food sources, followed by some vegetables, such as cauliflower, nuts, and legumes. In general all other meats, dairy products, and cereals are considered poor sources. Human milk has only one tenth the amount of biotin of cow's milk.

Most diets contain 150 to 300 μg. of biotin, which is supplemented by some from the intestinal synthesis by bacteria that is stimulated on a sucrose-containing diet. No evidence exists on which to justify the inclusion of biotin in the formula for a multivitamin supplement.

In addition to the biotin provided by the diet, a considerable amount is synthesized by intestinal bacteria. Conditions that reduce the number of microorganisms in the intestine may reduce the amount of biotin synthesized. Sulfonamides and oxytetracycline are known to reduce the number of biotin-synthesizing organisms. Some of the symptoms that develop with the use of sulfonamides may be evidence of biotin deficiency, since biotin administration seems to counteract them.

Deficiency

The effects of a biotin-deficient diet in animals are many and varied but seem to be characterized by early changes in the skin. Dermatitis, characterized by either scaliness or hardening, which frequently starts in the region of the eye, is common. This is often followed by loss of hair and evidence of muscular atrophy.

In a study in which four human subjects became deficient on a diet devoid of biotin and high in avidin, the symptoms observed were similar to those of a thiamin deficiency and included dermatitis, loss of appetite, nausea, muscle pains, and high blood cholesterol levels, among many other symptoms. In both cases a derangement of the metabolic enzyme system occurs.

Although no evidence exists of a natural biotin deficiency in human adults, recent evidence has suggested that two types of dermatitis—Leiner's disease and seborrheic dermatitis, which occur in infants—may be caused by a lack of biotin. They respond rather dramatically to biotin therapy, although similar conditions in adults are not responsive.

SELECTED REFERENCES

Ascorbic acid

Abt, A. F., von Schuching, S., and Enns, T.: Vitamin C requirements of man re-examined, Amer. J. Clin. Nutr. 12:21, 1963.

Baker, E. M.: Vitamin C requirements in stress, Amer. J. Clin. Nutr. 20:583-590, 1967.

Grewar, D.: Infantile scurvy, Clin. Pediat. (Phila.) 4:82, 1965.

Hodges, R. E., Baker, E. M., Hood, J., Sauberlich, H. E., and March, S. C.: Experimental scurvy in man, Amer. J. Clin. Nutr. 22:535, 1969.

King, C.: Present knowledge of ascorbic acid, Nutr. Rev. 26:33, 1968.

Lorenz, A. J.: The conquest of scurvy, J. Amer. Diet. Ass. 30:665, 1954.

Ossofsky, H. J.: Infantile scurvy, Amer. J. Dis. Child. 109:173, 1965.

Pauling, L.: The common cold and vitamin C,

San Francisco, 1970, W. H. Freeman & Co., Publishers.

Schwartz, F. W.: Ascorbic acid in wound healing—a review, J. Amer. Diet. Ass. **56**:497, 1970.

Shaffer, C. F.: Ascorbic acid and atherosclerosis, Amer. J. Clin. Nutr. **23**:27, 1970.

Sherlock, P., and Rothschild, E. O.: Zen diets and scurvy, J.A.M.A. **199**:794, 1967.

Szent-Györgyi, A.: Lost in the twentieth century, Ann. Rev. Biochem. **32**:1, 1963.

Udenfriend, S.: Formation of hydroxyproline in collagen, Science **152**:1335, 1966.

Uhl, E.: Ascorbic acid requirements of adults: 30 mg. or 75 mg.? Amer. J. Clin. Nutr. **6**:146, 1958.

Thiamin

Bradley, W. B.: Thiamine enrichment in the United States, Ann. N. Y. Acad. Sci. **98**:602, 1962.

Brin, M.: Thiamine deficiency and erythrocyte metabolism, Amer. J. Clin. Nutr. **12**:107, 1963.

Brozek, J.: Psychologic effects of thiamine restriction and deprivation in normal young men, Amer. J. Clin. Nutr. **5**:109, 1957.

Dreyfus, R. M., and Victor, M.: Effects of thiamine deficiency on the central nervous system, Amer. J. Clin. Nutr. **9**:414, 1961.

Latham, M. C.: Present knowledge of thiamine: In Present knowledge of nutrition, ed. 3, New York, 1967, Nutrition Foundation, Inc.

Lipmann, F.: The biochemical function of B vitamins, Perspect. Biol. Med. **13**:1, 1969.

Requirements of vitamin A, thiamin, riboflavin and niacin, Report of Joint FAO/WHO Expert Group, Techn. Rep. Ser. No. 362, 1967.

Salcedo, J.: Experience in the etiology and prevention of thiamine deficiency in the Philippine Islands, Ann. N. Y. Acad. Sci. **98**:568, 1962.

Sauberlich, H. E.: Biochemical alterations in thiamine deficiency—their interpretation, Amer. J. Clin. Nutr. **20**:528, 1967.

Wurst, H. M.: The history of thiamine, Ann. N. Y. Acad. Sci. **98**:385, 1962.

Riboflavin

Lane, M., Alfrey, C. P., Mengel, C. E., Doherty, M. A., and Doherty, J.: The rapid induction of human riboflavin deficiency with galactoflavin, J. Clin. Invest. **43**:357, 1964.

Mayersohn, M., Feldman, S., and Gebaldi, M.: Bile salt enhancement of riboflavin and flavin mononucleotide absorption in man, J. Nutr. **98**:288, 1969.

Revlin, R. S.: Riboflavin metabolism, New Eng. J. Med. **13**:626, 1970.

Windmueller, H. G., Anderson, A. A., and Mickel-

son, O.: Elevated riboflavin levels in urine of fasting subjects, Amer. J. Clin. Nutr. **15**:73, 1964.

Niacin

De Lange, D. J.: Assessment of nicotinic acid status of population groups, Amer. J. Clin. Nutr. **15**:169, 1964.

Goldsmith, G. A.: Niacin-tryptophane relationship in man and niacin requirement, Amer. J. Clin. Nutr. **6**:479, 1958.

Goldsmith, G. A.: Niacin, antipellagra factor; hypocholesteremic agent, J.A.M.A. **194**:167, 1965.

Goldsmith, G. A., Miller, O. N., and Unglaub, W. G.: Efficiency of tryptophane as a niacin precursor in man, J. Nutr. **73**:172, 1961.

Snydenstricker, V. P.: History of pellagra; its recognition as a disorder of nutrition and its conquest, Amer. J. Clin. Nutr. **6**:409, 1958.

Pyridoxine

Baker, E. M., Canham, J. E., Nunes, W. T., Sauberlich, H. E., and McDowell, M. E.: Vitamin B_6 requirement for adult men, Amer. J. Clin. Nutr. **15**:59, 1964.

Bunnell, R. H.: Vitamin B_6, Science **146**:674, 1964.

Committee on Nutrition, American Academy of Pediatrics: Vitamin B_6 requirements in man, Pediatrics **38**:75, 1966.

Coursin, D. B.: Vitamin B_6 requirements, J.A.M.A. **189**:27, 1964.

Drenick, E. J., Vinyard, E., and Swendseid, M. E.: Vitamin B_6 requirements in starving obese males, Amer. J. Clin. Nutr. **22**:10, 1969.

Kelsay, J., Baysal, A., and Linkswiler, H.: Effect of vitamin B_6 depletion on the pyridoxal, pyridoxamine, and pyridoxine content of the blood and urine of men, J. Nutr. **94**:490, 1968.

Linkswiler, H.: Biochemical and physiological changes in vitamin B_6 deficiency, Amer. J. Clin. Nutr. **20**:547, 1967.

Orr, M. L.: Pantothenic acid, vitamin B_6 and vitamin B_{12} in foods, Home Economics Research Report No. 36, Agricultural Research Service, Washington, D. C., 1969, U. S. Department of Agriculture.

Polansky, M. M., and Murphy, E. W.: Vitamin B_6 in fruits and nuts, J. Amer. Diet. Ass. **48**:109, 1966.

Polansky, M. M., Murphy, E. W., and Toepfer, E. W.: Components of vitamin B_6 in grains and cereal products, J. Ass. Agricult. Chem. **47**:750, 1964.

Review: Pyridoxine and dental caries; human studies, Nutr. Rev. **21**:143, 1963.

Shriver, C. R., and Hutchison, J. H.: The vitamin B_6 deficiency syndrome in human infancy:

biochemical and clinical observations, Pediatrics 31:240, 1963.

Trimpter, G. W., Andelman, R. J., and George, W. F.: Vitamin B_6 dependency syndromes: new horizons in nutrition, Amer. J. Clin. Nutr. **22:** 794, 1969.

Williams, M. A.: Present knowledge of vitamin B_6: In Present knowledge of nutrition, ed. 3, New York, 1967, Nutrition Foundation, Inc.

Pantothenic acid

Bean, W. B.: Present knowledge of pantothenic acid: In Present knowledge of nutrition, ed. 3, New York, 1967, The Nutrition Foundation, Inc.

Nelson, R. A.: Intestinal transport, coenzyme A and colitis in pantothenic acid deficiency, Amer. J. Clin. Nutr. **21:**495, 1968.

Zook, E. G., MacArthur, M. S., and Toepfer, E. W.: Pantothenic acid in foods, Agricultural Handbook No. 97, Washington, D. C., 1956, U. S. Department of Agriculture.

Folacin

Girdwood, R. H.: Abnormalities of vitamin B_{12} and folic acid metabolism—their influence on the nervous system, Nutr. Soc. Proc. **27:**101, 1968.

Herbert, V.: Biochemical and hematologic lesions in folic acid deficiency, Amer. J. Clin. Nutr. **20:** 562, 1967.

Metz, J., Festenstein, H., and Welsh, P.: Effect of folic acid and vitamin B_{12} supplementation on tests of folate and vitamin B_{12} nutrition in pregnancy, Amer. J. Clin. Nutr. **16:**472, 1965.

Rosenberg, I. H., Streiff, R. R., Godwin, H. A., and Castle, W. B.: Absorption of polyglutamic folate: participation of deconjugating enzymes of the intestinal mucosa, New Eng. J. Med. **280:** 985, 1969.

Santini, R., Brewster, C., and Butterworth, C. E.: The distribution of folic acid active compounds in individual foods, Amer. J. Clin. Nutr. **14:**205, 1964.

Streiff, R. R., and Little, A. B.: Folic acid deficiency in pregnancy, New Eng. J. Med. **276:**776, 1967.

Vilter, R. W., Will, J. J., Wright, T., and Rullman, D.: Interrelationships of vitamin B_{12}, folic acid and ascorbic acid in the megaloblastic anemias, Amer. J. Clin. Nutr. **12:**130, 1963.

Vitale, J.: Present knowledge of folacin, Nutr. Rev. **24:**289, 1966.

Cobalamin

Armstrong, B. K.: Absorption of vitamin B_{12} from the human colon, Amer. J. Clin. Nutr. **21:**298, 1968.

Baker, S. J.: Human vitamin B_{12} deficiency, World Rev. Nutr. Diet. **8:**63, 1967.

Chow, B. F.: Nutritional significance of vitamin B_{12}, World Rev. Nutr. Diet. **1:**127, 1960.

Herbert, V.: Nutritional requirements for vitamin B_{12} and folic acid, Amer. J. Clin. Nutr. **21:**743, 1968.

Heyssel, R. M., Bozian, R. C., Darby, W. J., and Bell, M. C.: Vitamin B_{12} turnover in man, Amer. J. Clin. Nutr. **18:**176, 1966.

King, C. G.: Practical and novel advances in relation to vitamin C, J. Nutr. Educ. **1:**19, 1969.

Schweigert, B. S.: The role of vitamin B_{12} in nucleic acid synthesis, Borden Rev. Nutr. Res. **22:** 19, 1961.

Sullivan, L. W., and Victor, H.: Studies on the minimum daily requirement for vitamin B_{12}, New Eng. J. Med. **272:**340, 1965.

Wilson, T. H.: Intrinsic factor and B_{12} absorption—a problem in cell physiology, Nutr. Rev. **23:** 33, 1965.

Biotin

Baugh, C. M., Malone, J. H., and Butterworth, C. E., Jr.: Human biotin deficiency. A case history of biotin deficiency induced by raw egg consumption in a cirrhotic patient, Amer. J. Clin. Nutr. **21:**173, 1968.

Bridgers, W. F.: Present knowledge of biotin, Nutr. Rev. **25:**65, 1967.

13

Other nutrient factors

In addition to the nutrients that have already been definitely established as vitamins, several other vitamin-like substances exist that, on the basis of current information, fail to meet all the criteria necessary to be classed as vitamins but still have some properties of vitamins. In some cases they are present in larger amounts than vitamins; in others the body can synthesize sufficient amounts to meet body needs if precursors are present; and for still others it has been impossible to determine any essential biological role.

Because these dietary factors are sometimes given vitamin status, it is believed that a brief discussion of present knowledge of their status is warranted here. Undoubtedly, some will in the future be established definitely as vitamins, whereas others will definitely be dropped from this classification.

MYOINOSITOL

Myoinositol, which is also known as muscle sugar and mesoinositol, is one of nine 6-carbon compounds closely related chemically to glucose. Of these nine, only myoinositol is biologically active. It was first recognized in 1928 as a growth-promoting factor for yeast and as a cure for alopecia in mice.

It is present in practically all plant and animal tissues in concentrations higher than those normally associated with vitamins. In animal cells it occurs primarily as a phospholipid, which is sometimes referred to as liposital. In grains it is present as a more complex water-soluble compound, phytic acid, the organic acid that binds both calcium and iron in an insoluble complex and prevents their absorption. It also occurs in nucleated erythrocytes. In soybeans it occurs in a free form, and in other plant and animal tissues it occurs as an unidentified complex. Some evidence exists that sharks and certain other fishes store carbohydrate as inositol rather than as glycogen.

Methods of analyzing for inositol are tedious and relatively inaccurate, but from available data it appears that heart muscle, brain, and skeletal muscle contain more inositol than do other tissues. Fruits, meat, milk, nuts, vegetables, and whole-grain cereals are the best food sources.

The biological significance of inositol in human nutrition is unknown, although several roles have been attributed to it. It may act as an intermediary product between carbohyrate and aromatic compounds, or it may retard the loss of vitamin C in scorbutic guinea pigs. It is believed to lead to a decrease in RNA synthesis, but none of these possible roles has been clearly established. It has, however, been found essential for the growth of liver and bone marrow cells.

Human beings apparently consume about 1 gm. of inositol a day in food. In addition, the body is able to synthesize sufficient amounts to meet its needs from glucose. Synthesis occurs within the individual cell rather than by intestinal organisms. The amount excreted in the urine is small and variable, averaging 37 mg. per day with a range from 8 to 144 mg., although diabetics excrete much more. Normal blood levels range from 0.37 to 0.67 mg. per 100 ml.

CHOLINE

Choline was identified in 1937 as a dietary factor that prevented the accumulation of fat in the liver of dogs. Since then it has been determined that the effectiveness of choline is due to three methyl (CH_3) groups present in its molecule, which are available to other biological compounds. As a methyl donor, choline provides one of the substances necessary to mobilize fat from the liver to be transported in the bloodstream to other cells of the body. Methyl groups are exchanged in a wide variety of biological reactions, and as a source of these, choline facilitates many reactions.

Choline can be readily synthesized in the body from the amino acid glycine, providing another source of the methyl group is available. These methyl groups may be provided by another amino acid, methionine; they can be synthesized in the presence of adequate folic acid or cobalamin; or they may be obtained from a variety of other sources. Thus it appears that choline cannot be considered a vitamin, since the human is not solely dependent on a dietary source of either choline or a direct precursor. In animals such as the guinea pig or fowl, choline is a dietary essential, since it cannot be synthesized at a sufficient rate to meet their needs.

In the body, choline occurs as a constituent of the fat-related substance lecithin, a form in which much fat is transported, and sphingomyelin, which occurs in nerve tissue. As such, it is a structural part of fat and nerve tissue and does not catalyze any reactions or act as part of a coenzyme. In addition, choline reacts with acetyl CoA to form an acetylcholine that is responsible for transmitting nerve impulses from one nerve ending to the next.

Choline is widely distributed in food, being present in relatively large amounts in all foods that contain fat, as shown in Table

Table 13-1. Choline content of representative foods

Food	Choline content (gm./100 gm.)
Egg yolk	1.7
Beef liver	0.6
Soybeans	0.2
Fish	0.2
Cereal	0.1

13-1. With the exception of legumes, fruits and vegetables contain virtually no choline. The average diet provides about 500 to 900 mg. per day.

The need for dietary choline has not been established since it is small or nonexistent when the diet contains sufficient methionine to provide methyl groups for the synthesis of choline or adequate amounts of folacin and cobalamin to stimulate the synthesis of methyl groups.

Choline is not associated with any specific deficiency disease in human beings. It does, however, exert a protective action in cirrhosis of the liver among alcoholics. In rats and dogs the symptoms associated with choline deficiency are aggravated by a pyridoxine deficiency, whereas in chickens and turkeys the perosis induced by choline deficiency can be cured by folic acid, manganese, or choline.

COENZYME Q (ubiquinone)*

The most recently discovered (1961) nutritional factor is coenzyme Q, a lipidlike substance that is somewhat similar in its

---

*Folkers in a review "Survey of Nutritional Aspects of Coenzyme Q" (Int. J. Vitamin Res. 39:334, 1969) suggests that the definition of a vitamin be modified to include substances produced by intestinal biosynthesis in mammalian cells. Since coenzyme Q synthesis depends on the availability of the amino acids tyrosine and phenylalanine and the vitamins niacin, folic acid, cobalamin, pyridoxine, and pantothenic acid, Folkers suggests that coenzyme Q should be considered a vitamin.

chemical makeup to both vitamin K and vitamin E. It was recognized simultaneously by two different groups, one studying vitamin A and the other studying electron transport in the cell mitochondrion. It belongs to a group of compounds known as ubiquinones, and the forms that appear to be biologically important have from 30 to 50 carbon atoms in a side chain attached to the basic quinone structure. The 50-carbon side chain occurs exclusively in higher animals.

Coenzyme Q is found in practically all living cells and appears to be concentrated in the mitochondria. Here it apparently operates as an essential link in the respiratory chain in which energy is released from energy-yielding nutrients as the high-energy compound ATP. It appears to be reversibly oxidized and reduced readily. Without this substance one would anticipate incomplete release of energy.

The ubiquinones are likely to be synthesized readily in the body, the ring structure from amino acids such as phenylalanine and the side chain from acetate available as an intermediary in carbohydrate and fat metabolism. A pantothenic acid deficiency has been shown to depress coenzyme Q synthesis by 50%, likely because of decreased availability of acetate. Ubiquinones therefore are of little dietary significance and cannot be truly classed as vitamins. In contrast to other fat-soluble vitamins, they can be excreted in the urine.

Ubichromenol, which is similar to vitamin E in structure and biological activity, can be formed from ubiquinone. Both vitamin E and selenium operate to maintain high tissue concentration of coenzyme Q.

Coenzyme Q–type compounds are widely distributed in food, being found in soybeans, vegetable oils, and a wide variety of animal tissues.

BIOFLAVONOIDS

The bioflavonoids were first suggested as dietary factors in 1936 when it was observed that extracts of both red pepper and lemon increased the antiscorbutic effect of ascorbic acid. A wide range of chemical substances, mostly belonging to the flavine and flavonoid compounds, were believed to exert a favorable influence in reducing capillary bleeding caused by the increased permeability of the cell membrane. For a while these compounds, of which *hesperidin* was one of the most active, were designated vitamin P, but the use of this term was dropped in 1950.

So far, scientists have been unable to ascertain any specific biological role for this group of compounds, although it is agreed that they may have some pharmacological effects. In addition, no proof has been found of clinical usefulness of the compounds that have been advocated at various times as therapeutic agents in the treatment of a range of unrelated conditions, such as cerebral accidents, arthritis, abortions, common colds, and retinal hemorrhages. Many suggestions have been made regarding the mode of action of the bioflavonoids, but none have been substantiated.

Bioflavonoids occur in highest concentration in the peel and juice of citrus fruit, in tobacco leaves, in buckwheat, and in some other fruits and vegetables. No evidence exists at the present time of a dietary need for bioflavonoids and certainly no justification for their inclusion in nutritional supplements; nor is there a justification in the promotion of certain foods on the basis of a high concentration of the substance. Several bioflavonoids are being investigated as potential low-calorie sweetening agents.

LIPOIC ACID

Lipoic acid is a water-soluble factor known to be essential for the growth of several microorganisms. It has been isolated from liver and yeast, and several aspects of its biochemical role have been elucidated. At the present time there is some question whether it should be considered a vitamin for humans, since no evidence has yet been established that humans or other mammals require a dietary source of the substance. Although it does participate in biochemical reactions in mammalian tissues, the amounts needed to meet these needs are likely synthesized in the body.

Lipoic acid is now identified in five distinct forms; three forms are fat soluble; one is a water-soluble complex; and one, which is bound to protein, has been known as factor 11 and 11A, pyruvic oxidation factor, thioctic acid, and protogen. Lipoic acid, the official name, and thioctic acid, indicative of the sulfur found in the molecule, are the names most frequently used now. The fat-soluble lipoic acid can be reversibly oxidized to the water-soluble beta-lipoic acid.

Function

Lipoic acid is essential along with the thiamin-containing enzyme, pyrophosphatase for the reactions in carbohydrate metabolism that convert pyruvic acid to acetyl coenzyme A. This is the point at which it joins the intermediary products of protein and fat metabolism in the Krebs cycle for the reactions involved in liberating energy from these nutrients. In its active form, lipoic acid is bound to a protein in a reaction requiring energy in the form of ATP and a metal ion, such as calcium or magnesium. In plant cells it may be involved in catalyzing some of the reactions of photosynthesis.

Several attempts have been made to relate lipoic acid nutrition to metabolic disorders in animals and humans, but most of the results have been contradictory. Some evidence showed that lipoic acid limited the plasma lipid formation on cholesterogenic diets in rabbits; other evidence showed that it stimulated tumor growth; and still other evidence showed that it led to a reduction in voluntary alcohol consumption. But none of the evidence is clear cut. In humans lipoic acid has been beneficial in the liver disease hepatic coma.

SELECTED REFERENCE

Roels, O. A.: Present knowledge of coenzyme Q, Nutr. Rev. **25**:97, 1967.

PART II

Applied

NUTRITION

14

Selection of an adequate diet, dietary standards, and tables of food composition

The recommended dietary allowances (RDA) provide a useful guide for nutritionists, dietitians, and agricultural experts in planning and evaluating diets of population groups and in planning food production programs. They are, however, of little value to the average individual or homemaker, who may become confused by the many units—milligrams, grams, International Units, and kilocalories—in which requirements are expressed. In addition, she seldom has access to tables of food composition or the inclination or ability to make the involved calculations necessary to evaluate a particular diet pattern in relation to recommended allowances.

If we believe that the standards set forth in the RDA are desirable and worthwhile goals, they must be interpreted in terms of the foods or food groups around which a homemaker plans her family's meals. This food guide must be sufficiently simple to make it practical for use by the average homemaker and yet sufficiently detailed to make it consistent with scientific facts and to accomplish its purpose within the framework of accepted food patterns of the country. The members of the Food and Nutrition Board, which developed the first dietary standards, emphasized that it was possible to achieve the level of nutrition they advocated through a well-chosen diet of natural foods. They also pointed out that it was possible to achieve this optimal nutrition through an unlimited number of combinations of foods—the choice of which may be determined by the availability of foods in a local market, socioeconomic

status of the family, and the cultural background, physical condition, and food preferences of the individual.

A sound nutrition program involves ascertaining the nutritive value of available foods and their contribution to meeting nutritional needs, and educating and motivating the public to make a wise choice of foods.

FOOD SELECTION GUIDES
Basic seven food groups

To translate the recommended allowances into familiar diet patterns, the Bureau of Home Economics of the United States Department of Agriculture recommended that certain classes of foods be included in the diet in specified amounts so that a person with no scientific knowledge of nutrition could select an adequate diet. Their recommendations became known as the *Basic Seven*, developed as part of the National Wartime Nutrition Program of the Research Administration of the Department of Agriculture in 1943. This familiar guide, presented in Table 14-1, was the basis of practically all nutrition education programs from 1943 until its revision in 1956. Other plans, differing only in minor details, had been promoted by special trade groups, but the basic seven remained the standard. It served a major purpose in providing a guide that would lead to the consumption of a diet adequate in most nutritional factors. This was accomplished through the use of the so-called protective foods—foods that provided a larger proportion of the needs for two or more nutrients than for energy. However, the complexity of a seven-group

283

plan coupled with the lack of specificity about what constituted a serving limited its effectiveness in many nutrition education situations.

Although the United States was promoting the seven-group plan, many other countries were developing plans that were designed to accomplish the same educational objective and that involved three, four, or five groups, based on their particular food patterns.

Basic four food groups

In 1956 the United States Department of Agriculture recommended that the complex seven-group plan be replaced by a simpler, less detailed four-group plan, which they termed *Essentials of an Adequate Diet*. This plan, shown in Table 14-1, differed from the basic seven only in that the three fruit and vegetable categories were grouped as one and the fat group was eliminated entirely. The elimination of the fat group was justified on the grounds that the consumption of foods from the other groups usually led to the use of fat to im-

prove the flavor and palatability of the food. In addition, the change was made at a time when there was concern about the increase in fat consumption by the American public and its possible role in the development of atherosclerosis. The Department of Agriculture did not want to find itself encouraging the consumption of a food that might later be proved to be the villain in a degenerative disease.

Food plans

As an aid to persons with a limited amount of money to spend on food, the Department of Agriculture publishes food plans that indicate the amounts of eleven types of foods to purchase per week for each member of the family. The three plans are based on different income levels—low, moderate, and liberal cost. When followed, they ensure a satisfactory level of nutrition for the whole family, assuming reasonably good practices in food preparation. The distribution of food to various family members is, however, the responsibility of the homemaker.

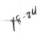

Table 14-1. Comparison of food guides—Basic Seven (1943) and Essentials of an Adequate Diet (1958)

Food group	Basic Seven	Essentials of an Adequate Diet
Milk and milk products	Children, 3-4 cups Adults, 2 cups	Children, 3-4 cups Adults, 2 or more cups
Fruits and vegetables		4 servings
Green and yellow vegetables	1 serving	
Citrus fruits or raw cabbage	1 serving	
Potatoes, other vegetables, and fruits	2 servings	
Meat, poultry, fish, and eggs	1 serving 1 egg (at least 4 per week)	2 or more servings
Bread, flour, cereal (enriched or whole-grain)	3 servings	4 or more servings
Butter or fortified margarine	Equivalent of 2 tablespoons	

NUTRITIVE CONTRIBUTION OF FOOD GROUPS

Each of the four food groups in the Essentials of an Adequate Diet is chosen because of a unique contribution it makes to the nutritive value of the diet. The contribution of each of the groups is shown graphically in Figs. 14-1, 14-3, 14-5, and 14-7. The values shown in the graphs represent a typical selection of foods within each category. It must be recognized that by differing the choices within the framework of the guide, wide variations may result in the nutritive quality of the diet. For instance, the choice of foods represented in the graphs represents approximately 1400 kcal. It is possible to stay within the framework of the plan and to choose foods ranging in caloric value from 800 to 1800. Likewise, the choice of vegetables may result in a diet providing less than 1000 or more than 10,000 I.U. of vitamin A.

Milk and milk products

The recommendation that the equivalent of 2 cups of milk be used by an adult can be met in many ways, as may be seen by the list of equivalents in Table 14-2. The use of nonfat milk, with less than 0.5% fat, in place of whole milk, with at least 3.2% fat, possibly will reduce the energy value by half and eliminate the vitamin A alto-

gether. Neither of these is necessarily undesirable. Most persons have no difficulty in obtaining sufficient calories, and the vitamin A in one serving of a vegetable such as carrots will make up for the loss of vitamin A in 20 cups of nonfat milk. In addition, an increasing proportion of the nonfat milk and nonfat dried milk solids reaching the market is being fortified with both vitamins A and D. Thus, if it is desirable to restrict calories, the use of nonfat milk is equally as desirable as whole milk. Chocolate milk has a higher caloric value but otherwise has the same nutritive value as whole milk.

Cottage cheese may be a poor substitute for whole milk, since calcium will be reduced if the cheese has been prepared by acid coagulation rather than rennin coagulation. It is a good source of protein in either case.

As shown in Fig. 14-1, the major contributions of the milk group are high-quality protein, present primarily as casein and lactalbumin, containing all eight essential amino acids; calcium, which is difficult to obtain in sufficient amounts from other sources alone; and riboflavin. The contribution of various dairy products to the intake of calcium is shown in Fig. 14-2. The riboflavin available from milk depends on the conditions under which it is stored. Since exposure to sunlight may reduce the ribo-

Table 14-2. Amount of milk substitutes needed to provide the amounts of calcium and protein in 1 cup of whole milk

	Amount required to provide 280 mg. calcium		Amount required to provide 9 gm. protein	
	gm.	Measure	gm.	Measure
Nonfat milk	231	1 cup	250	1 cup
Cheddar cheese	36	1⅓ ounces	36	1⅓ ounces
Cottage cheese	298	1⅓ cups	66	⅓ cup
Ice cream (10% fat)	220	1½ cups	220	1½ cups
Cream cheese	451	30 tablespoons	113	9 tablespoons

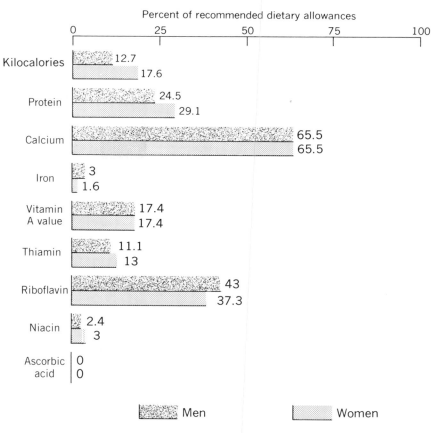

Fig. 14-1. Nutritive contribution of 2 cups of milk to diet of an adult.

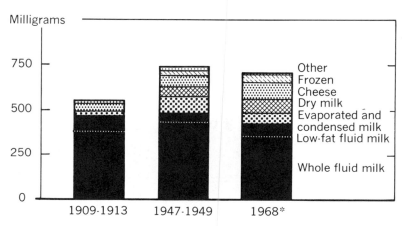

Fig. 14-2. Contribution of various forms of dairy products to total calcium intake. Calcium from dairy products (excludes butter) from 1909 to 1968, per capita per day.°Preliminary. (From Agricultural Research Service, U. S. Department of Agriculture, 1969.)

flavin content by as much as 50%, many dairies have taken some responsibility in helping to reduce this loss by selling milk in brown glass bottles or paper cartons or providing insulated boxes to cut down light exposure. Many times this has been done in the face of consumer opposition.

The limiting nutritional factors in milk are iron and ascorbic acid. Both of these are present in small amounts in a form that is available, but it has been well established that a milk diet alone is incapable of providing adequate iron to regenerate hemoglobin in infants after 6 months of age. The small amount of ascorbic acid normally found in milk is reduced still further by the process of pasteurization so that it is an undependable source of the vitamin.

Ice cream is a good substitute for milk as a source of calcium on the basis of weight but contains only half as much calcium on the basis of calories. Cheese is a popular substitute for milk. It has the same nutritive value as the milk from which it is made. As in the case of milk, the protein, calcium, and riboflavin content decreases, and the energy content increases proportionately as the fat content increases.

Milk is available to the consumer in many forms at widely varying prices determined primarily by the perishability of the product rather than by nutritive considerations. The relative costs of various forms of milk of essentially equal nutritive value are presented in Table 14-3. By choosing the least expensive form that meets a particular need, it is possible to reduce the cost of milk in the diet by an appreciable sum. In any case, milk is a relatively inexpensive source of protein.

Fruits and vegetables

The United States Department of Agriculture in *Essentials of an Adequate Diet* recommends that the diet contain four servings of fruits and vegetables, but to keep the plan simple includes no suggestion regarding the choice to be made within this group. Since foods in this group are so diverse in nutritional value, persons who use this guide as a basis for a nutrition education program urge people to consume one serving of a citrus fruit or another fruit or vegetable high in ascorbic acid every day and a serving of dark green, yellow, or orange vegetable as a source of vitamin A every other day. In this way the major contribution of this group in providing vitamins C and A will be satisfied, as shown in Fig. 14-3. Fig. 14-4 shows the pattern of consumption of vegetables and fruits in the United States.

A 4-ounce serving of fruit juice is considered an average serving. Citrus juices are generally rich sources, but other fruit juices vary considerably in their ascorbic acid content, as shown in Table 14-4. In using the guide, emphasis should be placed on those juices that provide at least 30 mg. of vitamin C in a 4-ounce portion, especially if the diet contains no other rich source. Many juices naturally low in vitamin C are now enriched at this level. An analysis of samples of fruit juices enriched with ascorbic acid shows a wide variation in the amount present, regardless of the declaration on the label.

In other fruits and vegetables the amount

Table 14-3. Relative costs of other forms of milk compared to fresh whole milk

Form	Relative cost*
Fresh whole milk	$1.00
Fresh homogenized whole milk	$1.04
Fresh homogenized chocolate milk	$1.08
Fresh nonfat milk	$ .76
Evaporated whole milk	$ .56
Evaporated nonfat milk	$ .52
Dried whole milk	$1.12
Dried nonfat milk	$ .20-.40
Yogurt	$4.00

*Based on prices in northeastern United States, spring, 1970.

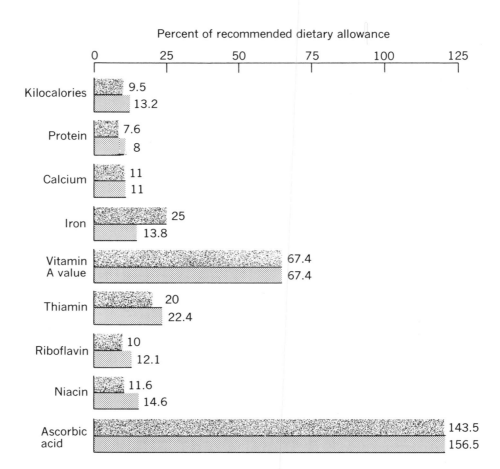

Percent of recommended dietary allowance

Kilocalories — 9.5 / 13.2

Protein — 7.6 / 8

Calcium — 11 / 11

Iron — 25 / 13.8

Vitamin A value — 67.4 / 67.4

Thiamin — 20 / 22.4

Riboflavin — 10 / 12.1

Niacin — 11.6 / 14.6

Ascorbic acid — 143.5 / 156.5

Men   Women

Fig. 14-3. Nutritive contribution of four servings of fruit or vegetables to diet of an adult.

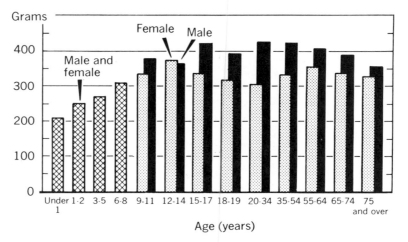

Fig. 14-4. Consumption of fruits and vegetables (quantity per person per day) related to age in the United States—spring 1965; 28 gm. = 1 ounce. (From Agricultural Research Service, U. S. Department of Agriculture, 1969.)

Table 14-4. Comparison of ascorbic acid content of different fruit juices[*]	
Juice	*mg. of ascorbic acid per 100 gm.*
Orange, fresh	50
Orange, frozen	45
Grapefruit	38
Tomato	16
Pineapple	9
Apple	1
Prune	1
Grape	Trace
Commercially enriched juices	25

*Based on Watt, B. K., and Merrill, A. L.: Composition of foods—raw, processed and prepared, U. S. Department of Agriculture Handbook No. 8, Washington, D. C., 1963.

Table 14-5. Vitamin A content of representative vegetables[*]	
Vegetable	*Vitamin A per 100 gm. (I.U.)*
Carrots, cooked	10,500
Kale	8,900
Spinach, cooked	8,100
Sweet potatoes, cooked	8,100
Mustard greens	7,000
Winter squash, baked	4,200
Endive	3,300
Asparagus, cooked	900
Green beans, cooked	540
Peas, cooked	540
Yellow corn, cooked	400
Lima beans, cooked	280
Leaf lettuce	264
Celery, raw	240
Head lettuce	175

*Based on Watt, B. K., and Merrill, A. L.: Composition of foods—raw, processed and prepared, U. S. Department of Agriculture Handbook No. 8, Washington, D. C., 1963.

of vitamin C present varies with the variety, the degree of maturity, the season, climatic conditions, and the length and conditions of storage. In apples, for instance, ascorbic acid values range from 5 to 19 mg. per 100 gm., depending on the variety, and these values fall to almost half after several months of storage. The loss of nutrients that occurs in fruits and vegetables begins right after harvest and may be rapid in the first few hours. In addition to biochemical losses, further loss is attributable to the removal of parts of the plant during preparation to make the product more palatable. The wilted outer leaves of lettuce, the leaves of broccoli, the skin on potatoes, and the bitter dark green leaves of endive, all of which are parts often discarded in preparation, have higher concentrations of some nutrients than do the parts consumed. The fact that ascorbic acid is a relatively unstable nutrient, being readily destroyed by heat, oxidation, and alkali, suggests the use of methods of preparation and harvesting that minimize the loss of nutrients. These include limiting exposure to air, especially at high temperatures; cooking in a minimum amount of water for the shortest period of

time; keeping the period of storage to a minimum; and serving immediately after cooking.

Other seasonal fruits rich in ascorbic acid are strawberries, cantaloupe, and cherries; among vegetables, broccoli, asparagus, spinach, and cabbage are important sources, especially when they are prepared in a way that minimizes losses.

Since relatively few of the dark green or yellow fruits and vegetables that are rich sources of carotene are popular items in the diet, a realistic approach to a food guide suggests the use of these every other day. This was additionally justified because of the stability of vitamin A and the fact that those foods that are rich sources usually provide more than the day's allowance in one serving, which means that the excess will be stored for future use. Thus a daily intake of foods high in vitamin A value is not absolutely necessary, although it may be desirable. The vitamin A value of some typical dark green and yellow vegetables is given in Table 14-5, where the relationship between degree of pigmentation and vitamin A values become apparent.

Aside from the unique contributions of carotene and ascorbic acid, the fruit and vegetable group contributes about 25% of the day's intake of iron. The amount varies with the foods and parts chosen, iron content being higher in leaves than in stems, fruit, or underground portions. Calcium intake from this group is small compared to that from the milk group but will assume more importance if milk intake is low. If peas or beans are chosen, a rich source of thiamin is provided, and if dark green leafy vegetables such as spinach are used, riboflavin will be high.

Generally speaking, fruits and vegetables are poor sources of protein and that present is of low biological value because of a lack of some essential amino acids. Roots and tubers contain 2% protein and 20% carbohydrate, whereas legumes such as peas and beans have 4% protein and 13% carbohydrate. Of the latter group, soybeans have a high biological value, and although they have been promoted extensively in underdeveloped countries as a source of protein, the production of soybean oil is the major use of the product in the United States. The energy contribution of the fruit and vegetable group is generally low because of the high proportion of cellulose and water and low fat content. Immature seeds such as peas and beans and starchy tubers such as potatoes contribute two to eight times as many calories per serving as do celery, carrots, spinach, and cabbage, which are high in cellulose and water but low in starch. One must remember, however, that the caloric contribution of a fruit or vegetable may double or triple, depending on the way it is served or the type of product in which it is incorporated, as shown in Table 5-4.

Data from an Agricultural Research Service study shows that fruits and vegetables contribute a higher percentage of the intake

Table 14-6. Percentages of various nutrients provided by fruits and vegetables*

Nutrient	Percentage
Energy	8.6
Protein	7.1
Calcium	8.7
Iron	19.7
Vitamin A value	52.4
Thiamin	20.2
Riboflavin	9.0
Niacin	18.1
Ascorbic acid	92.4

*From Stiebeling, H. K.: Foods of the vegetable-fruit group—their contributions to nutritionally adequate diets, Borden Rev. Nutr. Res. **25:**51, 1964.

of the seven nutrients than they do of calories (Table 14-6). Thus they can truly be called protective foods.

Another important nutritional benefit from the use of fruits and vegetables is attributed to the bulk provided by cellulose. This promotes normal gastrointestinal motility and greatly facilitates the passage of food through the digestive tract, helping to prevent constipation.

One should not overlook the value of many fruits in stimulating the appetite. They also serve as sources of an organic acid in the stomach and facilitate calcium and iron absorption in persons with a reduced secretion of hydrochloric acid. If fruits, sometimes described as "detergent food," are eaten at the end of a meal, they help remove carbohydrate that may have adhered to the tooth surface, thus having a beneficial effect on dental health.

Meat, fish, and poultry

The inclusion of meat and meat substitutes as a separate group is justified on the basis of the amount of high-quality protein it provides. As shown in Fig. 14-5, the meat group contributes about 45% of the protein in the diet as well as 35% of the iron and

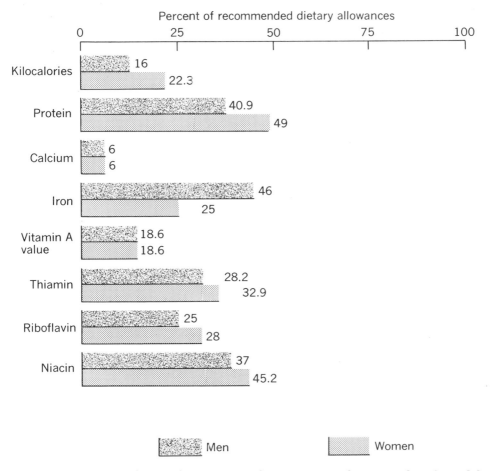

Percent of recommended dietary allowances

Fig. 14-5. Nutritive contribution of two servings of meat or meat substitute to diet of an adult.

40% of the niacin. One average 3- to 4-ounce serving should contribute about 20 gm. of protein, but the amount will vary slightly with the type of meat. Table 14-7 expresses the approximate composition of different meats, and Table 14-8 shows the amount needed to provide 20 gm. of protein. Meat substitutes, such as eggs, cheese, peas, beans, or peanut butter, may contain somewhat less per average serving. However, since they are usually consumed in combination with cereal protein, as in cheese or peanut butter sandwiches, cereal and milk, or eggs on toast, the combined protein values will approach that of a meat and will usually cost less. The quantity of

meat, fish, and poultry consumed in the United States in 1965 is shown in Fig. 14-6.

The lipid content of meat is variable, ranging from 1% to 40%; it depends on the type of animal, its condition at the time of slaughter, the cut, the extent to which the meat is trimmed, and the method of preparation. The higher the grade of meat, the more fat marbled throughout the muscle fiber and the higher the caloric value. Prime grade beef may have 25% lipid compared to 16% in standard grade and even less in utility grade. Fish and shellfish contain high-quality protein that is easily digested, and at the same time they are relatively low in lipid content.

Table 14-7. Approximate composition of meat and meat substitutes

Food	Moisture (%)	Protein (%)	Fat (%)	kcal./100 gm.
Beef	60.3	18.5	21.0	263
Pork (medium fat)	48.5	12.7	38.5	401
Veal	68.0	19.1	12.0	190
Lamb	56.0	13.4	27.1	310
Chicken	63.8	31.6	3.4	166
Egg (whole)	73.7	12.9	11.5	163
Salmon	63.4	27.0	7.4	182
Cod	64.6	28.5	5.3	170
Lobster	76.8	18.5	1.5	95
Scallops	73.1	23.2	1.4	112
Sardines	70.7	19.2	8.6	160

Table 14-8. Amount of meat or meat substitutes needed to provide 20 gm. of protein

Food	gm.
Chicken	67
Cod	70
Veal	74
Beef liver	77
Peanut butter	80
Lamb	90
Dried peas	90
Pork	90
Salmon (pink)	100
Luncheon meat	105
Frankfurters	160
Eggs	160

Dried peas and beans, with a protein content ranging as high as 35%, and nuts, with 15% protein, are frequent substitutes in the meat group, but as seen from Fig. 4-8 have less protein per 100 kcal. Two to three eggs, with 6 gm. of protein each, are also a good substitute for meat.

The amount of iron depends on the meat chosen, being low in chicken and fish but high in glandular organs. Pork liver is the richest source of iron and also one of the least expensive. Muscle meats high in both hemoglobin and myoglobin plus liberal amounts of iron-containing enzymes are good iron sources.

Since phosphorus is a component of most proteins, meat is one of the best sources of phosphorus in the diet.

The vitamin content of the general classes of meat is shown in Table 14-9. If pork is chosen, the meat group becomes the major source of thiamin.

Because of its high protein and hence tryptophan content, the meat group becomes a major contributor of niacin in the diet, two servings providing about 50% of the recommended allowance; veal and poultry are the richest sources.

The vitamin A, calcium, and ascorbic acid contents of meat are low. Liver is a rich source of vitamin A and a good source of ascorbic acid, but since it is not a consistent item in the diet, meat makes a limited contribution of these nutrients in the diet.

Meat is often the most expensive single item on the menu, accounting for 36 cents of every food dollar, thus we have come to plan our meal around the meat or protein dish. The cost of a serving of meat may range from a low of 8 cents for pork liver to a high of 60 cents for filet mignon for a 3- to 4-ounce serving.

Table 14-9. Content of B complex vitamins in 100 gm. of meat and eggs°

Food	Thiamin (mg.)	Riboflavin (mg.)	Nicotinic acid (mg.)	Vitamin B_6 (mg.)	Pantothenic acid (mg.)	Folic acid (μg.)	Vitamin B_{12} (μg.)
Beef	0.08	0.15	4.5	0.35	0.7	14	2.5
Veal	0.17	0.35	7.0	0.35	0.7	20	1.2
Pork	0.80	0.18	4.1	0.45	0.7	7	1.0
Lamb	0.15	0.20	4.6	0.35	0.7	7	2.8
Poultry	0.08	0.16	7.0	0.50	0.8	3	3.2
Eggs	0.10	0.35	0.1	0.25	1.3	8	0.7

*From Siedler, A. J.: Nutritional contributions of the meat group to an adequate diet, Borden Rev. Nutr. Res. **24:**29, 1963.

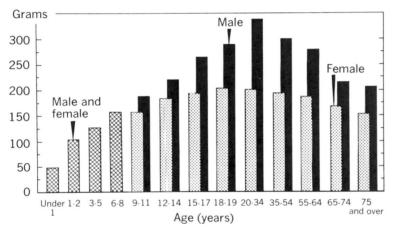

Fig. 14-6. Consumption of meat, fish, and poultry (quantity per person per day) as related to age in the United States—spring, 1965; 28 gm. = 1 ounce. (From Agricultural Research Service, U. S. Department of Agriculture, 1969.)

Cereal and cereal products

Four servings of enriched or whole-grain cereal products are recommended primarily for their contribution to the day's intake of thiamin, riboflavin, niacin, and iron (Fig. 14-7). The contribution of this group to the protein intake may be significant. Although most cereal products, with 7% to 14% protein, contain incomplete or low-quality protein, they are so frequently served in conjunction with a complete protein that will provide the essential amino acid lacking that the quality of the cereal protein is improved. Examples are macaroni and cheese, rice with chicken, poached egg on toast, or cereal and milk. In addition, two vegetables, cereals, or legumes served at the same time can supplement each other. The current practice of using dried milk solids in commercially prepared bakery products enhances their protein quality. The enrichment of both wheat and rice with lysine is being used as a means of improving the quality of these two relatively inexpensive

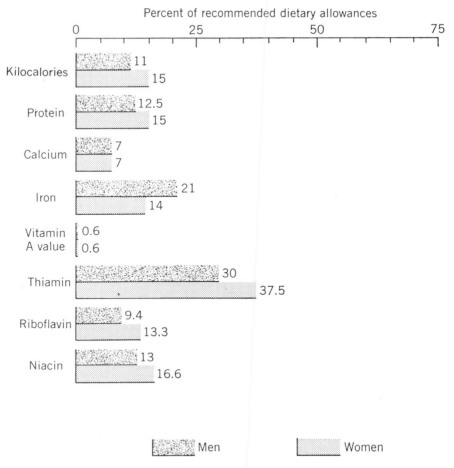

Percent of recommended dietary allowances

Kilocalories 11 / 15

Protein 12.5 / 15

Calcium 7 / 7

Iron 21 / 14

Vitamin A value 0.6 / 0.6

Thiamin 30 / 37.5

Riboflavin 9.4 / 13.3

Niacin 13 / 16.6

Men   Women

Fig. 14-7. Nutritive contribution of four servings of whole-grain or enriched cereal to diet of an adult.

cereal proteins. The addition of methionine and tryptophan may further enhance the quality of some cereal proteins. This technique has the greatest potential for developing countries in which staple cereals may provide as much as 80% of the calories and for people on limited incomes who consume a relatively high proportion of cereals and relatively less animal protein.

The concept that only such products as bread, rice, macaroni, and dry or cooked cereal would satisfy the recommendation for four servings of cereal has been modified so that any product made primarily of flour will be considered in the group. Although only 30 states have compulsory enrichment of bread and flour, over 90% of the flour now sold in the United States is enriched, and it is believed that most products made from flour contain appreciable amounts of the B vitamins and iron. Thus waffles, muffins, pancakes, pastry, cakes, and cookies can all be considered part of the cereal group. Commercially prepared mixes are unfortunately not made with enriched flour, although the food industry is now considering more universal use of enriched flour. The use of milk or nonfat milk solids in many of these products increases the calcium to significant levels and supplements the cereal protein. The value of iron in enriched cereals depends on the form in which it is

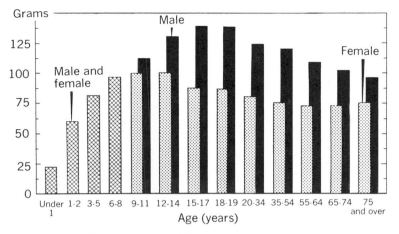

Fig. 14-8. Consumption of grain products (flour equivalent, quantity per person per day) as related to age in the United States—spring 1965; 28 gm. = 1 ounce. (From Agricultural Research Service, U. S. Department of Agriculture, 1969.)

added, the specific cereal, and the method by which it is prepared. One of the major justifications for the inclusion of cereal products is the contribution of relatively significant amounts of many nutrients at minimum cost.

One ounce of cereal, dry weight, is considered as one serving. Thus 1 ounce of a prepared cereal such as bran flakes or 1 ounce of oatmeal cooked constitute an average serving. The volume of 1 ounce of puffed cereal is usually so large that only ½ ounce will be used as a serving. Fig. 14-8 shows the pattern of consumption of grain products in the United States.

There has been a trend in the highly competitive breakfast cereal business to promote a cereal product enriched with any number of nutrients in addition to thiamin, riboflavin, niacin, and iron (which must be added to enriched cereals) and vitamin D and calcium (which are optional nutrients). Little justification can be found for adding ascorbic acid or vitamins A and D to cereal products. None of these are nutrients normally present in whole-grain cereal, nor are they generally lacking in the Western diet; therefore their addition seems only to raise the cereal to the status of a glorified vitamin

pill, which apparently gives it some trade advantage. The charge that some breakfast cereals are devoid of nutritional value is not justified. Nor is it of major concern, except on the basis of cost, that the manufacturer rather than the consumer adds sugar.

Converted rice is prepared by parboiling the rice kernels prior to polishing. During this process the nutrients normally concentrated in the outer husk are driven into the kernel, where they remain when the husk is removed. Thus we have a refined cereal that has been enriched with its own nutrients. This process has been used in India for many years.

FOUNDATION OF AN ADEQUATE DIET

As can be seen from Fig. 14-9, the inclusion of 2 cups of milk or its equivalent, two servings of meat or meat substitutes, four servings of fruit and vegetables, and four servings of enriched or whole-grain cereals will assure an intake of over 75% of the NRC recommended daily allowances of all nutrients except calories for the adult man and iron for the adult woman. With this foundation little need for guidance exists in the selection of additional foods to provide the calories needed to meet indi-

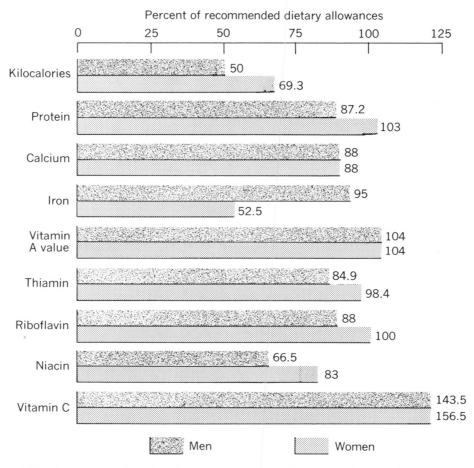

Percent of recommended dietary allowances

Fig. 14-9. Contribution of all four food groups of essentials of an adequate diet to nutritive intake of an adult.

vidual requirements. In many cases it will be met at least partially through additional servings of the four food groups. The use of the visible fats and oils, which are natural accompaniments to the cereals and vegetables and which constitute about one third of the total fat intake, will provide about 15% of the total calories. The use of carbohydrate-rich foods, which is advocated by some trade groups as the least expensive way of obtaining the additional calories, does not receive the wholehearted endorsement of nutritionists because of the adverse effect that sugar, especially in the form of icings or sticky candies, has on dental health.

For women, need exists to stress the use of foods high in iron as sources of the additional calories, since women are most likely to have an intake inadequate in iron. In fact, it is virtually impossible to obtain the recommended 18 mg. of iron on a diet of less than 3000 kcal., which is considerably more energy than is required by this group.

The number of calories provided by the four basic food groups will depend on the selection of foods made within each category. To illustrate the range possible within the specifications of the four-group plan, the caloric value of two extremes is calculated in Table 14-10. Admittedly dif-

Table 14-10. Caloric value of two diet patterns meeting requirements of essentials of an adequate diet°

Food group	Diet I foods	kcal.	Diet II foods	kcal.
Milk	Nonfat milk (2 cups)	160	Whole milk (1½ cups)	290
			Ice cream (1 cup)	145
Meat	Chicken, broiled (3 ounces)	185	Chicken, fried (3 ounces)	245
	Salmon, canned (3 ounces)	120	Ham (3 ounces)	340
Fruit and	Tomato juice (½ cup)	25	Sweet potatoes, baked	155
vegetable	Carrots (½ cup)	22	Lima beans (½ cup)	75
	Apple (1 medium)	70	Grape juice (½ cup)	82
	Green beans (½ cup)	12	Figs (4)	120
Cereal	Puffed wheat (1 cup)	50	1 waffle	240
	Bread, thin-sliced (3 slices)	135	2 cookies (3-inch diameter)	220
			Oatmeal (1 ounce)	115
			Muffin	135
Total		879		2162

*Calculations are based only on energy value of the food prepared and served without any flavor adjunct, such as butter, sugar, syrup, sauces, etc. Based on Nutritive value of foods, Home and Garden Bulletin No. 72, Washington, D. C., 1970, U. S. Department of Agriculture.

Table 14-11. Estimate of nutrients available per person per day on the retail markets in the United States compared to NRC recommended allowances for the adult male°

Nutrients	Amount available	Recommended allowances
Energy (kcal.)	3170	2800
Protein (gm.)	97	65
Fat (gm.)	147	
Carbohydrate (gm.)	371	
Calcium (gm.)	0.96	0.8
Phosphorus (gm.)	1.51	0.8
Iron (mg.)	16.6	10
Vitamin A (I.U.)	7700	5000
Thiamin (mg.)	1.83	1.20
Riboflavin (mg.)	2.26	1.70
Niacin (mg.)	21.5	17
Ascorbic acid (mg.)	99	60

*From Nutritive value of food available for consumption, United States, 1909-1964, Agricultural Research Service, Publication No. 62-14, 1966, U. S. Department of Agriculture.

ferences will exist in the level of other nutrients also, but the selection was made within the framework of the plan.

As the Food and Nutrition Board of the National Research Council emphasized with the publication of its first dietary standards, the level of nutrition they advocated as a goal in planning the food supplies of the nations could be met in innumerable ways by an unlimited combination of foods. The suggestions made in the basic four groups represent but one pattern that reflects dietary practices acceptable to a large number of people living in the United States. Although adherence to such a plan will usually ensure at least a minimal level of nutritional adequacy, failure to follow such a plan must never be construed as evidence of dietary inadequacy. It should, however, prompt a more careful evaluation of the nutritive content of the diet. Such a guide does provide a quick and easy basis for evaluating the adequacy of a prescribed or popular diet. If the minimum recommendations are met, one can be reasonably confident that the diet has a sound nutritional basis.

That the food supply available to the American public has the potential for meeting the nutritional needs of all citizens is evident in Table 14-11, in which estimates of the amount of each nutrient available per person at the retail level are tabulated.

DIETARY STANDARDS

Although the concept that food contained more than the energy-yielding nutrients was well established by 1920 and a knowledge of the role and need for many other nutrients had been ascertained by 1935, not until 1940 was any formal effort made in the United States to evaluate existing knowledge and to establish dietary standards. Previous efforts on the part of individuals and groups had attracted little attention. The economic depression of the 1930's focused attention on some nutritional deficiencies, and effort was made to incorporate the then-current knowledge of nutrition in programs of food subsidization. Only in the face of threat of war in 1940, however, did any strong feeling develop that nutritional science could make a contribution to the national security. The country had been appalled at the very high rejection rate among young service recruits for reasons that could be attributed to suboptimal nutrition. Against this background

twenty-five scientists met in 1940 as the first Food and Nutrition Board of the National Research Council, charged with the responsibility of establishing dietary standards that could be used to evaluate the dietary intake of large population groups and to provide a rational guide for practical nutrition and for the planning of agricultural production schedules. It was recognized that insufficient evidence of the nutritional needs of humans had been compiled to propose exact requirements but that a need did exist for a standard that reflected more than minimum needs. It was believed that even if the standards based on the available information should later prove to be inaccurate, they were very necessary. Indeed, it was with the belief and hope that they would soon be revised that the first standards were proposed.

National Research Council recommended allowances

The task of determining dietary standards was not an easy one. In the case of some nutrients very little information was available, for others little agreement was found among the fifty or more scientists consulted, and for still others it was recognized that such a wide range of requirements for the individual made it difficult to arrive at an acceptable figure. The data on which judgments were made were obtained from surveys of large groups of individuals to determine presence or absence of disease in relation to nutritive intake, from controlled feeding experiments with limited numbers of individuals, and from critical metabolic studies on several species of animals. The group did, however, agree in 1941 on the first National Research Council recommended dietary allowances (RDA), which were published in 1943. These allowances were numerical expressions of the quantities of certain nutrients believed to be needed by individuals classified into several age and sex categories for essentially all healthy persons in the

United States under the existing conditions. They did not represent average requirements, which would be adequate for only half the population, but figures that would include the whole range of requirements and would maintain good nutrition in practically all healthy persons in the United States. As such, they became goals to be used in planning national food supplies and meals for large groups. The term *allowance* was purposely chosen to avoid any implication of finality and to encourage a reevaluation of the figures as more information on which to base judgments became available. To allow for nutrient losses that might occur in cooking and storage of food, to cover the wide range of requirements in the population, and to provide a buffer under stress conditions a margin of safety of from 10% to 50% was added to the minimum requirements for each nutrient. The amount added varied from one nutrient to another, depending on the body's ability to store the nutrient, the range of observed requirements, the availability of the nutrient in the American diet, the possible hazards from an excessive intake, and the difficulties involved in establishing precise requirements.

It was emphasized that the allowances did not provide a criterion for judging the nutritional status of an individual but were a valuable guide for persons involved in feeding a population group. For individuals they served as a point of reference for judging nutritional adequacy, but only when an individual showed clinical, physical, or biochemical evidence of a dietary lack in addition to the suboptimal intake could he be considered deficient in the nutrient.

The original recommended dietary allowances have undergone six revisions, the latest being published in 1968. These are presented in Appendix C. The philosophy on which the allowances are based has remained essentially the same, but improved analytical techniques and increased knowl-edge of the biological importance of most nutrients has led to some change and to an increasing level of confidence in the recommended allowances, although complete agreement among nutritionists has not been reached. It is believed that the allowances provide sufficient buffer in cases of nutritional stress but will not meet the additional requirements of persons depleted by disease. The major goal of the allowances is to permit and to encourage the development of food practices by the population of the United States that will provide the greatest dividends in health and resistance to disease. The 1968 allowances differed from previous ones in that the age categories were expanded to include 18- to 22-year-olds as a separate category and that recommendations were made for an additional seven nutrients. Since revisions appear approximately every five years as research provides more information on which to base recommendations, the reader should be alerted to look for the next revision in about 1973.

Although the RDA have never been assumed to represent either a minimal or optimal level of intake, they have served several useful purposes. They have provided a yardstick for groups such as the Quartermaster Corps in planning diets. They have been widely accepted as a basis for evaluating diets; as an official guide for practically all nutrition projects, such as the school lunch program and cereal enrichment; and as a basis for formulating regulations governing the composition of foods, dietary supplements, and drugs. They are admittedly high for use under conditions of economic stringency or national emergencies but under normal conditions are a worthwhile goal.

In addition to the seventeen nutrients for which discrete recommendations are made, many other nutrients are discussed in the light of our current knowledge of their requirements and major biological roles. Among those discussed are carbohydrate, fat, alcohol, water, several micronutrient elements, choline, pantothenic acid, biotin, and vitamin K. It is hoped that the lack of information on requirements for these nutrients will stimulate research.

Other dietary standards

Many other countries have established dietary standards for their populations. However, comparison or evaluation of these is not valid until one recognizes the philosophy behind them. Care must be taken to distinguish among terms such as standards, requirements, and allowances, which must be defined before an interpretation of proposed nutrient intake can be made.

The British Medical Association, in establishing the British dietary standards, chose levels they believed represented the needs of the average healthy individual; these levels were never intended, as were the American standards, to cover the needs of all persons. British standards tend to be lower for some nutrients than American standards, although in a few instances they are the same in spite of the differences in philosophy behind them. The Canadian standard of 1964 is based on a sufficient excess above minimum requirements for the maintenance of health among the majority of Canadians. Previously they had considered their standards a nutritional floor below which adequate nutrition cannot be assumed but one well above the level required to prevent clinical deficiency symptoms.

The Food and Agricultural Organization (FAO), charged with devising a standard to meet the needs of fully active, healthy individuals that is equally applicable in all cultures under vastly different agricultural and climatic conditions, has thus far proposed practical allowances for kilocalories, calcium, protein, thiamin, riboflavin, niacin, vitamin A, and iron. A comparison of the

Table 14-12. Comparison of United States, British,° Canadian, and FAO dietary standards for the adult male and adult female

Classification	kcal.	Protein (gm.)	Calcium (gm.)	Iron (mg.)	Vitamin A (I.U.)	Thiamin (mg.)	Riboflavin (mg.)	Ascorbic acid (mg.)
United States								
Female (128 pounds, 64 inches)	2000	55	0.8	18	5000	1.0	1.5	55
Male (154 pounds, 69 inches)	2800	65	0.8	10	5000	1.3	1.7	60
Britain†								
Female	2200	55	0.5	12	750†	1.0	1.3	30
Male	2750	80	0.8	12	750†	1.0	1.7	30
Canada								
Female (124 pounds)	2400	39	0.5	10	3700	0.70	1.2	30
Male (158 pounds)	2850	50	0.5	6	3700	0.90	1.4	30
FAO								
Female	2300	39	0.4-0.5	18	750†	0.90	1.3	—
Male	3200	46	0.4-0.5	10	750†	1.30	1.8	—

*Department of Health and Social Security: Recommended intakes of nutrients for the United Kingdom, Reports on Public Health and Medical Subjects, No. 120, London, 1969, Her Majesty's Stationery Office.

†μg. retinol equivalents (1 μg. retinol equivalent = 1 μg. retinol = 3.3 I.U.)

American, Canadian, British, and FAO standards is given in Table 14-12.

Minimum daily requirements

A second set of dietary standards is used in the United States by the Food and Drug Administration for labelling purposes. These are known as minimum daily requirements (MDR) and provide a standard legally acceptable for use by food processors in making claims for the nutritive content of their product in advertising. They do not bear a consistent relationship to RDA but are invariably lower. This is frequently a source of confusion to consumers who do not recognize the difference in the two standards. Thus one finds the distributor of a fruit juice containing 30 mg. of ascorbic acid per 4-ounce serving advertising that one serving will provide 100% of the adult MDR. This is not, however, 100% but only 50% of the RDA of 60 mg. for an adult. The Food and Drug Administration has been hearing testimony since 1966 relative to a proposal to abolish the MDR. A comparison of minimum daily requirements (MDR) and recommended dietary allowances (RDA) is given in Table 14-13.

TABLES OF FOOD COMPOSITION

Although the use of food composition tables as applied to food intake records provide our least expensive and most widely used tool in estimating the nutrient intake of an individual or group, only with an understanding of the method by which the tables were developed can one recognize their limitations and make an intelligent interpretation of the results. The food composition tables in Appendix F are based on values in the standard publication for food composition in the United States, U. S. Department of Agriculture Handbook No. 8, *Composition of Foods— Raw, Processed and Prepared.* Originally published in 1950 and revised in 1963, this publication presents food values in terms of 100 gm. edible portion (E.P.) and 1 pound as purchased (A.P.) of the foods. Information is given about the energy value and contribution of 16 different nutrients for 2483 food items in the 1963 edition, which represents an expansion from values on energy and eleven nutrients for 751 foods in 1950. In Appendix F, as in the U. S. Department of Agriculture Home and Garden Bulletin No. 72 (1970), food values are expressed in terms of average servings

Table 14-13. Comparison of minimum daily requirements (MDR) and recommended daily allowances (RDA) for several nutrients

Nutrient	MDR (adults)	RDA (adult man)	MDR (children 6-11 years)	RDA (boys 10-12 years)
Vitamin A (I.U.)	4000	5000	3000	4500
Thiamin (mg.)	1.0	1.4	0.75	1.3
Riboflavin (mg.)	1.2	1.7	0.9	1.3
Ascorbic acid (mg.)	30	60	20	40
Vitamin D (I.U.)	400	—	400	400
Calcium (gm.)	0.75	0.80	0.75	1.2
Iron (mg.)	10	10	10	10

or common household units. Differences in values for the same foods in these two editions may reflect changes in marketing and processing techniques as well as improved analytical techniques. For instance, breeding of poultry has produced a product with a reduced fat content, the use of dried milk solids in bread has led to an increase in its calcium content, and the use of cooking oils with higher percentages of unsaturated fatty acids has changed the character of fat in many food products.

Although the details of the biological and chemical techniques by which the values are derived are beyond the scope of this discussion, some mention of the methods by which the data were compiled should provide a rational basis on which to evaluate the values obtained in dietary calculations.

Great variation exists in the amount and specificity of data available for different foods and different nutrients. Much data that was potentially useful could not be used because of lack of an adequate description of the product, the source of the product, the method of processing, or the basis on which data were presented. Most of the data was obtained from published and unpublished analyses made by laboratories of government agencies, colleges, universities, and private industry. Only data on food samples adequately identified were usable. In some cases very few or only a single analytical report was available. In other cases data were available on several varieties of the same food at several seasons of the year and from various geographical areas. An example of the last is the ascorbic acid in oranges. The single value appearing in the table represents a weighted average obtained by making use of marketing information on the extent to which each variety was consumed, the percentage of the domestic production coming from each geographical area, and the size of the crop in each season. Thus, although the value may not be accurate for any one

specific orange, it does provide a value representative of all oranges consumed in the United States.

Similarly, values for other foods and nutrients take into account varietal, seasonal, and geographical differences in the nutrient content of foods and loss or gain of nutrients through harvesting, handling, commercial processing, packaging, storage, home practices of preparation, cooking and serving, and consumption statistics. The factors that result in changes in the content of important nutrients vary with both the food and the nutrient. The vitamin A value of sweet potatoes varies with the variety, the ascorbic acid in potatoes with the maturity and conditions of storage, vitamin A in butter with the season, ascorbic acid in oranges with the site of production and the time of harvesting, and vitamin A in plants with the part used.

In addition to Handbook No. 8, many other food composition tables in wide use today are based on sound analytical data. The beginning student is cautioned not to be concerned over differences between values from different tables, since they often merely represent slightly different interpretations of the same analytical data. Usually the differences are small when one considers the errors in the methods of collecting data. To be concerned over minor differences is to attribute an unwarranted degree of accuracy to the tables.

The nutrients for which values are presented in the table are those for which data were available for a sufficient number of foods to justify their inclusion. For nutrients such as pantothenic acid, folic acid, pyridoxine, amino acids, vitamin B_{12}, and magnesium tables have been published separately. As more precise analytical methods become available, tables for other nutrients will undoubtedly be published.

For those nutrients currently tabulated, a brief explanation of the derivation of the values follows.

Energy value expressed as kilocalories is

calculated by a modification of a method used by Atwater in 1899 when the first table of chemical composition of food was published. In this an energy equivalent is determined for each gram of carbohydrate, fat, and protein in a range of separate food groups such as eggs, milk, meat, fruits and vegetables, and cereals. These are based on the heat of combustion (as measured in the bomb calorimeter) for each of these energy-yielding nutrients and the coefficients of digestibility for each of these in each general class of food. From data on the carbohydrate, fat, and protein in a food, it is then possible to calculate its energy value.

The values of 4, 9, and 4 kcal. per gram of carbohydrate, fat, and protein respectively are widely used to represent their physiological fuel values. Their use is justified when applied to whole diets, but because these values vary from one food to another, they must be used with reservation for individual foods. For instance, the physiological fuel value of protein for which the widest variation is found is 4.35, 4.25, 3.70, 3.20, 3.15, and 2.90 kcal. from eggs, meat, cereals, legumes, fruits, and vegetables, respectively. The calculations shown in Table 14-14 illustrate variations in heat of combustion, coefficients of digestibility,

and hence physiological fuel values observed with different foods.

Protein is determined by measuring the nitrogen in a food; from knowledge of the percentage of nitrogen in a specific protein, it is possible to calculate the amount of protein. Many proteins, such as eggs, meat, corn, and beans, contain 16% nitrogen, but others, such as milk contain less, and nuts and many cereals slightly more. Assuming an average of 16% nitrogen in protein, a factor of 6.25 has been widely used to convert nitrogen values to protein values, especially in mixed diets, but if a more precise figure is needed, factors of 6.38 for milk, 5.7 for refined flour, 5.8 for whole-wheat flour, and 5.3 for nuts give more accurate estimates. The fact that all foods, especially vegetables, contain some non-protein nitrogen is a source of error in protein calculations.

Fat values are admittedly difficult to determine and have been obtained largely by simple solvent extraction methods. These methods may overestimate by including nonfat material and may underestimate by failing to separate the fat from a protein-fat or carbohydrate-fat complex in which it frequently occurs in food.

Carbohydrate values are obtained by subtracting the total percentage of water,

Table 14-14. Calculations of physiological fuel value of energy-yielding nutrients in two classes of foods

Food	Heat of combustion	Coefficient of digestibility	Physiological food value
Eggs			
Carbohydrate	3.75	98	3.68
Fat	9.50	95	9.02
Protein	4.50	97	4.36
Potatoes			
Carbohydrate	4.20	96	4.03
Fat	9.30	90	8.37
Protein	3.75	74	2.78

mineral, protein, and fat from 100. This is known as *carbohydrate by difference* and is used because no satisfactory method exists for determining carbohydrate by direct analysis. The values for carbohydrate include sugars, starches, fiber, and other complex forms of carbohydrate, some of which are not available to the human as a source of energy. The values reported for indigestible fiber, or cellulose, are based on methods that now appear to yield low values as new procedures suggest values three to four times as high.

The food composition tables record values for vitamin A in food and the potential vitamin A from the precursor carotenoids. In foods such as oranges and corn, in which cryptoxanthine, a biologically active precursor of vitamin A, is present in large amounts, the vitamin A values may be underestimated, since methods for determining carotenes do not include cryptoxanthine. On the other hand, some yellow- and red-pigmented foods have carotenoids that are not physiologically available but that will be measured. Even when it is accurately measured, the extent to which carotene is utilized varies from 33% to 100%. Some vitamin A values are obtained by biological assay and others by physiochemical means.

Thiamin values are determined by chemical or microbiological methods but make no allowances for the losses that may occur through solution or destruction by heat or alkali during home preparation and storage. Riboflavin is generally determined by fluorometric and microbiological methods, but no method has been developed to assess the increase in riboflavin that occurs with cooking, which may reflect the liberation of bound riboflavin not measured by current methods. Methods of determining niacin involve the conversion of the amide form that occurs in many foods to the acid form. Although it has been well established that tryptophan in excess of the body's needs for protein synthesis can be converted into

niacin (60 mg. tryptophan yielding 1 mg. niacin), the values in the tables report only niacin content and not niacin equivalent (niacin content plus niacin that could be formed from tryptophan). It is suggested that niacin equivalents will be about 50% higher than the niacin values recorded in the tables even after subtracting about 500 mg. of tryptophan to meet the needs for protein synthesis.

The National Research Council, on the other hand, has recognized that the body does not discriminate between niacin that is preformed in food and niacin obtained from tryptophan and has established its allowance in terms of niacin equivalents. It is possible then that the calculated niacin values for a diet may be considerably lower than the actual niacin available so that failure of a calculated diet to meet an established standard cannot be considered evidence of an inadequate intake of the nutrient.

One interesting aspect of the niacin content of foods is the presence of a biologically inactive form of the vitamin, trigonelline, in many seeds and nuts. The roasting process for coffee beans tends to convert it into an active form so that coffee beverage provides some niacin in the diet.

A similar situation exists in regard to the data for ascorbic acid in food composition tables. We know that the body uses both reduced ascorbic acid and dehydroascorbic acid. However, the limited data available on dehydroascorbic acid and total ascorbic acid values had led to the inclusion of only reduced ascorbic acid values in the current food composition tables for raw, canned, and dehydrated fruit and vegetables. For some foods this may lead to markedly low values, whereas for others the differences may be insignificant. It is highly possible that for such a labile nutrient any underestimate caused by failure to include the variable dehydroascorbic acid values will merely compensate for losses during storage and preparation or for the measurement of other reducing substances as ascorbic acid. It is also possible that some dehydroascorbic acid undergoes further oxidation to an inactive form. The data for frozen foods include the total for dehydroascorbic acid and reduced ascorbic acid and were obtained on foods under rather ideal conditions, permitting almost complete retention of the vitamin. These values may be high, since much storage of frozen foods is under less than ideal conditions and treatment of the food during thawing and serving may cause considerable loss.

In spite of their recognized limitations, the food composition tables allow estimates of the nutritive content of diets that approximate those determined by direct chemical analysis but at a much lower cost in time, equipment, and money. These tables represent an indispensable tool for people concerned with evaluating national food supplies, developing programs of food distribution, planning and evaluating food consumption surveys, and estimating the nutritive intake of individuals. The availability of the information from food composition tables on cards and magnetic tapes for use in computers has greatly facilitated the use of this information in menu planning and the analysis of dietary intake and has increased tremendously the scope of calculations that can be reasonably made with this information.

SELECTED REFERENCES

Food selection guides

Maynard, L. A.: An adequate diet, J.A.M.A. **170**:457, 1959.

Phipard, E. F., and Page, L.: Meeting nutritional needs through foods, Borden Rev. Nutr. Res. **23**:31, 1962.

Siedler, A. J.: Nutritional contributions of the meat group to an adequate diet, Borden Rev. Nutr. Res. **24**:29, 1963.

Stiebeling, H. K.: Foods of the vegetable-fruit group—their contributions to nutritionally adequate diets, Borden Rev. Nutr. Res. **25**:51, 1964.

Dietary standards

Dietary standards for Canada, Canad. Bull. Nutr. **6**:1, 1964, rev. 1968.

Food and Agricultural Organization: Calorie requirements, FAO Nutr. Stud., No. 15, 1957.

Food and Agricultural Organization: Protein requirements, FAO Nutr. Stud., No. 16, 1957.

Food and Agricultural Organization: Calcium requirements, FAO Nutrition Report Series No. 30, 1962.

Food and Agricultural Organization: Requirements of vitamin A, thiamine, riboflavin and niacin, FAO Nutrition Report Series, No. 41, 1967.

Food and Nutrition Board: Recommended dietary allowances, ed. 7, Publication No. 1694, Washington, D. C., 1968, National Academy of Sciences–National Research Council.

Food and Agricultural Organization: Requirements of ascorbic acid, vitamin D, vitamin B_{12}, folate and iron, WHO Techn. Rep. Ser., No. 452, 1970.

Hegsted, D. M.: Establishment of nutritional requirements in man, Borden Rev. Nutr. Res. **20**:13, 1959.

Roberts, L. J.: Beginnings of the recommended dietary allowances, J. Amer. Diet. Ass. **34**:903, 1958.

Tables of food composition

Fatty acid content of foods, Home Economics Research Report No. 7, Washington, D. C., 1959, U. S. Department of Agriculture.

Folic acid content of foods, U. S. Department of Agriculture Handbook No. 29, Washington, D. C., 1951, U. S. Department of Agriculture.

Food and Agricultural Organization: Amino acid content of foods, Nutr. Stud., No. 24, 1967.

Hardinge, M. G., and Crooks, H.: Lesser known vitamins in foods, J. Amer. Diet. Ass. **38**:240, 1961.

Harris, R. S.: Reliability of nutrient analyses and food tables, Amer. J. Clin. Nutr. **11**:377, 1962.

Leung, W. T. W.: Problems in compiling food composition data, J. Amer. Diet. Ass. **40**:19, 1962.

Mayer, J.: Food composition tables: basis, uses, and limitations, Postgrad. Med. **28**:295, 1960.

Pantothenic acid, vitamin B_6 and vitamin B_{12} in foods, Home Economics Research Report No. 36, Washington, D. C., 1969.

Watt, B. K.: Concepts in developing a food composition table, J. Amer. Diet. Ass. **40**:297, 1962.

Watt, B. K., and Merrill, A. L.: Composition of foods—raw, processed and prepared, U. S. Department of Agriculture Handbook No. 8, Washington, D. C., 1963, U. S. Department of Agriculture.

15 Evaluation of nutritional status

Just as it is relatively easy to identify individuals who are markedly obese or markedly undernourished from casual observations, it is a simple matter to diagnose severe nutritional deficiency states, such as beriberi, pellagra, or scurvy, without the aid of any sensitive biochemical assessment technique. However, these deficiency diseases are encountered relatively infrequently, especially in developed countries. As a result, nutritionists are concerned with developing techniques of evaluating nutritional status sufficiently sensitive to identify individuals who have a marginal nutritive intake, which fosters a low level of vitality and health and which may eventually result in subclinical nutritional deficiency symptoms. It is important to identify these people in the early stages of undernutrition so that preventive measures can be taken before the deficiencies result in overt functional or anatomical changes. The severe deficiency state will often become evident only when the deficiency has persisted for a long period of time or when it is precipitated by a severe stress, such as surgery, prolonged fever, or infection. Although primary and secondary causes of nutritional deficiencies lead to the same results, it is important to identify the cause. For instance, the symptoms developing on a strict vegetarian diet devoid of vitamin B_{12} and those resulting when a genetic defect in the gastric mucosa prevents vitamin B_{12} absorption will be the same, but the conditions will be treated differently.

Because of the multiple causes of nutritional deficiencies and the diverse ways in which deficiencies of various nutrients manifest themselves, no one method of assessing nutritional status has proved completely satisfactory. As a result, several techniques are used to identify individuals whose limited nutritive intake or inability to absorb or utilize a nutrient have resulted in biochemical changes in tissues, which, if continued sufficiently long, will lead to clinically observable symptoms. The techniques by which attempts are made to assess the nutritional status of an individual include clinical observations, biochemical analyses, physical or anthropometric measurements, and dietary evaluations. In addition, some information of nutritional adequacy of population groups can be elucidated from the vital statistics of a country. The general features and unique advantages and limitations of each of these methods will be discussed.

The ways in which nutritional deficiencies develop are outlined in Fig. 15-1. The techniques for detecting the changes are shown in boxes.

CLINICAL OBSERVATIONS

Clinical observations lend themselves to use in nutritional surveys of population groups because they involve an assessment of the health of those parts of the body that can be observed in a relatively short period of time in a routine physical examination and do not involve obtaining blood, urine, or tissue samples. The most commonly observed tissues are the eyes, mucous membranes, skin, hair, mouth, teeth, tongue, thyroid gland, and lower extremities. Although many of the changes in these tissues are often specific for a single nutrient,

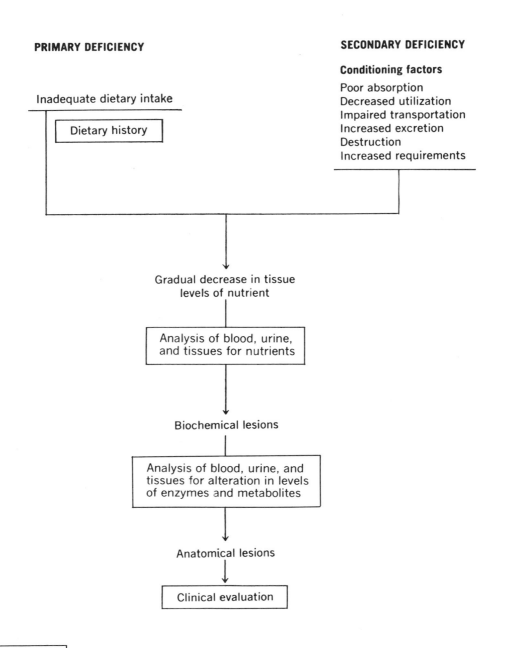

PRIMARY DEFICIENCY   **SECONDARY DEFICIENCY**

                                          Conditioning factors

Inadequate dietary intake   Poor absorption
                                          Decreased utilization
| Dietary history | Impaired transportation
                                          Increased excretion
                                          Destruction
                                          Increased requirements

Gradual decrease in tissue
levels of nutrient

| Analysis of blood, urine,
and tissues for nutrients |

Biochemical lesions

| Analysis of blood, urine, and
tissues for alteration in levels
of enzymes and metabolites |

Anatomical lesions

| Clinical evaluation |

| | Method of evaluation

Fig. 15-1. Development and evaluation of nutritional deficiencies. (Adapted from Krehl, W. A.: Med. Clin. N. Amer. 48:1129, 1964.)

they do not occur until the deficiency is well advanced. In other cases the same changes may be caused by the lack of several nutrients. Even though clinical observations are of limited value in the early diagnosis of a deficiency state or in identifying marginal intakes that prevail for short periods, they are widely used to confirm biochemical and dietary data. Because of the subjective nature of the judgment in a clinical evaluation, it is extremely unreliable even when used by highly skilled observers.

The most useful findings in each of these tissues will be discussed.

Eyes. The most commonly observed symptom is a dryness of the cornea and conjunctiva usually associated with a lack of vitamin A. An increase in severity of vitamin A deficiency shows up as Bitot's spots (Fig. 11-9), or foamy spots in the cornea, followed by a complete opacity in the cornea in a condition known as xerophthalmia. Infiltration of the cornea by blood vessels is associated with a low intake of riboflavin.

Membranes. The color of the mucous membranes in which the blood supply is close to the surface provides an opportunity to observe the pigmentation of the blood. A pale mucous membrane is suggestive of anemia, whereas a more highly colored membrane usually occurs in persons with adequate hemoglobin levels.

Skin. The condition of the skin is often a reflection of the nutritional state of the individual, although all skin changes are by no means of nutritional origin. Deficiencies of some of the vitamins manifest themselves in varying forms and degrees of dermatitis. Skin lesions on areas of the skin exposed to sunlight occur in niacin deficiency, and a roughness and hardness of the papillae at the base of the hair follicle is associated with a lack of vitamin A. The latter occur primarily on the arm, chest, back, and thighs. Pyridoxine deficiency sometimes causes a dermatitis in the area surrounding the nose (nasolabial area). In infants,

eczema may indicate an essential fatty acid deficiency. A dry inelastic skin is most frequently observed after dehydration. The presence of small pinpoint hemorrhages under the skin after the application of either positive or negative pressure is indicative of fragility in the capillary wall, often a manifestation of ascorbic acid deficiency.

Mouth and teeth. Cracks at the corners of the mouth, referred to as angular stomatitis, and vertical cracks followed by redness, swelling, and ulceration in other than the corners of the lips reflect a lack of riboflavin. Loss of the papillae on the tongue and a scarlet and raw appearance of the tongue is associated with a niacin deficiency. A magenta color reflects a riboflavin deficiency. Similar changes have been observed in folacin and cobalamin deficiencies Soft, spongy, and bleeding gums observed in people with teeth are indicative of a lack of ascorbic acid. The presence of mottling on the tooth enamel results from a high intake of fluorine. The incidence of dental caries reported as a DMF index may be an indication of nutritional status but usually reflects diet during the early years of life when the teeth were forming.

Other tissues. One of the first clinical observations to be correlated with a nutritional factor was the enlargement of the thyroid gland associated with a deficiency of the mineral iodine or an intake of food goitrogens. Other clinical observations that may be significant are edema, especially of the lower extremities, which accompanies thiamin deficiency and protein inadequacies; the lack of luster, depigmentation, and decreased hair diameter in protein deficiency; the cupping of the nails when iron is inadequate, and the beading of the ribs, especially at the junction with the breastbone, with a lack of vitamin D.

BIOCHEMICAL ANALYSES

The biochemical evaluation of nutritional status involves quantitative determinations of nutrients or related metabolites in such tissues as the blood and urine. Occasionally analysis will be made of a biopsy sample of liver or bone, but the use of this rather hazardous and involved technique is not justified in routine nutritional evaluations. The potential of the analysis of hair as an indicator of nutritional status, especially for micronutrient elements, is now being investigated. Since variations in composition of the blood and other tissues often reflect recent changes in quantity and composition of the diet, an understanding of the metabolism of the nutrient is necessary to interpret the findings. In many instances the homeostatic mechanisms of the body will mask changes that would otherwise reflect nutritional status. Biochemical data serve either to confirm findings from clinical observations and dietary studies or to identify subclinical deficiencies before clinical symptoms are evident. They can be used for some nutrients to assess the range from frank deficiency levels through adequate, optimal, and excessive levels of nutritive intake.

The interpretation of findings from biochemical data is complicated by the fact that the levels of many nutrients and metabolites in the blood and urine vary sufficiently throughout the day that the use of values from a single determination may be misleading. In addition, only when the body's ability to compensate for deficiencies is overwhelmed will diagnostic changes occur in the nutrient or metabolite levels in the blood and urine. The causes of the observed deviations—whether dietary, genetic, environmental, or physiological—cannot always be identified on the basis of biochemical data.

Many of the analytical techniques for evaluating the constituents of the blood and urine have been adapted for use on very small samples. These microtechniques enable biochemists to be able to make determinations for as many as 15 or 20 nutritional factors or metabolites with a sample of blood as small as 1 ml., which may be collected in capillary tubes from a fingertip puncture.

A discussion of some of the information that can be obtained biochemically follows.

Blood levels of nutrients

The determination of either blood serum or blood plasma nutrient level may reflect the most recent intake of a nutrient or may be indicative of the body's reserves. For instance, levels of ascorbic acid in the blood reflect recent intake. After about six weeks of a deficient diet, however, normal vitamin C serum levels of 0.5 mg. will drop to zero when reserves are only 50% depleted. The level of the vitamin in the white blood cells, however, will drop only when tissue saturation is down to 20% of normal, which will occur only at the time other symptoms of scurvy are about to appear. On the other hand, blood levels of calcium are of little value in assessing nutritional status; the body has so many mechanisms that operate to maintain normal blood levels that only when these mechanisms fail or body reserves are depleted will any change occur in blood calcium levels. The large reserves of vitamin A maintained in the liver similarly make blood levels of vitamin A rather meaningless as an indicator of current intakes. Recently use has been made of serum lipid values, especially cholesterol, triglycerides, and lipoproteins, to screen persons who may be potential victims of coronary heart disease. It is desirable to know if the blood sample was a fasting one.

Blood levels of metabolites

In many cases the absence of a vitamin leads to a block in the normal series of reactions in the metabolism of carbohydrate, fat, or protein. An accumulation of one of the intermediary products in the blood often indicates a lack of the nutrient required for metabolism to proceed beyond that point. For instance, an increase in the pyruvic acid in the blood occurs when insufficient thiamin is available to form the enzyme necessary to decarboxylate pyruvic acid formed in carbohydrate metabolism.

Blood enzyme levels

Since many vitamins act as parts of enzymes or as coenzymes, it is frequently possible to determine the level of enzyme as a measure of the amount of the nutrient available. For instance, the level of the enzyme transketolase in the red blood cells is a sensitive indicator of the available thiamin, which is part of a coenzyme that works in conjunction with transketolase in the metabolism of glucose. Transketolase values are easily determined, and a drop in the level precedes any other signs of a deficiency. As such, they are a valuable diagnostic tool in detecting subclinical thiamin deficiency.

An increase in the amount of another enzyme, alkaline phosphatase, occurs in a vitamin D deficiency. On the other hand, a drop in the level of this enzyme has also been reported in protein deficiency so that these two forces in some instances may counteract one another. Since all enzymes are protein in nature, a drop in all enzyme levels could be expected when labile protein reserves are depleted.

Urine analysis

Biochemical determinations of the nutrients or metabolites in the urine often give valuable information about the nutritional status of an individual. Not only is the amount of a nutrient found in the urine significant, but the presence of substances not normally found in the urine is also informative.

In a saturation test the urine is analyzed to determine the proportion of a large test dose of a water-soluble vitamin that is excreted. It is assumed that an individual whose tissues are saturated with the nutrient will retain little and excrete most of the dose, whereas a person who has had low intakes will retain more in an effort to raise

tissue levels to normal. This test has been widely used in efforts to assess the ascorbic acid status. Test doses of 200 to 1000 mg. are used.

A variation of this is a load test, such as the tryptophan load test. This amino acid requires the vitamin pyridoxine if it is to be metabolized and excreted in a normal manner as N-methyl nicotinamide. If insufficient pyridoxine is available, an abnormal urinary constituent, xanthurenic acid, appears. The level of xanthurenic acid in the urine is low when pyridoxine reserves are high and high when little pyridoxine is available for tryptophan metabolism. Similarly, histidine load tests are used to evaluate folic acid nutriture. In the absence of folic acid, formiminoglutamic acid (FIGLU), an intermediary product of histidine metabolism, accumulates and appears in increased amounts in the urine. Hydroxyproline appears in the urine only as the result of the breakdown of the protein collagen. Determination of hydroxyproline in the urine is a useful indicator of the extent of collagen metabolism. High levels are considered desirable and low ones undesirable.

The amount of creatinine in the urine is a direct reflection of the muscle mass of an individual and has been assumed to be constant. Such information is helpful in determination of body composition, in which it is desirable to know the percentage of body weight represented by fat or muscle tissue. Some other urinary data may be more meaningful when expressed in terms of the amount of creatinine excreted at the same time. This is especially true when data are obtained from a casual urinary sample rather than from a complete 24-hour specimen. For instance, urinary nitrogen in relation to creatinine excretion in a 4-hour specimen has been used as one of the best indicators of protein nutrition, although its value is now being questioned. The excretion of several vitamins is routinely recorded as a function of creatinine excretion. However, interpretation of such data is often difficult because of observed diurnal and day-to-day variations in both creatinine and vitamin excretion.

The excretion of riboflavin reflects fairly accurately the daily intake of the vitamin. An excretion of 50 μg. or less per day is usually associated with other riboflavin deficiency symptoms. Since about 10% of the intake under 1 mg. is excreted, an excretion as low as 50 μg. would result from an intake of less than 0.5 mg., generally regarded as a suboptimal intake.

Other biochemical tests

The rate of hemolysis, or breakdown, of the red blood cell membrane is sufficiently influenced by the amount of vitamin E available that it has become an adequate test for vitamin E status. The analysis of tissues such as hair for mineral composition is being used with increasing frequency.

The routine determinations of hemoglobin as an indication of iron nutriture and hematocrit (blood solids or packed cell level) as an indication of red blood cell formation reflect the amount of available iron and protein in the diet. Plasma albumin levels are maintained by synthesis of protein within the body and will be normal when adequate amounts of amino acids are available. However, the serum levels usually fall only after other signs of protein deficiency are evident. The free amino acid pool in the blood drops in a protein deficiency.

The types of biochemical tests used in the evaluation of nutritional status in the *National Nutrition Survey* are listed in the following outline:

Blood analysis
  Hemoglobin
  Hematocrit
  Total serum
    protein
  Serum albumin
  Plasma vitamin A
    and carotene
  Serum vitamin C

Blood analysis—cont'd
  Total serum iron
    and iron-binding
    capacity
  Serum and whole
    blood folic acid
  Serum globulin ⎫
  Serum cholesterol ⎪
  Transketolase ⎬ Optional
  Plasma amino acid ⎪
    ratio ⎭

Urine analysis
  Creatinine
  Thiamin
  Riboflavin
  Iodine
  Albumin
  Glucose
  Urea nitrogen
  N-Methyl ⎫
    nicotinamide ⎪
  Hydroxyproline ⎬ Optional
  Creatine ⎭

Although a set of standards for evaluating these biochemical data has been proposed, interpretation of much of the data is difficult. The need for improved methodology for the biochemical evaluation of nutritional status is being increasingly recognized.

ANTHROPOMETRIC DATA

Scientists have attempted for years to establish a criterion of nutritional adequacy that involves the use of simple body measurements, such as height, weight, chest circumference, ankle circumference, and skinfold thickness. So far their efforts have met with only limited success. This is partly caused by the difficulties of standardizing the techniques by which the measurements are obtained. Height and weight measurements can be obtained fairly readily, but the others involve a high degree of skill if they are to be useful. Techniques for employing calipers to measure bone structure are difficult to master, especially if measurements are made on persons with an appreciable amount of fat obscuring the bony framework. A second problem is that with improved medical and nutritional knowledge larger and healthier mothers are giving birth to larger and healthier babies whose growth is accelerated. The question, then, is whether or not standards developed twenty to thirty years previously are still valid.

Height and weight tables, long used as a growth standard, have many limitations. If they fail to recognize differences in body build for persons of the same age and sex they are assuming too high a degree of hereditary homogeneity in the population. On the other hand, the use of tables based on different body builds with no basis on which to choose the proper category—small, medium, or large frame—requires a subjective evaluation.

Two general types of tables have been used. The first type merely records the average weight for height and age based on insurance statistics. The most recent table of this type was released in 1959 by the Society of Actuaries in a publication entitled *Build and Blood Pressure Study* and was based on measurements of nearly 5 million insured persons from ages 15 to 69 in ordinary indoor clothing and shoes. Values in this table tended to be lower for women and higher for men than earlier tables published in 1912 and 1952.

The second type of table, which is more useful in evaluating nutritional status, is one giving "ideal" or desirable weights for height. These tables ignore age and use three classifications of body build—small, medium, and large frame. In each of these is presented the range of weights that is associated with the lowest mortality. These weights are essentially the average weights at age 27 for men and age 23 for women. Unfortunately, again no criterion is given on which to base a judgment of body size. The original tables of ideal weights published in 1942 were replaced in 1960 by tables designating desirable weights based on the 1959 *Build and Blood Pressure Study* in which the same classifications of body frame types were used but in which the

desirable weights believed compatible with lowest mortality were about 4 pounds lower for men and 1 to 2 pounds lower for women. It is these tables that are presented in Appendix E. Desirable weights were generally 15 to 25 pounds below average weights for both sexes. All these standards have been criticized because they represent only people who buy insurance, who may not be a representative population group, and also because they imply that overweight is a cause of early mortality, whereas their data show only the relationship.

In adults the body chest breadth as measured on roentgenograms of the thoracic area provide a good measure of stature, but the cost of such a procedure limits its usefulness to research studies and precludes its use in large populations. A weight of 3.4 kg. per centimeter of chest breadth is an acceptable standard for weight.

For evaluating the growth of children Faulkner has developed a chart giving the fifth, fiftieth, and ninety-fifth percentile heights and weights for children from birth to 18 years. He suggests that children falling outside the range from the fifth to the ninety-fifth percentile should be evaluated further to determine if their deviation in growth is cause for concern. His standards are presented in Appendix D.

A parental midpoint scale has been advocated by Garn for use with children. In this he proposes that the most acceptable standard for growth of a child is one that recognizes the role of hereditary factors and reflects the stature of the parents. He has developed tables, one for boys and one for girls, in which he establishes height standards for children of known parentage from birth to age 18 based on the average height of both parents. He believes that his parent-specific scales are much more individualized than are tables based on height for age, irrespective of the hereditary growth capacity of the child. The Fels parent-specific standards for boys and girls are reproduced in Table 15-1.

*Table 15-1. Fels parent-specific standards for height: children's stature by age and midparent stature in inches**

| | Midparent stature† | | | | | |
| | 64.0 inches | | 66.5 inches | | 69.0 inches | |
Age	Boys	Girls	Boys	Girls	Boys	Girls
1-0	29.0	29.0	29.5	29.0	30.5	29.5
2-0	33.6	33.0	34.5	33.5	35.0	34.5
3-0	36.5	35.5	37.5	37.0	39.0	38.0
4-0	39.0	38.0	40.5	41.0	42.0	41.0
5-0	41.5	40.5	43.5	43.0	44.5	43.5
6-0	43.5	43.5	45.5	45.5	47.0	46.0
7-0	45.7	46.0	48.0	47.5	49.0	49.0
8-0	48.0	48.0	50.0	49.5	51.5	51.0
9-0	50.0	50.5	52.0	52.0	53.5	54.0
10-0	52.0	53.0	54.0	54.0	55.5	56.5
11-0	54.5	55.5	56.0	56.5	58.0	59.0
12-0	57.0	58.0	58.5	59.0	60.0	61.5
13-0	59.5	60.5	61.0	62.0	63.0	63.5
14-0	62.5	62.5	63.5	63.0	66.0	65.5
15-0	65.5	63.0	66.0	64.0	69.0	66.5
16-0	66.5	63.0	68.0	64.0	69.5	67.0
17-0	67.5	63.5	69.0	64.5	70.0	67.5

*Age-size tables for Ohio white children whose midparent stature (or parental midpoint) is the average of the stature of the two parents. All values rounded off to the nearest half inch. (From Garn, S. M.: The applicability of North American growth standards in developing countries, Canad. Med. Ass. J. **93:**914, 1965.)
†Average of maternal and paternal statures.

A widely used growth standard based on successive height and weight measurements for a child is the Wetzel grid. In this the child serves as his own control. A typical grid is reproduced in Fig. 15-2. The child's weight in relation to height is plotted and falls in one of the nine developmental channels ranging from channel B4 for a tall, thin person to channel A4 for an obese individual. In subsequent measurements the growth progress is determined by advancement within a developmental channel. Deviations on successive measurements into channels away from the median channel are often diagnostic of some medical or nutritional abnormality. A trend in the direction of channel A4, which is indicative of excess weight for height, may serve as a warning to initiate caloric restriction and to try to determine the underlying cause of the

developing obesity. Trends in the other direction toward channel B4 may signal infection or other conditions that have resulted in loss of appetite and weight. Again the value of the grid is in presenting a visual record of a growth trend. Such records have proved useful in medical evaluations in developing countries.

With the increasing incidence of obesity in the population and the need to recognize those individuals with excess body fat as distinct from those with above-average body weights, attempts have been made to find a method of assessing body fatness. Determination of body density, which involves a comparison of the weight of the body under water with that in air and correcting for the air in the lungs, is the most precise way of estimating body fat but is impractical for use on large groups. Special skin-

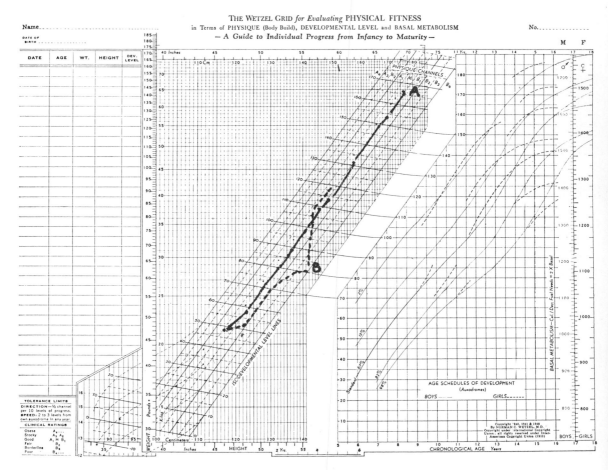

THE WETZEL GRID *for Evaluating* PHYSICAL FITNESS
in Terms of PHYSIQUE (Body Build), DEVELOPMENTAL LEVEL and BASAL METABOLISM
— *A Guide to Individual Progress from Infancy to Maturity* —

Fig. 15-2. The Wetzel grid. Grid is used to assess growth and physical fitness on the basis of successive weight measurements. Growth curve **A** represents a normal growth pattern. Growth curve **B** represents simple growth failure with subsequent recovery. (Courtesy Dr. Norman Wetzel and the National Education Association, Cleveland Heights, Ohio.)

fold calipers that exert a specific pressure on a specific area of skinfold have been developed to measure the thickness of a skinfold in various parts of the body as an indication of the amount of subcutaneous fat. The most satisfactory sites are the upper arm over the triceps, midway between the tip of the scapula and the elbow, and below the tip of the right scapula. It is generally believed that this device is useful only for normal or moderately fat persons and is not equally useful in all body parts. However, Selzer has postulated that the

single skinfold measurement of the triceps is useful in diagnosing obesity (Fig. 15-3).

X-ray films have also been used to assess the amount of subcutaneous fat in various areas of the body. By this technique it has been possible to measure body fat in such areas as the hips, where caliper measurements of skinfold thickness are of little value. This technique has been standardized to the extent that each millimeter of outer fat is believed to represent 1 to 2 kg. of total body fat.

The difficulties of making accurate an-

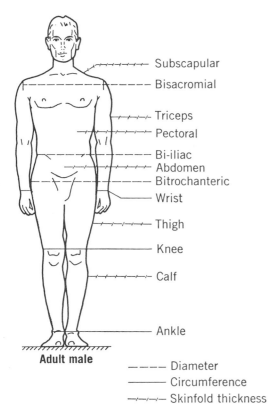

Subscapular
Bisacromial
Triceps
Pectoral
Bi-iliac
Abdomen
Bitrochanteric
Wrist
Thigh
Knee
Calf
Ankle

Adult male

- - - - Diameter
——— Circumference
-/-/-/- Skinfold thickness

Fig. 15-3. Anthropometric measurements used in various formulas for evaluating nutritional status.

thropometric measurements of body structure in very obese people impose limitations on the usefulness of some of the anthropometric indices. In addition to wishing to know something of body composition for purposes of identifying obese persons, doctors use fat-free weight estimates to determine drug dosages. Body fat may also be estimated from the relationship between body weight and lean body mass based on the whole body counter assessment of potassium 40, as discussed in Chapter 7.

A formula using four of the anthropometric measurements shown in Fig. 15-3 has been devised for estimating body fat, which reportedly correlates well with other methods of estimating body fat. It involves measurement of arm and thigh circumferences, abdominal skinfold, and weight. The for-

mula for calculating body fat in Caucasian females between 25 and 34 years of age, for example, has been established as follows:

kg. of body fat = arm circumference (cm.) × 0.354 + thigh circumference (cm.) × 0.403 + abdomen skinfold (mm.) × 0.159 × weight (pounds) × 0.083 − 26.189

In developing countries the single measure of arm circumference has been used to identify undernourished children.

In the National Nutrition Survey, the following anthropometric measurements have been obtained to provide a basis for the evaluation of nutritional status: height, weight, knee height, knee, wrist and shoulder diameter, calf, arm, shoulder and head circumferences, and triceps and subscapular skinfolds. In addition, a wristbone x-ray film is routinely taken. The relative usefulness of these data will become known only after it has been possible to correlate them with other evidence of nutritional status.

DIETARY EVALUATION

An evaluation of nutritional status by an assessment of nutritive intake is not in itself sufficient evidence to suggest that a person is well or poorly nourished. However, when a low dietary intake of a specific nutrient is found in conjunction with biochemical and clinical signs of a deficiency, the dietary data serve to confirm the diagnosis and provide a basis on which to build a dietary treatment. An apparently adequate diet may be taken by a person exhibiting deficiency symptoms, and, conversely, persons with apparently suboptimal intakes may show no evidence of deficiency symptoms. In these cases the discrepancy can often be explained on the basis of the wide individual variability in nutritive needs resulting from differences in ability to absorb a nutrient or in efficiency of utilization. In addition, a dietary evaluation reflects only the immediate intake, whereas much of the biochemical and clinical evidence reflects long-term nutritive intake. A recently improved diet would not immediately result in relief of the symptoms so that a discrepancy between dietary and clinical findings can be explained on the basis of the continuation of deficiency symptoms after the initiation of a better diet.

Dietary evaluations are carried out in a number of ways, each with its own merits and limitations. In a general way they can be categorized as *indirect* and *direct*.

Indirect methods

Food balance sheet or food disappearance data. The most common of the indirect methods is the national food balance sheet. In this the records of agricultural productivity and of the export and import of food products of a country and estimates of food wastage are used to obtain a measure of the kinds and amounts of food and hence of nutrients available to a country. Adjustment must be made for food directed to animal feeding. Since no information is provided on the distribution of food within a country, this is in no way an assessment of the nutritive intake of individuals, nor does it provide information of the variation of intake that occurs with socioeconomic status, cultural background, age, occupation, or sex. It is, however, useful in detecting year-to-year trends of the availability of nutrients, in providing a basis for planning the emphasis that should prevail in agricultural production and processing, and in pinpointing possible nutritional shortages.

Vital statistics. The vital statistics of a country provide a second indirect method of assessing nutritional adequacy. Records of the ages and cause of illness and deaths provide a measure of the extent and nature of morbidity and mortality of a population. Where the incidence of nutritionally related conditions such as beriberi or kwashiorkor is high, malnutrition is undoubtedly present. Where the incidence is low, it may reflect adequate nutrition in regard to these nutrients, but it is equally possible that the

recording of mortality and morbidity statistics has not been sufficiently accurate to reflect these less well known causes of death. Instead, they may only reflect the ultimate cause of death, such as heart failure or tuberculosis. The incidence and death rate from infectious diseases, such as measles or tuberculosis, is often higher in a malnourished population that lacks the ability to combat the infection. In these cases, however, it is difficult to distinguish the role played by nutrition from that of environmental hygiene and medical practices. When used with a recognition of their limitations, vital statistics or public health indices provide a useful tool in evaluating trends on the nutritional status of a population.

Not until 1970 was malnutrition considered a reportable disease in the United States and then only in a few states.

Direct methods

Direct methods involve an evaluation of the dietary intake of a much smaller unit, such as an institution, a family, or an individual. These methods will be discussed in increasing order of specificity of data obtained.

Food inventory. The food inventory method is used with either a socially homogeneous group such as residents in an institution or members of a family who are fed from a common kitchen. A record is made of all the foods available at the beginning of the study, all food purchased or grown for consumption during the period of the study (usually two weeks to a month), the food remaining in the inventory at the end, and an estimate of the waste of food occurring during the course of the study and the food used in feeding animals. From this information an approximation of the nutritive value of the food available to those eating in the group during the period is calculated. This method has several limitations. First, with no indication of who consumes the food, it is quite possible that some members of the group are adequately nourished or even overnourished, whereas others may lack one or more nutrients even though the amount consumed by the group would have been adequate for all had it been properly distributed.

Second, studies on small family units have shown that the homemaker modifies her habits of purchasing food during a time when she is made more conscious of her buying habits. The mere presence of a person recording the food inventory creates a situation in which food habits may vary from normal. It may also increase the reluctance of families, especially in higher income groups, to participate.

Individual food intake. No matter what standard of evaluating an individual's dietary habits is used, whether it be a dietary score or nutritive value calculated from tables of food composition, it is necessary to have as complete a record as possible of the food intake for a specified period of time or to have typical food patterns. These are obtained in several ways.

Twenty-four–hour recall. The subject is interviewed by a trained interviewer who asks him to recall and describe the kinds and amounts of food consumed in the previous 24 hours. The subject is often given food models, measuring cups, or a ruler to help him describe the amounts of food consumed. This method has two major advantages. Since it is a retrospective account taken at an unannounced time, it reduces the possibility of the subject modifying his food habits during a time when he knows they are being assessed. The use of the immediately past 24 hours does not involve an appreciable memory span, thus increasing the likelihood of obtaining a complete record. Since it does not require written records, it is suitable for use in illiterate populations. By asking appropriate questions, the trained interviewer is able to probe further and elicit information that might otherwise have been overlooked.

However, individual interviews are a rather costly method of obtaining dietary information. If data are desired on a group such as school children, 24-hour diet records are sometimes obtained as written records.

Comparison between diet records from 24-hour recall and seven-day written records show the 24-hour recall tends to be higher, which has been interpreted to reflect a desire of the subject to make a good impression on the interviewer.

Dietary history. A dietary history is an effort to obtain qualitative rather than quantitative information on long-standing food habits that influence the appearance of clinical signs and symptoms. Used in conjunction with the 24-hour recall of food intake, it is considered by many as a very effective method of assessing nutritive adequacy. The subject is asked for information on his past dietary habits—the number and type of meals he normally eats, the frequency and extent to which he uses the various food groups (green and yellow vegetables, milk or milk substitutes, meat, eggs, cereals, etc.), his food likes and dislikes, food allergies, and seasonal variations in intake. From this data it is possible to establish whether the pattern observed in the 24-hour record represents a typical or an atypical food intake. Much of the success of this method depends on the cooperation of the subject and the effectiveness of the interviewer. It is relatively costly in time and money, a typical interview requiring at least 45 minutes. Estimates of dietary intake from a dietary history tend to be low compared to those from other means.

Food intake records. When evaluating the diets of large groups of literate subjects, the use of written food intake records has proved an inexpensive and relatively satisfactory method of obtaining data. The question not yet answered satisfactorily is how many and which days should be used. In a country such as the United States, with a varied food supply and a tradition for consuming a varied diet, a one-day food record is considerably less representative of usual dietary patterns than in a country where the diet seldom varies. It is recognized that for many people dietary patterns on weekends differ from those on weekdays. Yet experience has shown that persons asked to keep a seven-day food record lose interest in the task as the period progresses and keep progressively less satisfactory records or stop entirely. Some investigators have found three weekdays and one weekend day provide a more accurate picture. If no provision is made to see that records are kept daily, there is always the possibility that the task will be put off until the end of the period, leading to errors from incomplete or inaccurate recall. Many investigators have chosen to use the three-day

written food record as the one giving sufficiently useful information within a period of time in which one could expect to maintain the cooperation of subjects. Some studies in a highly selected group have made use of 28-day records at four seasons of the year, but this involves a strong commitment and a high degree of cooperation on the part of the subjects.

Weighed food records. When a precise individual dietary analysis is required, the weighed food record provides the most accurate means of obtaining it. All food taken by the subject must be accurately weighed and corrected for any plate waste. This involves training the subject to keep accurate records or assigning an investigator to be present at all times to help. In either case the problem exists that the work involved in record keeping and/or the presence of a

Table 15-2. Food selection check sheet

Food	Credits	Daily score						
Milk								
One cup of milk	10							
Second cup of milk	10							
Third cup of milk or more	10							
	30							
Fruits and vegetables								
One serving of green or yellow vegetables	10							
One serving of citrus fruit, tomato, or								
cabbage	10							
Two or more servings of other fruits and								
vegetables, including potato	10							
	30							
Breads and cereals								
At least two servings of whole-grain or								
enriched cereals or breads	15							
Meats								
One serving of egg, meat, fish, poultry,								
or cheese (or dried beans or peas)	15							
One or more additional servings of egg,								
meat, fish, poultry, or cheese	10							
	25							
	100							

stranger may lead to a modified eating pattern.

Evaluation of food intake records

Dietary score. Several dietary scores similar to the one in Table 15-2, proposed by the United States Department of Agriculture, are used to give a rapid evaluation of the adequacy of the diet. Most are based on the *Essentials of an Adequate Diet* or other dietary guides. A maximum score of 100 indicates that the diet is based on a sufficient variety of protective foods that it will provide an adequate foundation of most of the nutrients. Scores less than 100 represent diets that lack one or more food groups, with the increased possibility of an inadequacy of one or more nutrients. This scoring system is one that can be readily used by a homemaker to evaluate the quality of the meals she serves.

Calculations from tables of food composition. Many tables based on chemical analyses of food composition are available. The standard reference is the United States Department of Agriculture Handbook No. 8, which has been compiled after a careful analysis of data available from many research laboratories. Consideration was given to variety, method of preparation, sources in terms of climates and soil environment, degree of maturity, and many other factors that influence the nutritive value of foods as consumed by the American public. An abbreviated and updated version of this table published as Home and Garden Bulletin No. 72, *Nutritive Value of Foods* (1970) is reproduced in Appendix F.

The rapid rate at which the food industry is marketing new food products and imitation foods has complicated the task of providing an accurate, up-to-date compilation of the nutritive contribution of available foods. Much of this information is included in the most recent revision of Home and Garden Bulletin No. 72 reproduced in Appendix F. However, if exact

information on the composition of new foods is essential, as in therapeutic diets, it is wise to obtain the information from the manufacturer or processor.

With an accurate description of the kind and amount of food eaten, it is possible to use tables to calculate the amount of various nutrients present in a diet. This method assumes that the food consumed can be represented by the food described in the table. One of the major limitations to the analysis of diets from food records is the variations and limitations in an individual's estimate of the amount of food eaten and his failure to describe the food in sufficient detail. Tables for a short method of dietary calculation have been developed in which similar foods are grouped in broad categories, and one figure is given for the nutritive value of the whole group. Estimates of nutritive content using the short method agree rather closely with those obtained from the long method and may be satisfactory for the analysis of diets in which the amount of food has been estimated in the first place. Persons using data derived from calculations from diet records should be cautioned against reporting the values as precise figures (that is, protein to 0.1 gm. or thiamin to 0.01 mg.), since this represents a degree of accuracy not justified within the limitations of the method of collecting the data.

Chemical analysis. In research situations, when it is essential to know as exactly as possible the intake of a nutrient, the food intake is weighed accurately and a representative or aliquot sample is saved for chemical analysis in the laboratory. The cost of such a means of determining nutritive value of a diet precludes its use in routine dietary studies. It is useful when a carefully prescribed diet is being consumed but has many limitations on a freely selected diet.

Standards for evaluating dietary intake. Knowledge of the nutritive content of a diet is meaningless unless it can be com-

Table 15-3. Suggested Guide to Interpretation of Nutrient Intake Data[*]

	Deficient	*Low*	*Acceptable*	*High*
Protein (gm./kg.)	<0.5	0.5-0.9	1.0-1.4	>1.5
Iron (mg./day)	<6.0	6-8	9-11	>12
Calcium (gm./day)	<0.3	0.30-0.39	0.4-0.7	>0.8
Vitamin A (I.U./day)	<2000	2000-3499	3500-4999	>5000
Ascorbic acid (mg./day)	<10	10-29	30-49	>50
Thiamin (mg./100 kcal.)	<0.2	0.20-0.29	0.3-0.4	>0.5
Riboflavin (mg./day)	<0.7	0.7-1.1	1.2-1.4	>1.5
Niacin (mg./day)	<5	5-9	10-14	>15

[*]From Manual for nutrition surveys, ed. 2, Washington, D. C., 1963, Interdepartmental Committee on Nutrition for National Defense.

pared to some standard. In the United States the most commonly used standard is the daily recommended allowances prepared by the Food and Nutrition Board of the National Research Council. These standards, shown in Appendix C, were established as the result of careful evaluation of evidence of nutritional needs for various nutrients by various population groups and of an evaluation of figures on agricultural productivity, imports, and exports to determine the availability of nutrients in the food supply. These standards do not represent minimum requirements, and any failure to consume the recommended amounts must *not* necessarily be interpreted as evidence of dietary deficiencies. In fact, a large segment of the population can maintain a high level of health on intakes below half the recommended amounts, although a small group may require the full amounts. In most studies of dietary adequacy, intakes of two thirds the recommended allowances have been considered

Table 15-4. Dietary standards used by the U. S. Public Health Service in evaluating dietary intake in the National Nutritional Survey, 1970

Age	Energy (kcal./kg.)	Protein (gm./kg.)	Calcium (mg.)	Iron (mg.)	Thiamin	Riboflavin	Vitamin A (I.U.)	Ascorbic acid (mg.)
6-7 years	82	1.3	450	10	0.4 mg./1000 kcal.	0.55 mg./1000 kcal.	2500	30
10-12 years								
Male	68	1.2	650	10	0.4 mg./1000 kcal.	0.55 mg./1000 kcal.	2500	30
Female	64	1.2	650	18	0.4 mg./1000 kcal.	0.55 mg./1000 kcal.	2500	30
17-19 years								
Male	44	1.1	550	18	0.4 mg./1000 kcal.	0.55 mg./1000 kcal.	3500	30
Female	35	1.1	550	18	0.4 mg./1000 kcal.	0.55 mg./1000 kcal.	3500	30
Adults								
Male	38	1.0	400	10	0.4 mg./1000 kcal.	0.55 mg./1000 kcal.	3500	30
Female	38	1.0		18	0.4 mg./1000 kcal.	0.55 mg./1000 kcal.		
Pregnant	+200	+20	800	18	0.4 mg./1000 kcal.	0.55 mg./1000 kcal.	3500	30
Lactating	+1000	+25	900	18	0.4 mg./1000 kcal.	0.55 mg./1000 kcal.	4500	30

adequate and those below this level as indicative of a possible but not necessarily a suboptimal state of nutrition. Because of the wide individual variation in need for a specific nutrient, a great deal of caution must be observed in comparing the intake of an individual to that of the recommended allowances.

The Interdepartmental Committee on Nutrition for National Defense (ICNND) has developed a *Suggested Guide to Interpretation of Nutrient Intake Data* to apply to 25-year-old physically active males 67 inches tall and 143 pounds in weight. It is reproduced in Table 15-3. To interpret dietary data from the *National Nutritional Survey,* yet another standard has been developed. It is outlined in Table 15-4.

Unless low dietary intakes are accompanied by some clinical or biochemical abnormalities associated with a lack of the nutrient, it is dangerous to assume that the intake is below the need of that individual. However, low intakes should prompt an evaluation of nutritional status.

SELECTED REFERENCES

Arroyave, G.: Biochemical evaluation of nutritional status on man, Fed. Proc. **20**:39, 1960.

Beal, V. A.: The nutritional history in longitudinal research, J. Amer. Diet. Ass. **51**:426, 1967.

Bridgforth, E. B.: Statistics in clinical appraisal of nutritional status, Amer. J. Clin. Nutr. **11**:433, 1962.

Brin, M.: Erythrocyte as a biopsy tissue for functional evaluation of thiamine adequacy, J.A.M.A. **187**:762, 1964.

Byron, A. H., and Anderson, E.: Retrospective dietary interviewing, J. Amer. Diet. Ass. **37**:558, 1960.

Cinnamon, A. D., and Beaton, J. R.: Biochemical assessment of vitamin B_6 status in man, Amer. J. Clin. Nutr. **23**:696, 1970.

Committee on Procedures for Appraisal of Protein-Calorie Malnutrition, International Union of Nutritional Science: Assessment of protein nutritional status, Amer. J. Clin. Nutr. **23**:807, 1970.

Dewhurst, W. G., and Morgan, H. G.: Importance of urine volume in assessment of thiamin deficiency, Amer. J. Clin. Nutr. **23**:379, 1970.

Ferro-Luzzi, G.: Rapid evaluation of nutritional level, Amer. J. Clin. Nutr. **19**:247, 1966.

Garn, S. M.: The applicability of North American growth standards in developing countries, Canad. Med. Ass. J. **93**:914, 1965.

Harris, R. S., editor: Symposium on recent advances in appraisal of nutritional intake and nutritional status in man, Amer. J. Clin. Nutr. **11**:331, 1962.

Hollingsworth, D.: Dietary determination of nutritional status, Fed. Proc. **20**:50, 1960.

How to control your weight, supplement (based on 1959 Body build and blood pressure study), New York, 1960, Metropolitan Insurance Co.

Howells, G. R., Wharton, B. A., and McCance, R. A.: Value of hydroxyproline indices in malnutrition, Lancet **1**:1082, 1967.

Hunscher, H. A.: Pertinent factors in interpreting metabolic data, J. Amer. Diet. Ass. **39**:209, 1961.

Hutson, E. M., Cohen, N. L., Kunkel, N. D., Steinkamp, R. C., Rourke, M. H., and Walsh, H. E.: Measures of body fat and related factors in normal adults, J. Amer. Diet. Ass. **47**:179, 1965.

Kelsay, J. L.: A compendium of nutritional status studies and dietary evaluation studies conducted in the United States, 1957-1967, J. Nutr. **99** (supp. 1, part II):123, 1969.

Klevay, L. M.: Hair as a biopsy material. Assessment of zinc nutriture, Amer. J. Clin. Nutr. **23**:284, 1970.

Krehl, W. A.: The evaluation of nutritional status, Med. Clin. N. Amer. **48**:1129, 1964.

Krehl, W. A., and Hodges, R. E.: The interpretation of nutrition survey data, Amer. J. Clin. Nutr. **17**:191, 1965.

McGavack, T. H.: Optimal weight determination —experiences with a method of Willoughby as a guide to reduction, Metabolism **14**:150, 1965.

Medical assessment of nutritional status, Report of the Joint FAO/WHO Expert Committee, WHO Techn. Rep. Ser. No. 258, 1963.

Nutritive value of foods, Home and Garden Bulletin No. 72, Agriculture Research Service, Washington, D. C., 1970, U. S. Department of Agriculture.

O'Neal, R. M., Johnson, O. C., and Schaeffer, A. E.: Guidelines for classification and interpretation of group blood and urine data collected as part of the National Nutrition Survey, Pediat. Res. **4**:103, 1970.

Pearson, W. N.: Biochemical appraisal of the vitamin nutritional status in man, J.A.M.A. **180**:49, 1962.

Phipard, E. P.: The recommended allowances in assessing diets, J. Amer. Diet. Ass. **36**:37, 1960.

Plough, I. C., and Bridgforth, E. B.: Relations of clinical and dietary findings in nutrition surveys, Public Health Rep. **75**:699, 1960.

Pollack, H.: Creatinine excretion as an index for estimating urinary excretion of micronutrients or their metabolic end products, Amer. J. Clin. Nutr. **23**:865, 1970.

Rao, M. V. R.: Clinical evaluation of vitamin and mineral status in man, Fed. Proc. **20**:32, 1960.

Selzer, C. C., Goldman, R. F., and Mayer, J.: The triceps skinfold as a predictive measure of body density and body fat in obese adolescent girls, Pediatrics **36**:212, 1965.

Wadsworth, G. R.: Nutritional surveys—clinical signs and biochemical measurements, Proc. Nutr. Soc. **22**:72, 1963.

Walker, A. R. P.: Interpretation of biological data on one ethnic or regional group may not be equally applicable to other groups, Amer. J. Clin. Nutr. **20**:1025, 1967.

Wilson, C. S., Schaeffer, A. E., Darby, W. J., Bridgforth, E. B., Pearson, W. N., Combs, G. F., Leatherwood, E. C., Greene, J. C., Teply, L. J., Plough, I. C., McGanity, W. J., Hand, D. B., Kertesz, Z. I., and Woodruff, C. W.: A review of methods used in nutrition surveys conducted by the Interdepartmental Committee on Nutrition for National Defense (ICNND), Amer. J. Clin. Nutr. **15**:29, 1964.

Young, C. M.: Body composition and body weight: criteria of overnutrition, Canad. Med. Ass. J. **93**:900, 1965.

16 Nutrition in pregnancy and lactation

PREGNANCY

From a nutritional point of view the nine months of pregnancy must be considered a period of stress during which the nutrient demands of the developing fetus are superimposed on those for normal maintenance of the adult woman. For the pregnant teenager the needs are even greater, as maternal tissue is also experiencing a period of rapid growth with high nutritional requirements. The needs of the growing fetus necessitate an increased dietary intake on the part of the mother but one considerably less than the combined needs of the mother and fetus. The mother experiences a series of physiological adjustments that result in an increased efficiency in the absorption of nutrients, a decrease in the excretion or loss of nutrients, or, in many cases, alterations in metabolism that result in conservation of nutrients. The extent and nature of the adjustments are determined to a large extent by the nutritional status of the mother at the time of conception and may vary from one nutrient to another. The capacity of the mother to adjust to the nutritional demands of pregnancy is sufficient that a mother whose diet has been reasonably adequate prior to pregnancy is usually able to bear a full-term viable infant without any extensive modification in her diet. It is however, strongly recommended that the mother's food intake be of sufficiently good quality that the fetus will be able to grow without causing depletion of the mother's reserves of nutrients.

The recommended increase over the normal nutrient needs of the mother to meet the demands of pregnancy varies from one nutrient to another, as shown in Table 16-1. Since the question of the pregnant teenager is one of more recent concern, we have practically no evidence on which to determine the level of nutrient intake that will be adequate to meet the stress of both maternal growth and reproduction. For some nutrients, such as iron and vitamin A, the infant accumulates sufficient amounts to establish a storage supply to last through the early stages of infancy. For others, such as vitamin D, ascorbic acid, and calcium,

Table 16-1. Increase in nutritional requirements during pregnancy and lactation

Nutrient	Percentage increase over normal	
	Pregnancy	Lactation
Energy	10	50
Protein	18	36
Vitamin A	20	60
Vitamin D	++	++
Vitamin E	20	20
Ascorbic acid	11	11
Folacin	100	25
Niacin	15	54
Riboflavin	20	33
Thiamin	10	50
Pyridoxine	25	25
Cobalamin	60	20
Calcium	50	62
Phosphorus	50	62
Iodine	25	50
Iron	0	0
Magnesium	50	50

++ = No requirement for adult woman except during pregnancy and lactation.

virtually no storage occurs in the infant's body at birth so that the mother need provide only enough for fetal growth.

Rate of growth

The rate of fetal growth is very slow in the first half of pregnancy. At a gestational age of 25 weeks the growth increment is only 6 gm. per day, whereas at 34 weeks it is estimated at 40 gm. per day and by term has dropped again to 13 gm. The fetal weights at various ages of gestation are shown in Table 16-2. The relatively slow development of the human fetus means that nutritional deficiencies must prevail over a long period of time if they are to have a marked effect on fetal development. In contrast, many animals used in nutrition investigations develop at a very rapid rate, produce litters of larger size relative to maternal size, and thus are much more responsive to short-term dietary deviations. A comparison of the rate of development and the relationship of litter size to maternal weight is shown in Fig. 16-1. It will be observed that mice produce a litter weighing 30% of maternal weight in three weeks,

---

Table 16-2. Fetal weight at different ages in gestation*

Age (weeks)	Total weight (gm.)
10	5
12	30
24	900
28	1240
30	1484
32	1750
34	2278
36	2750
38	3052
40	3230
42	3310

*Adapted from Lubchenko, L. O., Hansman, C., Dressler, M., and Boyd, E.: Intrauterine growth as estimated from liveborn birth weight data at 24 to 42 weeks of gestation, Pediatrics **32:**793, 1963.

---

whereas the human mother takes nine months to develop a fetus, representing 5% of her weight.

Physiological stages of pregnancy

Implantation. Pregnancy can be divided into three main phases, each with specific nutrient needs, from a physiological point of view. The first two weeks of gestation is a period of *implantation*, during which the fertilized ovum becomes embedded in the wall of the uterus. At this time the fetus is nourished from the outer layers of the germ plasm and from the secretions of the uterine glands, known as *uterine milk*.

Organogenesis. The next six weeks (from 2 to 8 weeks of age) are known as the period of organogenesis, during which the developing fetal tissue, known as the embryo, undergoes differentiation. During this period, nourishment is obtained from the blood and degenerating cells in the space between the embryo and the maternal tissue. The beginnings of the individual organs and the various aspects of skeletal formation are established during this period, and the presence or absence of many nutrients may be crucial for the continued growth of a normal fetus. Considerable evidence exists in animal studies linking the absence of certain nutrients during specific periods of organogenesis with specific congenital abnormalities in the newborn. For instance, riboflavin deficiency has been associated with poor skeletal formation, and niacin and folic acid deficiency with cleft palate. It has been difficult to demonstrate such a relationship in human nutrition because any dietary information must come from retrospective accounts and not from experimental manipulation of the diet. Once the abnormality is observed, however, it is sometimes possible to implicate nutritional factors. A nutritional inadequacy with its potential hazards to the fetus during organogenesis is possible, since this rather critical period occurs at an earlier stage in pregnancy than it is customary for

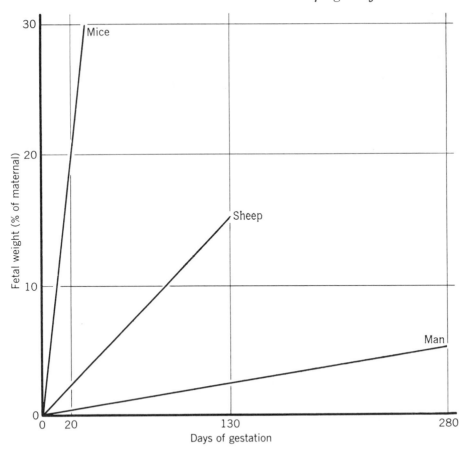

Fig. 16-1. Products of conception of three mammalian species in percentage of maternal weight. (From Smith, C. A.: Pediatrics **30:**145, 1962; based on data from McCance, R. A., and Widdowson, E.: Brit. Med. Bull. **7:**297, 1951.)

a pregnant woman to seek medical advice, which, it is assumed, includes some guidance in selecting an adequate diet. In addition, many women experience nausea of pregnancy that depresses appetite and food intake and in many cases reduces the amount of food available for absorption to a critically low level. It is under such conditions that the mother who has had good dietary habits prior to conception has an advantage over her less well-fed counterpart who may not have entered pregnancy with such good reserves.

Growth. The remaining seven months of pregnancy are known as the growth period. During this time the differentiated tissues

continue to grow until they reach a functional size capable of supporting the extrauterine life of the infant. The needs for nutrients at this time are high both quantitatively and qualitatively, although a deficiency will usually result only in a premature birth or smaller infant, rather than the serious deficiency symptoms observed as a result of a dietary lack during organogenesis.

Early in this growth stage the placenta develops and takes over its role in providing nourishment for the fetus. The placenta, which weighs from 325 to 1000 grams at birth, is the tissue through which the nutrients and oxygen needed for fetal growth are transferred from the maternal tissue to the fetus and through which fetal waste is excreted. No direct circulatory connection between the fetus and the mother occurs, but in the placenta the two independent circulatory systems come in sufficiently close contact with one another that nutrients are able to pass from one to another. In the placenta, which regulates the flow of nutrients to the fetus, approximately 13 square meters of contact exist between the two circulations. For some nutrients, such as iron, cobalamin, folacin, pyridoxine, and vitamin C, the placenta allows the passage of sufficient amounts to meet the demands of the growing fetus even at the expense of maternal reserves. For others, such as thiamin, riboflavin, and vitamin D, it allows the maternal and fetal tissue to compete. Vitamins A and E are present in lower amounts in fetal than in maternal blood. Thus the placenta becomes the regulator of fetal nutrition, the success of which depends not only on the nutrients available in the bloodstream of the mother but also on the way in which the placenta governs their transfer. In addition to promoting the active transfer of nutrients, the placenta is capable of synthesizing some body compounds. It is postulated that nutritional failure is as often the result of an inadequate supply of blood to the placenta as of a low level of nutrients in the maternal blood.

From studies on animals it is evident that the stage in pregnancy at which the deficiency occurs determines susceptibility to the deficiency and the way in which it is manifest. If the inadequacy occurs in the very early stages, the result may be a failure in pregnancy, reflected in a spontaneous abortion; at certain stages during differentiation, it may show up in a variety of forms of congenital abnormalities, such as cleft palate, harelip, malocclusion, or defective tooth formation; and again, there are stages, especially after differentiation is complete, at which a deficiency will have virtually no effect on the developing fetus.

Different animals will vary in their susceptibility to deficiencies depending on their genetic makeup. In human studies it has not been possible to implicate deficiencies in the formation of congenital abnormalities, since in severe deprivation mothers either become sterile or abort or deliver stillborn, premature, or smaller but normal children.

Physiological adjustments

During pregnancy many physiological, biochemical, and hormonal changes occur that influence the need for nutrients and the efficiency with which the body uses them. Total blood volume is known to increase about 33% above normal levels and plasma volume 50% in primiparas and higher in multiparas. This is—partially, at least—a response to the need to carry nutrients to the fetus and metabolic waste, such as carbon dioxide and nitrogenous end products, away from the fetus. This hemodilution results in decreased hemoglobin and plasma protein values as well as a lowered per unit volume concentration of red blood cells, which increase only 18%, and of many nutrients, observations often erroneously interpreted as evidence of a deficiency. Frequently the total amount may have increased, although the per unit measurement will have dropped.

The decrease in gastric motility common in pregnancy has the advantage of slowing the passage of food through the gastrointestinal tract and enhancing the possibility of absorption of nutrients. On the other hand, it may be a factor in nausea of pregnancy and may lead to considerable discomfort when it results in an inability to empty the gastrointestinal tract in the latter part of pregnancy.

The observed decrease in the secretion of hydrochloric acid reduces gastric acidity, which could have a depressing effect on calcium and iron absorption, in which the ionization of the element from its complex depends on acid. However, any such effect is counterbalanced by other factors that lead to an increased absorption of these two elements in the last trimester of pregnancy.

The 60% increase in rate of filtration in the kidney, the 33% increase in blood flow, the increase in blood enzymes, especially alkaline phosphatase, and the increase in cardiac output are other physiological adjustments that have nutritional implications during pregnancy.

Nutritive needs

The change of nutrient intake recommended to meet the nutritional stresses of pregnancy varies with the nutrient, depending on many factors, such as the body's mechanism for adjusting to increased demands, the nature of the metabolic changes of pregnancy, and the nutrient reserves of the mother. The National Research Council recommended dietary allowances are based on rather scanty information regarding quantitative needs during pregnancy. For a better understanding of the kind of dietary adjustment that may be necessary during pregnancy, the needs for each nutrient will be discussed separately.

Energy. During pregnancy caloric needs

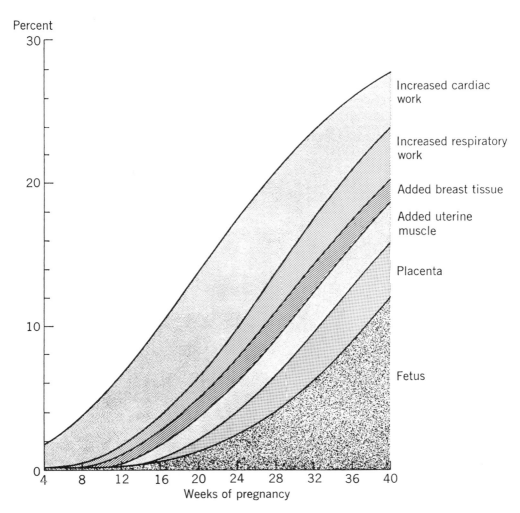

Fig. 16-2. Components of increased oxygen consumption in pregnancy. (From Hytten, F. E., and Leitch, I.: The physiology of human pregnancy, Philadelphia, 1963, F. A. Davis Co.)

are influenced by several forces. On one side, the growth of the fetus, although very slow at first, calls for additional energy, as does the growth of the placenta, the normal increase in maternal body size, including fat reserves of 35,000 kcal., the additional work of carrying the growing infant, and the steady but slow rise in basal metabolism while the decreased activity of the mother depresses the caloric requirement. It is estimated that the growth of the fetus and maternal tissue and their maintenance calls for approximately 80,000 kcal., but normal energy requirements are reduced by 40,000 kcal. through decreased activity. This results in a net increased requirement of 40,000 kcal. Fig. 16-2 shows the components of the increased energy need of pregnancy. For some mothers who greatly reduce their activity a demand for an increase in energy may never occur in spite of the increased basal energy requirement and fetal growth needs of the last trimester.

Along with the growth of the developing fetus itself, a concurrent increase in the size of supporting maternal tissues occurs. The nature of maternal weight gain shown in Table 16-3 indicates that a normal pregnancy calls for considerable weight gain over and above that represented by size of the fetus. Thus, if the net gain in maternal

Table 16-3. Nature of maternal weight gain in pregnancy

Tissue		Weight (pounds)
Fetus	7	(Range, 5-10)
Placenta	1.5	
Amniotic fluid	2	
Uterus	2	
Breasts	1	Relatively constant
Increase in blood volume	3	
Tissue fluids	3	
Fat	9	
Total		28.5

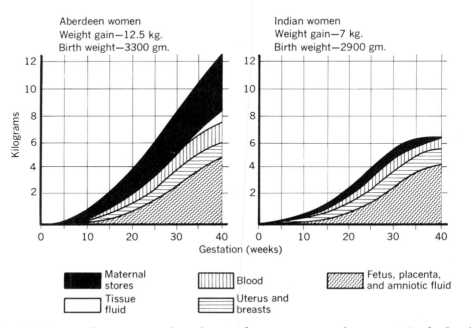

Fig. 16-3. Estimated components of weight gain during pregnancy of women in Scotland and in India. (From Hytten, F. E.: Proceedings of the Sixth International Congress on Nutrition, Edinburgh, 1963, E. & S. Livingstone, Ltd.)

weight is less than 25 to 30 pounds, one must assume that the growth of the child as a parasite on the mother has caused a depletion of the mother's tissue reserves. A failure in the development of mammary structures and fat reserves during pregnancy may preclude a normal and successful lactation period. The distribution of the components of weight gain during pregnancy is shown in Fig. 16-3.

Energy stored as fat in the maternal tissue is concentrated almost exclusively in fat depots, with virtually none occurring in the reproductive tissues other than the mammary gland. Fat that is deposited throughout the whole period of pregnancy acts as a buffer against food deprivation and prevents the catabolism of the mother's tissue. The increase in ketones that appear in the urine in late pregnancy suggest that fat reserves are being utilized to take care of the high energy needs of the rapidly growing fetus and to spare protein for tissue growth. The increase in body fat during pregnancy represents storage of sufficient energy to subsidize lactation at 300 kcal. per day for four months.

In the first trimester the fetus accumulates no fat other than that which is part of the essential lipids in the cell wall and the nervous system. At 20 weeks the fetus contains only 0.5% fat, but this rises steadily to 3.5% at 28 weeks, 7.5% at 34 weeks; and 16% of body weight at term. Fat is synthesized by the fetus from glucose, which crosses the placental barrier readily. The only fatty acids to be transferred from the mother to the child are the essential fatty acids, the rest being synthesized from glucose.

There has been much conflict in the literature regarding what constitutes a desirable gain in weight for a pregnant woman. The practice of allowing the mother unrestricted weight gain on the theory that she was "eating for two" was widely accepted in the early part of the century. The undesirable consequences of this regime, such as toxemia, difficulties of labor with increased risk to the mother, and the birth of large babies who suffered many complications in early life, soon became evident. The proponents of unlimited weight gain were replaced by a group recommending caloric restriction sufficiently severe to limit weight gain to 10 to 12 pounds, a regimen that resulted in equally undesirable consequences. Mothers who fail to gain weight in the second trimester are very likely to have premature deliveries, with increased risk to the health of the baby, and to experience toxemia or preeclampsia, with its symptoms of proteinuria, blood pressure elevated above normal, headache, blurred vision, and edema. Some edema, especially in the ankle region is normal and in the absence of other symptoms is not considered suggestive of toxemia. Eclampsia with convulsive seizures is more common among women who are overweight at conception and those who gain excessively in the latter half of pregnancy. It is most severe, however, in women who are underweight at conception and who fail to gain weight. Women at greatest risk are those who experience a sudden and excessive weight gain, especially after the twenty-fourth week. Mothers who experience eclampsia are the ones who gain less than 15 pounds or over 29 pounds during gestation. The relationship between weight gain and complications of pregnancy is shown in Fig. 16-4. Research data showed that women consuming less than 1800 kcal. per day were unable to maintain a positive nitrogen balance, which means that if the fetus continued to grow, it did so at the expense of maternal tissue that would not be replaced as fast as it was depleted. In addition, the restriction in energy intake seldom led to the birth of a smaller baby with less strain on the mother during labor. In fact, it is believed that the birth weight of the infant is more closely correlated with the weight of the mother at conception than to the weight gain of the mother during pregnancy. It would appear, then, that caloric restriction prior to pregnancy so that

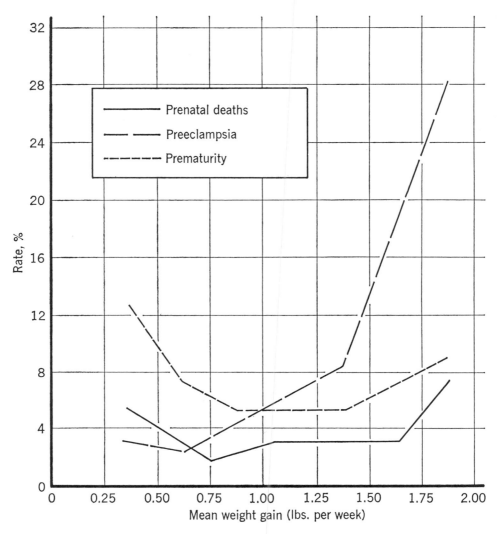

Fig. 16-4. Incidence of three major obstetrical complications by mean weight gain between 20 weeks and delivery. (From Hytten, F. E., and Leitch, I.: The physiology of human pregnancy, Philadelphia, 1963, F. A. Davis Co.)

the mother enters the reproductive period at normal body weight will do more to assure the birth of a child of average weight than will caloric restriction during pregnancy.

Many women restrict their weight gain in fear that a gain may remain a permanent weight increment. Studies show that about 8 pounds of weight gained during pregnancy remains immediately after birth and only 4 pounds at six weeks postpartum. All

the gained weight is usually lost in six to eight months.

Although some workers maintain that the woman who is obese at the onset of pregnancy can successfully reduce her own body size without jeopardizing the health of the infant or herself if the qualitative aspects of the diet are guarded carefully, the preponderance of the evidence suggests that any major adjustments in the mother's weight should be undertaken under normal circumstances rather than during a period of nutritional stress such as pregnancy. Aside from the physiological stress produced by caloric restriction, the emotional tension accompanying it, especially in the face of a stimulated appetite, may have even more adverse effects. If weight gain is to be controlled, however, the only effective way to do it is through caloric restriction rather than by a restriction of salt or water intake.

The Food and Nutrition Board of the Committee on Maternal Nutrition of the National Research Council has concluded that a gain of 25 to 30 pounds minimizes the risks of pregnancy and is most desirable in terms of the health of both the mother and baby.

After a careful evaluation of all relevant data the National Research Council has suggested that an additional 200 kcal. per day in the last half of pregnancy will take care of the energy demands of pregnancy and will lead to the desirable weight gain.

Protein. The growth of the infant makes heavy demands for protein of high biological value. If two thirds of the protein comes from animal sources, an additional 10 gm. of protein per day will be adequate to meet the needs for the increase in maternal tissue and also to support the growth of the fetus. Protein intake of the mother influences the birth length of the fetus within the limits determined by heredity, taller babies being born to mothers with high-protein diets than to those with limited protein intake. The smaller babies born to mothers on diets inadequate in protein are more susceptible to the hazards of early life and have a decreased chance of survival.

Although total weight gain during pregnancy includes 2 pounds of protein, a 7½-pound infant will have almost a pound of it. The greater part of this protein has been deposited in the fetal tissue at a rate of 4.5 to 5.7 gm. per day during the last half of pregnancy when the growth hormone produced during pregnancy stimu-lates the retention of nitrogen. Protein is transferred to the fetus in the form of amino acids. Since the fetus cannot oxidize amino acids, it appears that they are used exclusively for protein synthesis.

There is little storage of protein in maternal tissues other than reproductive tissues. When dietary protein is restricted, it is the amount in storage that is reduced, rather than the amount transferred to the fetus. The reserve of energy in the form of fat helps to spare protein during rapid fetal growth.

Protein restriction during fetal life is associated with a decrease in the number of cells in tissues at the time of birth. This is particularly serious in the case of the brain, which is relatively well developed in prenatal life and may be irreversibly stunted. This is in contrast to other tissues that undergo less growth in the prenatal period and relatively more in postnatal development.

Studies on rats and humans suggest that a protein and caloric deficiency during gestation results in poor utilization of food by the offspring after birth and a failure to ever compensate for early food deprivation.

In addition to the amino acids that are transferred to the fetus, large protein molecules such as antibodies also cross the placental barrier and give the infant passive immunity to the antigens to which the mother has been exposed.

Calcium. Although the infant's bones are poorly calcified at the time of birth, a demand still exists for an appreciable amount of calcium for fetal development. The demand of approximately 7 mg. a day for the first trimester increases to 110 mg. per day in the second trimester and jumps to 350 mg. in the last trimester. This leads to the deposition of approximately 30 gm. of calcium in the body of the newborn infant. Although the mother has more than 1000 gm. of calcium to draw on, she becomes more efficient in absorbing calcium. The decrease in absorption that occurs under conditions of emotional stress, such as may prevail among unwilling mothers, may counterbalance the increased absorption that is a normal response to the demands of pregnancy. It is estimated that about 30% of fetal calcium has been obtained from maternal stores. The amount of dietary calcium needed is reduced if vitamin D is available and is increased if it is not. Ideally, there should be a storage rather than a depletion of calcium in the mother's tissues during pregnancy to help anticipate the demands for calcium, which are particularly high during lactation, but we have no evidence to confirm this.

Iron. Since infants are born with high hemoglobin levels of 18 to 22 gm. per 100 ml. of blood and with a supply of iron stored in the liver to last from three to six months, the maternal organism is called upon to transfer about 300 mg. of iron to the fetus during gestation. In addition to this need for fetal growth, 70 mg. are required for the placenta and 280 mg. for the formation of hemoglobin, which is the result of the increase in red cell mass associated with the increase in blood volume. Of this total of 650 mg. that represents almost the total iron reserves of the adult female, a saving of 100 to 200 mg. is effected by the absence of menstrual losses. In addition, about 230 mg. of the iron in the extra hemoglobin will be returned to the iron pools when the blood volume returns to normal after delivery. A need still occurs however, for about 1 mg. per day of iron over and above the needs of the nonpregnant woman. If dietary iron is not available to meet this need, iron stores will be depleted, and there will be reduction in the expansion of red cell mass, rather than an impairment of fetal iron reserves. If the mother has no iron reserves, as appears to be the case in many young women, especially teen-agers, maternal hemoglobin levels will drop and may reach the level of 10 gm. per 100 ml., which is considered indicative of anemia in the pregnant woman. Assuming that the usual rate of iron absorption of 10% of dietary intake increases in response to the demands of pregnancy, the Food and Nutrition Board saw no reason to raise the recommended dietary allowance above the 18 mg. suggested for the nonpregnant woman to maintain maternal reserves and to meet fetal requirements during pregnancy. An increase in the amount of the protein transferrin, which influences the capacity for iron absorption, is observed during pregnancy. This suggests that the capacity for iron absorption is increased. An absorption as high as 40% of dietary iron has been observed in the last trimester of pregnancy when as much as 3.5 mg. of iron is retained by the fetus each day. As under normal conditions, the amount of iron absorbed is influenced by the need for it and the food source. Iron from cereals is poorly absorbed and that from muscle is readily available. Such observations are of special significance in countries where cereals are the staple item in the diet.

It is believed that the best method of combatting iron deficiency in pregnancy is to promote high intakes of available iron by the nonpregnant woman so that she enters pregnancy with adequate stores. Some investigators have found that the injection of a single large dose of iron at the beginning of pregnancy builds iron stores and protects against iron depletion throughout pregnancy. Such a procedure may be justified in the light of the finding that patient cooperation in taking iron may be an important consideration in failure in treating iron deficiency in pregnancy. The Committee on Maternal Nutrition of the National Research Council, recognizes that women normally ingest only 10 to 12 mg. of iron per day, an amount well below the 18 mg. recommended, and may have entered pregnancy with suboptimal stores. They suggest a supplement of 30 to 60 mg. of iron per day in divided doses during the second and third trimesters.

Evidence that hemoglobin levels do not necessarily reflect the adequacy of the iron supply and that the maintenance of normal bone marrow levels of iron and of iron-containing enzymes in the liver and kidneys are more sensitive criteria is accumulating.

Macrocytic (large cell) anemia, which frequently occurs in pregnancy, is believed to be caused by a relatively inadequate intake of dietary folate. There are indications that iron deficiency puts additional stress on folate metabolism and may convert a subclinical folate deficiency into a megaloblastic anemia.

Iodine. Levels of iodine that will prevent goiter under normal circumstances frequently prove inadequate in pregnancy, leading to goiter in the mother, especially an adolescent mother. The relative deficiency may be due in part to the increased urinary losses of iodine observed in pregnancy. When the mother has goiter, the chances that the child will develop goiter are increased ten times. In addition, the incidence of cretinism, the severe form of iodine deficiency, among infants rises to 1% when the incidence of goiter among mothers reaches 55%.

In many parts of the country, diets are adequate in iodine only when iodized salt is used in cooking. Should salt intake be restricted in an attempt to control toxemia of pregnancy, the woman is deprived of her only reliable source of iodine and should be encouraged to use some other supplementary source as a protection against goiter

Other mineral elements. Little work has been done to determine quantitative needs for other mineral elements during pregnancy, but it seems reasonable to suggest that the body's ability to adapt to a state of stress by improved absorption and decreased excretion will take care of some but not necessarily all of the additional needs for mineral elements. Evidence that infants develop teeth with increased resistance to dental caries when the mother's

diet contains adequate fluorine is controversial. Considerable evidence now exists that, contrary to early opinion, the need for sodium is increased above that for normal maintenance and that sodium restriction may have many adverse effects. This has been borne out by the successful use of diets high in salt rather than the usual salt-restricted diet in the treatment of toxemia of pregnancy in a group of 1000 pregnant women. Evidence from animal studies has also shown need for increased intakes of sodium during reproduction. The National Research Council maintains that there is no justification for routine salt restriction in pregnancy and is especially concerned that diuretics not be used along with salt restriction.

Low levels of zinc, magnesium, and manganese have all been associated with undesirable changes in the developing fetus. Excessively high levels also have adverse consequences. Although levels used in experimental studies far exceed those found in normal dietaries, these findings should be kept in mind when dietary supplementation or food enrichment is considered.

Fat-soluble vitamins. Although it is fairly well established that the pregnant animal has a series of adaptive mechanisms to cope with increased demands for minerals during pregnancy, no evidence has been compiled that such a system of adaptation exists for vitamins.

Vitamin A. Aside from the fact that animals on vitamin A–deficient diets have a poor reproductive performance, little is known about the need for vitamin A during pregnancy. The National Research Council, however, has suggested that a small increase to 6000 I.U. per day should be adequate, especially if some is preformed vitamin A. Lack of vitamin A during the early stages of fetal development in animals has been implicated in cleft palate and skeletal and eye defects. Similar relationships in humans have not been established.

Vitamin D. The need for vitamin D is set at 400 I.U. per day to promote the absorption and utilization of calcium and phosphorus, which are so essential in bone formation. Unless milk fortified with vitamin D or a combination of other foods to which vitamin D has been added is used, a normal diet cannot be relied upon to provide adequate amounts for women living in the temperate zone. Supplements providing 400 I.U. per day are recommended. However, evidence linking arteriosclerosis, mental retardation, and renal acidosis in infants with excessive intakes by the mother during pregnancy suggests caution in the use of supplements along with fortified foods if overdoses and the resultant toxic effects are to be avoided. If milk fortified with 400 I.U. of vitamin D per quart is used, no need exists for an additional source of the nutrient; in fact, it should be avoided.

Vitamin E. The observation of a role of vitamin E in promoting normal reproduction and reducing the number of abortions and stillbirths in animals led to many studies to elucidate a similar role in humans. So far scientists have been unable to determine any unique role of the tocopherols in human reproduction in spite of some evidence that they may be beneficial to women who have experienced repeated abortions or a failure to conceive. No evidence of any increased need for vitamin E in pregnancy has been found, and, as under normal conditions, the requirement appears to be adequately met by a normal diet, with little likelihood of a deficiency unless the diet contains abnormally high amounts of polyunsaturated fatty acids. Little vitamin E crosses the placenta so that the human infant has low tissue concentrations. Although the effect of pregnancy on vitamin E requirements has not been established, the RDA are set at 30 I.U. per day, an increase of 5 I.U. above normal requirements.

Vitamin K. As the vitamin concerned with the synthesis of prothrombin necessary for normal coagulation of the blood, vitamin K has long been considered to play a role in preventing neonatal hemorrhaging, which was often fatal to either the mother or the fetus. It became routine practice to give menadione orally to the mother in the last several weeks of pregnancy or even by injection during labor to prevent hemorrhage. Evidence of some adverse effects, such as hyperbilirubinemia, especially in premature infants from the use of large doses of the synthetic form have led to the recommendation that if a synthetic analogue is given it should be given in a controlled dose to the mother at a level sufficiently high to prevent hemorrhage but low enough to preclude adverse reactions. The inclusion of menadione in over-the-counter supplements for pregnancy is prohibited. Similar and safe protection is afforded by giving vitamin K_1, the natural form of the vitamin, either by injection or orally to the infant or to the mother.

Water-soluble vitamins. Since water-soluble vitamins are not stored to any appreciable extent, the pregnant woman must rely on a daily intake sufficiently high to meet the added requirements of pregnancy.

Thiamin. The relationship between thiamin needs and caloric intake remains the same during pregnancy as under normal circumstances, thus calling for a slight increase of 0.1 mg. The normal urinary excretion of thiamin drops in pregnancy, indicating that more is being retained and used by the tissues. Some investigations have shown that thiamin helps relieve the nausea of pregnancy.

Riboflavin. The increase in body size with the growth of the fetus and accessory tissues calls for an increase in riboflavin of 20%.

Animal studies have shown that a lack of riboflavin in the thirteenth and fourteenth embryonic days interferes with cartilage formation, resulting in skeletal malformations such as shortening of the long bones and a fusion of the ribs.

Pyridoxine. Women under the normal

stress of pregnancy exhibit an altered tryptophan metabolism and a decreased ability to handle sodium, both of which can be corrected by additional pyridoxine.

There is an active transport of pyridoxine to the fetus to maintain a level in fetal blood five times that in maternal blood. Although no experimental evidence exists to indicate the exact amount required to meet the needs of pregnancy, the RDA has been increased by 0.5 mg. above that recommended for the nonpregnant woman.

Pyridoxine has been used experimentally to help control the nausea of pregnancy, but the results, though encouraging for some individuals, have not been conclusive, and no satisfactory theory explains this phenomenon.

Folic acid. Folate intake during pregnancy has been associated primarily with the promotion of normal fetal growth and the prevention of a macrocytic anemia of pregnancy. The need for folic acid in pregnancy is known to increase, and the recommended daily allowance is twice that of nonpregnant women. In iron deficiency, need increases further.

Although this level of intake may prevent the diagnosis of pernicious anemia, the incidence of undiagnosed cases is believed to be sufficiently low that the problem is minor. Evidence exists of a marked decrease in folate absorption and an increase in urinary excretion during pregnancy, which may contribute to the depletion of maternal reserves. Scientific opinion suggests that folic acid deficiency is a major cause for concern in pregnancy, with abruptio placenta, hemorrhage, fetal malformation, and absorption among the frequently observed complications. Not all studies have confirmed these reports of pregnancy wastage associated with low serum folate levels, nor have they established that folic acid supplements alleviate any of the problems other than megaloblastic anemia.

The importance of folic acid in promoting a normal pregnancy is emphasized by the fact that the use of a folic acid antagonist, aminopterin, induces the resorption of fetuses in animals. Its use in human beings does not lead to resorption or abortion of a fetus but rather to the birth of a child with congenital malformations such as harelip, cleft palate, or hydrocephalus.

Cobalamin. It has been confirmed that the infant is parasitic on the mother for cobalamin, as evidenced by the higher vitamin B_{12} levels found in fetal blood than maternal blood even when maternal levels are depleted. The capacity to absorb cobalamin is increased in pregnancy, but a large amount is transferred to the fetus. The recommended daily intake of cobalamin to maintain constant serum cobalamin levels is 8 μg. If these amounts are not supplied, the serum vitamin B_{12} levels drop but return to normal without supplementation after pregnancy.

Ascorbic acid. The NRC recommended allowances for ascorbic acid are increased by 5 mg. during pregnancy, although there is little evidence on which to base this figure. Ascorbic acid does pass the placental barrier freely, and serum values of a fetus have been established at two to four times that of the mother. Some evidence has been established to indicate that the placenta is capable of synthesizing ascorbic acid, which could account for the higher levels in fetal tissues. Low maternal intakes of ascorbic acid are associated with premature rupture of fetal membranes and increased neonatal death rates.

Role of nutritional supplements during pregnancy

The reproductive period is one in which heavy demands are made on the mother to provide the nutrients needed for normal fetal development. It has been shown that the increase in need varies from one nutrient to another with a small increase for calories. To provide the amounts of protein, minerals, and vitamins recommended

Table 16-4. Proposed Food and Drug Administration regulations for supplements for pregnancy, 1966

Nutrient	Mini- mum	Maxi- mum	Units
Vitamins			
Mandatory			
Vitamin A	1250	8000	I.U.
Vitamin D	100	400	mg.
Vitamin C	18	100	mg.
Thiamin	0.3	1.2	mg.
Riboflavin	0.5	1.9	mg.
Niacin	5	21	mg.
Optional			
Vitamin E	8	30	mg.
Vitamin B_6	0.5	2	mg.
Folic acid	0.03	0.1	mg.
Pantothenic acid	2.5	10	mg.
Vitamin B_{12}	2	5	μg.
Minerals			
Mandatory			
Calcium	200	1300	mg.
Iron	4	20	mg.
Optional			
Phosphorus	200	1300	mg.
Magnesium	75	300	mg.
Iodine	0.04	0.15	mg.
Copper	0.05	2	mg.

*From Dietary supplements and vitamin- and mineral-fortified foods, Federal Register **31:** 15730, Dec. 14, 1966.

without exceeding the caloric allowance, a woman must choose her food carefully and almost exclusively from protective foods (i.e., those that provide as high a percentage of the day's requirements of at least two nutrients as they do of calories). The selection of a diet adequate for pregnancy is relatively easy if one is concerned with an isolated day or two, but the pregnant woman must maintain this high level of nutritive intake for the 280 days of the normal gestation period. To do this, she must constantly be conscious of her food choices. The woman who takes such a responsibility seriously is subjecting herself to a constant stress during a period that is frequently characterized by at least some degree of emotional stress. To allow her a little more freedom in the selection of food and an occasional indulgence in a favorite

food, it may be reasonable to suggest that she use a supplement that provides a balanced formula at protective levels—possibly 25% of the day's recommended allowance. Because of the competitive nature of the drug market most manufacturers find it necessary to market supplements providing an excessive amount of the nutrients needed, to include many for which there is little likelihood of a deficiency occurring even in pregnancy, or to include ineffectual amounts of others. The use of such supplements is not only an economic waste and unnecessary from a nutritional point of view but also a practice that could produce nutritional imbalances, especially if the product contains mineral elements, and could adversely affect the fetus if the fat-soluble vitamins reached toxic levels. The Food and Drug Administration (FDA) maintains that there is justification for the inclusion of only eleven vitamins and six minerals in dietary supplements. The FDA proposed in 1966 that nutritional supplements be restricted to eleven vitamins and six minerals for which they believed some evidence of need had been established. Their proposal, which is still under consideration, is presented in Table 16-4.

Table 16-5 gives the composition and cost of several supplements promoted in the retail trade in the fall of 1970. From this it is obvious that some supplements contain amounts of some nutrients in excess of total needs of pregnancy and also of the levels suggested by the FDA, while making insignificant contributions of others. The money spent on some of these may do much more toward promoting a satisfying pregnancy if it were spent on some form of recreation, an additional dress, or domestic help!

Supplements may be especially useful for a woman experiencing nausea of pregnancy whose dietary pattern may be disturbed, but again, they should be restricted to protective levels.

Iron supplements, often not incorporated

Table 16-5. Nutritive composition and cost of several nutritional supplements used during pregnancy

Brand		A	B	C	D	E	F	G
Vitamin A	(I.U.)	5000	4000	6000	4400	4000	6000	2500
Vitamin D	(I.U.)	400	400	400	500	400	400	1000
Thiamin	(mg.)	2	1.5	3	10	3	1.5	1
Riboflavin	(mg.)	1	2	3	10	2	2.5	1.5
Niacin	(mg.)	6	12	20	100	10	15	6
Pyridoxine	(mg.)		1	2	2	1	3	
Calcium pan-tothenate	(mg.)		2.5	0.5	20		0.5	
Ascorbic acid	(mg.)	100	60	75	300	50	100	25
Cobalamin	(μg.)		3	12	4		2	2
Calcium	(mg.)	125		100	50	230	250	
Iodine	(mg.)			0.15	0.15	0.01		
Iron	(mg.)			45	10	30	40	30
Magnesium	(mg.)			6	6			
Zinc	(mg.)			1.5	1.5	0.085		
Manganese	(mg.)				1	0.05		
Copper	(mg.)			1	1	0.15		
Potassium	(mg.)				5	0.835		
Cost per day	(cents)			4.0	7.0	4.6	4.8	

in the multivitamin-mineral preparations, are recommended for women whose hemoglobin drops below 10.5 gm. per 100 ml., a level indicative of depletion of iron reserves as well as hemodilution. Therapeutic iron in doses of 30 to 60 mg. as ferrous sulfate or ferrous gluconate are most frequently recommended. Calcium to meet the needs of the growing fetus can be provided in calcium supplements, but the amounts in routine vitamin-mineral preparations are seldom significant.

One additional basis for caution in the use of high-level nutritional supplementation during pregnancy has been brought to light recently with the observation that animals may become conditioned to a high intake during fetal life if the intake of the maternal organism is high and may reflect this in an increased need in the postnatal period. This has been advanced as a possible explanation for the increase in infantile scurvy among infants in technically advanced countries. The toxic effects of too much of the fat-soluble vitamins A and D have been well documented.

Research workers at Vanderbilt University believe that the mother can adapt to such a wide range of nutrient intake during the stress of pregnancy that there is no need for supplementation.

Dietary modifications in pregnancy

In addition to a need to modify the normal diet pattern to take care of the quantitative needs for nutrients, other modifications may have value. During the early part of pregnancy when appetite may be disturbed, the consumption of smaller and more frequent meals has been helpful to many women. The same pattern is helpful in the latter part of pregnancy when the problem is one of discomfort after large meals because of crowding of the abdominal cavity.

Between the fourth and seventh months particularly, many women experience an insatiable appetite. To control this to help limit weight gain to a desirable level, the practice of eating a small meal slightly before the time when hunger sensations become most severe has been found a useful method of controlling the total intake.

The use of a diet relatively high in bulk may be helpful in maintaining normal gastric motility at a time when a tendency toward constipation occurs.

The way in which the nutritive needs of pregnancy are met will vary with the preferred food habits or likes and dislikes of the women. Usually a diet containing three cups of milk or its equivalent, two servings of meat, fish, or poultry, one egg, a dark green or yellow vegetable, and a generous serving of a citrus fruit daily will provide a foundation for a nutritionally adequate diet.

EFFECT OF NUTRITION ON PREGNANCY

It has been fairly well established that the nutritional status of the mother at the time of conception is as important for the outcome of pregnancy as is the diet during the period of gestation. The nutritional status of the mother at conception is generally a reflection of long-standing food habits that change in relatively few people during pregnancy in spite of the motivation one would expect to prevail at this time. Because of the influence of many factors, such as the maternal age, birth rate, birth interval, and metabolic interrelationships, it is difficult to delineate specific dietary effects.

The impact of the nutrition of the mother on the course of pregnancy and the condition of the infant at birth has been the subject of many investigations, but not all have led to the same conclusions. The now classic study of Burke, which has been described in the introductory chapter, points most conclusively to a relationship between maternal diet and well-being of the infants, the chances of a child with a high pediatric rating being born to a mother with a good or excellent diet being much better than when the maternal diet is rated as poor or very poor. Studying Canadian women, Ebbs found a similar relationship, with mothers on good diets experiencing few complications during pregnancy and giving birth to infants with a greater chance of surviving the neonatal period. More recently, however, a group of investigators at Vanderbilt University failed to demonstrate a relationship between the quality of maternal diet and the course and outcome of pregnancy. They believed that complications of pregnancy led to suboptimal intakes rather than the converse. Although they found a relationship between diet and the course of pregnancy only at dietary intakes of less than 1500 kcal. and 50 gm. of protein, they emphasized that these findings should not be interpreted to mean that good nutritional practices should not be encouraged. None of the subjects in their study had markedly suboptimal diets so that they may have entered pregnancy in sufficiently good nutritional status to provide a buffer against the stress of pregnancy.

Thomson in England in 1959 was unable to demonstrate any difference in the diet of mothers who had a normal clinical history during pregnancy and those who experienced some clinical abnormality. No relationship was found between diet and the duration of gestation, the birth weight of the infant, fetal malformation, perinatal deaths, or failure of lactation. In this study one can conclude that the abnormalities of reproduction were not caused by dietary deficiencies. However, this must not be interpreted to mean that dietary inadequacies could not cause abnormalities of pregnancy.

In 1963 after reviewing 4300 obstetrical cases, Thomson and Billewicz found that the incidence of prematurity, cesarean section, and perinatal deaths increased as the dietary rating of the maternal health fell. Their results are shown in Table 16-6.

Other investigators have indicated a re-

Table 16-6. Incidence of obstetric abnormalities in Aberdeen primigravidas by maternal health and physique, as assessed at the first antenatal examination (twin pregnancies excluded)

| | Maternal health and physique | | | |
	Very good	Good	Fair	Poor; very poor
Prematurity† (%)	5.1	6.4	10.4	12.1
Cesarean section (%)	2.7	3.5	4.2	5.4
Perinatal deaths per 1000 births	26.9	29.2	44.8	62.8
Number of subjects	707	2088	1294	223
Percentage tall (5 feet, 4 inches or more)	42	29	18	13
Percentage short (under 5 feet, 1 inch)	10	20	30	48

*From Thomson, A. M., and Billewicz, W. Z.: Nutritional status, maternal physique and reproductive efficiency, Proc. Nutr. Soc. **22:**55, 1963.
†Birth weight of baby 2500 gm. or less.

lationship between specific dietary factors and specific complications of pregnancy. Toxemia of pregnancy is often associated with diets low in protein or pyridoxine, failure to gain enough weight, or too large a weight gain. The incidence of abortion in early pregnancy among women with low-protein diets is almost twice as high as it is in women with high-protein diets.

The effect of diet prior to pregnancy can be illustrated from data on babies born during a period of wartime starvation in two different countries—Holland and Russia. In Holland the children born during a hunger period had been conceived prior to the period by mothers whose previous diet had been good. The babies were shorter and 10% lighter than babies born to mothers whose diets were adequate throughout pregnancy, but there was a decrease in stillbirths (5%), prematurity, and congenital malformation, all indications of the protective effect that a good diet prior to pregnancy may exert during the course of pregnancy. In contrast, mothers whose babies were born during the siege of Leningrad and whose diets had been poor prior to pregnancy experienced a stillbirth rate double the normal rate, a 41% inci-

dence of prematurity among live births, and a 31% incidence of neonatal deaths among low–birth weight infants. A reduced rate of conception also occurred.

Additional evidence suggesting that the lifetime diet habits of the mother influence the outcome of pregnancy is advanced by Thomson, who found a prematurity rate of 32 per 1000 births and a neonatal death rate of 19 per 1000 births in children born to mothers over 64 inches tall. These, he assumed, represented women who had been relatively well nourished throughout their lives. Similar statistics on women under 61 inches tall who may have been less well nourished during their own growth period showed a threefold increase in prematurity, with 91 per 1000 infants weighing less than 2500 gm. and a doubled incidence of neonatal deaths. Many other studies have suggested that the better the state of nutrition of the mother prior to or at the time of conception, the greater the chance of normal pregnancy leading to the birth of a healthy child.

LACTATION

The decision to breast- or bottle-feed an infant is one often surrounded with much emotion. The advantages of breast-feeding will be discussed in greater detail in Chapter 17, but some of the more cogent considerations are that it represents a very satisfying emotional experience for the mother, provides a source of nourishment uniquely suited to the growth demands and physiological capacity of the human infant, is a foolproof method that can be duplicated only by intelligent, constant, carefully guarded, artificial feeding, and seldom, if ever, causes allergic reactions—an especially important consideration for parents with a family history of allergy. The decision to breast-feed is generally made early in pregnancy or even before conception. Once the decision has been made the likelihood of success depends to a large extent on the mothers attitude toward breast-feeding, her understanding of the process of lactation, and the support and encouragement she receives from medical personnel and the family in her efforts to initiate a successful experience.

Nutritive needs

The nutritive demands on the mother during lactation far exceed those of pregnancy, although she may actively cease to feel the responsibility of "eating for two." A normally developing infant doubles its birth weight accumulated in nine months of pregnancy in five months of life—evidence of the demands that the breast-fed infant makes on the mother. Milk secreted in one month represents more kilocalories than the net energy costs of pregnancy. This same milk contains 240 gm. of protein. The infant synthesizes more tissue each day in postuterine life than during fetal life and in addition, must provide for its own temperature regulation, more extensive body movements, and must take care of many more intermediate steps in the utilization of food.

The health of the mother who is lactating successfully can be assured only if her own nutritive intake is satisfactory. In most cases a severe deficiency of a nutrient in the maternal diet will be reflected in a decreased secretion of milk, but in a few instances a milk of inferior quality will be produced. The NRC recommendations for dietary intakes during lactation are based on even less data on quantitative needs than are those for pregnancy. It is fairly well established that these levels will support the average production of 850 ml. of milk, but it is entirely possible that satisfactory lactation can be maintained on somewhat lower levels of intake. Evidence also exists that many women produce much more than 850 ml. of milk. For instance, one study among Budapest mothers of 19 to 23 years of age showed an average secretion of 1029 ml. at three weeks, 1263 at seven weeks, and 1492 at 14 weeks, with some mothers secreting over 2500 ml.

Recommended allowances

An adequate diet during pregnancy is one of the best bases for the initiation of breast-feeding, but the nutritional goals for successful continuation of lactation are less obvious. Lack of clear-cut information on the nutritive composition of milk, the volume of milk produced, and the efficiency of milk production has complicated the task of arriving at recommended levels of nutrients in the maternal diet to allow adequate milk production. Lack of agreement is found regarding what constitutes a normal composition of either colostrum, transitional, or mature milk, but just as cows of different genetic makeup secrete milks of different nutritive composition, human mothers with still greater heterogeneity of heredity can be expected to produce milks of varying compositions. The fact that many mothers, especially in developing countries, are able to maintain a prolonged and satisfactory lactation period on diets well below currently accepted standards suggests a reappraisal of nutritional goals for lactating women. Since it is possible that in these cases lactation has been carried on at the expense of maternal reserves, which may be depleted to the point of endangering the maternal health, high standards are likely justified for the maintenance of a satisfactory level of milk production. The basis for current standards will be discussed for individual nutrients. Table 16-1 shows the suggested increase in nutritive intake for lactation over that required under normal conditions. The increase suggested can be met by the equivalent of an additional meal of approximately 1000 kcal. of protective foods each day.

Energy. The energy required to take care of the needs for lactation is proportional to the amount of milk produced and will vary considerably from one woman to another. In general 120 kcal. are required for every 100 ml. of milk produced. Thus, for the woman who secretes the typical 850 ml. per day, energy needs are increased by 1000 kcal. Of this, 400 kcal. represent the energy required in the synthesis and secretion of the milk and the remaining 600 kcal. the energy content of the milk itself. This longstanding belief that the mammary gland is only 60% efficient in transferring energy to milk has been challenged by data suggesting 90% efficiency from 49 women in Scotland. In addition to the energy needed to produce sufficient milk to meet the demands of a rapidly growing baby, the mother may have an increased energy requirement created by her return to a more active routine in caring for a small child.

Protein. Since human milk contains 1.2 gm. of protein per 100 ml., the secretion of 850 ml. of milk calls for about 10 gm. of protein and 1200 ml. for 15 gm. This is based on a protein of high biological value. To make allowances for consumption of less than ideal protein, the recommended dietary allowances have been set at 20 gm. above normal needs. The FAO in proposing practical allowances recommends that intake be increased by 15 gm. Increasing the protein content of the mother's diet above a certain low level (approximately

35 gm.) does not result in an increased protein content of the milk secreted. Its effect on the quantity of milk produced has not been ascertained.

Fat. No recommendations are made regarding the level of fat in the diet of a lactating woman. The amount of fat in the milk is not influenced by the amount in the mother's diet, but the character of the fat does reflect composition of the ingested diet about 8 hours later. Medium-chain saturated fatty acids appear when the diet is high in carbohydrate and decrease when a large percentage of the calories comes from fat. Longer-chain and polyunsaturated fatty acids are derived from ingested fat. Human milk contains mostly medium-chain fatty acids and, in contrast to cow's milk, has virtually none with less than 10 carbon atoms. Human milk provides from 6% to 9% of its calories in the form of linoleic acid, most of which comes from the polyunsaturated fatty acids in the mother's diet.

Calcium. Although human milk contains only one fourth the level of calcium of cow's milk, the mother needs to increase her own intake by 500 mg., or 62% above normal, if she is to prevent a depletion of her own calcium stores. Although the calcium content of milk will vary from one mother to another, it is not influenced by the level of calcium in her diet.

Iron. Since relatively little iron is transferred to the infant through milk, the need for iron in the maternal diet does not increase above that for pregnancy. The amount that does occur in human milk is well utilized and may delay the normal drop in hemoglobin levels in early infancy.

Vitamin A. Although most infants have a fair reserve of vitamin A stored in their liver at the time of birth, human milk provides both vitamin A and carotenoids. An intake of 8000 I.U., easily achieved by the mother's regular use of green and yellow vegetables, allows production of milk with 170 I.U. per 100 ml., which is sufficient to meet the needs of the infant. In one study of vitamin A supplementation of the diet of poor Indian women, no increase in the vitamin A in the milk was observed. The investigators hypothesized that once the mother's reserves have been restored, the levels in the milk would increase. The amount of vitamin A in human milk decreases throughout the first twenty weeks of lactation. A single large dose of the vitamin will cause a rapid but transitory increase in the amount in the milk.

Thiamin. Thiamin is one nutrient for which a deficiency in the mother's diet is reflected in the production of a milk low in the nutrient rather than in a diminished output of milk. In addition, a mother whose diet is very low in thiamin may secrete a substance, glyoxal, which accumulates in thiamin deficiency. The presence of this potentially toxic substance along with a low thiamin content in milk is associated with infantile beriberi. An intake of 0.5 mg. per 1000 kcal. is recommended for the production of a milk with adequate thiamin levels. Although cow's milk may have a higher content than human milk, the fact that this heat-labile vitamin is destroyed during pasteurization and sterilization of the formula makes human milk a more dependable source.

Riboflavin. Milk is one of the most dependable sources of riboflavin in the adult diet, and human milk provides high levels for the infant. The mean content of 0.04 mg. per 100 ml. of milk would require that 0.34 mg. be transferred to human milk each day. Since about 70% of this additional riboflavin is assumed to be utilized, it is recommended that the nursing mother increase her intake by 0.5 mg. above normal.

Ascorbic acid. The amount of ascorbic acid in human milk is higher than that in cow's milk, which, because of losses during heat processing, is incapable of meeting the needs of the infant after the first two weeks. The transfer of ascorbic acid to human milk calls for an intake of 60 mg., which is easily obtained from a serving of citrus fruit. An analysis of human milk has revealed a seasonal variation in its ascorbic acid content, reflecting changes in maternal intake.

Vitamin D. Vitamin D is transferred to a limited extent to the milk so that even breast-fed infants require a supplementary source of the vitamin for maximum utilization of calcium and phosphorus for bone formation. Even so, an intake of 400 I.U. per day is recommended for the lactating woman.

Other nutrients. The transfer of the micronutrient elements iodine and fluorine through the mother's milk to the infant is efficient and contributes appreciably to the intake of the infant when the mother's intake is adequate, protecting against goiter and reducing tooth decay. Ingested sodium is rapidly transferred to the milk, appearing within 20 minutes. On the other hand, vitamin K given to the mother is not transferred to the milk until the fourth day postpartum, which is too late to give the infant the immunity to postnatal hemorrhages during the critical first few days of life.

The effect of drugs, pesticides, herbicides, and other contaminants on the composition of mother's milk and on the infant is poorly understood. Some concern exists that DDT may reach questionably high levels in mother's milk or that the effect of the oral contraceptives on milk composition may be detrimental to the infant. Infants of mothers who are taking sedatives suck less vigorously than normally.

• • •

These relatively high nutritional requirements of lactation require a significant increase in the quantity of food consumed and also dictate that the qualitative aspects of the food be carefully controlled. The use of an extra serving of meat, green and yellow fruits or vegetables, citrus fruit, and the equivalent of 2 cups of milk over and above a normal adequate diet will take care of the additional nutrients required. Obviously this quantity of food cannot be incorporated into three regular meals without taxing the capacity of the stomach. Since most lactating women have very good appetites, it is feasible to suggest an eating pattern that includes five or six meals a day. If between-meal snacks are kept relatively low in satiety value, the appetite for regular meals shows little decrease.

Dietary supplements

In light of the very high level of nutritional intake prescribed for normal lactation, it is likely sound practice to recommend the use of a dietary supplement that provides protective levels of the nutrients for which the possibility of a dietary lack exists. This does not imply the endorsement of a supplement providing therapeutic levels of some nutrients and insignificant amounts of others.

Stimulation of lactation

Many techniques have been suggested to stimulate a satisfactory level of lactation. Likely none are as effective as a constant stimulation of the mammary gland by the vigorous sucking of an infant and the presence of adequate nutritive reserves in the mother's tissues as a result of an adequate diet before conception and during pregnancy to initiate milk production. The first fluid secreted by the human breast, colostrum, is a thin, yellowish, watery fluid that bears little physical resemblance to milk and has its own unique nutritional composition, as shown in Table 16-7. The flow of colostrum may not begin for two to four days postpartum—a delay that is often erroneously interpreted as a failure of lactation.

Oxytocin, a hormone of the pituitary

Table 16-7. Composition of colostrum; immature and mature human milk and cow's milk per 100 ml. of milk*

| | Human | | | |
| | Colostrum | Transitional | | Mature |
Nutrient	(1-5 days)	(6-10 days)	Mature	cow's milk
Energy (kcal.)	58.0	74.0	71.0	69.0
Fat (gm.)	2.9	3.6	3.8	3.7
Lactose (gm.)	5.3	6.6	7.0	4.8
Protein (gm.)	2.7	1.6	1.2	3.3
Casein (gm.)	1.2	0.7	0.4	2.8
Lactalbumin (gm.)		0.8	0.3	0.4
Calcium (mg.)	31.0	34.0	33.0	125.0
Phosphorus (mg.)	14.0	17.0	15.0	96.0
Iron (mg.)	0.09	0.04	0.15	0.10
Vitamins				
A (I.U.)	296	283	176	113
Carotene (I.U.)	186	63	45	63
D (I.U.)			0.42	2.36
E (mg.)	1.28	1.32	0.56	0.06
Ascorbic acid (mg.)	4.4	5.4	4.3	1.6
Folic acid (μg.)	0.05	0.02	0.18	0.23
Niacin (mg.)	0.075	0.175	0.172	0.085
Pantothenic acid (mg.)	0.183	0.288	0.196	0.350
Pyridoxine (mg.)			0.011	0.048
Riboflavin (mg.)	0.029	0.033	0.042	0.157
Thiamin (mg.)	0.015	0.006	0.016	0.042

*Based on Food and Nutrition Board: The composition of milks, Publication No. 254, Washington, D. C., 1953, National Academy of Sciences–National Research Council.

gland, has been effective in stimulating lactation through stimulation of the letdown reflex in which the smooth muscles surrounding the alveoli of the nipple contract to allow the release of milk. It helps counteract the inhibition of the reflex, which is often caused by pain, emotional conflict, and embarrassment. Although large amounts of estrogens suppress lactation, small amounts appear to have a stimulating effect by preventing an abnormal engorgement of the breast. Almost every culture has its own medicinal or food galactogogues, substances believed to stimulate lactation. These include garlic, cottonseed, candy, beer, ale, and large quantities of milk.

The relationship between fluid intake and volume of mammary secretion has not been established. Even when fluid intake is low, the volume secreted remains constant although urine volume drops, indicating that the mother has had to concentrate her urinary excretions. A decreased intake of fluids will limit milk production only when total intake is less than the volume of milk produced. Drinking water beyond the level of natural thirst suppresses milk secretion through its action on the hormones of the pituitary that regulate milk production. Although high intakes do not stimulate milk production, liberal fluid intake is suggested to preclude the necessity of the formation of a highly concentrated urine.

Success and duration of lactation

Many attempts have been made to predict the success of lactation. Some evidence has been established that the output of milk is directly proportional to the metabolic size of the mother and also that a strong positive correlation exists between rise in temperature of mammary skin due to nursing and milk supply. Other studies have shown that the course of lactation is established by the end of the first week, at which time the output should reach 500 ml. A positive attitude on the part of the mother is a determining factor not only in the decision to breast-feed but also in success once it is undertaken. Although a great many undernourished women do succeed in breast-feeding satisfactorily, the woman who was severely malnourished in childhood may have impaired development of secondary sex characteristics, resulting in inadequate mammary tissue.

The period of time for which lactation is continued varies with a great many factors, both social and physiological. In many cultures, breast-feeding is carried on for two to three years with milk being the sole source of food for a year or more. In other cultures, breast milk may be supplemented with other foods as early as three or four weeks. The latter case is believed to lead to less vigorous sucking, which in turn leads to a reduction in milk output and usually early weaning. Some evidence has been found that this same group experiences an earlier return to a regular pattern of ovulation with subsequent pregnancies occurring sooner. The observed trend for a longer lactation period in lower socioeconomic groups now appears to be reversing itself, with mothers of higher socioeconomic and educational status breast-feeding their infants for six months or more.

For some mothers, lactation is terminated when the amount of milk produced declines to a point at which such extensive supplementary feeding is required that it is no longer feasible to continue breast-feeding.

SELECTED REFERENCES

Pregnancy

Alpern, J. B., Haggard, M. E., and McGanity, W. J.: Folic acid, pregnancy and abruptio placentae, Amer. J. Clin. Nutr. **22:**1354, 1969.

Beaton, G. H.: Some physiological adjustments relating to nutrition in pregnancy, Canad. Med. Ass. J. **95:**622, 1966.

Burke, B. S., Stevenson, S. S., Worcester, J., and Stuart, H. C.: Nutrition studies during pregnancy. V. Relation of maternal nutrition to condition of infant at birth: study of siblings, J. Nutr. **38**:453, 1949.

Clements, F. W.: Nutrition in maternal and infant feeding, Fed. Proc. (no. 1, part 3) **20**:165, 1961.

Chow, B. F., Blackwell, R. Q., Blackwell, B. N., Hou, T. Y., Anilane, J. K., and Sherwin, R. W.: Maternal nutrition and metabolism of the offspring: studies in rats and man, Amer. J. Public Health **58**:668, 1968.

Committee on Maternal and Child Health: Maternal nutrition and the course of pregnancy, Publication No. 1761, Washington, D. C., 1970, National Academy of Sciences—National Research Council.

Ebbs, J. F., Tisdall, F. F., and Scott, W. A.: Influence of prenatal diet on mother and child, J. Nutr. **22**:515, 1941.

Gold, E. M.: Interconceptional nutrition, J. Amer. Diet. Ass. **55**:27, 1969.

Hafez, E. S. E.: Reproductive failure, Science **154**:546, 1966.

Hancock, K. W., Walker, P. H., and Harper, T. H.: Mobilization of iron in pregnancy, Lancet **2**:1055, 1968.

Holly, R. G.: Dynamics of iron metabolism in pregnancy, Amer. J. Obstet. Gynec. **93**:370, 1965.

Jackson, H. N., Burke, B. S., Smith, C. A., and Reed, D. E.: Effect of weight reduction in obese pregnant women on pregnancy, labor, and delivery and on the condition of the infant at birth, Amer. J. Obstet. Gynec. **83**:1609, 1962.

Kodicek, E.: Nutrition of the foetus and the newly born, Proc. Nutr. Soc. **28**:17, 1969.

Larson, R. H.: Effect of prenatal nutrition on oral structures, J. Amer. Diet. Ass. **44**:368, 1964.

McCollum, E. B.: Symposium on prenatal nutrition, J. Amer. Diet. Ass. **36**:236, 1960.

McGanity, W. J., Bridgforth, E. B., and Darby, W. J.: Vanderbilt cooperative study of maternal and infant nutrition; effect of reproductive cycle on nutritional status and requirements, J.A.M.A. **168**:2138, 1958.

Macy, I. G.: Metabolic and biochemical changes in normal pregnancy, J.A.M.A. **168**:2265, 1958.

Pike, R. L.: Sodium intake during pregnancy, J. Amer. Diet. Ass. **44**:176, 1964.

Seifert, E.: Changes in beliefs and food practices in pregnancy, J. Amer. Diet. Ass. **39**:455, 1961.

Smith, C. A.: Prenatal and neonatal nutrition, Pediatrics **30**:145, 1962.

Stearns, G.: Nutrition status of mother prior to conception, J.A.M.A. **168**:1655, 1958.

Stevens, H. A., and Ohlson, M. A.: Nutritive value of the diets of medically indigent pregnant women, J. Amer. Diet. Ass. **50**:290, 1967.

Thomson, A. M.: Diet in pregnancy. 3. Diet in relation to the course and outcome of pregnancy, Brit. J. Nutr. **13**:509, 1959.

Thomson, A. M., and Billewicz, W. Z.: Nutritional status, maternal physique and reproductive efficiency, Proc. Nutr. Soc. **22**:55, 1963.

Thomson, A. M., Hytten, F. E., and Billewicz, W. Z.: The epidemiology of oedema during pregnancy, J. Obstet. Gynaec. Brit. Comm. **74**(1):1, 1967.

Nutrition in pregnancy and lactation, Report of the Joint FAO/NRC Expert Committee, Techn. Rep. Ser. No. 302, 1965.

Widdowson, E. M.: How the foetus is fed, Proc. Nutr. Soc. **28**:17, 1969.

Lactation

Bigwood, E. J.: Nitrogenous constituents and nutritive value of human and cow's milk, World Rev. Nutr. Diet. **4**:95, 1963.

Gopalan, C., and Belavady, B.: Nutrition and lactation, Fed. Proc. (part 2) **20**:177, 1960.

Gunther, M.: Diet and milk secretion in women, Proc. Nutr. Soc. **27**:77, 1968.

Macy, I. G., Kelly, H. J., and Sloan, R. E.: The composition of milks, National Research Council Publication No. 254, Washington, D. C., 1953, National Research Council.

Mayer, J.: Nutrition and lactation, Postgrad. Med. **33**:380, 1963.

Meyer, H. F.: Current feeding practices in hospital maternity nurseries, Clin. Pediat. **8**:69, 1969.

Newton, M., and Newton, N.: The normal course and management of lactation, Clin. Obstet. Gynec. **5**:44, 1962.

Newton, N., and Newton, M.: Psychologic aspects of lactation, New Eng. J. Med. **277**:1179, 1967.

Thomson, A. M., Hytten, F. E., and Billewicz, W. Z.: The energy cost of human lactation, Brit J. Nutr. **24**:565, 1970.

Williams, H. H.: Differences between cow's and human milk, J.A.M.A. **175**:104, 1961.

Woody, D. C., and Woody, H. B.: Management of breast feeding, J. Pediat. **68**:344, 1966.

17 | *Infant nutrition*

The adequacy of nutrition in infancy is crucial to the well-being of the individual throughout life. The infant who is adequately nourished undergoes a normal rate of physical and mental development. On the other hand, one who is inadequately nourished in respect to one or more nutrients may experience a stunted growth and other biochemical changes associated with undernutrition. Some of these may be reversed if the inadequacy is corrected while the growth response is still present. Brain and neurological development may be more seriously affected, and some concern exists that a depressed brain development caused by severe dietary restriction at a critical period in very early infancy may result in a permanent stunting of brain size. Thus, in light of future development, both mental and physical, the importance of an adequate nutritive intake in early infancy cannot be overemphasized. A relationship between depressed brain size and depressed mental development has not been demonstrated, however.

BREAST-FEEDING

The incidence of breast-feeding in the United States, which underwent a decline from an almost universal practice at the turn of the century to 38% incidence in 1946, declined still further to 21% in 1958 and 18% in 1966. In some regions the incidence was as low as 9% of all babies leaving the hospital and in others as high as 27%. Studies since that time have indicated increased interest in breast-feeding among the more educated, higher socioeconomic groups. One report shows that 50% of mothers in a college town are breast-feeding successfully. Similarly, a study of 2233 mothers in the Boston area showed that, although only 22% of the total group were breast-feeding, 69.3% of those married to students breast-fed and that 39.8% of the upper social class and only 13.6% of the lower social class breast-fed. College-educated women tended to choose to breast-feed. No relationship was found between a daughter's decision and her mother's. The pattern of feeding used by the better-educated group is frequently followed several years later by less educated mothers and those of lower socioeconomic status in a wavelike sequence, with the lower socioeconomic group emulating the higher. Whether such a trend prevails will not be ascertained for several years.

In a few cases, when the mother has tuberculosis or breast cancer, breast-feeding is precluded. But in most cases the decision will be made after a consideration of the relative merits of the two types, since, for all intents and purposes, either should be possible and successful in a Western culture. In developing countries, on the other hand, breast-feeding is almost essential if the child is to survive the neonatal period.

Considerations favoring breast-feeding

Nutritional. In general, it is believed that the nutrient composition of the milk of each species is the one best suited to the growth needs of its offspring, and when possible it should be used. If this is not possible, the

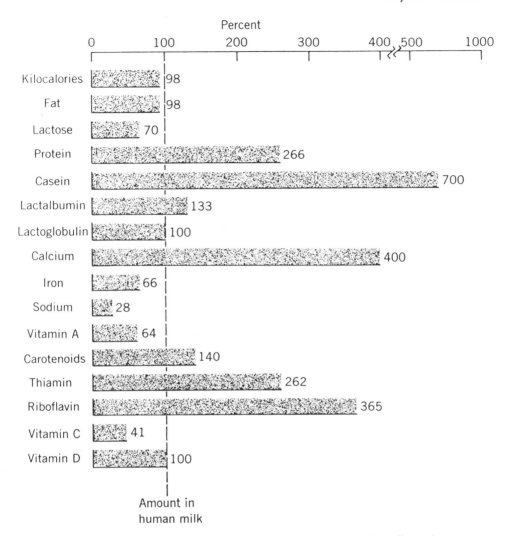

Fig. 17-1. Relative amounts of various nutrients in human and cow's milk, with amount in human milk represented as 100% and solid bars representing amount in cow's milk. (Based on data from Composition of human milk, Publication No. 254, Washington, D. C., 1953, National Academy of Sciences–National Research Council.)

milk of another species should be modified to approximate the composition of the maternal milk.

The difference in nutritive composition of human and cow's milk is well documented and is presented in Fig. 17-1. These data show that breast milk contains more of some nutrients and less of others. The absolute amounts for some nutrients are given in Table 16-7, which includes a comparison of colostrum and mature milk. The lower

concentration of some nutrients, such as calcium and protein, in breast milk is believed to reflect the differing growth needs between the human infant and the calf. The latter doubles its birth weight in two months, compared to the human infant, which takes five months. Not only does the total amount of some nutrients differ but also the physicochemical properties of the form in which they exist. For instance, human milk, in which the protein is predominately lactalbumin, contains only half as much protein as cow's milk, in which most of the protein is in the form of casein. Casein forms a hard curd when subjected to the action of rennin in the stomach, whereas lactalbumin forms a soft flocculent curd on which digestive enzymes act freely and which leaves the stomach faster. Fatty acids in human milk are less saturated, have 10 to 14 carbon chains, and are utilized more effectively than are the short-chain, more saturated fatty acids in cow's milk. Ninety-five percent of human milk fat is retained compared to 61% of butterfat. The caloric value of the two milks is similar, as is the total fat content. The lower protein is compensated for by a higher amount of lactose in human milk. Fat provides 50%, protein 7%, and carbohydrate 43% of the calories in human milk compared to 50%, 20%, and 30%, respectively, in cow's milk.

The disaccharide lactose found in both human and cow's milk is present at a higher level in human milk. Lactose has several advantages in infant feeding over other carbohydrates in that it facilitates the absorption of calcium and magnesium and favors amino acid absorption and nitrogen retention. The addition of lactose to modified cow's milk formulas is generally not practical because of its high cost and low solubility. Some evidence exists also that lactose favors riboflavin and pyridoxine synthesis, although it may be of little benefit to the infant if it occurs in the lower gastrointestinal tract.

Infants fed human milk are afforded a high degree of protection against the accumulation of strontium in the body. Cow's milk, with a strontium content six times that of human milk, leads to doubling of body strontium by 1 month.

The amount of the heat-labile vitamins thiamin and ascorbic acid found in human milk is almost completely available to the infant, whereas the amount available from cow's milk may be substantially reduced from the application of heat in the pasteurization of milk and sterilization of the formula.

One unidentified factor in human milk has been designated as the *Lactobacillus bifidus* factor, since it creates a medium in the gastrointestinal tract conducive to the growth of the microorganism *Lactobacillus bifidus*. This microorganism, by producing acetic or lactic acid from lactose, depresses the growth of pathogenic organisms, thus decreasing the susceptibility to infection. It is postulated that the factor in human milk is lactulose, a derivative of lactose known to occur in large amounts in breast milk and in higher amounts in heat-treated than untreated cow's milk. The growth of *L. bifidus* is enhanced on a high-lactose, low-protein diet with a lactose-protein ratio of 7:1 to 4:1.

The presence of a protein-splitting enzyme in breast milk reduces proteins to the less complex peptone stage, on which digestive enzymes act more effectively. These enzymes in cow's milk are destroyed by the heat of pasteurization.

Colostrum, the secretion of the breast that precedes the secretion of mature milk, differs from milk in appearance and nutritional properties. This watery yellowish fluid is believed to contribute a high degree of *passive immunity* to the infant consuming it because its antibodies are absorbed intact during the first few days of life. Considerable evidence indicates that it contains a poliomyelitis antibody. Agreement is not universal regarding the nutritive value of colostrum. Between the fifth and tenth day, colostrum undergoes changes in chemical and physical composition until by the tenth day it has usually assumed the characteristics of mature milk.

Psychological. The psychological advantages of breast-feeding have been freely discussed but are poorly documented. The consensus of opinion is that the infant derives a sense of security and belonging in the early mother-child relationship from the warmth of the mother's body and from the comfort of being held rather than from the feeding process per se. Harlow, in a classical study with monkeys, showed that those fed by a surrogate mother (a bottle inserted in a wire screen covered with warm terry cloth) were equally as well adjusted as those fed by the real mother. Monkeys fed by a bottle alone showed more evidence of emotional instability. Research with dogs and ducks has identified a critical period during the first few days of life when imprinting or learning, which is remarkably resistant to modification, occurs. It may be that the impact of the mother on the child in this critical period will have implications for later development. Although psychologists so far have been unable to elucidate consistent differences in personality between bottle-fed and breast-fed infants, it has been demonstrated that breast-feeding increases a mother's feeling of competence in dealing with her child. It is conceivable that more carefully controlled studies may show effects on personality that have so far largely evaded detection. There is some feeling that the greatest psychological advantages accrue to the mother who feels that she is involved in a unique relationship with the child and is fulfilling her true maternal role.

Other factors. Various other advantages have been attributed to breast-feeding. Since the work of obtaining milk from the breast is much more difficult than from most bottles, it is believed that the use required of muscles of the mouth leads to the development of the jaw and reduces the incidence of crowded dentition in later years. Others maintain that the hormonal balance, especially the secretion of oxytocin that exists in lactation, favors the contraction of the uterus, thus speeding the return of the mother's abdomen to normal size. The reduced likelihood of contamination, the elimination of the possibility of mistakes in mixing the formula, or the necessity of finding a satisfactory formula are

more salient factors favoring breast-feeding among the less well-educated segment of the population and in developing countries than they are for the intelligent middle-class mother. However, a mistake in the preparation of infant formula in a hospital when salt was used instead of sugar became a tragic example of the possibility of human error in preparing a formula. The incidence of infection is generally lower in breast-fed than in bottle-fed infants, as reflected in lower morbidity rates.

The growth rate of breast-fed infants exceeds that of bottle-fed infants for the first four to five months of life, after which bottle-fed infants experience a more rapid growth rate. No differences between the two groups can be ascertained at 2 years of age. The use of breast milk virtually eliminates the possibility of a milk allergy, whereas reports on the incidence of cow's milk allergy range from 0.3% to 7% of artificially fed infants. One explanation of the increased incidence of "cot deaths" among infants is that it represents an allergic reaction after the aspiration of cow's milk protein regurgitated during sleep by a bottle-fed infant who apparently was sensitized to cow's milk protein in the first few months.

Considerations favoring bottle-feeding

Available substitute. The availability of safe and satisfactory preparations in which cow's milk has been modified to provide a satisfactory substitute for human milk leads many mothers to choose bottle-feeding. To be most satisfactory, cow's milk must be modified so that it resembles human milk as closely as possible in composition and in physiochemical properties. The dilution of cow's milk to provide a concentration of protein similar to that of human milk also causes a reduction in curd tension and leads to the formation of a softer, more flocculent curd that can be more readily handled by the proteolytic enzymes in the gastrointestinal tract of the infant. Other methods of modifying the character of the curd that are sometimes used in place of or in addition to dilution include the use of pancreatic enzymes, heat treatment, the addition of an acid such as citric acid or acid-producing microorganisms, or the addition of alkali in the preparation of infant formulas. One method seems to have little advantage over another. The dilution of milk has the advantage of creating a calcium concentration more nearly approximating human milk and the disadvantage of reducing the caloric value from a normal level of 22 kcal. per ounce. The addition of a soluble and readily utilizable carbohydrate such as dextromaltose or sucrose can raise the caloric value to that of human milk. The lower level of sodium deemed desirable to reduce the burden on the kidney through which sodium is excreted in the urine can be achieved by removing much of the electrolyte by dialysis, a method sometimes employed in commercial formula preparation. This is especially important when fluid losses are high due to excessive heat or diarrhea. Other processors have attempted to simulate the higher linoleic content of human milk by replacing the butterfat (short-chain saturated fatty acids) with corn oil (long-chain unsaturated fatty acids). Fat in this form is tolerated better by the infant and provides more adequate levels of the essential fatty acid linoleic acid. Substitution of butterfat with coconut oil is no improvement. The use of too high a level of polyunsaturated fatty acids, however, increases the need for vitamin E. No satisfactory substitute for the colostrum provided by the human breast has been found.

The safety of bottle-feeding has increased with increasing awareness of the importance of aseptic techniques in the preparation of infant formula. Sterilization of feeding equipment and formula has reduced the transmission of pathogenic organisms and the resulting disease. Prior to the discovery of microorganisms as the cause of disease, the hazards of bottle-feeding were so great that infant mortality and morbidity rates were considerably higher than those for breast-feeding. Some reports still indicate a markedly higher mortality and morbidity rate in bottle-fed infants than in breast-fed infants, but among infants born to middle-class mothers in technologically developed countries there generally is no significant difference. The use of expensive but bacteriologically safe preprepared sterilized formulas in disposable bottles is increasing, offering advantages of convenience and safety to those who can afford them.

Psychological. Many mothers experience psychological blocks concerning breast-feeding. These range from considering it a bovine function to considering it a form of "uneating." Others are unwilling to risk breast-feeding for fear that their figures may become permanently distorted and that it will take longer to return to a prepregnancy weight. Neither belief has been adequately documented. If the mother lacks the desire to breast-feed, the chances of it succeeding are greatly reduced. Positive maternal attitudes are highly correlated with successful lactation. Some studies found that mothers chose bottle-feeding because they needed to see the amount of milk the child was consuming.

Economic. According to a study conducted by the Maternal and Child Health section of the American Public Health Association, the cost of the increased amount of food required by the mother to provide the recommended 1000 kcal., 0.5 gm. of calcium, and 40 gm. of high-quality protein needed over and above that suggested for the nonpregnant, nonlactating woman is higher than the cost of the 1 quart of milk needed by the infant. On a moderate-cost diet they believed that the addition of a quart of milk, 6 ounces of orange juice, 2 slices of whole-wheat bread, ½ ounce of butter, and an egg would provide the added nutrients at a cost of 41 cents. On a low-cost food budget they considered the use of ¼ pound of nonfat milk solids, 2 ounces of cooking oil, an ounce of enriched cornmeal, ⅓ pound of turnip greens, and a vitamin supplement every other day at a total cost of 15 cents. The cost of these relatively simple additions to the diet is about equal to the 15 cents suggested by the same committee as the cost of a modified evaporated milk formula. Commercially prepared formulas in which the milk has been adequately modified to simulate human milk cost approximately 25 cents per day. The cost of equipment such as bottles and sterilizers has not been included.

Social. For many mothers the freedom and flexibility for professional and social life that bottle-feeding affords is an overriding consideration in the choice. In fact, among 55 mothers who had had a satisfying breast-feeding experience, the loss of freedom and restriction of their social life were considered disadvantages by 29. Most of these mothers had found, however, that an occasional bottle could be substituted

with no adverse reaction from the child, although the mother may have experienced physical discomfort from the engorgement of the breast.

Disadvantages of breast-feeding

Since a fairly high percentage of mothers choose not to breast-feed, there must be some objections or disadvantages to it. Among these are the failure of the mother to secrete adequate milk, the constant fatigue reported by many mothers, the lack of freedom, the impossibility of turning the responsibility over to someone else, the possibility of breast infection, and a desire to quickly restore the mother's figure to normal.

From a physiological point of view the transmission of the hormone pregnanediol through the mother's milk, resulting in hyperbilirubinemia in the infant has been reported. Recent reports express concern over high levels of DDT and other environmental contaminants in human milk.

For some mothers a failure to recognize

Table 17-1. Recommended dietary allowances for infants°

Nutrient	Age (months)			
	0-2	2-6	6-12	12-24
Kilocalories	wt. (kg.) × 1.20	wt. (kg.) × 110	wt. (kg.) × 100	1100
Protein (gm.)	wt. (kg.) × 2.2	wt. (kg.) × 2.0	wt. (kg.) × 1.8	25
Calcium (mg.)	0.4	0.5	0.6	0.7
Iron (mg.)	6	10	15	15
Iodine (μg.)	25	40	45	55
Magnesium (mg.)	40	60	70	100
Vitamin A (I.U.)	1500	1500	1500	2000
Vitamin D (I.U.)	400	400	400	400
Vitamin E (I.U.)	5	5	5	10
Ascorbic acid (mg.)	35	35	35	40
Folacin (mg.)	0.05	0.05	0.1	0.1
Niacin (mg.)	5	7	8	8
Riboflavin (mg.)	0.4	0.5	0.6	0.6
Thiamin (mg.)	0.2	0.4	0.5	0.6
Pyridoxine (mg.)	0.2	0.3	0.4	0.5
Vitamin B$_{12}$ (μg.)	1	1.5	2	2

From Food and Nutrition Board: Recommended dietary allowances, ed. 7, Publication No. 1694, Washington, D. C., 1968, National Academy of Science–National Research Council.

that the onset of lactation may be delayed until three to five days after birth and that the physical appearance of colostrum is different from milk and that their milk has not "turned to water" may explain their decision to abandon attempts at breast-feeding. The desire of mothers for either economic or psychological reasons to leave the hospital as soon as possible after birth can mean that if lactation is not established shortly after birth, the mother will give up her plans in the interest of taking the infant home on a functioning feeding routine, that is, bottle-feeding.

Adequacy of milk diet

The NRC recommended allowances for infants are shown in Table 17-1. A diet composed solely of human or cow's milk consumed at a level of approximately 850 ml. per day will provide recommended amounts of all the nutrients needed except ascorbic acid and vitamin D up to 3 months of age. At 3 to 6 months when fetal iron reserves are depleted, milk is incapable of providing sufficient iron to maintain hemoglobin level.

Ascorbic acid is a limiting factor only for bottle-fed infants whose formula is subjected to high heat during processing. These infants should receive a supplementary source of ascorbic acid by the tenth day of life. After the discovery of antiscorbutic properties of oranges, orange juice was fed as a source of vitamin C, starting with 1 teaspoon of juice diluted with an equal amount of water and building up to about 2 tablespoons of juice. With an increasing number of reports of allergic reactions, apparently from the oil of the orange rind which was extracted with the juice, a trend occurred toward the use of a synthetic source of ascorbic acid that minimized any sensitizing reaction. This is a general practice in the first few months of life, after which the child can be given a fruit juice high in ascorbic acid. Evidence exists that infants born to mothers who had

an extremely high ascorbic acid intake during pregnancy have a conditioned need for a high level of the vitamin.

The amount of vitamin D in either human or cow's milk is to some extent a function of the diet of the mother or cow but even under ideal conditions does not approach the 400 I.U. recommended by the Food and Nutrition Board of the National Research Council. Thus, unless a child has regular exposure to sunlight, it is necessary to provide a vitamin D supplement, preferably by 5 days of age. Cod-liver oil, the most popular source after the discovery of its antirachitic properties in promoting normal calcification of bones and teeth, has been replaced by water-miscible preparations to avoid the danger of lipoid pneumonia from the aspiration of the oily particles of cod-liver oil into the lungs. If, however, a bottle-fed infant is given a prepared formula or a formula made with evaporated or homogenized milk, which is normally fortified with 400 I.U. of vitamin D per quart, no supplementation is necessary. In the light of current reports of toxic reactions caused by the use of diets high in vitamin D such supplementation is likely undesirable.

The low level of iron in milk is not a cause of concern, since infants are born with a reserve of iron in the liver to meet their needs for three to six months. It does, however, seem appropriate to add some source of iron to the diet by 3 to 6 months of age to prevent a drop in hemoglobin levels to a level of less than 10 gm. per 100 ml. of blood—a level considered indicative of anemia. Many commercial formula preparations are now fortified with iron. Since a drop in hemoglobin level from the 18 gm. characteristic of birth levels is normal and the body absorbs virtually no iron until a need for it occurs, the supplementation of formula in the early weeks of life appears unnecessary. One study of the use of a formula supplemented with vitamins and iron (12 mg. per 32 ounces) produced no differences in growth and development, in number of illnesses, or in hemoglobin, hematocrit, or serum iron levels up to 3 to 3½ months of age. The blood values were higher after this time when the iron-fortified formula was used. Another extensive study of the use of iron-enriched formula from birth suggests that its use does provide a protection against subsequent drop in hemoglobin levels by maintaining hemoglobin levels 1 to 1.5 gm. higher at 9 months of age. Whether the infant's mechanism for regulating iron absorption is sufficiently sensitive to prevent the uptake of excess iron that leads to iron overload when it is fed prior to a time of need has not been investigated.

Temperature of milk

The question of the temperature of a milk feeding has been raised. Several investigators have contended that formula from the refrigerator is well tolerated by 50% of very young infants and 75% of older infants and gives as good a growth response as that which has been warmed to body temperature. Research indicates that feeding ice-cold milk lowered gastric temperature for at least an hour, decreased the activity of proteolytic enzymes, and hence delayed digestion.

Concentration of milk

Human milk in which fat provides about 50% of the calories can be consumed in sufficient volume to meet the energy needs of the infant. When fat provides less than 15% of the energy, the infant cannot take sufficient milk, and if he does, he may be susceptible to water intoxication when his fluid intake exceeds the kidney's capacity to excrete it. When the caloric concentration of the feeding increases, the infant is unable to decrease its intake accordingly and may eat in excess of its needs. If less than 20% of the calories come from fat, an increased proportion will come from protein. This may result in an excessive renal solute load because of the need to excrete the urea formed from the deamination of the protein.

Nutritive needs of infants

Precise information on the nutritive needs of infants is available for only a few nutrients, but the National Research Council has suggested levels of intake that appear to support growth in healthy infants.

Energy. An intake of 120 kcal. per kilogram of body weight or 54 kcal. per pound appears to be adequate to meet the needs for maintaining body temperature, for growth, and for activity for the first two months. Since the body surface area of infants per unit of body weight is twice as great as that of adults, the insensible heat loss from the surface is twice as great. A very placid infant is reported to need as few as 70 kcal. per kilogram, whereas a crying infant may need as many as 130 kcal. By 6 months energy needs have decreased to 100 kcal. per kilogram.

An excessive intake of calories leading to a rapid gain in weight is equally as undesirable in infants as in adults. MacKeith, in discussing the question "Is a big baby a healthy baby?", suggested that a baby who weighs 27 pounds at 1 year of age is more likely to grow up to be an obese adolescent or adult than is one weighing less. Bakwin has raised the question of a relationship between early feeding of solids, with consequent increase in calories, and subsequent obesity. Hirsch has postulated that the number of adipose, or fat, cells is determined early in life and is proportionately larger in the overfed infant who has a greater need for more cells to store fat. For these infants the regulation of weight in later life is more difficult because of a tendency for these cells to remain filled with fat.

For a newborn infant, milk provides all the calories. Filer reports that by 6 months of age 70% of the energy is still provided by milk, with fruit, providing 10%, and cereal, meat, egg, and vegetables each 5%.

Protein. The needs for protein during the period of very rapid skeletal and muscular growth of early infancy are relatively high. An intake of 2.2 gm. of protein of high biological value per kilogram of body weight supports a nitrogen retention of about 45%, sufficiently great to allow normal growth. The need for protein remains 1.8 gm. per 100 kcal. the level found is breast milk, throughout the first year of life. When this is calculated on the basis of body weight, the requirement drops to 2 gm. from 2 to 6 months and to 1.8 gm. from 6 months to a year. Both these recommendations assume a protein of high biological value such as milk protein. If the child gets an increasing proportion of its protein from sources of lower biological value, as happens when the child receives a progressively higher proportion of his protein from cereal, the total intake should increase. A protein intake providing from 6.5% to 8% of the total dietary calories is capable of meeting the protein requirement, but if it should drop below this, it is very difficult for the child to get enough food to meet his requirement. This is essentially what happens in many developing countries when the child is weaned to a high carbohydrate–low protein diet. There was no difference in nitrogen retention in a group of infants receiving 10% of their calories from protein and a group receiving 15%. Nor were there any differences in the composition of fat-free tissues on low- or high-protein intakes.

There is no evidence of advantages of protein intakes above these levels, and some evidence of disadvantages has been compiled. Infants receiving whole unmodified cow's milk have suffered from a hypochromic macrocytic anemia caused by gastric bleeding leading to large blood losses in the feces, apparently the result of an allergy to the cow's milk protein. The frequency with which other manifestations of a cow's milk allergy are also reported indicates that the high protein content of cow's milk may lead to a protein sensitivity. Protein in excess of the body's need for growth and repair of tissue must undergo deamination in the liver so that the non-amino portion of the amino acids can be used as a source of energy. The nitrogenous NH_2 group must be converted to urea and must be excreted through the kidney. Since the infant has a limited capacity to concentrate metabolites in the urine, the excretion of more wastes requires a larger volume of water. If the necessary water is not available, urea will accumulate and the infant ironically suffers from protein edema. In addition, the need for the liver to produce the enzymes (deaminases) that are necessary to remove the amino group may lead to an undesirable hypertrophy or increase in size of the liver.

It is also postulated that the higher rate of infection in infants fed cow's milk may occur because mechanisms that may normally be concerned with the formation of antibodies are used to combat foreign milk protein.

In rats it was found that the animals on a high-protein diet who had had hypertrophy of the liver were less able to adjust to a low-protein diet than were those that had previously been on a moderate- or low-protein diet.

Studies to evaluate the relative biological value of meat and milk proteins have shown similar protein efficiency ratios (gain per unit of protein). Both meat and milk protein are well tolerated in the digestive tract, and infants appear to have adequate proteolytic enzymes to handle meat protein and milk protein if the curd tension is adequately reduced.

The amino acid requirements of infants are proportionately higher than those in adults. In addition to the eight amino acids needed by adults, histidine is required by infants at < 35 mg. per kilogram of body weight per day, a level surpassed in both breast- and bottle-feeding.

In one study of 6-month-old infants it

was found that 70% of the protein in the diet came from milk, 15% from meat, and 3% each from egg, cereal, and vegetables.

Thiamin. Although studies based on the thiamin intake from human milk or formula and on urinary excretion data indicate that the minimum requirement is 0.2 mg. per 1000 kcal., the recommended dietary allowance has been set at 0.5 mg. per 1000 kcal. Breast milk is usually adequate if the mother's diet is adequate, but thiamin is one nutrient for which the mother does not reduce the quantity of milk rather than produce a milk of lower nutritional quality. This has been observed primarily in developing countries where cereals and starchy roots are eaten, where the diet of the mother is high in carbohydrate and very low in thiamin, and where infants are solely breast-fed for a year or more. Infants fed such milk low in thiamin failed to gain weight, were constipated, and vomited frequently. In bottle-fed infants the possibility of a deficiency of heat-labile thiamin occurs when the formula is subjected to high heat.

Attempts to show that thiamin is beneficial as an appetite stimulant have failed to reveal any value in infant feeding, nor have scientists been able to demonstrate any benefit from thiamin supplementation on height, weight, manual dexterity, or retentive memory. It is conceded that once the metabolic defect caused by a thiamin deficiency has been corrected, the appetite improves.

In infants from 6 months to 2 years of age, diet records showed that those infants whose diets were adequate in thiamin were receiving enriched cereals, whereas those who did not receive adequate thiamin were not receiving enriched cereals.

Riboflavin. The recommendation that infants receive 0.1 mg. riboflavin per unit (weight in kg. ¾) of metabolic size to maintain tissue saturation means that an infant up to 2 months of age needs 0.4 mg. and by 6 to 12 months needs 0.6 mg. Human milk with 0.04 mg. per 100 ml. will provide slightly below this amount in the usual 850 ml. available for the newborn.

Niacin. The recommended intake of 5 to 8 niacin equivalents for the infant can be met by human milk, which provides 0.17 mg. of niacin and 22 mg. of tryptophan, or a total of 0.5 niacin equivalents per 100 ml. of milk. This amounts to slightly more than the 6.6 equivalents per 1000 kcal. recommended for adults.

Pyridoxine. The National Research Council recommends an intake of 0.2 mg. up to 2 months of age, 0.3 mg. from 2 to 6 months of age, and 0.4 mg. from 6 to 12 months. They are not concerned about the fact that human milk contains only 0.02 mg. per 1000 ml. by the end of the first month of life, increasing to 0.1 mg., since the infant has a sufficient store of pyridoxine at birth to protect him against a diet practically devoid of the nutrient. If the pyridoxine content of mother's milk fails to increase above 0.06 or 0.08 mg. per liter, as will happen if the mother is undernourished, then clinical and biochemical abnormalities may appear as the protein content of the diet continues to increase to the point where it overtaxes the infant's supply of pyridoxine to metabolize it. The fact that infants are susceptible to a vitamin B_6 deficiency became evident when infants receiving proprietary preparations that had been subjected to very high heat (which destroyed the pyridoxine) developed convulsive seizures. As a result, the pyridoxine content of infant formulas is now maintained at a level to provide either 0.015 mg. per gram of protein or 0.04 mg. per 100 kcal., which will satisfy the metabolic requirements of the infant. An evaluation of commercially prepared infant foods showed that they contained a sufficient proportion of the vitamin in relation to the amount of protein that they provided.

Folacin. The National Research Council states that the infant probably needs from 0.005 to 0.02 mg. of folacin per day but sets the recommended dietary allowance at 0.05 mg. for the newborn and 0.1 mg. for the

6- to 12-month-old baby. Since folic acid deficiency is considered rather general among pregnant women, the reserves with which the infant enters life may be minimal.

Cobalamin. It appears that the infant is parasitic on the mother in respect to cobalamin, since the infant at birth has blood levels approximately twice that of the mother. Although the daily intake of vitamin B_{12} from human milk is only 0.15 to 0.25 μg., the recommended dietary allowance during the first year of life ranges from 1 to 2 μg. per day. However, because of the reserves established during the prenatal period, little likelihood of a deficiency exists.

There have been several reports and many claims in advertising that cobalamin acts as a growth stimulant. The Academy of Pediatrics, in reviewing the literature on the subject, found that in thirteen studies involving 546 "normal children," only two studies involving 69 children reported a significant and stimulating effect on growth with either oral or intramuscular doses of cobalamin. In all these the children were underweight at the beginning.

Ascorbic acid. Infant needs for ascorbic acid have been set at 35 mg. per day, although many studies suggest that a much lower level will provide protection against scurvy, and others suggest that the infant may be conditioned to even higher levels. Breast-fed infants usually receive adequate amounts, but because of the destruction of heat-labile ascorbic acid during pasteurization, infants fed cow's milk usually rely on a dietary supplement during the first few months.

Vitamin A. It is assumed that the human infant, like the young of other species, enters life with a reserve of the fat-soluble vitamin A stored in its liver. The amount, however, will be dependent to a large extent on the vitamin A status of the mother. Since little information exists on the vitamin A requirements of infants, the Food and Nutrition Board of the National Research Council recommends that the infant receive the 1500 I.U. of vitamin A, the amount normally supplied in 850 ml. of mother's milk—an amount that is apparently adequate to meet the needs of the first few months of life.

Vitamin D. The need for vitamin D during infancy is well documented. Although as little as 100 I.U. per day will prevent rickets and 300 I.U. per day will cure the condition, the ingestion of 400 I.U. per day promotes good calcium absorption and skeletal growth. Intakes above this apparently have no advantage, and at levels beyond 1800 I.U. a decrease in calcium utilization may occur. Since human milk does not provide the recommended level of vitamin D, a supplement should be provided in the first week of life. For bottle-fed babies the supplement will be necessary only if the milk or formula is not itself fortified with the vitamin. In fact, concern is being expressed for the infant who consistently receives in excess of 2000 I.U. per day, since excess intake leads to such symptoms as depressed appetite, vague aches and pains, and retarded growth.

Vitamin E. Since little vitamin E crosses the placenta, human infants are born with low concentrations in the tissues. An intake of 5 mg. of vitamin E is advised during the first year of life. Only when large amounts of unsaturated vegetable fats are substituted for the butterfat will the need for vitamin E increase.

Calcium. Because of the rapid rate of calcification of bone to provide the rigidity and strength needed to support the weight of the body by the time the baby walks, a very rich dietary source of calcium is needed in early infancy. Milk, the staple item in the diet at this time, is capable of providing the infant's needs, but the efficiency with which it is used is greatly enhanced when vitamin D is available simultaneously. Although some calcification of teeth has begun in the prenatal period, the availability and utilization of calcium in the postnatal period is a crucial factor in adequate tooth formation.

Breast milk provides about 60 mg. of calcium per kilogram, which is apparently adequate because the high retention may amount to as much as two thirds of the intake. The recommended allowances of 400 to 600 mg. per day are intended only for the bottle-fed infant who receives about 170 mg. per kilogram of weight but retains only one third to one half of it.

Phosphorus. The calcium to phosphorus ratio of 1.2:1 found in cow's milk is considered too low for the young infant, who has difficulty excreting the relatively high phosphorus. This imbalance may result in a hypocalcemic, neonatal tetany, an even greater problem if the retention of calcium is depressed. Thus it is recommended that the calcium to phosphorus ratio in an infant's diet at least be kept at 1.5:1, gradually decreasing in later infancy to a ratio closer to that in cow's milk. On the other hand, studies by Widdowson have shown beneficial effects on the absorption of calcium and magnesium when breast-fed infants were given supplements of 120 mg. of phosphorus per day, suggesting that the calcium to phosphorus ratio of 2:1 in breast milk may limit calcification of bone and growth of soft tissue at an early age.

Iron. The infant's need for iron is determined to a large extent by his gestational age. Normally a full-term infant has benefitted from the transfer of a significant amount of iron from the mother to the fetus. If such reserves from fetal life are present, the infant will need virtually no dietary iron for at least 3 months. In fact, if it is added to the milk, very little will be absorbed before 3 to 4 months of age, when a drop in hemoglobin level reflects depletion of reserves in the liver. By that time an intake of 10 mg. per day is recommended. This may be obtained from enriched cereal or egg yolk and later on from meat.

The premature infant with a shorter gestational period is deprived of these fetal reserves and will need a dietary source earlier. The same is true of twins, who must compete for maternal reserves and share that available. As much as 2 mg. per kilogram may be needed shortly after birth by low–birth weight infants (less than 2500 grams).

Dietary allowances are based on an average need of 1.5 mg. per kilogram per day, although evidence exists that a normal full-term infant can maintain optimal hemoglobin levels on an intake of 1 mg. per kilogram. The intake of 15 mg. recommended from 6 to 12 months of age can be obtained only through the use of fortified food products. Infant cereals have traditionally been fortified at a level of about 12 mg. per ounce. More recently the use of iron-fortified formulas has been advocated.

Fluorine. Fluorine, which has been established as a dietary essential, is mentioned in a discussion of infant feeding because of the beneficial effects in providing resistance to tooth decay that accrue when fluorine is present during the period of calcification of dental tissues. If the mother is using fluoridated water, it will be reflected in the level of fluorine in the breast milk. Bottle-fed babies whose formulas are diluted with fluoridated water will also receive protection. Since infants normally consume little water in the first few months, it is likely desirable to provide it in some supplement.

Water or fluid. Although the intake of water is crucial at all stages in the life cycle, it receives a little more attention in infancy than at other times because the demands are relatively greater then. The surface area per unit of body weight is twice that of the adult, which leads to a heat and water loss through the skin at a rate almost double that of the adult. Because of the high basal metabolic rate (two times that of an adult) proportionately more metabolic wastes occur, which calls for more water so that the kidney can adequately excrete them. This, coupled with the fact that the kidney of an infant does not have the ability to concentrate urine to the extent that a mature kidney does, means that relatively more water is required in the elimination of the same amount of metabolites. The metabolic waste is higher on a diet high in protein when the nitrogen from the deamination of amino acids in excess of needs for growth must be eliminated. More water is also required if the diet contains excess electrolytes such as sodium and potassium. An infant receiving a diet of human milk requires 20 ml. of water per kilogram of body weight to provide a sufficient amount for the kidney to handle excretory products. If undiluted cow's milk is used, 87 ml. is required, and if cow's milk, with one third of the calories coming from added carbohydrate, is used, 61 ml. At a normal room temperature of 70° F., any one of these formulas would provide enough water, but at 93° F. the cow's milk would not provide enough when proportionately more water is lost through the skin. If normal excretion of metabolic waste is to occur, additional water should be given. Even with a formula providing the normal 20 kcal. per ounce, parents should offer the child additional water when the environmental temperature is high. Body water will be reduced to 70% of normal before influencing the renal excretion of water.

INTRODUCTION OF SOLID FOODS

At the turn of the century, pediatricians were recommending that the milk diet of infants be supplemented with a food such as meat or cereal after 1 year of age. By 1917 Dr. Emmett Holt was suggesting that a meat broth could safely be introduced at 8 or 9 months of age but that solid foods should be withheld until 1 year. By 1956 the pendulum had swung so far in the opposite direction that some pediatricians were recommending that an infant could be put on solid foods and be expected to adhere to three meals a day by 2 or 3 weeks of age. The Academy of Pediatrics, recognizing a trend in infant feeding practices toward progressively earlier introduction of solid foods in the absence of any evidence of a nutritional or physiological need, surveyed practicing pediatricians to determine their recommendations and the bases for them. It found that the physicians were indeed suggesting the use of cereal by 3 to 6 weeks of age, followed by other foods so that by 4 or 5 months the child had received a full diet of meat, eggs, fruit, vegetables, and cereal. Their reasons for this practice reflected their response to the demands of mothers that they follow this "progressive" procedure rather than to any belief that the infant needed the solid food. The advertising by commercial companies marketing special infant foods is also a contributing factor to the mother's anxiety to conform to what she believes to be sound eating habits.

A rational approach to the question of the timing and sequence of additions to the infant's diet should involve consideration of the nutritional needs of the infant, his physiological readiness to use foods other than milk, his physical capacity to handle them, and the relative advantages and disadvantages of adding semisolid or solid foods.

Nutrition. From a nutritional standpoint it has been established that the nutritive needs of an infant can be readily met for the first three months by a milk diet supplemented with sources of ascorbic acid and vitamin D. Since these are normally provided by the use of a vitamin preparation or by the addition of orange juice and cod-liver oil, the provision of these nutrients involves only the use of liquids. By 3 months of age it is desirable to provide some rich source of iron, since milk is a poor source and fetal reserves begin to be depleted at this age. This may be provided in several foods. The most usual method is to use an iron-enriched cereal, which contributes 12 mg. per ounce, or 0.92 mg. per tablespoon. If fed as a single-grain cereal, these cereals are minimally allergenic, and the consistency can be readily adjusted to the infant's ability to handle it. Egg yolk, a rich source of iron (1 mg.), vitamin A, protein, and riboflavin, is recommended by many investigators, although there is no consistent evidence that it promotes hematopoiesis more effectively than cereal does. It is likely unwise to use egg for infants with a family history of allergy, since the high protein may evoke a reaction in sensitive individuals. Meat, providing 0.23 mg. per tablespoon, has also been recommended, but again, in the absence of any evidence of unique benefits it is generally conceded that meat should be added later. Fruits and vegetables (0.05 to 0.32 mg. per tablespoon) may be used as a source of iron, although the concentration is lower than that in meat, cereal, or egg yolk. Some efforts are being made to promote the iron enrichment of milk on the theory that the iron should be provided by the major source of calories, especially among poor families who may be able to provide only a limited variety of foods.

With the increase in size of the infant it becomes increasingly difficult to meet the protein needs for growth on a diet of milk alone. By 6 months of age most infants are able to tolerate whole milk with its protein content of 3.2%. In addition to this, other dietary sources of complete protein are recommended; egg yolk with 33% protein, meat with 20%, and cottage cheese with 17% are considered suitable additions to the diet by 6 months of age.

Foods that provide the additional iron and protein needed by the growing child usually meet any additional needs for thiamin and niacin.

Physical development. Infants vary in the rate at which the normal rooting, sucking, and extrusion reflexes inherent at the time of birth are replaced by the ability to swallow; and as these changes occur,

an infant must learn to use them in the eating process, just as he learns to walk or talk. The lower jaw is very poorly developed at birth to facilitate sucking, but as the infant matures, he becomes better developed and better prepared for chewing functions. The swallowing reflex involves sufficient innervation of the tongue to enable it to form any solid food placed at the tip of the tongue into a ball and throw it to the back of the mouth, where first gravity and then the peristaltic action of the esophagus take over to convey it to the stomach. This ability usually develops at 3 months of age, but before this the extrusion reflex that causes the infant to forcibly reject food or objects placed at the front of the tongue must diminish in strength. Since the ability to move food from the tip of the tongue to the throat normally develops at 2½ to 3 months of age, any effort to feed solid or semisolid foods prior to that time means that some other way must be employed to convey the food to the esophagus. Either it must be placed sufficiently far back in the mouth that it can reach the esophagus by gravity, or the consistency of the product must be so thin that it is merely a semisolid food and the infant is able to suck it from the spoon as a liquid, rather than using a swallowing mechanism. Many times the infant who cannot manipulate the tongue to swallow cannot use it to reject objects or food placed in his mouth either. Thus it is not uncommon to have mothers report that infants who had apparently accepted solid food at 3 to 6 weeks of age appear to reject it at 10 to 12 weeks. Developmentally few infants are ready to handle anything but liquid food until 10 to 12 weeks of age. Any effort to force them earlier may result in a frustrating and unhappy feeding experience for both the mother and the child.

Physiological development. The ability to handle foods other than milk also depends on the physiological development of the infant. All the secretions of the digestive tract contain enzymes especially suited to the digestion of the complex nutrients of milk but few needed for other foods.

For instance, the secretion of the salivary glands is minimal at birth but increases in volume until it becomes sufficiently copious to cause drooling by 2 or 3 months. This is evident in the infant who has not developed the innervation of the outer part of the lips necessary to prevent it. Since salivary enzymes are involved only in the digestion of the complex starches, they are unnecessary as long as the child is receiving only milk with the disaccharide lactose as the only carbohydrate. The appearance of salivary amylase in the saliva between 2 and 3 months of age marks the time when the infant is first ready to handle more complex carbohydrates such as the starch in cereals.

The proteolytic enzymes are present in adequate amounts to digest milk protein as long as it is sufficiently dilute to produce a soft flocculent curd on which the enzymes can act. As the child matures, the secretion of proteolytic enzymes in the intestinal juice increases this capacity of the infant to digest nonmilk proteins. By 4 to 6 months of age, most infants are able to handle most proteins.

The kidney function of the full-term infant is not completely mature. The well-developed glomeruli satisfactorily filter the blood presented to the kidney, but the tubules, which are functionally less mature, are unable to resorb water and some solutes adequately. The tubules become efficient by 6 to 8 weeks, after which there is less concern over the use of a high-protein, high-sodium diet.

Other considerations. Many reasons have been advanced either to support or to reject the introduction of solid foods from 2 to 8 weeks of age. The belief of many mothers that they can hasten the time at which the infant sleeps through the night has not been corroborated by experimental data when the criterion of 8 consecutive hours of sleep was considered "sleeping through the night."

One must also consider that if the infant does sleep through the night at an early age, he must either experience a reduction in total food intake or consume larger amounts at each of the remaining feedings, thus taxing the capacity of the stomach. Some scientists have expressed fear that such a pattern of overeating at an early age may persist throughout life and be a possible factor in obesity of children and adolescents. Such obesity of early onset is one of the most difficult types to treat.

One study to determine the effect of the addition of solid foods on the nutritive intake of infants showed that in the first two months solid foods were consumed in such small amounts that they had little influence on the nutritive adequacy of the diet. Later, when more food was eaten, it tended to replace milk rather than be used in addition to it. This corresponds with the findings that showed the volume of milk increased with body weight from 3 to 5 kg. but remained stationary as weight increased from 5 to 7 kg. after 3 months of age.

Since the nutritive value of the solid food consumed in the first few months is usually of minimum significance, the major argument in favor of its use is that the child becomes accustomed early to a wider variety of flavors and textures of food and continues to accept these as he matures. Beal found that the age at which a child accepted solid foods did not parallel an advancement in the age at which the food was offered. As a result, she reported a period during which the child and mother experienced an unpleasant feeding relationship, with the mother trying to feed an infant who was not yet ready for the food. She believed that the forcible feeding of semisolids before the ninth to twelfth weeks tended to increase the incidence of feeding problems and food dislikes in the infant. The relationship between the age of intro-

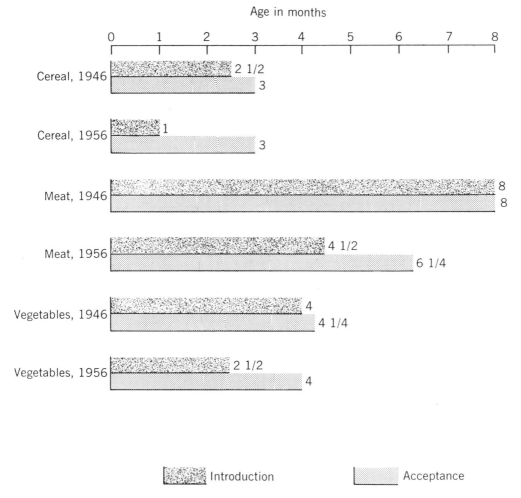

Age in months

Cereal, 1946 — 2 1/2 / 3
Cereal, 1956 — 1 / 3
Meat, 1946 — 8 / 8
Meat, 1956 — 4 1/2 / 6 1/4
Vegetables, 1946 — 4 / 4 1/4
Vegetables, 1956 — 2 1/2 / 4

Introduction   Acceptance

Fig. 17-2. Comparison age of introduction of solid food and acceptance between 1946 and 1956. (Based on Beal, V. A.: Pediatrics **20**:448, 1957.)

duction of solid foods and their acceptance is shown in Fig. 17-2.

Although findings in the literature are not unanimous, many studies report an increased incidence of food allergy among infants who are introduced to a variety of foods at an early age. This is an especially important consideration among infants with a family history of allergy. For these, allergists suggest delaying the time of initial introduction of solid foods and choosing foods that are minimally allergenic, such as vegetables, fruits, and rice cereal. They

also advise feeding each food for a relatively short time and then switching to another to avoid the sensitization that may arise from prolonged exposure to one food.

As discussed earlier, if the added food is high in protein, deaminating the protein in excess of needs and excreting the urea are necessary, which calls for an increase in urine volume. This can be a problem, especially at high environmental temperatures; if it fails, the electrolytes will be retained with resulting edema.

Gyorgy recognizes that the extrusion or

"thrust" reflex is innate to normal infants, but that it may be suppressed by prolonged spoon-feeding. He suggests that the inhibition of this natural defense mechanism might lead to frustration and mental insult, finally manifesting itself in a neurotic reaction.

In addition to an immaturity of secretion of digestive enzymes, the young infant has low levels of many cellular enzymes. One that has been known for some time is phenylalanine hydroxylase, which is required for the metabolism of phenylalanine. A diet high in protein in the neonatal period will tax the infant's ability to tolerate the amino acid phenylalanine.

Concern over the safety of food additives in infant foods has focussed on the use of salt (sodium chloride) and monosodium glutamate. Both are added to many commercially prepared infant foods, primarily to make them more palatable to the mother who is feeding them, rather than to the child who is eating them. Since no physiological or nutritional reason exists for adding them, as long as the question regarding their safety remains unresolved, in 1970 the National Academy of Sciences recommended to the Food and Drug Administration that the level of salt in infant foods be restricted to 0.25% in contrast to the 1% found in many commercially prepared products. The concern about the use of salt centers around the theory that the young infant with an immature kidney cannot cope with the increased electrolyte that must be excreted and retains it, with the resultant increase in fluid volume and the potential of becoming predisposed to hypertension. The sodium intake of an infant of 4 months of age may be three times the recommended level if he is eating a full complement of baby foods, many of which have salt added or to which mothers add salt. The earlier he begins eating solid foods, the earlier his intake will reach these levels. Studies of the preferences of infants showed that they ate the same amount of food regardless of whether or not salt was added. In the case of monosodium glutamate, a flavor enhancer, the concern arises from reports that mice fed high intakes developed brain tumors. So far there is no evidence of potential danger in the amounts consumed by the young infant.

Additions to the diet. In spite of current trends in infant feeding practices, which show that 90% of infants in the United States are fed solid food before 3 months of age, the Academy of Pediatrics, after a careful consideration of all the factors involved, recommends that the optimal time for introducing solid foods into the infant's diet is 2½ to 3 months of age. They agree that no nutritional or psychological benefit results from any earlier introduction.

Once the child is physically and physiologically capable of handling solid foods, the sequence and timing with which they are introduced should be determined by the nutritional needs of the child. Single-grain cereals are frequently used first because of their iron content, their ease of preparation and storage, and relatively low cost. This is usually followed by a variety of strained fruits and vegetables, with care being taken to avoid those that may be irritating to the gastrointestinal tract either through roughage or the production of gas. Egg yolk, which provides vitamin A, iron, and riboflavin, is frequently used as an early source of protein. By 6 months of age most infants will also be receiving meat. The order of use of foods is not crucial, as is evidenced by the number of patterns on which children thrive. More important is the provision of the nutrients needed to supplement a milk diet in a form suited to the digestive capacities of the child and the formation of a set of eating habits that will lead to good nutrition throughout childhood.

In most infants the eruption of the first teeth and the physical readiness to chew both occur at approximately 5 to 6 months of age. It is very important that the infant be given an opportunity to chew at this critical time in order that this capacity be developed. Dry bread is the most acceptable food to stimulate chewing. Caution should be exerted to avoid the use of hard flintlike materials such as crisp bacon and certain commercial biscuits, which may irritate the throat.

As the infant's digestive capacities de-

velop, the strained foods of early infancy can be replaced by less finely chopped foods, with a final transition to table foods. A wide range is found in the age at which this transition is made in a normal child, and failure of a child to keep up with the neighbor's child in this regard must not be considered prognostic of success in college or on the gridiron.

SELECTED REFERENCES

Andelman, M. B., and Sered, B. R.: Utilization of dietary iron by term infants, Amer. J. Dis. Child. 111:45, 1966.

Athreya, B. H., Coriell, L. L., and Charney, J.: Poliomyelitis antibodies in human colostrum and milk, J. Pediat. 64:79, 1964.

Bakwin, H.: Feeding programs for infants, Fed. Proc. 23:66, 1964.

Beal, V. A.: On the acceptance of solid foods and other food patterns of infants and children, Pediatrics 448, 20:1957.

Beal, V. A.: Breast- and formula-feeding of infants, J. Amer. Diet. Ass. 55:31, 1969.

Beal, V. A., Myers, A. J., and McCammon, R. N.: Iron intake hemoglobin and physical growth during the first two years of life, Pediatrics 30:518, 1962.

Butler, A. M., and Wolman, I. J.: Trends in the early feeding of supplementary foods to infants, Quart. Rev. Pediat. 9:63, 1954.

Call, J. D.: Emotional factors favoring successful breast feeding of infants, J. Pediat. 55:485, 1959.

Cameron, M. E.: The effect of the addition of foods to human milk on the protein value of the infant's diet, Proc. Nutr. Soc. 27:8A, 1968.

Committee on Nutrition, American Academy of Pediatrics: On the feeding of solid foods to infants, Pediatrics 21:685, 1958; Trace elements in infant nutrition, Pediatrics 26:715, 1960; Infantile scurvy and nutritional rickets, Pediatrics 29:646, 1962; The prophylactic requirement and toxicity of vitamin D, Pediatrics 31:512, 1963; Vitamin D intake and the hypercalcemic syndrome, Pediatrics 35:1022, 1965; Proposed changes in Food and Drug Administration regulations concerning formula products and vitamin-mineral dietary supplements for infants, Pediatrics 40:916, 1967; Iron balance and requirements in infancy, Pediatrics 43:134, 1969.

Dahl, L. K., Kesanen, A., and Peltonen, T.: High salt content of western infant's diets, Nature (London) 198:1204, 1963.

Ezekiel, E.: Intestinal iron absorption by neonates and some factors affecting it, J. Lab. Clin. Med. 70:138, 1967.

Farquhar, J. D.: Iron supplementation during first year of life, Amer. J. Dis. Child. 106:201, 1963.

Filer, L. J., Jr., and Martinez, G. A.: Intake of selected nutrients by infants in the United States, Clin. Pediat. 3:633, 1964.

Fomon, S. J., Filer, L. J., Thomas, L. N., Rogers, R. R., and Proksch, A. M.: Relationship between formula concentration and rate of growth of normal infants, J. Nutr. 98:241, 1969.

Fomon, S. J., Owen, G. M., and Thomas, L. N.: Milk or formula volume ingested by infants fed ad libitum, Amer. J. Dis. Child. 108:601, 1964

Fomon, S. J., Thomas, L. N., and Filer, L. J.: Acceptance of unsalted strained foods by normal infants, J. Pediat. 76:242, 1970.

Fraser, D.: The relation between infantile hypercalcemia and vitamin D—public health implications in North America, Pediatrics. 35:1022, 1965.

Grunwaldt, E., Bates, T., and Guthrie, D.: The onset of sleeping through the night in infancy, Pediatrics 26:667, 1960.

Gryboski, J. D.: The swallowing mechanism of the neonate, Pediatrics 35:445, 1965.

Guthrie, H. A.: Nutritional intake of infants, J. Amer. Diet. Ass. 43:120, 1963.

Guthrie, H. A.: Effect of early feeding of solid foods on nutritive intake of infants, Pediatrics 38:879, 1966.

Guthrie, H. A.: Infant feeding practices—a predisposing factor in hypertension? Amer. J. Clin. Nutr. 21:863, 1968.

Gyorgy, P.: Orientation in infant feeding, Fed. Proc. 20(supp. 7):169, 1961.

Gyorgy, P.: The late effects of early nutrition, Amer. J. Clin. Nutr. 8:344, 1961.

Hansen, A. E., Wiese, H. F., Boelsche, A. N., Hoggard, M. E., Adam, D. J., and Davis, H.: Role of linoleic acid in infant nutrition, Pediatrics 31:171, 1963.

Heiner, D. C., Wilson, J. F., and Lahey, M. E.: Sensitivity to cow's milk, J.A.M.A. **189**:563, 1964.

Heseltine, M. M., and Pitts, J. L.: Economy in nutrition and feeding of infants, Amer. J. Pub. Health **56**:1756, 1966.

Hirsch, J., and Knittle, J. L.: The cellularity of obese and nonobese human adipose tissue, Fed. Proc. (In press.)

Holt, L. E., and Snyderman, S. E.: Protein and amino acid requirements of infants and children, Nutr. Abstr. Rev. **35**:1, 1965.

Illingworth, R. S., and Lister, J.: The critical or sensitive period, with special reference to certain feeding problems in infants and children, J. Pediat. **65**:839, 1964.

Jusko, W. J., Khanna, N., Levy, G., Stern, L., and Yaffe, S. J.: Riboflavin absorption and excretion in the neonate, Pediatrics **76**:549, 1970.

MacKeith, R. C.: Is a big baby healthy? Proc. Nutr. Soc. **22**:128, 1963.

Matoth, Y., Pinkas, A., and Stroka, C.: Studies in folic acid in infancy. 3. Folates in breast-fed infants and their mothers, Amer. J. Clin. Nutr. **16**:356, 1965.

Meyer, H. F.: Breast feeding in the United States, Clin. Pediat. **7**:708, 1968.

Nammacher, M. A., Willemin, M., Hartmann, J. R., and Gaston, L. W.: Vitamin K deficiency in infants beyond the neonatal period, J. Pediat. **76**:549, 1970.

Mott, G. A., Ross, R. H., and Smith, D. J.: A study of vitamin C and D intake of infants in the metropolitan Vancouver area, Canad. J. Pub. Health **55**:341, 1964.

Owen, G. M.: Modification of cow's milk for infant formulas. Current practices, Amer. J. Clin. Nutr. **22**:1150, 1969.

Rueda-Williamson, R., and Rose, H. E.: Growth and nutrition in infants; the influence of diet and other factors on growth, Pediatrics **30**:639, 1962.

Salber, E. J., and Feinlieb, M.: Breast feeding in Boston, Pediatrics **37**:299, 1966.

Snyderman, S. E., Boyer, A., Roitman, E., Holt, L. E., Jr., and Prose, P. H.: The histidine requirement of the infant, Pediatrics **31**:786, 1963.

Stitt, G., and Heseltine, M. M.: Some practical consideration of economy and efficiency in infant feeding, Amer. J. Pub. Health **52**:125, 1962.

Tomarelli, R. M., Meyer, B. J., Weaber, J. R., and Bernhart, F. W.: Effect of positional distribution on the absorption of fatty acids of human milk and infant formulas, J. Nutr. **95**:583, 1969.

Widdowson, E. M.: Effect of giving phosphate supplements on the absorption and excretion of calcium, strontium, magnesium and phosphorus to breast-fed babies, Lancet **2**:1250, 1963.

Widdowson, E. M.: The experimental approach to some pediatric problems, Proc. Nutr. Soc. **22**:121, 1963.

Williams, H. H.: Differences between cow's and human milk, J.A.M.A. **175**:104, 1961.

18 | *Nutrition from infancy to adulthood*

In discussing the nutritive needs during infancy in Chapter 17, we dealt with the character of the diet and the gradual change in both variety and quality of the dietary intake that occurs as the child's nutritive needs increase and as his ability to handle a greater variety and complexity of foods improves during the first year of life. The age at which an infant makes the transition from bottle- or breast-feeding and from pureed or chopped baby foods to drinking from a cup and eating selected items from the regular family diet varies greatly from one child to another. Some make the adjustment as early as 8 months of age, whereas others may not reach this stage of maturity until 2 years of age or later. Aside from encouraging the child to chew when the ability to chew is established and to feed himself when he has the manual dexterity to manipulate a spoon, there is little reason to push the change. Indeed some evidence suggests that the infant should not be denied the work of sucking from either the breast or bottle at too early an age, as this omission may predispose to poorly developed jaws with attendant problems of crowded dentition or to thumb-sucking in early childhood. This chapter will deal with the nutritive needs and special considerations in adapting food to the child's needs after the pattern of feeding of early infancy has been modified to include the use of table foods.

CHILDHOOD

As one would expect, the rapid and constant increase in body size that occurs dur-

ing the growth period is unique and calls for an increase in the intake of practically all nutrients. The dietary standards proposed by the Food and Nutrition Board of the National Research Council represent the level of intake they believe will provide optimal health benefits to practically all children in each age group. The recognition that growth of children occurs in spurts—with a period of rapid increase in skeletal height followed by a slow increase in height but a more rapid increase in weight—should suggest that these values may represent an excessive margin of safety at one time and a realistic goal at another. They do remain, however, the standard against which to assess dietary adequacy and the nutritional goal used in planning food intakes. Although the total nutritional need increases with age, the requirement on the basis of body weight declines.

Fig. 18-1 represents the percentage change in nutritive needs over a base of 2 to 3 years that occurs with increasing age. It is obvious that the suggested increment varies from one nutrient to another. Fortunately, in terms of ease of diet planning the increment for calories in the majority of cases is as large or larger than the increment for other nutrients. As one would expect, the increase in energy needs represents the amount of energy needed for basal metabolism, activity, and the amount stored as new muscle or adipose tissue. Requirements for basal metabolism and activity will increase proportionately with body size, whereas that for growth will vary with the rate of growth and deposition of

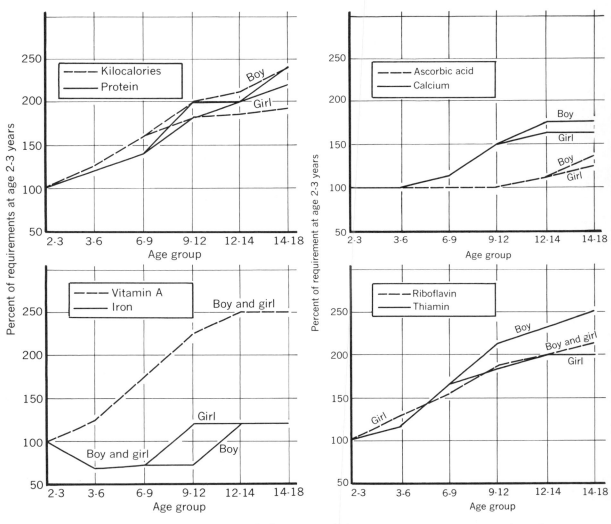

Fig. 18-1. Increase in nutritive needs during growth from age 2-3 years to 18 years. (Based on Food and Nutrition Board: Recommended dietary allowances, ed. 7, Publication No. 1694, Washington, D. C. 1968, National Academy of Sciences—National Research Council.)

new tissue. Since many of the water-soluble vitamins, such as thiamin, niacin, and pantothenic acid, are involved primarily in energy metabolism, it is not surprising to find their requirements increasing in proportion to total energy needs. Pyridoxine, involved in the utilization of dietary protein and in the synthesis of tissue protein, will be required in greater amounts during periods of rapid muscle growth. Any increase in muscle mass that must accompany bone growth requires a positive nitrogen balance that is met by protein intakes of 1.5 to 2 gm. per kilogram of body weight. The increase in total body size necessitates a larger vascular system to transport nutrients to the tissues and waste products away, thus making demands for nutrients needed in blood formation—iron, protein, and folacin. Bone growth increases the need for protein, calcium, phosphorus, and vitamin D. Although the biological roles of vitamin A and ascorbic acid have not been elucidated, adequate evidence indi-

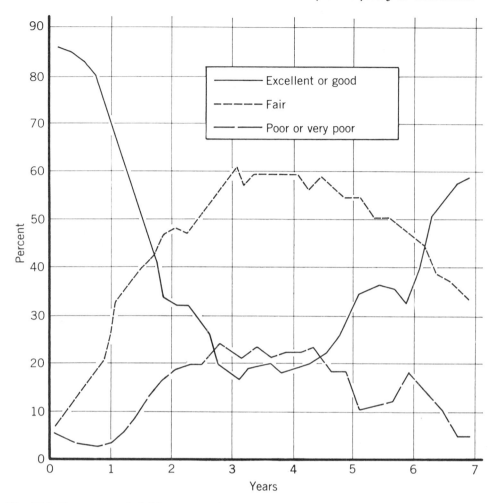

Fig. 18-2. Percentage of children 6 months to 7 years whose appetites were rated excellent, fair, or poor by their mothers. (From Beal, V. A.: Pediatrics **20**:448, 1957.)

cates that the amount needed increases with body size.

Although we know that the overall need for nutrients increases throughout the growth period, there will be periods when growth is slow, with needs for certain nutrients reduced proportionately. Children frequently reflect these fluctuations in need by fluctuations in appetite, a phenomenon that may be the cause of much anxiety to the parents. It is common and natural for a child who has a hearty appetite to go through a period in which both the appetite and food intake are noticeably reduced.

Unless such a period is very prolonged and is accompanied by signs of undernutrition, such as lethargy, fatigue, and increased susceptibility to infection, it should be no basis for concern. The unnecessary concern of some mothers over their children's food habits is exemplified in a study in Minnesota that showed that several mothers rated their children's food habits as poor when they met all criteria for nutritionally adequate meals. Fig. 18-2 represents the fluctuations in appetite with age as reported by mothers of Colorado children.

In response to concern over appetite variations, promoters of dietary supplements have recommended both thiamin and cobalamin to stimulate appetite and growth in children, but experimental evidence indicates that thiamin is of value for only the most severely deprived human and that cobalamin is of no value as an appetite stimulant, although both play significant roles in metabolism.

Transitional foods

In supervising the change from an infant diet to regular adult-type diet, several factors about a child's reaction to food should be kept in mind to facilitate the transition and to minimize the trauma of the experience for both the mother and the child. Lowenberg, on the basis of extensive observations of the reaction of children to food, suggests that their acceptance of food represents a favorable reaction to the color, flavor, texture, and temperature of the food as well as to the size of the servings and the attitude and atmosphere in which it is presented. A rejection of food may be attributed to an unfavorable reaction to one of these. She advises that the wise mother will try to analyze the reactions and determine their cause.

Children favor foods that are soft in texture and are less accepting of foods that are dry or flintlike, have tough or stringy parts, or are too thick. For instance, they prefer thin to thick puddings, celery with the strings removed, stewed tomatoes with the fibers cut, soft mashed potatoes to baked potatoes, moist ground meats to dry fish, and soft bread to coarse bread. This preference for moist foods may reflect the absence of a copious supply of saliva to provide a natural lubricant for the food. In terms of temperature they prefer foods that are lukewarm to those that are very cold or very hot. By serving a child's food first, one finds that it is at the right temperature by the time others at the table are served. Removing milk from the refrigerator sufficiently long before serving to warm it

slightly increases its acceptance. The tendency of a child to dawdle over ice cream until it is semisolid reflects his distaste for very cold foods. Children are very sensitive to flavors, reacting to off-flavors that may go undetected by adults, although experimental evidence does not support the notion that children are more sensitive to flavor variations than their parents are. Their sensitivity to flavor has been observed when they reject milk with a slight taint or recognize when food has been only slightly scorched. In the case of vegetables, children will often refuse vegetables of the cabbage or onion families when they are cooked in such a way as to maximize the retention of nutrients and the flavor but will accept them when cooked in a larger amount of water or when served with a cream sauce to modify the flavor. Once the mild flavor of the vegetable has been accepted it can be presented gradually in a more intensified form until it approaches normal flavor concentration, which also maximizes the retention of nutrients.

The quantity of food offered a child at one time influences his reaction to it. It is more satisfactory from a psychological point of view to offer a child less than you anticipate he will eat and have him return for more than to present him with such a large quantity that he is defeated before he begins to eat it. The use of small 6-ounce glasses that can be easily grasped in the child's chubby hands is preferable to a large 8- to 10-ounce glass that overtaxes his manual dexterity and the capacity of his stomach. Allowing the child to serve himself so that he can determine the amount of food on his plate or the preparation of food in bite-size pieces may produce greater acceptance of the meal.

Visually the child is responsive to a colorful meal whether the color is provided by the plate and setting, the combination of foods, or the judicious use of edible garnishes. Care should be exercised to avoid unnatural food shapes, inedible material, or colors not normally found in food, such as blue or purple, in an attempt to give the meal eye appeal.

Young children in their curiosity about their environment like to experience the feel of food. They also find that many foods are more easily manipulated with the hands than with utensils. Thus the preparation of foods such as strips of meat, wedges of lettuce, or raw vegetables as finger foods allows the child to experience the feel of foods and is certainly justified if it encourages their use. The age at which a child develops sufficient manual dexterity to handle the utensils to manipulate food is again an individual matter, but until the child reaches the stage of motor development when he is skilled in their use, food should be presented in a way that requires a minimum of manipulation for its enjoyment. It should be kept in mind that children are just as individual in their reactions as are adults. Therefore it is to be expected that the reader could point to many examples of children whose food preferences do not conform to the patterns that we are suggesting in the above generalizations.

Snacks. Snacks in the diet of young children have been encouraged by some and condemned by others. During periods of high nutritive needs the small child may be unable to take in sufficient food to satisfy his needs in three meals without overtaxing the capacity of his stomach. On the other hand, if snacks of high satiety value are taken too near regular meal hours, they may reduce the food intake at mealtimes. Munro found that snacks given 2½ hours before lunchtime had no effect on the appetite for lunch. They did, however, reduce the caloric intake at lunch, although the combined intake from lunch and snacks was greater than from lunch alone. A cogent argument in favor of well-chosen snacks is provided by research showing that smaller, more frequent meals are utilized in such a way that depresses the formation of adipose tissue and stimulates muscle for-

mation, as desirable during growth as in the prevention of obesity.

Food jags. Although it is deemed desirable to educate children to accept a wide variety of foods and to develop an accepting attitude toward new foods, it is recognized that it is common for young children to go on food jags in which they accept a very limited number of foods and reject all others. Should the accepted foods represent a nutritionally adequate, albeit monotonous, diet, as is often observed, there is little evidence that these preferences should provoke undue concern, since they seldom persist for prolonged periods nor is there evidence that they lead to bizarre food habits in adulthood. It has been observed, however, that the quality of the diet of 12- to 14-year-old girls was positively correlated with the number of different food items eaten during the day, thus emphasizing the importance of encouraging the use of a variety of foods during the years when food habits are forming.

Food preferences. Several studies to determine food preferences of children, which represent their reaction to the taste, texture, and temperature of food, have all led to similar conclusions. Only 37% to 41% of the children studied liked vegetables, whereas over two thirds liked fruits. The fact that vegetables are generally unpopular may reflect the many and possibly unsatisfactory ways in which they are prepared. Meat, milk, and bread ranked next to fruit in popularity. Food likes of youngsters appear to be related to those of other family members, especially the father, whose food preferences influence the frequency with which specific foods are served and hence the extent to which the child is familiar with them.

Adequacy of diets of infants and children. The findings on dietary adequacy of 9-month-old to 2-year-old infants are illustrated in Fig. 18-3, which shows clearly that iron, ascorbic acid, and thiamin are the nutrients most likely to be provided in less than recommended amounts.

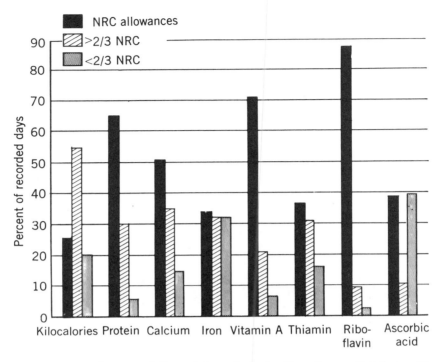

Fig. 18-3. Nutritive adequacy of diets of forty 9-month-old to 2-year-old infants. (Based on data from Guthrie, H. A.: J. Amer. Diet. Ass. **43:**120, 1963.)

Relatively few studies have been concerned with the nutritive intake of young children, but in practically all studies the results have shown that the most common nutrient deficiencies are calcium, iron, vitamin C, and vitamin A, with protein and riboflavin the ones most likely to be present at recommended levels. A relatively small number of children, about 20%, have intakes of one or more nutrients of less than two thirds of recommended amounts, but an equally small number have intakes for all nutrients that either meet or exceed these levels. Since the standards involve such a wide margin of safety, these deficiencies are not a major concern unless there is some evidence of impaired physiological function.

EVALUATION OF NUTRITIONAL STATUS

Since childhood is a period of active growth and a well-nourished child can be expected to have a growth pattern characterized by regular increments in both height and weight, physical growth has become a readily available standard on which to assess nutritional status. Children in this generation are achieving a more rapid rate of growth and are reaching maturity at an earlier age than did those a few decades ago. This is a function not only of improved nutrition but also of favorable environmental factors and the advances in medical science that have reduced or eliminated many of the diseases that depressed growth in the earlier period. It is important that any growth standard used in evaluating nutritional status be one derived from recent data. Falkner has developed such a standard (Appendix D), in which he presents height and weight data for the fifth, fiftieth, and ninety-fifth percentile for boys and girls of different ages on the theory that a range of values is more valuable than norms. He emphasizes that although data from standards will give a smooth curve, those from individuals will be characterized by peaks and valleys. He also presents data on yearly growth increments in both height and weight as a guide for assessing growth rates and stresses the importance of assessing the pubertal stage as the child approaches this age. These standards are not as genetically specific as are those of Garn, shown in Chapter 15, which are based on the parental midpoint size. The assessment of body composition has also proved useful in evaluating growth in children. The percentage of body weight represented by fat declines up to 7 years of age. For girls the proportion of body weight as fat increases steadily until maturity, whereas for boys it declines from puberty until maturity. Techniques for measuring both cell number and cell size are making it possible to assess the nature of growth and the effect of specific deficiencies on the composition of tissues.

Nutritional inadequacies in childhood

Severe malnutrition in childhood in the United States is seldom encountered now because of the availability of medical services to practically everyone and the improvement of techniques for identifying abnormalities before they develop into a full-fledged deficiency syndrome. Pellagra and beriberi are virtually unknown, and only an occasional case of scurvy is recorded. The *National Nutrition Survey* has revealed a 2% incidence of rickets in Texas children, however. As many as 18% of the children enrolled in Head Start programs fall below the third percentile on height and weight standards. Such a growth retardation is associated with high morbidity and mortality rates. Of all manifestations of malnutrition, anemia and obesity are the most common, in addition to varying degrees of subclinical deficiency states. Dental caries incidence may also reflect nutrient intake.

Anemia, primarily the result of a lack of dietary iron, is encountered most often among children in lower socioeconomic groups, in whom the reported incidence of hemoglobin levels below 10 gm. per 100 ml. of blood ranges from 20% to 40%. In most cases the lack of dietary iron reflects either parental ignorance of the importance and sources of iron or poverty, which restricts the amount and variety of foods available. In some cases the situation is aggravated by the presence of intestinal parasites. A few instances are recorded of anemia resulting from the exclusive use of a milk diet after the first 6 months of life. Treatment of anemia of childhood usually involves the therapeutic use of iron salts at levels providing 30 to 100 mg. of iron per day, often in conjunction with ascorbic acid, until the hemoglobin levels have been restored to normal levels. This is followed by the use of a diet high in iron-rich foods such as meat, green leafy vegetables, and enriched cereals. The child who suffers from anemia is usually lethargic, fatigues easily, and is highly susceptible to infection.

Obesity, a form of overnutrition, represents the other end of the nutritional spectrum. Childhood or juvenile obesity is a particular problem because it is very refractory to treatment and tends to persist into adulthood. This increasing problem may be attributed to several factors. Many mothers, in their concern over the child's food habits, unwittingly establish a pattern of overeating when they introduce solid foods at a very early age, equate weight gain with good health, or use food as a reward for good behavior. The situation is further complicated by inactivity, as discussed in Chapter 20. The syndrome of the pale flabby child who spends his summers in an air-conditioned house, immobilized in front of a television set and drinking calorie-laden carbonated beverages to keep cool, is frequently observed and is a cause for concern. The importance of preventing obesity in childhood through an education program involving both sound food selection and exercise cannot be overstressed.

Nutrition and dental health

During childhood, dietary factors may influence dental health through their effect on both tooth formation and on the character of the oral environment. Before tooth decay will occur, three conditions must be present—a caries-susceptible tooth, a fermentable carbohydrate, and microorganisms to ferment the carbohydrate. The susceptibility of the tooth to decay may be determined genetically, but few children are endowed with caries-resistent teeth. Beyond this, the integrity of the tooth structure may be a function of the nutrients that are available at a critical point in tooth formation. Vitamin A is necessary for the formation of the enamel layer; vitamin C for the dentin layer; and calcium, phosphorus and vitamin D for the process of calcification. In addition, the availability of fluorine during the time the tooth is calcifying will greatly decrease the susceptibility of the tooth to decay. Once the tooth has erupted, the presence or absence of a sticky carbohydrate to adhere to the tooth surface is the major dietary factor influencing tooth decay. It is not the nutrient content of the diet but rather the extent to which candy and other carbohydrates are consumed under conditions that allow them to become embedded on the tooth surface that determines the cariogenic character of the diet. Of all dietary factors that can help control tooth decay, fluorine has the greatest effect and shows the most promise as a preventive.

ADOLESCENCE

The period of transition from childhood to adulthood, commonly called adolescence, is a relatively short stage in the life cycle characterized by accelerated physical, biochemical, and emotional development. Adolescence has an effect on both nutritional needs and the absorption and utilization of nutritive intake. This period witnesses a rapid enlargement of organs and tissues and changes in physiological functions in response to hormonal changes. As reflected in the National Research Council recommended dietary allowances, this phase of the life cycle is the one of highest nutritive needs in the life of a male and for girls is surpassed only during pregnancy and lactation. These allowances represent the needs for the increase in body size and the maturation of organs. Since the 13- to 19-year-olds numbered 24 million in the United States in 1970 and since they are at a vulnerable age when the dietary patterns and attitudes they develop toward food are going to influence the health of their children and dictate the food patterns of the next generation, they are a prime and challenging target for nutrition education programs.

Adequacy of diets

Evaluations of the nutritive adequacy of the diets of young adults between 12 and 18 years of age in various regions in the United States have all yielded essentially the same results, although differences in degree are found. In all instances it was observed that the diets of boys were more adequate and less variable than were those of the girls. This can be explained in part by the fact that the extra quantity of food required to meet the energy needs of boys (1100 kcal.) dictates at least a minimal level of other nutrients, whereas girls, with lower caloric intakes, are forced to make more judicious choices of foods to meet the needs for all other nutrients. In general, the diets of girls provided a higher proportion of their needs for ascorbic acid and calories than did those of boys, although ascorbic acid was often low for both. Girls' diets were generally low in iron, but this was not accompanied by a higher incidence of anemia. Calcium was more frequently low in the diet of girls than of boys, and vita-

Table 18-1. Percentage of boys and girls with nutrient intakes below two thirds of the NRC recommended dietary allowances°

Nutrient	Boys (%)	Girls (%)
Calcium	10–42	15–70
Iron	0–18	10–45
Ascorbic acid	10–65	20–60
Thiamin	3–30	8–50
Vitamin A	3–38	5–45
Riboflavin	2–25	10–45
Niacin	2–30	5–22

*Based on Morgan, A. F.: Nutritional status U.S.A., California Agricultural Experiment Station Bulletin 769, 1959.

min A was low in both, a reflection of a general rejection of vegetables. Protein and niacin intakes, which paralleled the use of meat, were most often adequate.

Table 18-1 presents data on the percentage of adolescents in various studies in the United States whose intake of different nutrients fell below two thirds of the NRC recommended dietary allowances. In general, the subjects with the poorest diets were those who skipped more meals, ate smaller quantities of food at meals, and ate fewer snacks.

In using the findings of dietary studies, one should bear in mind the edition of the recommended dietary allowances on which the evaluation was based. Since the recommendations have shown a downward trend for all nutrients except calcium, which has been unchanged, and iron, which has been increased in recent revisions, diets that were assessed as inadequate on earlier standards may now be considered adequate. In the case of iron, a reevaluation of the data may show an even higher incidence of suboptimal intakes.

Factors influencing food habits

Few attempts have been made to determine the attitudes that influence the selection of a diet. Young girls who were concerned about their health, who were emotionally stable and conforming, and who came from homes characterized by good family relationships chose better diets than did those motivated by considerations of group status, sociability, independence from parental control, or enjoyment of eating. Criticism of their eating patterns led girls to skip meals more frequently, and skipping breakfast was found to be common. Better meals were selected in winter than in summer because of the regularity of schedules. The more meals eaten away from home, the less likely an adolescent is to consume meals of adequate nutritional content, which no doubt represents a response to the habits of the peer groups. This is especially true when lunch money is used to buy lunches outside the school, a practice that is becoming less frequent with the trend toward short lunch periods in high schools and lack of freedom to leave the school building. School lunches that qualify for federal and state subsidies are selected to provide one fourth to one third of the nutritive needs of the schoolchild. Packed lunches are found to be somewhat less adequate, and those purchased outside the school are poor. It is obvious that many factors contribute to the poor food habits observed during the teen years, but the most frequently observed causes are failure to eat breakfast (or less frequently some other meal of the day), lack of time or companionship for regular meals, drinking no milk (which may be a rebellion against parental influence), lack of supervision in the selection of meals eaten away from home, an overriding fear of obesity, especially among girls, and a concern that certain foods will aggravate adolescent acne.

Obesity

Studies indicate that 30% to 35% of teenagers are overweight, although not necessarily obese. Teen-agers, especially girls, are either fat or fearful of becoming fat. Because of their idol of the fashion model in a size six dress, girls often adopt an unrealistic and unhealthy standard of body size to which they aspire. Hence they embark on a self-directed program of weight reduction that can easily be hazardous to health because of inadequate levels of nutrients at a time when there are still high nutrient demands for growth. The problem is even greater when weight reduction is carried out spasmodically, with a period of weight loss followed by one of weight gain.

As will be discussed in Chapter 20, the major cause of caloric imbalance among adolescents is a depressed level of activity rather than an excessive food intake. Whether the cause of this inactivity is physiological or psychological or both has not been determined. It has been observed that obese youngsters have significantly lower serum iron with normal hemoglobin levels than do nonobese youngsters. The low serum iron levels could be indicative of low levels of myoglobin and other iron-containing pigments, which may cause an unconscious reduction in activity when the oxygen available to the cells is reduced. This situation, characterized by reduced activity, can be better handled by a program of consistent moderate exercise than by one of spasmodic and vigorous activity. The nature of activity patterns that are developed in late adolescence often prevails throughout adulthood so that to develop habits of active exercise at an early age becomes important in terms of preventing obesity in adulthood. Equally important is the observation that the earlier a person learns to respond to satiety signals, the more likely he is to be able to adjust his food intake to correspond to his needs in response to a sensitive satiety mechanism.

Breakfast

The importance of breakfast for any group is well documented, and there is likely no nutritional substitute for a good breakfast. Having a good breakfast has two major advantages. First, it generally provides nutrients, especially ascorbic acid, calcium, and riboflavin, that may not be provided in adequate amounts by the foods typically consumed at other meals. Second, the availability of a readily utilizable carbohydrate results in a rapid increase in blood glucose levels and the concurrent decrease in reaction time so that performance is improved and accident rate declines.

Since adolescence is a time when skipping breakfast hits a peak and a time during which dietary habits that may persist for life are formulated, this is a period when attention should be directed toward the problem. Studies show that the calcium and ascorbic acid intakes of persons who omit breakfast are reduced by about 40% and the intakes of iron and thiamin by 10%. Leverton also found that 17- to 19-year-old college women who skipped breakfast obtained 18% of their energy intake from snacks, whereas those who ate breakfast snacked less frequently and obtained only 7% of their energy intake from snacks. Since the snacks chosen were characteristically high in calories relative to other nutrients, those who snacked more had diets that were less adequate nutritionally than did those of persons who had breakfast.

Boys report eating breakfast more frequently and eating breakfasts that provide more nutrients than do girls. Many rationalizations are presented for failure to eat breakfast, including lack of time, lack of appetite, preference for sleep, spending time over personal appearance, or fear of becoming fat.

In one study it was observed that the availability of someone with whom to eat breakfast, someone to prepare it for them, the availability of prepared foods, and the acceptance of the breakfast-eating habit in the peer group all influenced the extent to which breakfast was eaten.

It should be pointed out that breakfast

need not be the conventional fruit, cereal, toast, and beverage pattern but can be any combination of foods, either liquid or solid, that provides its nutritional equivalent, at least 300 kcal., and sufficient protein and fat to provide a sense of satiety until the next meal.

Concern over teen-agers' diets

Nutritionists express concern over the nutritional habits of the 12- to 19-year-old group for many reasons. This is a period marked by a level of physical and emotional growth that often results in stress and anxiety, which in turn influence physiological, psychological, and social behavior, all of which affect nutritional behavior.

The incidence of dietary inadequacies is higher during adolescence, which is a stage at which the results of nutrient lack are far reaching, especially for girls, than at any other stage of the life cycle. Second, many relationships between physical abnormalities and dietary practice have been observed.

The incidence of tuberculosis is highest in adolescence, and some evidence suggests a relationship between nutritional status and onset of tuberculosis, speed of recovery, and rate of reinfection.

Emotional instability, noted especially among girls who mature early, influences the utilization of nutrients. Negative nitrogen and calcium balances have been observed among both young girls and older persons who are under extreme emotional stress.

With 53% of girls between 15 and 19 years of age married, the possibility that a girl will bear a child before she is fully matured herself is a reason to focus special attention on her nutritional status. One out of 4 mothers bearing her first child is less than 20 years old, and 6% of all deaths among 18- to 19-year-old girls result from the complications of pregnancy. If the nutritive intake of a girl has been inadequate prior to conception, she is less able to cope with the added physical stress of pregnancy and the demands of the growing fetus and is unable to make up for her own nutritive deficits. As a result, babies of teen-agers are more often born prematurely, have more congenital defects, and have inadequate nutritive stores to carry them through the initial period of extrauterine life. In all respects the malnourished mother is a poor obstetrical risk. Whether a concern over the welfare of their yet unconceived children will provide sufficient motivation to teen-age girls to modify their food habits remains to be tested, but the concern of nutritionists over the present status of the diets of adolescents has prompted a concerted effort to reach this group.

ROLE OF SNACKS IN DIETARY INTAKE

Until recently nutritionists tended to stress the importance of three "good" meals a day and to ignore the possibility that snacks could provide anything other than empty calories. With the recognition that smaller more frequent meals may have many physiological and nutritional advantages, and that snacking is a way of life with teen-agers, there has been concern about improving the quality of snacks. Data on food intake patterns show that snacks provide from one fourth to one third of the caloric intake of adolescents. The extent to which snacks contribute to the intake of other nutrients is a function of the nature of the snacks. Once the adult has accepted the fact that snacking is not necessarily detrimental and need not spoil the appetite for well-planned meals, he can do much to see that snacks are beneficial by monitoring the kinds of foods that are available. The most likely places for the adult to make his influence felt are through access points such as the school lunch program, the home refrigerator, and the offerings of vending machines. Studies have shown that as long as the teen-ager had three meals a day, little difference in nutrient intake was found with increased frequency of meals. Snacking can be encouraged when it becomes an integral part of the total eating pattern but must be condemned if it constitutes overeating in disregard of the total food pattern. Snacking that is confined to the evening hours in what is described as the "night-eating syndrome" has been implicated as a factor in obesity.

SCHOOL LUNCH

With 20 million of the nation's school children participating in the National School Lunch Program, it can be considered an important factor in the nutrient intake of schoolchildren. The program was originally conceived to "safeguard the health and well-being of the nation's children and to encourage the domestic consumption of nutritious agricultural commodities and other foods."* From its inception in 1946 the School Lunch Act required that a type A lunch provide one third or more of the daily nutrient intake of the 10- to 12-year-old child with adjustments made for both younger and older children. To encourage the preparation of nutritious lunches the United States Department of Agriculture provided subsidies in the form of technical advice, surplus agricultural commodities or those purchased as part of the price support programs, and a cash subsidy if the food service adhered to certain requirements. Specifically the School Lunch Act required that each participating school operate on a nonprofit basis, serve meals at a regular meal hour, provide lunches free or at reduced cost to those unable to pay, and serve meals meeting specified nutritional standards. In 1970 about 20% of the children participating received free or reduced-

---

*National School Lunch Act, Public Law 396, Seventy-ninth Congress, June 4, 1946.

price lunches. A 1970 amendment has authorized schools to make contracts with food service management companies to provide school lunches. They must, however, keep records available for inspection and must use federally donated commodities only for the benefit of the participants. To qualify for reimbursement, a school has to serve as a plate lunch a meal containing at least the following:

½ pint of fluid whole milk
2 ounces of a meat or alternate such as fish, poultry, dried beans, peanut butter, eggs, or cheese
¾ cup of two or more fruits and/or vegetables
1 serving of enriched or whole grain cereal
1 teaspoon butter or fortified margarine

With the publication of the 1968 revision of the recommended dietary allowances, concern has developed that the lunches are failing to provide one third of the requirement for magnesium and pyridoxine. There are proposals to modify the type A lunch pattern to assure desirable intakes of these nutrients. Consideration is also being directed toward modifying the provisions of the act to allow for satellite feeding operations in which food is provided to several schools from a central facility, not necessarily a nonprofit organization. The necessity of providing a hot lunch for every child is also being questioned, especially in this era of well-heated schools and school buses.

The Special Milk Program supplements the School Lunch Program and provides a subsidy for each half pint of whole milk served in a school. Under the Child Nutrition Act of 1966 some pilot school breakfast programs have been instituted. The selected schools participating in this part of the feeding program are primarily those with many needy pupils or pupils who travel great distances from their homes. Seventy-three percent of the 0.5 million children participating in 1970 received free or reduced-price breakfasts. Schools provide at cost one serving of fruit or juice, ½ pint of whole milk, and one serving of cereal prior to the regular school hour. This program has been promoted as a means of dealing with the serious nutritional deficits of the lower socioeconomic groups in the country. Although the evidence is subjective, it is suggestive of better school performance and improved attention among children who have this breakfast before coming to school.

Other innovative, intervention programs are being investigated as possible means of improving the nutritional intake of the nation's schoolchildren, especially those from economically deprived groups.

ATHLETES

Although the principles of good nutrition are the same for athletes as they are for others, adolescent athletes participating in varsity and intramural sports frequently receive dietary advice from coaches. As a result, many theories exist regarding the role that nutrition may play in maximizing the performance of the athlete. Diet, however, is no substitute for aptitude, training, and motivation.

Contrary to general opinion, muscular exercise does not require an increased intake of protein but rather involves only an expenditure of energy. This is more readily available from carbohydrate foods than from foods rich in fat or protein. It is, however, common practice for coaches to arrange a pregame meal that is relatively high in protein and almost invariably has a generous serving of meat. This is included for psychological rather than for physiological reasons.

Coaches are concerned about the digestibility of the pregame meal when the athlete is under emotional stress. Many are recommending a liquid pregame meal. It is less expensive, can be taken closer to game time, and in addition is associated with reduced incidence of pregame vomiting and muscle cramps. By feeding a meal that is completely digested by game time,

the competition between the muscles and the digestive system for simultaneous use of the blood pool is reduced. Such competition could result in a compromised efficiency of both. The pregame meal is usually eaten 3 to 5 hours before competition. High levels of protein or fat should be avoided to be sure that the food is digested by the time of competition. Gas-producing foods and foods high in bulk are usually considered undesirable.

There has been much concern over the effect of milk on athletic performance. Although many enthusiastically recommend it, others recommend that it be eliminated, mainly on the basis of some unfounded beliefs. Some controlled studies of the effect of varying levels of milk on performance showed that there were no differences in training response or all-out performance when an intake of 3 pints of milk per day and 2 pints of ice cream per week was compared to a diet without any milk.

The capacity for prolonged strenuous exercise is enhanced when the carbohydrate stores of glycogen are large. Research has shown that the normal reserve of about 800 to 1000 kcal. in the form of glycogen in the liver and muscle can be almost doubled by a dietary regimen in which the athlete consumes a diet low in carbohydrate and high in fat and protein for several days prior to the meet while in training. The day before the contest the diet is supplemented with carbohydrate, which is preferentially stored in the liver at a level exceeding that which normally occurs. This type of regimen may be especially useful for the track man, who may require large amounts of energy in a short period of time.

The American Medical Association is concerned over hazards of indiscriminate and excessive weight reduction to which adolescents are frequently subjected to meet a specific weight requirement for participation. Required weight loss can be accomplished through the use of hot boxes, rubberized or plastic clothing, and induced vomiting, none of which are recommended. Since premature fatigue is associated with even a minimal water loss of 3% of body weight, such a fluctuation in weight may be accompanied by a depressed level of performance that will undo the benefits of training. Dehydration is less serious if it is confined to 2 to 3 hours before weigh-in and is followed by immediate rehydration. The practice of withholding water and inducing severe dehydration over a several-day period may cause severe problems such as the excretion of a reduced and highly concentrated urine, deposits of calculi, or stones, in the kidney, and the retention of urea, leading to uremia. Many substances believed to be ergogenic (strength producing) have been recommended, but their effectiveness has not been demonstrated. Any value seems to be psychological rather than physiological.

To compensate for the salt loss that accompanies water loss and sweating, many coaches are using flavored electrolyte solutions containing, in addition to salt, other electrolytes and sugar. The products currently on the market provide the equivalent of 1 gm. of salt (the amount in 2 salt tablets) per liter of solution and will compensate only for low sodium losses. So far no studies indicate improved athletic performance with their use.

IMPROVING NUTRITIONAL HABITS

It has been well documented that nutrition knowledge is not necessarily reflected in food habits. The key to the application of sound nutritional principles to eating patterns appears to be motivation. In adolescence the most effective motivation is the hope for vitality, good looks, and popularity. Concern over long-term effects of malnutrition or undernutrition on health has relatively little impact on the high school student or even the college student. Of the various methods attempted, the use of group sessions during which the group accepts certain standards of eating and then helps provide the incentive and backing to implement them has been most effective. In some cases it is necessary to "unlearn" sets of habits, but in others it is merely a case of modifying or improving the current set of habits. A positive approach that builds on the prevailing habits rather than a negative one that involves pulling all the props out from under a person is preferable and more effective. It is important to start with the present habits of the individual, reinforce the good aspects and replace the poor with new habits and to recognize that good diets do not just happen but are planned.

SELECTED REFERENCES
Childhood
Breckenbridge, M. E.: Food attitudes of five- to twelve-year-old children, J. Amer. Diet. Ass. **35:**704, 1959.
Bryan, M. S., and Lowenberg, M. E.: The father's influence on young children's food preferences, J. Amer. Diet. Ass. **34:**30, 1958.
Committee on Nutrition, American Academy of Pediatrics: Appraisal of the use of vitamins B_1 and B_{12} or supplements promoted for the stimulation of growth and appetite in children, Pediatrics **21:**860, 1958.
Committee on Nutrition, American Academy of Pediatrics: Factors affecting food intake, Pediatrics **33:**135, 1964.

Dierks, E. C., and Morse, L. M.: Food habits and nutrient intakes of preschool children, J. Amer. Diet. Ass. **47:**292, 1965.
Hathaway, M. L., and Sargent, D. W.: Overweight in children, J. Amer. Diet. Ass. **40:**511, 1962.
Haughton, J. G.: Nutritional anemia of infancy and childhood, Amer. J. Public Health **53:**1121, 1963.
Kerrey, E., Crispin, S., Fox, H. M., and Kies, C.: Nutritional status of preschool children. I. Dietary and biochemical findings, Amer. J. Clin. Nutr. **21:**1274, 1968.
Lantis, M.: The child consumer—cultural factors influencing his food choices, J. Home Economics **54:**370, 1962.

Lowenberg, M. E.: Food preferences of young children, J. Amer. Diet. Ass. 24:430, 1948.

Metheny, M. Y., Hunt, F. E., Patton, M. B., and Heye, H.: The diets of preschool children. I. Nutritional sufficiency findings and family marketing practices, J. Home Economics 54:297, 1962.

Munro, N.: How do snacks affect total caloric intake of preschool children, J. Amer. Diet. Ass. 33:601, 1957.

Norman, F. A., and Pratt, E. L.: Feeding of infants and children in hot weather, J.A.M.A. 166:2168, 1958.

Owens, G. M., Garry, P. J., Kram, K. M., Nelson, C. E., and Montalvo, J. M.: Nutritional status of Mississippi preschool children—a pilot study, Amer. J. Clin. Nutr. 22:1444, 1969.

Woodruff, C.: Nutritional anemias in early childhood, Amer. J. Clin. Nutr. 22:504, 1969.

Adolescence

American Medical Association Committee on Medical Aspects of Sports, Wrestling and weight control, J.A.M.A. 201:541, 1967.

Astrand, P.: Something old and something new—very new, Nutr. Today 3(2):9, 1968.

Christakis, G., Sajecki, S., Hillman, R. W., Miller, E., Blumenthal, S., and Archer, M.: Effect of a combined nutrition education program and physical fitness program on the weight status of obese high school boys, Fed. Proc. 25:15, 1966.

Everson, G. J.: Bases for concern about teenagers' diets, J. Amer. Diet. Ass. 36:17, 1960.

Gallagher, J. R.: Weight control in adolescence, J. Amer. Diet. Ass. 40:519, 1962.

Heald, F. P.: Natural history and physiological bases of adolescent obesity, Fed. Proc. 25:1, 1966.

Hinton, M. A., Eppright, E. S., Chadderdon, H., and Wolins, L.: Eating behaviour and dietary intake of girls 12-14 years old. Psychologic, sociologic and physiologic factors, J. Amer. Diet. Ass. 43:223, 1963.

Leverton, R. M.: The paradox of teen-age nutrition, J. Amer. Diet. Ass. 53:13, 1968.

Ohlson, M. A., and Hort, B. P.: Influence of breakfast on total day's food intake, J. Amer. Diet. Ass. 47:282, 1965.

Peckos, P. S., and Heald, F. P.: Nutrition of adolescents, Children 11:27, 1964.

Roth, A.: The teenage clinic, J. Amer. Diet. Ass. 36:27, 1960.

Steele, B. F., Clayton, U. U., and Tucker, R. E.: Role of breakfast and of between-meal foods in adolescents' nutrient intake, J. Amer. Diet. Ass. 28:1054, 1952.

Tipton, C. M., and Tcheng, T. K.: Iowa Wrestling Study, J.A.M.A. 214:1269, 1970.

Wharton, M. A.: Nutritive intake of adolescents, J. Amer. Diet. Ass. 42:306, 1963.

White, H. S.: Inorganic elements in weighed diets of girls and young women, J. Amer. Diet. Ass. 55:38, 1969.

19 | _Nutritional considerations in aging_

Geriatrics, the branch of medicine concerned with the care of the aging as well as the aged, is concerned with prolonging the prime of life, delaying the onset of the severely degenerative aspects of aging, and treating the diseases of the aged. Gerontology is the broader branch of science dealing with the psychological, sociological, economic, and physiological as well as the medical aspects of aging. Both fields of study have witnessed a surge of activity in the last two decades. This increasing concern over the problems of the aging population has been motivated by the increase in both the total numbers and proportion of the population who are living beyond retirement age. Advances in medical technology, environmental hygiene, and nutrition have meant that more people are living longer with greater freedom from disease and in many cases with better health for a longer period of time. The extension of life has meant also that more of the complications of aging, both physiological and psychological, have become evident, calling for more thorough studies of the problem. As has been frequently stated, both medical and social scientists are concerned with adding life to years as well as years to life. There were over twice as many people living to 65 years of age in 1960 as in 1900, representing 10% instead of 4% of the population. By 1985 the number of persons over 65 will have reached 25 million. A large number of these will be over 70 years of age. Public responsibility for the care of the aged has been reflected in the passage of many pieces of legislation concerned with their health care.

A similar change in the life expectancy at the time of birth has occurred, as shown in Table 19-1. Figures for women are higher and for men are lower than the average presented here.

NATURE OF AGING PROCESS

The human being is the product of his genetic heritage as well as his past and present environment, including the injuries, infections, stresses, fatigues, nutritional imbalances, and emotional trauma associated with them. It therefore stands to reason that the longer a person lives, the more complex he becomes and that the physical and physiological variations found in 70-year-old persons, each of whom has been subjected to widely different environments, make them a heterogeneous group. Thus it is much more dangerous to generalize about all older people from studies on a few than it is to do so for newborn infants, whose environments by comparison have been relatively homogeneous.

Table 19-1. Life expectancy at birth

Year of birth	Life expectancy (years)
1850	40
1900	47
1940	63
1950	68
1960	70
1970	70

Since the nutritional status of an individual at any age is a reflection of his previous as well as his present dietary habits, Shock has suggested that the best preparation for a healthy old age begins in the office of the pediatrician. As with any biological process, aging occurs at different rates in different individuals even under similiar environmental conditions. A person with a chronological age of 80 may have a biological age of 50 and vice versa. One factor believed to be responsible for delaying the onset of the senile process is a high but not excessive level of nutritive adequacy in the presenile years in the presence of adequate but not excessive caloric intake.

In aging, as at any other time, the state of nutrition of the body is determined by the state of nutrition of the individual cells. Cells will be less than adequately nourished under conditions of dietary deficiencies or excesses, impaired digestion, incomplete absorption, inefficient distribution and utilization of nutrients, and accumulation of waste products. Many of these situations are likely to occur as the body ages.

The stresses that affect aging may be subtle and insidious, but when allowed to accumulate over a period of years, they become cumulative and detrimental. This can be most vividly illustrated by a caloric imbalance of as little as 10 kcal. per day, which at the end of a year amounts to a gain or loss of 1 pound of weight. When accumulated over a 40-year period this represents an appreciable change in body size. Similarly, rather small stresses in individual cells or organs that accumulate over the years may become sufficiently great to cause impaired cellular functioning.

Physiologists have been seeking an answer to the question of the nature of the degenerative changes that occur with aging. Aging, in theory, begins with conception, but during the period of growth the anabolic, or building-up, processes exceed the catabolic, or degenerative, changes so that the net result is one of growth and increased

functional capabilities of the organs and tissues of the body. Once the body has reached physiological maturity, the process is reversed, slowly at first, until the rate of degenerative changes outweighs the growth changes. Along with this comes impaired functioning of many organs of the body. The difficulties of studying one person through the 50 or 60 years of aging are obvious. It is a question whether the subject or the investigator is lost first. So far we have relied on data from many different people at different ages, but there is at least one longitudinal study designed to assess the biochemical and physiological changes that occur in a group of men to be studied for twenty years. Such an investigation should shed considerable light on the biochemistry and physiology of the aging process.

The concensus of opinion now maintains that a decrease in the efficiency of any organ is caused more by a loss of cells than by a change in the functioning level of the remaining cells. It is postulated that with aging the cells form defective RNA from the DNA, which appears to be damaged with age. The defective RNA then calls for the synthesis of defective enzymes, which are not capable of performing normal cellular functions. This, of course, leads to death of the cell. When many cells fail

Table 19-2. Percentage of functions or tissues remaining in a 75-year-old man compared to a 30-year-old man°

Tissue	Percent remaining in 75-year-old man
Brain weight	56
Number of glomeruli in kidney	69
Number of nerve trunk fibers	63
Number of taste buds	36
Body water content	75

*Adapted from Shock, N. W.: Physiology of aging, Scient. Amer. **206:**100, 1962.

to reproduce effectively or to function, the number of cells of an organ and hence its size and functional capacity are reduced, although each remaining cell is functional. The percentage of various tissues remaining in a 75-year-old man compared to those in a 30-year-old man is shown in Table 19-2. A decrement of 10% to 15% in cellular function was found to lead to decrements of 40% to 60% in organ function. Thus the changes caused by aging are believed to be due to loss of cells rather than to a depressed level of functioning. Some workers,

however, have reported a 15% decrease with age in the number of mitochondria, the site of energy metabolism, in cells from heart and liver tissue suggesting that the capacity of a cell to release energy may be diminished.

The rate of decline in the functioning capacity differs in various systems of the body. Shock has studied and measured the change in 50- and 70-year-old men compared to a 30-year-old man. Some of his results are summarized in Fig. 19-1.

In addition to the decrease in the num-

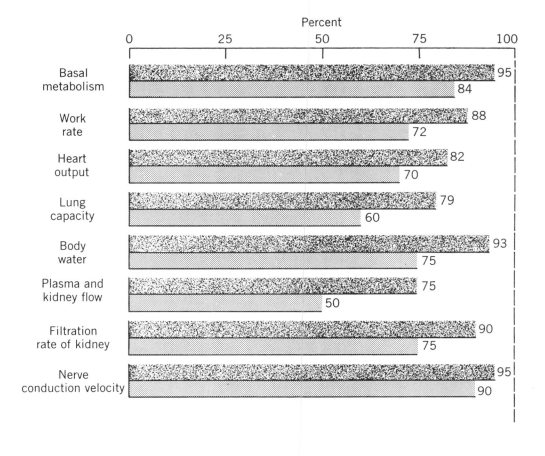

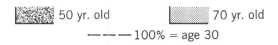

Fig. 19-1. Percentage of certain physiological functions remaining at ages 50 and 70 compared to age 30. (Adapted from data from Shock, N. W.: Scient. Amer. **206**:100, Jan., 1962.)

ber of cells of the body in aging, there are structural changes associated with collagen, the noncellular protein substance that binds the cells together. Collagen, in which the rate of protein turnover is slow, becomes less elastic and more fibrous as the cell ages. Some evidence has been established that the connective tissue or collagen replaces some of the more active cells lost from an organ so that the decline in functional capacity of an organ may be greater than that represented by the decrease in organ weight. In muscle tissue, muscle fibers may be replaced by connective tissue. The accumulation of collagen in the skin is believed to contribute to the aging appearance of the skin. Although complete agreement does not exist on the cause of aging, it is agreed that, generally speaking, the changes are irreversible.

NUTRIENT INTAKE

The factors that influence the nutritional habits and intake of older people can be classified as those that affect intake, digestion, absorption, storage, and metabolism of nutrients, and elimination of waste products. Requirements also change with age.

Factors affecting the ingestion of nutrients

Long-standing dietary habits. Patterns of eating are established early in life, and evidence has been found that people tend to prefer the type of foods they learned to eat when young. Nutrition education has had relatively little impact on the food habits of an individual; thus we find an older person is likely to choose and enjoy the foods he has eaten throughout his life that have become part of this cultural heritage. To him they may represent a certain form of security. Since many experiences with food are pleasant ones, the use of a specific food may conjure up pleasant memories. Many individuals now in their later years were forming their food habits in an era when the kinds and variety of

foods available the year round were much different from and fewer than those available in the markets fifty years later. As a result, they do not readily make use of the new marketing techniques that increase the variety of food available and may eat in the same way they learned to eat when the selection was more limited. An examination of dietary intakes of older people reveals that vitamin A and ascorbic acid are the nutrients most likely to be lacking. These, it will be recognized, are provided through ample use of fresh fruits and vegetables that were available only seasonally, unless home-preserved, sixty to seventy years ago.

In old age, as in other stages of life, one of the major deterrents to optimal nutrition is the established eating habits of the individual. Because the many meanings food has for older people may be more deeply ingrained and more intense, it is likely unwise to insist on any abrupt change in dietary habits without a thorough knowledge of the individual's reactions to food. A slower, more subtle approach in which modifications are made within the framework of individual's food preferences is more likely to be successful. When abnormal metabolic conditions, such as diabetes, ulcer, or obstruction of the bile duct, dictate regulated dietary patterns, the medical necessities of the changes are of primary concern and leave no alternative but a sudden modification of eating habits.

Loss of teeth. The longer one lives, the more likely he is to lose his teeth, and the lower his socioeconomic status, the less likely he is to replace them with satisfactory dentures. The American Dental Association estimates that of every hundred 70-year-olds, 28 men and 38 women have lost all their teeth and that 80% of these either fail to replace them or replace them with ill-fitting dentures. In either case the absence of a satisfactory method of chewing food leads to many modifications in eating patterns. Food that is inadequately chewed is difficult to swallow. Thus a tendency develops to substitute foods requiring little chewing, such as ground meat, for those requiring more, such as steaks and roast. When foods high in cellulose such as fruits and vegetables are eliminated from the diet, the bulk of the diet is reduced, with the resultant decrease in gastrointestinal motility and problems of elimination. If fluoridation of the water supply by reducing dental caries decreases the number of edentulous senior citizens, its benefits may be even greater in later years than in childhood.

Diminished sense of taste and smell. The noted decline in the number of taste buds at age 70 to 36% of those at age 30 may explain the observation that a decreased interest in food often develops with increase in age. With a diminished number and sensitivity of taste buds, it is understandable that much of the pleasure of eating is removed.

Loss of neuromuscular coordination. The ability to maintain fine neuromuscular coordination declines with the aging process, frequently manifesting itself as an inability to manipulate eating utensils. Rather than risk the embarrassment that would come with spilled food or inability to cut meat or eat soup, a person will avoid all such foods. This may lead to marked dietary changes and often nutritional inadequacies.

Physical discomfort. The discomfort that often accompanies ingestion of certain foods is more pronounced in older people. Some may cause heartburn, others cause gastric distention, and still others are incompletely digested. Efforts to avoid the offending foods may lead to the elimination of nutritious foods.

Economic considerations. The economic pressures to which many older people are subjected play an important role in determining their dietary adequacy. When it is recognized that 50% of persons over 65 years of age had an income of less than $1480 per year and 25% had less than $1000 in 1967, it is not surprising that they have restricted amounts for food expenditures. The necessity of living on a meager income to remain financially independent forces many older people to choose the least expensive foods that provide them with the energy for which they recognize a need. This frequently means substituting the relatively inexpensive carbohydrate foods, bread and cereal products, which are low in the protective nutrients, for the more expensive meat, milk, fresh fruits, and vegetables, which are normally dependable sources of protein, minerals, and most vitamins. The ease with which carbohydrates are obtained and stored enhances their appeal.

A study of the food consumption of older persons in Rochester, New York, who were beneficiaries of the Social Security program's Old Age Survivors and Disability Insurance showed that, although less than half the households had diets that furnished full amounts of NRC recommended dietary allowances for all nutrients, one fourth had diets that failed to meet two thirds of this standard for one or more nutrient. When the nutritive adequacy was related to the amount spent for food, it was found that 80% of those who spent more than the cost of the United States Department of Agriculture's liberal-cost food plan met the recommended allowances in full, whereas those who spent less than its estimate for the cost of a low-cost food plan failed to meet two thirds of the recommended allowance for one or more nutrients. Those with low incomes of less than $1000 per person per year had diets considered poor two and one half times as often as did those with high incomes ($2000 for one person or $3000 for two). The relationship between income and dietary adequacy in this study is shown in Fig. 19-2.

The disappearance of the corner groceries from the older residential and downtown areas and their replacement with large supermarkets in suburban shopping plazas have compounded the problem of

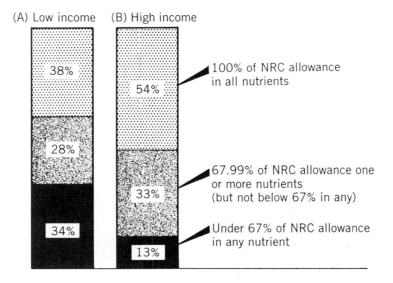

(A) Low income   (B) High income

100% of NRC allowance
in all nutrients

67.99% of NRC allowance one
or more nutrients
(but not below 67% in any)

Under 67% of NRC allowance
in any nutrient

(A) Under $1,000 for one and $2,000 for two members
(B) $2,000 and over for one, $3,000 and over for two members

Fig. 19-2. Diet quality as related to income among older households in Rochester, New York. (From LeBovit, C., and Baker, D. A.: Food consumption and dietary levels of older households in Rochester, New York, Home Economics Research Report No. 25, Washington, D. C., 1965, U. S. Department of Agriculture.)

the older citizen, who characteristically chooses to live in the more familiar, central, less expensive part of town. To take advantage of the lower prices at the larger market he must either pay for public transportation to and from the store or must become dependent on friends with cars. Once in the store, he may become overwhelmed and confused by the choices with which he is confronted and in the end may shop rather ineffectively or may return to the smaller delicatessen or service store at which prices are higher but which offer the familiar personalized service.

The pervading fear that they may become ill and be unable to look after themselves renders elderly people ready prey for the food faddist or purveyor of natural food and food supplements who promises them excellent health, eternal youth, increased vitality, and assurance that they will avoid the debilitating diseases so feared in old age. All too frequently they

are persuaded by door-to-door salesmen to invest a significant part of their income in all-but-worthless products, greatly overpriced, that cannot provide the protection they seek against conditions for which no cure is known.

Social factors. A person who preserves his independence by living alone may find that this in itself modifies his eating pattern. Lack of motivation to cook regular meals leads to the use of snack-type foods at irregular times, resulting in a poorly balanced meal nutritionally. Inexpensive living quarters may lack adequate cooking and refrigeration facilities. Swanson has observed that it is not unusual to find an older person showing a very erratic eating pattern—a day of nibbling followed by a day of overeating. In one instance she found a woman's daily intakes varying from 800 to 3700 kcal., accompanied by loss of nitrogen except on days when the intake was above 3000 kcal. and 100 gm. of protein.

Psychological factors. Conditions of emotional stress or deprivation often lead to modifications in attitudes toward food and in food habits. Persons who are anxious may experience loss of appetite and resultant undernutrition or, on the other hand, may indulge in compulsive nibbling, which leads to overnutrition. Their interest in food may represent emotional poverty or lack of other interests. Some older people who find their living situation intolerable escape it by relying on the sedative effect that occurs following a large meal. In spite of this tendency to overeat, obesity is rarely a problem in old age, although LeBovit found about one third of her subjects overweight. Others use food as an attention-getting device. The older person who is completely self-sufficient is often neglected by his relatives and friends. On the other hand, the person who does not eat adequate meals becomes a cause of concern and is often the recipient of attention and invitations. The same diet consumed under the emotionally unhappy condition of living alone compared to the pleasant atmosphere of companionship leads to a loss of nitrogen over a period as short as 30 days.

Factors affecting digestion and absorption

Changes in digestive secretions. With the degeneration in the size of the salivary glands that has occurred by 60 years of age there is a decrease in the secretion of saliva. The effect of this on carbohydrate digestion is minimal, since other enzymes are capable of complete carbohydrate digestion. However, the loss of saliva as a lubricant for food may have a more profound effect. With the decline in saliva, a trend develops toward the use of softer, more moist foods, such as creamed dishes, mashed potatoes rather than baked potatoes, and thinner starch-thickened products, possibly a means of compensating for the natural lubricants in the saliva.

The secretion of most digestive enzymes shows a decline with aging, but the extent of the decrease and the age at which it occurs has not been fully established. Depending on the extent of the decrease, food may be less completely digested or will require a longer time for complete digestion. Impaired liver function with a loss of bile secretion has been shown to influence fat digestion. Evidence reported earlier that a decline in hydrochloric acid secretion of 9% to 35% occurred in aging has been refuted in more recent work that failed to show a decline.

Factors affecting metabolism and excretion

Decline in physiological function. Many of the changes associated with aging occur in functions that require a coordination among various organ systems that decline at varying rates. The rate at which nerve impulses are conducted varies only slightly, but the amount of blood the heart can pump and the capacity of the lungs declines with age. Thus marked impairment occurs in the amount of physical exercise an older person can tolerate.

The rate of blood flowing through the kidney is decreased to 50% of the normal adult capacity. This means that less blood is presented to the filtering system of the kidney, through which the waste products of metabolism are eliminated and the nutrients are returned to the general circulation. Thus an increase develops with aging in the time required to excrete waste products.

The normal functioning of individual cells requires a definite chemical composition of the fluids bathing them. This varies directly with the composition of the blood so that a measure of blood composition reflects that of cell environment. No measurable difference is found between the blood of older and younger subjects, but if the composition is deliberately altered, as it could be by the ingestion of sodium bicarbonate, a person 70 years old requires from four to eight times as long as does a person 30 years of age to reestablish normal blood composition. This is only one example of changes in the rate at which the body can adjust to stress.

Alterations in the blood vessels, such as the narrowing of the lumen, loss of elasticity, thickening of the wall, and replacement of elastic muscle fibers with nonelastic material, reduce the capacity of the blood vessels to effectively nourish all parts of the body.

Hormonal secretions. Changes in hormonal secretions that exert a regulatory effect on a wide range of physiological processes have a direct or indirect effect on the nutrition of the cells and hence of the whole organism. By regulating the diameter of blood vessels, the endocrine glands regulate the amount of blood and hence the nutrients reaching the tissues. In aging persons there is a greater restriction in the size of the blood vessels leading to the kidney than in the size of those leading to the

brain, thus assuring more adequate blood supply to the more vital centers.

The adrenal gland, which normally responds to the stimulation by the pituitary hormone during stress, does not respond as rapidly in older people, indicating a reduced capacity to respond to stress. In contrast, the thyroid gland retains its ability to manufacture and secrete thyroxin, although a slight reduction occurs in the amount of protein-bound iodine, which indicates the level of the circulating thyroid hormone.

Nutritive needs

The information available on the nutritive needs of persons over 40 years old is scanty and is based primarily on studies of the intake of healthy persons, rather than on experimental balance studies designed to determine their needs. In general it is suggested that the nutritive intakes proposed for early adulthood be maintained throughout life. Except for calories, there is little

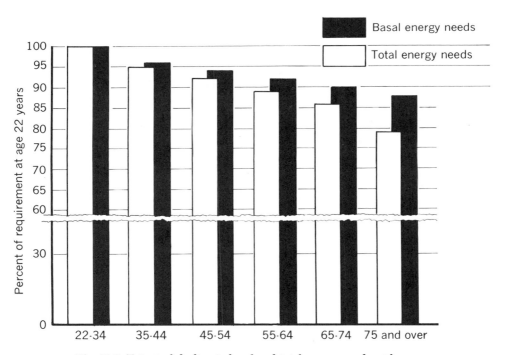

Fig. 19-3. Extent of decline in basal and total energy needs with age.

evidence that needs either diminish or increase. The extent of information available on each nutrient will be discussed.

Energy. The National Research Council has recognized the change in activity patterns and energy needs that occurs with aging. The trend from active sports to spectator sports, the decline in activity accompanying retirement, the decrease in the amount of housework for women, and the decline in basal metabolic needs as the number of cells in the body decreases with the loss of tissue mass—all contribute to this. They suggest that the average reduction in total energy needs with increasing age is 5% between 22 and 35, 3% per decade between 35 and 55, 5% per decade from 55 to 75, and a further decrease of 7% after 75. The change in basal and total energy needs is depicted in Fig. 19-3.

Studies on nutritive intake of older persons have shown intakes below 1400 kcal., representing either efforts to reduce weight, inability to buy or eat more, failure to eat regularly, or inability to chew food. In addition to failing to meet the individual needs for energy, such diets invariably are inadequate in some other nutrients, such as calcium, iron, and several vitamins. Even though the suggested amount of protein may be provided, much that should go into the synthesis of body proteins is diverted to be used as a source of energy, leading to negative nitrogen balance. This situation occurred experimentally in diets of less than 1800 kcal.

Failure to consume adequate calories and with it adequate levels of other nutrients may account for the fatigue, lassitude and lack of interest in life so often experienced by elderly people. The lassitude and fatigue may depress activity to the extent that the need for calories is reduced, leading to weight gain even on a low energy intake. It is conceivable that the use of nutritionally suboptimal low-calorie meals may be related to the premature signs of aging.

One study of 100 women 40 to 70 years of age established a relationship between caloric intake and general level of health. Those whose health was rated good consumed 1650 to 1825 kcal., whereas those whose health was rated as poor were consuming 1125 to 1475 kcal. This study confirmed that the number of symptoms and the likelihood of other nutrient deficiencies increased when the energy value of the diet was lower. It is difficult to separate cause and effect in such a situation, however.

Protein. The National Research Council recommends that an intake of 0.9 gm. of protein per kilogram of body weight be maintained throughout adulthood. Studies show that average intakes of elderly people are in the neighborhood of 45 gm. daily. This may occur for many reasons. A low protein intake almost always occurs with a low caloric intake. Inability to chew properly reduces the intake of protein-rich meat, and the rejection of milk as a food suitable only for infants or because of intolerance due to lactase deficiency eliminates another potentially good source of protein. Protein-rich foods are the most expensive group and may well be reduced for considerations of economy.

Some evidence has been established that the elderly have amino acid requirements that differ from those of younger adults. Specifically, the need for lysine and methionine is thought to increase.

Emotional state of a person influences nitrogen balance, with emotional instability depressing nitrogen and calcium retention.

In the adult, protein is used primarily for maintenance of cells and for the synthesis of enzymes needed for digestion and cellular metabolism. If cellular enzymes are not produced, the cell cannot function properly and ultimately dies, leading to a loss of cell mass reflected in decreased organ size and reduced organ function. This may account for the observation that as the amount of protein decreased, the number of symptoms reported went up.

Since iron, thiamin, riboflavin, and niacin occur together in many foods high in protein, a deficiency of protein will lead to a deficiency of these other nutrients as well. A reduction in thiamin to critically low levels depresses appetite, which further reduces total food intake and compounds the problem of dietary inadequacy.

Calcium. Early in the study of bone and tooth metabolism it was believed that these tissues were metabolically inert and that once they were formed, the need for a dietary source of calcium was drastically reduced. Although subsequent research has clearly established that bones are metabolically dynamic tissues calling for a constant source of dietary calcium, it has been very difficult to convince older people that they do not outgrow their need for calcium. The loss of 100 mg. of calcium per day, which can occur on a diet providing 400 mg. or less, would lead to a loss of 30% of the skeleton in 10 years. Such a loss would result in osteoporosis, a condition characterized by a decrease in bone mass but no change in bone quality. Older persons suffering from osteoporosis have a decreased stature and fragile bones that are slow to heal after a fracture. Factors other than diet are implicated in this condition that afflicts more women than men. However, evidence exists that an intake of calcium that leads to the formation of bones with a maximum density at maturity, coupled with an intake of 800 to 1000 mg. during adulthood, is the best protection against the development of osteoporosis in old age. Once osteoporosis has developed, one can only hope to inhibit its progress. Intakes of vitamin D as high as 1000 to 5000 I.U. have been shown to restore positive calcium balance in people with osteoporosis. The ingestion of fluorine throughout adult life is believed to have a beneficial effect in retarding the course of osteoporosis. Intakes of fat above 200 or below 50 gm. also inhibit calcium absorption. An inadequate intake of calcium rather than poor absorption is likely to be the cause of the lowered retention. The decreased use of milk products and the resultant decrease in calcium intake is evident from Fig. 19-4, based on data from 1965 survey of food consumption in households in the United States.

Pyridoxine. Although some reports indicate that the need for pyridoxine increases with age, this is most likely due to the effect of some medications such as isoniazid or penicillamine used in treating infections.

Ascorbic acid. The intake of vitamin C among older persons is frequently reported to be extremely low. Long-standing food habits have not established the practice of

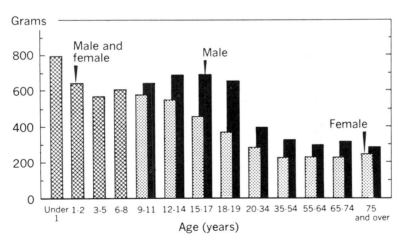

Fig. 19-4. Consumption of milk and milk products (calcium equivalent, quantity per person per day) as related to age—spring, 1965; 28 gm. = 1 ounce. (From Agricultural Research Service, U. S. Department of Agriculture, 1969.)

using fresh fruits and vegetables. The relatively high cost of these foods and the bulk that many provide may be some of the factors contributing to a restriction in their use. A beneficial effect from ascorbic acid (as replacement for hydrochloric acid in older people) on the absorption of calcium and iron has not been substantiated.

Iron. The need for iron does not change for men, but for postmenopausal women who no longer suffer iron losses in monthly menstrual flow, the recommended allow-

ances drop back to 10 mg. from 18 mg. The ability to absorb iron does not diminish, but with a decrease in caloric intake the iron intake frequently drops. This is especially true if protein content of the diet decreases.

Fat. Because of possible relationship between high fat intake and the development of atherosclerosis and heart disease, it is suggested that older persons, especially those who may be overweight, restrict their fat intake to a level providing 30% to 35%

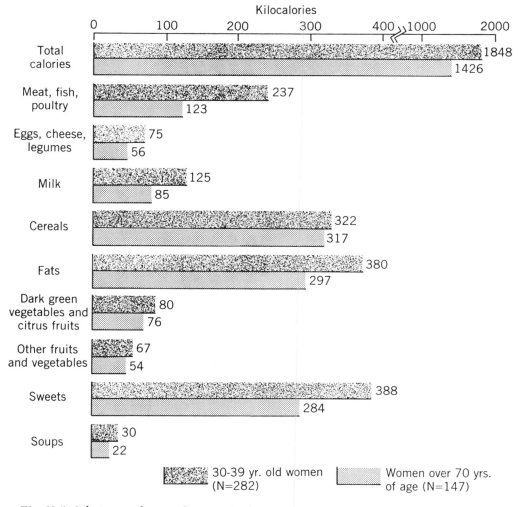

Fig. 19-5. Caloric contribution of various food groups in 30- to 39-year-old women and women per day) as related to age—spring, 1965; 28 gm. = 1 ounce. (From Agricultural Research **56**:728, 1964.)

of the calories. Age per se does not affect tolerance for fat.

ADEQUACY OF DIETS

The assessment of adequacy of diets of aging people is complicated by the difficulty in obtaining subjects. In one study only 13% of the people contacted agreed to participate, raising the question how representative they were of the original group. In spite of the difficulties of obtaining the cooperation of a sufficiently large group of aging people, several studies have been successfully completed to give some picture of prevailing dietary patterns. Although the majority have been confined to institutions to facilitate data collection, some have been carried out on groups of individuals living in their own homes.

Swanson, comparing the nutrient intake of Iowa women at 30 to 39 years of age with those of women over 70, reported a decrease in intake of calories, protein, ascorbic acid, and calcium. The relative and absolute amounts of meat, fish, and poultry, of sweets, of fats, and of milk products accounted for this decrease. The relationship between calories contributed by these groups in the two age groups is shown in Fig. 19-5. The amount of cereal products in the diet remained constant but constituted a higher proportion of the total calories as aging people reduced their total caloric content.

Kelly, in a study of food selection of 114 older Michigan women, also reported low intakes of calcium and ascorbic acid as well as vitamin A, with a higher mortality rate among those getting less than 40% of the recommended allowances of one or more nutrients. A large number of her subjects complained of tiredness, pains in joints, shortness of breath, constipation, and other signs of general malaise.

Fry, in a smaller study of 32 women over 65, found their diets to be reasonably adequate, with iron, calcium, and vitamin A the most likely limiting factors. But only 12%, 16%, and 9% of the women, respec-

tively, showed these specific deficiencies. Similarly, a study of low- and moderate-income elderly people in rural Pennsylvania showed vitamin A and calcium intakes below two thirds of RDA for 66% of the subjects and caloric, thiamin, riboflavin, and vitamin C intakes below two thirds for over 40%. Iron and protein were most often taken above this level. Those on low incomes had significantly lower iron and protein intakes than those on moderate incomes.

A study of 283 households in which homemakers were over 60 and were dependent on Old Age Survivors and Disability Insurance showed 44% with diets evaluated as good and 25% with poor diets, defined as those containing less than two thirds of the recommended allowances for one or more nutrients. It was observed that diets low in protein were low in at least four other nutrients. Thiamin, which was lacking in the diets of 40% of the households, and calcium and ascorbic acid, low in 30% of the cases, were the nutrients most often low.

Steinkamp was able to follow a group of 577 aging persons in California over a fourteen-year period. She found that the mean intake met the standards for all nutrients except calories for men, calcium for women, and ascorbic acid for both. However, one fourth of the men and one half of the women had less than two thirds of the recommended calcium allowances, and one fourth of both sexes had equally low intakes of ascorbic acid. They showed a slight downward trend for all nutrients with age, and a sharp downward trend after 75. She found that the decrease in calories was associated with a general decrease in the amount of food consumed, rather than a decrease in a particular food or food group.

DIETARY SUPPLEMENTS

The fact that older persons are concerned about their health and are highly motivated to take any steps that they believe will help maintain a sufficient level of health for them to maintain their independence means that the use of dietary supplements—especially multivitamin and mineral capsules—is widespread. In Rochester, New York, it was found that 37% of the households of people 55 or older were using supplements, 29% of which were ordered by the doctor. Of these 104, 48 were consuming diets adequate in all nutrients and needed no supplements, and 56 with fair or poor diets would have benefitted from the correct supplement. However, only 12 of this group used supplements that provided all the nutrients lacking in their diets, 31 used products providing some but not all of the nutrients they needed, and 13 supplemented their diets with nutrients they were already getting in adequate amounts in their regular diet but not with the nutrients they needed. A similar situation was noted in a study of men and women over 50 years of age in California

where Steinkamp found that 35% were using mineral, vitamin, or other food supplements. Of those taking vitamin supplements, 37% had diets already adequate in the vitamins taken. Of the 63 diets found low in vitamin A, 12 diets were supplemented; of 43 low in ascorbic acid, 11; for niacin, 8 of 45; for riboflavin, 4 of 29; and for thiamin, 3 of 11. In the case of minerals only 3 of 89 persons with suboptimal intakes of calcium took supplements including calcium, and none of the 23 needing iron received it. Since the amount spent on supplements may represent an appreciable proportion of the money available for food, one would hope that more guidance could be available to help those who would profit from supplements to choose the correct ones and to counsel those whose diets are already adequate against wasting their money.

SELECTED REFERENCES

Anderson, W. F.: Nutritional problems of the elderly, Proc. Nutr. Soc. 27:185, 1968.

Batchelder, E. L.: Nutritional status and dietary habits of older people, J. Amer. Diet. Ass. 33:471, 1957.

Berry, W. T. C.: Protein status of the elderly, Proc. Nutr. Soc. 27:191, 1968.

Bjorksten, J.: Aging: present status of our clinical knowledge, J. Amer. Geriat. Soc. 10:125, 1962.

Black, K., and Guthrie, H. A.: Dietary practices of the elderly in Bedford County, Pennsylvania. (In preparation, 1970.)

Brink, M. F., Speckmann, E. W., and Bailey, M.: Current concepts in geriatric nutrition, Geriatrics 23:113, 1968.

Curtis, H. J.: Biological mechanisms underlying aging process, Science 141:686, 1963.

Davidson, C. S., Livermore, J., Anderson, P., and Kaufman, S.: Nutrition of a group of apparently healthy aging persons, Amer. J. Clin. Nutr. 10:181, 1962.

Esposito, S. J., Vinton, P. W., and Rapuano, J. A.: Nutrition in the aged. Review of the literature, J. Amer. Geriat. Soc. 17:790, 1969.

Fry, P. C., Fox, H. M., and Linkswiler, H.: Nutrient intakes of healthy older women, J. Amer. Diet. Ass. 42:218, 1963.

Garry, R. C.: Symposium. Nutrition and the elderly, Proc. Nutr. Soc. 19:107, 1960.

Hovell, S. C., and Loeb, M. V.: Nutrition and aging, monograph, Gerontologist 9:1, 1969.

LeBovit, C.: The food of older persons living at home, J. Amer. Diet. Ass. 46:285, 1965.

Lutwak, L.: Nutritional aspects of osteoporosis, J. Amer. Geriat. Soc. 17:115, 1969.

Pelcovitz, J.: Nutrition in older Americans, J. Amer. Diet. Ass. 58:17, 1971.

Shock, N. W.: Physiologic aspects of aging, J. Amer. Diet. Ass. 54:491, 1970.

Steinkamp, R. C., Cohen, N. L., and Walsh, H. E.: Resurvey of an aging population—fourteen-year followup, J. Amer. Diet. Ass. 46:103, 1965.

Swanson, P.: Adequacy in old age. I. Role of nutrition, J. Home Economics 56:651, 1964.

Tappel, A. L.: Will antioxidant nutrients slow aging processes? Geriatrics 23:97, 1968.

Watkins, D. M.: New findings in nutrition of older people, Amer. J. Public Health 55:548, 1965.

Watkins, D. M.: The impact of nutrition on the biochemistry of aging in man, World Rev. Nutr. Diet. 6:124, 1966.

Williams, I., and Smith, C. E.: Home-delivered meals for the aged and handicapped, J. Amer. Diet. Ass. 35:146, 1959.

20 | *Weight control*

Weight control is a term generally applied to efforts to maintain body weight within the limits compatible with maximum level of health or to adjust body weight to conform to these established standards. For the vast majority of adults this control is readily achieved with little or no conscious effort. This is impressive when one considers that a daily error of 10 kcal. (0.5% of the caloric intake of a sedentary adult female) will accumulate to represent a change in body weight of 1 pound per year, and a daily 100 kcal. error, a change of 10 pounds. For a relatively small group of people the problem is one of keeping weight up to desired levels, and for a somewhat larger group, estimated as high as 25% of the population, the problem is one of restricting weight gain. Although the health hazards of being underweight may be equally as great as those of being overweight, persons in the latter group are more receptive to advice and more motivated to seek it. They are also the subject of vastly more research and are more ready targets for promoters of food supplements ready to capitalize on their desire for a panacea for weight problems. The underweight individuals are, comparatively speaking, totally ignored. This discussion will reflect the situation by drawing rather extensively on the vast literature available to discuss obesity and dealing with the problems of the underweight individual in a few paragraphs. This must not be interpreted to imply that the underweight individual does not warrant attention.

OBESITY

Obesity is generally defined as a condition in which there is an abnormal accumulation of fat in body tissue. When 20% of body weight of a man and 28% to 30% of the weight of a woman is composed of fat (normal values are 12% to 18% and 18% to 24%, respectively), the amount of fat is judged to be abnormally high, and the individual is described as obese. An increase in fat to these levels means the body cells that normally contain some fat have become saturated with fat. In addition, to accommodate the fat that must be formed to store energy intake in excess of expenditures, these are special fat, or adipose, cells capable of holding as much as 62% fat and possibly connective tissue cells that are converted into fat cells. This increase in body fat usually corresponds with a weight at least 15% above ideal or desirable weights and is evidenced by an increase in the bulk or size of the body, which may be either localized or distributed throughout the body. Formerly described as simple obesity, the condition is now recognized as a symptom of one or more disturbing influences—either physiological, psychological, or pathological. It is indeed a condition of multiple origins.

In addition to the segment of the population who can be theoretically described as obese, there is another group designated as merely overweight, whose body weight is above the level believed to be compatible with the optimal level of health but not sufficiently high to represent an excess accumulation of fat. Overweight individuals, of course, are very likely to become obese unless preventive measures are taken when the increments in weight begin.

Bruch suggests that the body may have a preferred weight that bears no relation to an accepted standard but one that the individual tends to maintain or to revert to after an attempt at weight adjustment.

Diagnosis

The absence of any single, effective technique for measuring body fat on which to base a diagnosis of obesity has led to the use of many methods.

Appearance. Diagnosis of severe obesity can be made reliably on the basis of physical appearance, but this criterion is useless in identifying cases of borderline obesity, since it does not distinguish between body size caused by an accumulation of fat and that caused by an accumulation of water or muscle. On the basis of appearance some persons may be judged to be obese at a body weight that cannot be considered unhealthy. One group, however, did show that visual observations of children were a valid means of differentiating the obese from the nonobese. These judgments correlated well with those based on body weight, skinfold, or growth patterns.

Skinfold measurements. Efforts to assess subcutaneous fat, which represents 50% of the total body fat, by measuring the thickness of a skinfold have been only moderately successful. Mayer believes that a single skinfold measurement on the triceps, located at the back of the right upper arm midway between the elbow and the shoulder, is adequate for diagnostic purposes. Others, however, maintain that they must be made in several parts of the body. Measurements must be made with a constant-pressure caliper (usually 10 gm. per square millimeter). These measurements must then be compared to an established standard for obesity. Generally the relation of skinfold thickness to body fat is independent of height. Ruffer has presented evidence that an index based on triceps skinfold and weight correlates well with body fatness and is a simple, useful tool for identifying obesity. The major drawback to this method is the difficulty of getting reliable measurements not only from different technicians but also from the same technicians on separate occasions. The wide variation noted under normal conditions is another complicating factor. For instance, in 12-year-old boys the median measurement of triceps skinfold was 9 mm., with a range of 4.5 to 22 mm.

X-ray measurement of body fat. A relatively new technique in which the thickness of fat is measured in various parts of the body as it shows up on an x-ray plate is useful in clinical studies but is of limited value for routine diagnostic purposes because of its high cost and the relative hazard of widespread use of x-ray technique.

Comparison of body weight to an established standard. In spite of the limitations of a comparison of the weight of an individual to established standards of weight for specific age and height, it remains the most widely used criterion available. Practically all standards are based on figures made available by insurance companies and are the ones associated with the lowest mortality rates. The current standards described as "desirable weights" at age 25, released by the Society of Actuaries, are reproduced in Appendix E. It will be noted that these weights are made with normal clothing, and heights are taken with 2-inch heels for women and 1-inch heels for men. Nude weights are 7 to 9 pounds less for men and 4 to 6 pounds less for women than are weights with clothing on. Moreover, the individual using these tables must arbitrarily classify himself in one of three body frame types—small, medium, or large. This makes it possible for an individual to place himself in the category that best suits his needs as he perceives them and is frequently the one that represents his present status in the most favorable light.

The use of standard height-weight tables

to determine presence or absence of obesity, considered 15% to 20% above desirable weight, can be very misleading when the individual is edematous (suffering from an excess accumulation of fluid in the tissues) or when his weight is composed of a low proportion of muscle and a high proportion of fat, or vice versa.

Determination of lean body mass. Three major techniques are available to determine the relative amounts of fat and lean body mass comprising body weight, but all require trained workers and expensive equipment. The measurement of specific gravity involves comparing the weight under water (corrected for residual air in the lungs) to the weight in air. When the proportion of fat is normal, the ratio of weight in water to weight in air, or specific gravity, will be approximately 1, indicating a normal distribution of musculature and fat. Adipose tissue has a specific gravity of 0.92, compared to 1.1 for the rest of the body. As the proportion of fat increases, the specific gravity decreases, since fat is lighter per unit of volume than lean body mass. The lower the specific gravity, the greater the proportion of fat in the body.

Since the amount of water in the body is known to be approximately 72% of lean body mass, knowledge of the amount of water in the body can be used to compute the amount of lean body mass. This in turn could be subtracted from the total body weight to determine the amount of body fat.

Another technique for measuring body water involves injecting a known amount of either of the chemicals, antipyrine or deuterium oxide, into the blood and removing a sample of blood after a prescribed period to determine the extent to which body water had diluted the chemical. From this determination total body water, then lean body mass, and finally body fat can be calculated.

A technique known as the *whole body counter* is based on the theory that potassium represents a fixed percentage of lean body mass or protoplasm and that potassium 40, a radioactive form of potassium, is a fixed percentage of the potassium in food consumed and hence of the potassium in body tissue. By measuring the radioactivity of potassium 40 in the whole body by subjecting an individual to a short period in front of a Geiger counter, it is possible to measure the amount of this substance in the body, and from this to calculate the total amount of potassium and then the lean body mass. Subtracting this from total body weight, one then calculates the amount of body fat present. Although the equipment is initially expensive and requires a skilled operator, the test subjects the individual to no discomfort or hazards and may have potential as a diagnostic tool.

Other techniques. The search for a simple method of recognizing obesity has led to the development of many gimmicks. For instance, Joliffe suggested the "ruler test," in which a ruler laid from the chest to the abdomen of a subject lying on his back will rise at the end toward the feet in an obese person and be flat or slanted downward in a person of normal weight. Another criterion, the "perfect 36" index, involves subtracting a person's waist measurement in inches from his height in inches. Values of 36 to 40 are considered characteristic of persons of normal body weight, whereas a value less than 25 represents obesity. The limitations of such methods are obvious.

Prevalence

The difficulty of arriving at a suitable criterion for diagnosing obesity has led to confusing reports on the incidence of obesity, even when one recognizes that marked differences may exist in various segments of the population. For instance, public health statistics suggest an incidence of 10% to 13%, insurance statistics based on a selected population 6% to 7%, and statistics from a study of Iowa women 25%. A weight at least 20% above standards, which represents a doubling of fat reserves, is found in millions of Americans, representing 3% of the population over 30 years of age, according to MacBryde. Duncan in Philadelphia, basing his figures on the *Build and Blood Pressure Study,* reports that 5% of the males (1 in 20) and 11% of women (1 in 9) are at least 20% over the desirable weights suggested by life insurance statistics as most conducive to longevity. Pollack and others in New York placed the figures at 30% for males and 40% for females over 40. One study of 12,000 schoolchildren showed 30% of them more than 20% overweight, based on standard height-weight charts, whereas another reported that 12.5% of adolescent girls and 9.5% of adolescent boys were overweight.

A study of 110,000 people in Manhattan showed seven times the incidence of obesity in the lower socioeconomic groups as in the middle and upper groups. The former continued to gain weight after 35 years of age, whereas the latter group did not. In contrast, another study reported that middle-class adolescents were more likely to be obese than either their lower- or upper-class counterparts.

Many of the discrepancies in the reported incidence of obesity can be attributed to differences in the social, cultural, and economic background.

Practically all studies agree that obesity becomes a progressively greater public health problem as the ability to regulate exercise and intake is lost from ages 20 to 60, with the gradual decline in energy requirements. At birth the infant requires 50 kcal. per kilogram of body weight for basal metabolism, at 5 years a child needs 45 kcal., and at 15 an adolescent needs 40 kcal., after which needs decline steadily at a rate approximating 1% per year. After 60 to 70 years of age the incidence of obesity declines, reflecting the higher mortality rates prevailing among younger obese people in the population so that the obese do not live to become a statistic at age 60.

Disadvantages

Before a person is motivated to correct a condition such as obesity, which calls for considerable willpower and perseverance over a long period, he must be convinced that the disadvantages of the condition are sufficiently great to warrant the self-discipline involved. There are many disadvantages from a health standpoint as well as physically, physiologically, economically, and socially.

Health hazards. It is well established that chronic illness is more prevalent among obese than nonobese and that even for people only 10% to 15% overweight mortality rates are higher. Table 20-1 shows the increase in mortality rates that occurs with progressively higher body weights and the

---

Table 20-1. Increase in mortality rates with severity of obesity

Percent overweight	Percent increase in death rate
10	10-15
20	20-25
30	40-45
40	70

Table 20-2. Mortality rates from various causes among overweight men and women—percent actual of expected deaths*

Causes of death	Men	Women
All causes	150	147
Cardiovascular-renal diseases	149	177
Diabetes	383	372
Cirrhosis of the liver	249	147
Appendicitis	223	195
Ulcers	67	—
Suicide	78	73
Tuberculosis	21	35
Pneumonia	102	129

*From Marks, H. H.: Influence of obesity on morbidity and mortality, Bull. N. Y. Acad. Med. **36:**15, 1960.

concomitant decrease in life expectancy. For each pound of weight above ideal weight, the death rate increases by approximately 1%. Table 20-2 shows the effect of obesity on mortality rates from specific diseases. It is evident that the risk of cardiovascular disease, cerebral hemorrhage, and nephritis is much higher among obese than nonobese persons. Even with greatly improved surgical techniques

the obese person subjected to surgery is still in considerable hazard. The relationship between heart disease and obesity can be appreciated when one recognizes that for every pound of added fat the heart must pump blood through an additional two thirds mile of blood vessels.

The relationship between obesity and diabetes may not be one of cause and ef-

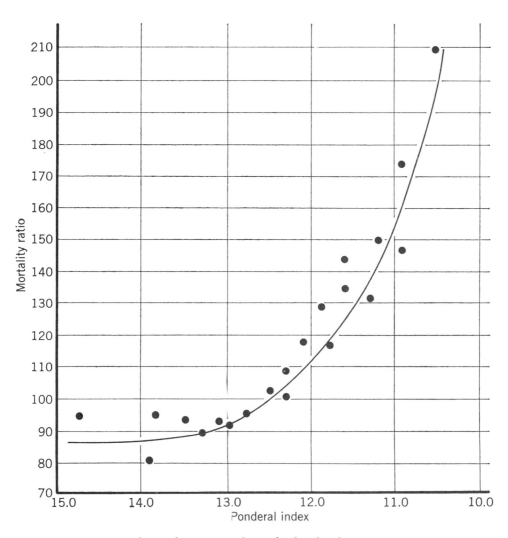

Fig. 20-1. Association of mortality ratio with ponderal index for men, issue ages 40 to 49. Ponderal index = height in inches divided by cube root of weight in pounds; issue ages = age at which insurance was issued. (Data derived from Build and blood pressure study, 1959; from Seltzer, C. C.: New Eng. J. Med. **274:**254, 1966.)

fect, since current theories suggest that obesity may be an early sign of adult-onset diabetes and may be caused by essentially the same metabolic defect. Obesity may be a stress factor in diabetes to precipitate diabetes in susceptible individuals.

Although the presence of some fat surrounding vital organs such as the kidney, heart, and lungs is desirable, excessive fat accumulation interferes with their mechanical efficiency.

Seltzer has found that in men a decrease in the ponderal index (height in inches divided by cube root of weight in pounds) below 12.5 is closely related to an increased mortality rate. This index represents body shape rather than body size, for which mortality precipitously rises at the lower end of the ponderal index range as shown in Fig. 20-1. This lower end of the index represents extreme endomorphs who have long been characterized as obese.

Social disadvantages. The obese person frequently finds himself caught in a vicious circle from a social point of view. Often the initial weight gain is a reflection of an unhappy social adjustment. The resultant obesity leads to social rejection, which in turn leads to more overeating, to increased weight, and to continued or more profound rejection. Adolescents in particular are victims in this chain of events. Excessive weight precludes their effective participation in many active sports, such as tennis, badminton, or swimming, and in social activities, such as dancing. The reduced activity often accompanied by a nibbling pattern of eating makes weight gain easier, again setting up a vicious circle. It has been demonstrated that obese girls have reduced chances of being admitted to college. This is further evidence that obesity can be considered a deterrent to advancement on the socioeconomic scale.

Economic disadvantages. The obese individual finds that certain occupations, such as airline stewardess, nursing, selling, receptionist, or other jobs in which public impressions are important or mobility essential are closed to him. Some employers are reluctant to train persons who are obviously health risks. This not only limits the vocational choices open but also curtails advancement in many occupations. In addition, this person may find that the cost of special clothes, furniture, or transportation will increase his cost of living well above normal. In considering economic factors, one may also consider the amount that may well be spent in potential cures or weight-reducing panaceas or the cost of his excessive food intake.

Psychological disadvantages. Although it has been impossible to attribute any particular personality traits to obese individuals, several studies have revealed some interesting relationships. It is difficult to determine if psychological factors are a cause or effect of obesity, but it may be easy to underestimate the psychological effects of obesity on an obese individual, especially an adolescent girl. For instance, Mayer observed that obese girls had personality characteristics similar to those of racial and ethnic minority groups—self-blame, withdrawal, passivity, inferiority feelings, and sensitivity about one's status. Lack of family support exposed obese adolescents to greater tension. Obese persons have been found to have "distorted body images," a preoccupation with weight, and a tendency to blame all failures and disappointments on their weight. It is possible that social pressures on obese juveniles affect their personalities permanently.

Causes

The development of the concept that obesity is a disease of multiple origins or a syndrome rather than a single disease entity does not represent any rejection of the long-established concept that fat will accumulate only when the intake, or consumption, of energy (measured in kilocalories) exceeds the output, or expenditure, of energy. It does, however, propose that the cause of a failure to make a successful adjustment in caloric intake may be found in diverse areas and even suggests that perhaps not all persons should reduce. It still holds true that when caloric intake exceeds caloric expenditure, the excess cannot be excreted and will be stored as body fat once the limited glycogen reserves of liver and muscle have been saturated. Nor is there any reason to believe that body fat arises spontaneously. It arises only as a storage form of energy. In the growing individual, however, energy will also be used in the increase in body musculature and bone. In short, the law of conservation of energy still holds. In general, the factors that influence the individual's ability to adjust caloric intake to expenditure will be classified as environmental, psychological, genetic, cultural, and physiological.

Environmental factors

Availability of food. Obesity is a significant problem for large segments of the population only in countries where the food supply exceeds the demand. It is, in essence, a disease of plenty. The middle and upper socioeconomic classes in most countries have always had plenty of food and hence have been the ones who have tended to become obese. This is depicted in medieval paintings in which the corpulent rich man is shown being waited on by lean servants. In many societies today one evidence of a successful man is a plump, well-fed wife.

Advertisers are constantly inducing us, especially our children, to buy more food; at the same time, another segment of the industry is promoting weight-reducing aids for those who have bought and consumed too much food.

Comfort of environment. Well-heated houses and warm, lightweight clothing have reduced the amount of energy needed to maintain normal body temperature in temperate climates, and the energy costs of procuring food have been decreasing constantly with the mechanization of the food and agriculture industries.

Food and hospitality. The use of food as an expression of hospitality does much to increase the energy intake of the population by having food more constantly available. People are offered food and drink in almost all social situations from the early-morning coffee klatsch to the late-evening buffet supper and midnight snack. Failure to offer food in a social situation may be interpreted as a lack of hospitality, and failure to accept food on the part of the guest may be interpreted as a rejection of hospitality. The more important the occasion, the greater the amount of food and drink offered. In many cultures even the very poor feel compelled to save or borrow for a special festive occasion such as a wedding or baptism to save face by providing a feast.

Family food habits. Long-standing family food habits, many of which were established when existence involved more strenuous physical activity and everyone worked harder with less protection against extremes of weather, have been retained in the current push-button, air-conditioned era. The daughter serves the same kind of meal to her family that her mother served several decades earlier in spite of marked changes that have occurred in family energy needs.

The pattern of food intake is a significant factor among overweight persons. In one group 75% consumed most of their food between 4 o'clock in the afternoon and midnight. Only 17% of the subjects reported eating only three meals a day.

Decreased activity. A decrease in the amount and intensity of physical activity tends to occur with increasing age, with the transition from active to spectator sports. In addition, for the woman often the activity associated with homemaking decreases. Not only does she exercise less in looking after the needs of her children and home but also expects them to take over some of the household tasks she formerly did herself. The increased availability of labor-saving devices and more readily available transportation has resulted in lower energy expenditures among succeeding generations. For instance, power steering in a tractor reduces the energy expenditure by 20% compared to regular steering. A secretary working 6 hours a day on an electric typewriter expends 450 kcal. less per week than her counterpart using a standard typewriter. Similarly, it has been estimated that the average man expends 210 kcal. in walking 1 mile, 171 kcal. in cycling the same distance, and 17 kcal. in driving an automobile. The telephone company claims that the installation of an extension in the home will save 70 miles of walking a year. This could account for 1½ pounds of weight a year. If traditional meal patterns are not adjusted accordingly, the likelihood of an undesirable weight gain is increased.

Mayer, in studying the activity patterns of obese and nonobese children, found that the obese exercised significantly less each day with less enthusiasm than did the nonobese. Even when they reportedly participated in an activity for a comparable period of time, their actual time of activity was as little as one third that of nonobese. They also ate less, but the adjustment was not sufficiently large to compensate for the lower caloric requirements. Because of their larger weight load, obese individuals are often less skilled in sports and may limit their participation even more. Mayer also observed that adolescent obesity usually began in the winter, traditionally a period of reduced activity in the temperate climate. For some persons, periods of forced immobility coupled with admonitions to eat to keep up strength may initiate an excessive weight gain. The widespread use of school buses, often for reasons of safety, in transporting children to and from school further deprives young people of a mild but consistent form of exercise. To compensate for such things, these people must make a conscious effort to increase their activity, since prescribed physical education programs in schools are much too short to substitute for this. It has been shown similarly that obese women walked only half as much as controls or 20 miles less during a week. In many cases they sought ways of reducing activity, such as use of elevators, efficient schedule planning to reduce activity, or choosing a mode of living that called for a minimum energy expenditure.

Response to external stimuli. Schachter observed that in contrast to nonobese persons, the obese ate in response to external stimuli, rather than to internal sensations of hunger. They were more likely to eat in response to the time on a clock, when food was readily available, or in response to stress than in response to hunger sensations associated with physiological changes.

Patterns of infant feeding. The tendency of mothers to consider large weight gains in early infancy as highly desirable and to compare the eating habits of their infants to those of other infants leads them to introduce solid foods at an early age and to force large quantities of food. Bakwin attributes some of the problems of obesity in adolescence to a pattern of eating in which the individual is trained to eat beyond the point where he experiences normal satiety signals to the point where he is overeating. He believes that such a situation can be conditioned by patterns of feeding in early infancy. Some infants have been encouraged to eat as much as they want as frequently as they want; at the same time, physical activity is often minimized.

Psychological factors

Investigations to determine whether psychological factors are causative or perpetuating in obese persons were begun in the late 1940's and have not yet identified any personality factors common to persons who experience difficulty in making a satisfactory weight adjustment. The psychological makeup of the individual influences not only the intake of food but also the level of activity and hence the energy expenditure.

An extensive review of the relationship between specific psychological factors and the incidence of obesity is well beyond the scope of the discussion, but some of the more established relationships will be discussed. Although obesity is compatible with normal personality factors, some characteristics occur more frequently in obese than nonobese subjects. According to Bruch, overeating may be a balancing factor in adjustment to life. If overeating is to be stopped, the individual must be helped to find some other form of emotional support. Failure to do so may result not only in unsuccessful weight reducing but may also produce trauma far worse than the obesity it was designed to cure. The threat of earlier mortality from many diseases is not a motivating factor for many. To them, the prospect of dying early and happy is much less threatening than is the prospect of an unhappy life adjustment that comes with an inability to reduce in the face of continuing efforts. Indeed, without his pattern of overeating he may be in danger of developing a form of mental illness. The need for individual therapy is evident. From a psychological point of view, overeating may be a response to nonspecific emotional tensions or a symptom of underlying emotional tensions, or it may represent an addiction to food.

Anxiety. An anxious person deprived for one reason or another of an outlet in physical activity may seek solace in food, the consumption of which represents a pleasureful pastime. The greater the level of anxiety, the more likely weight gain is to occur.

Substitute for love and security. To at least some obese individuals, overeating, a pleasant experience, is used as a substitute for love and affection or as an expression of self-pity. An overprotective mother may overfeed her child to reinforce her love for him. For others the strength symbolized by a large body is apparently a source of se-curity representing a bulwark against an unfriendly world.

Tenseness or frustration. In some persons food is a response to, compensation for, or defense against tension and frustration.

Genetic factors

Characteristics of an individual that determine his level of intake and pattern of utilization of food may be determined by heredity. Such factors may explain the different responses in different individuals in common environments or similar responses among identical twins in markedly different environments.

Somatotype. The anthropological classification of somatic body types as endomorphic (plump and round), mesomorphic (muscular), and ectomorphic (linear and fragile) is based on genetically determined traits. The endomorph is likely to become obese, whereas the individual with few of the endomorphic characteristics tends to remain slim, as does the individual with a high ectomorphic component in his body build. The mesomorph will become obese if his build includes more of an endomorphic than ectomorphic component. In a study of obese girls it was shown that none of them had an elevated ectomorphic component, whereas 40% of endomorphs of normal weight had a high ectomorphic component in their body structure. The endomorph tends to gain weight easily, whereas the ectomorph seldom does. Obese girls have been demonstrated to have broader, shorter hands than nonobese, which further points to a relationship between the fragile bony structure of the ectomorph and the absence of obesity. In Britain it was demonstrated that mesomorph-endomorphs had a ratio of 2.4:1 as many relatives in the same somatotype as ectomorphs.

Level of enzyme activity. Evidence has suggested that the rate of production of enzymes involved in either fat storage or fat mobilization can affect the formation of fat and the ease with which it can be used as a source of energy. An efficient or active enzyme system involved in fat formation (lipogenesis) may remove glucose from the bloodstream so rapidly that the normal satiety signals to reduce food intake do not operate quickly enough to regulate food intake, leading to an increased food intake and hence fat formation. This rate of lipogenesis in obese persons may be as much as five times greater than normal. Once fat has been deposited in adipose tissue primarily as triglycerides, it must be broken down into fatty acids and glycerol (lipolysis) before the fat can be released from the storage site to be transported in the bloodstream for use as a source of energy in tissues requiring energy. This lipolysis depends on the presence of a fat-splitting enzyme—a lipase. In obese people the level of activity of this enzyme may be low or inhibited so that they do not mobilize or release stored fat rapidly enough to meet the body's demand for a source of energy. To meet the need, the individual is forced to consume more food. It has also been established that once fat has been deposited in adipose tissue, the cell will again store fat more readily after its removal. Thus it is easier for a person who has been obese to become obese again than it is for one who has never been overweight.

Although each gram of carbohydrate or protein has the potential of yielding 4 kcal. in the body and each gram of fat 9 kcal., many enzymes are involved in the many steps in their conversion to carbon dioxide, water, and energy in the form of ATP. Since we have much evidence of biochemical individuality in many enzyme reactions in the body, it is logical to assume that wide individual differences exist in the degree of efficiency with which energy will be released from these potential sources and with which it will be converted to mechanical, chemical, osmotic, or electrical energy for vital body functions. Such differences are undoubtedly genetically determined and are encoded in the DNA of the cell nucleus. An individual with a low lipase activity or a very inefficient enzyme system for the release of energy may have more difficulty regulating his weight. Conversely, a person with an adequate lipase activity and a high efficiency rate in the release of energy will make a much more adequate weight adjustment. Aerobic metabolism is more efficient than anaerobic metabolism, in which it is necessary to expend energy to resynthesize glycogen. It is possible that the tendency toward aerobic metabolism, the more efficient type, may be genetically determined, leaving more energy to be stored. Such differences are well known to animal breeders; they choose animals whose genetic characteristics allow them to gain the most weight on the smallest amount of food, which facilitates the production of wool, milk, or eggs.

Genetically determined characteristics also influence a person's athletic aptitude and hence his participation in active sports.

The sensitivity of the appetite-regulating center of the brain, the hypothalamus, appears to be genetically determined. A sensitive hypothalamus responds quickly to an elevated level of arterial blood glucose relative to venous blood glucose and depresses appetite. A less sensitive hypothalamus will respond more slowly and will allow the individual to eat more before a feeling of satiety is reached.

Studies to determine the incidence of obesity in children of obese parents have shown that if both parents are obese, the chance is 73% that the children will be; if one parent is obese, the chance is 50%; and if neither parent is obese, the chance is only 9% that the children will be. When the children are reared in the same environment as the parents, the relationship is undoubtedly partially environmental and partially hereditary. However, Mayer, in studying the effect of environment on the incidence of obesity, found that infants adopted into families with one or more obese parents did not become obese, whereas those born into similar families did become obese.

Once genetic factors are recognized as determinants, it would be reasonable from a public health standpoint to encourage persons with a hereditary predisposition to obesity to participate in a preventative program based on a regimen of activity and a regulation of food intake begun at an early age. Genetically determined differences between individuals may be impossible to detect with the sensitivity of present analytical methods, but if even small differences accumulate, they become appreciable.

Cultural factors

The meaning of body size varies from one cultural group to another and influences attitudes toward obesity. To many groups a large body represents success; the man with the plump wife is one who is sufficiently successful to provide her with adequate food. The stereotype of the plump, successful nineteenth century businessman, an object of envy to his less successful contemporaries, is gradually being replaced by that of the sleek, well-dressed, efficient young executive. In certain primitive tribes young girls will be kept in, fed, and fattened into attractive young women. In many royal courts the women carried about on litters vie with one another to be the fattest and hence the most attractive to royalty.

Food assumes special meanings in various life situations; it is frequently offered in times of sickness or death; it is basic to the feasts used to celebrate births, marriages, and deaths in many cultures in which the provision of adequate food may involve incurring large debts.

Physiological factors

Decreased basal energy needs. The need for energy to carry on the vital body functions, known as basal metabolism, declines gradually with age. Although the difference in needs between one year and the next may be imperceptible and may call for no conscious adjustment in energy intake, failure to make a satisfactory adjustment of intake to needs over a period of years can lead to an appreciable positive caloric balance in old age.

Secretion of endocrine glands. The basal metabolic rate is determined by the level of secretion of the thyroid gland, thyroxin. In most individuals this is maintained within a normal range, but a small segment of the population may find their energy needs depressed because of a depressed secretion of thyroxin. Some persons experience an easy accumulation of fat and may find it easier to achieve caloric balance if either thyroxin or the closely related compound thyronine is administered. Because of the hazards from unsupervised use of the hormone, it is available only on prescription.

Insulin, the secretion of the pancreas that is necessary for the conversion of carbohydrate to fat as well as for the utilization of carbohydrate as a primary source of energy, can influence the rate at which adipose tissue is formed.

Some endocrine secretions influence the distribution of fat in various parts of the body, and abnormal distributions represent an abnormal endocrine balance.

Adaptation. A severe caloric restriction for a period of time activates an adaptive mechanism that leads to a lowered basal metabolic rate and a greater efficiency in energy expediture, thus conserving the energy available.

Regulation of food intake. The mechanisms by which the amount of food a person eats is regulated are still subject to much study, but it now appears that there is both a short-term and long-term regulation.

Short-term regulation. The meal-to-meal or short-term regulation of intake is controlled by the appetite-regulating center of the brain, the hypothalamus. The gluco-static theory suggests that the medial part of the hypothalamus is sensitive to the level of glucose but not of amino acids or lipids in the bloodstream. When the difference in glucose content of arterial and venous blood (A-V difference) is large, indicating that the tissues have more glucose available than they are removing, the hypothalamus stimulates a satiety response that depresses the appetite and feelings of hunger. When the A-V difference is small, the hypothala-mus responds by stimulating the hunger sensation, thus producing an increased in-take of food. Although it is generally agreed that the hypothalamus regulates food intake, there is not complete agree-ment that it responds to blood glucose levels, since some evidence exists that it may respond to the heat produced by the specific dynamic action of food. It is also suggested that an unidentified factor in blood plays a regulatory role in controlling food intake.

Long-term regulation. The long-term reg-ulation of food intake is governed by the reserves of fat in the adipose tissue cells of the body. It is hypothesized that a type of feedback mechanism operates whereby the food intake of one day reflects the intake of the previous days, with hunger being stim-ulated when low intakes have led to a depletion of fat reserves.

Persons who have difficulties in reducing weight have low, free–fatty acid levels in the blood after fasting compared to those in persons whose obesity responds to re-duced caloric intake. This suggests a differ-ence in their ability to mobilize fat reserves to supply energy during caloric restriction. These same persons respond slowly to the presence of a fat-mobilizing substance such as epinephrine. It may be the result of a metabolic defect that limits the breakdown of body fat stores or one that hastens the reformation of fatty acids and glycerol into fat depots or the presence of a lipase in-hibitor.

Classification

Obesity can be classified on several bases. One classification chooses to differ-entiate between *juvenile onset obesity,* which usually develops before the child is 10 years old, and *adult onset obesity,* which develops later in life. The former is gen-erally more severe than the latter, is more difficult to treat, has a poor response to therapy, and occurs twice as frequently in girls as boys. Frequently it is associated with a low intelligence and occurs among those with relatively little schooling. In some respects it may be an inherited con-dition caused by either more efficient use of energy or greater efficiency in energy ex-penditure. In contrast, adult onset obesity is characterized by a constant food intake in conjunction with a slowly declining en-ergy expenditure both for basal metabolism and for activity. It is the result of the slow insidious weight gain of as little as ½ to 1 pound per year, which may occur with aging but may go unrecognized until it is well advanced. Sometimes the reduction in cell mass that occurs with reduced ac-tivity masks the accumulation of fat, which signals the onset of obesity.

In another classification based on patho-genesis, obesity has been identified as either *regulatory,* in which there is either psychological or physiological defect in the regulation of food intake in relation to energy expenditure, or *metabolic,* in which there is an underlying metabolic de-fect in the handling of either carbohy-drate or lipid that can be enzymatic, hor-monal, or neurological in nature. It is suggested that juvenile onset obesity and metabolic obesity are the same and that adult onset and regulatory obesity are the same. Bruch, whose experience is primarily with persons seeking psychological help, has suggested that *constitutional obesity* due primarily to physiological causes, in which the person has a healthier per-sonality adjustment to obesity and may suf-fer some form of maladjustment if forced to reduce, can be distinguished from *reactive obesity,* most common in adults in which overeating as a response to tension or frustration is often accompanied by decreased physical activity. Episodes of grief or depression frequently correspond to weight gains. Persons with reactive obesity often experience a night-eating syndrome, a higher level of eating corresponding with periods of depression. These two forms in turn, she believes, are different from developmental obesity, which is common in children whose emotional development centers around eating as much as they want, at the same time avoiding physical activity and social contacts.

In general, the basis on which the classification is made reflects the perspective of the investigator. It may be that physiological factors mediate the psychological trauma that leads to overeating.

Treatment

The treatment of obesity involves the successful reversal of the positive caloric balance that caused the condition, that is, a caloric intake less than caloric expenditure. Because of the multiple origins of obesity and the many meanings of food to individuals, it is often difficult to find the cause of obesity. Until the cause is known, efforts to correct the condition are discouraging. Although the effectiveness of treatment depends on many factors, the motivation of the patient and the establishment of a realistic goal are of prime importance. In most cases the obesity is the result of a low caloric surplus over a long period of time. A small error in intake when accumulated over a period of years is reflected in a sizeable weight gain. Conversely, a constant intake of 100 kcal. less than daily expenditure will result in a 10-pound weight loss in one year.

The patient launching a weight-reducing regimen should be aware that for some persons no drop will occur in body weight for perhaps two or three weeks regardless of strict adherence to a diet known to be deficient in calories. The explanation is that as fat is withdrawn from storage sites, water may enter the cells to replace fat and may remain there for a period of time, after which it may be released rapidly. Unfortunately, this phenomenon occurs at the stage in weight reducing when a person is most in need of some evidence of success. Usually when weight loss is looked at over a longer period of two to three months, the predicted weight loss will be observed. It is common for a person to experience spurts of weight loss followed by a plateau, even with constant caloric intake and expenditure.

Studies on the prognosis of treatment have shown that success is more likely in adult onset than in juvenile onset obesity, in males than in females, in younger people than in older, in married people than in widowed, separated, or divorced, in single people (especially women under 30), in the higher socioeconomic groups, in those making their first attempt than those making subsequent attempts, among those less than 60% overweight, among emotionally mature and well-adjusted rather than anxious or depressed persons, and among those with a medical problem that is complicated by obesity. It should also be emphasized that success will be greater if attempts are made in early stages and if done under supervision of a physician who concerns himself with the underlying causes, rather than with a quack, charlatan, faddist, pseudoscientist, or well-meaning but misguided friends.

The reversal of the caloric balance involves setting the total caloric intake at a level less than that required to meet energy needs. This may be accomplished by either decreasing the intake or increasing activity or preferably both. The level of caloric intake that will accomplish this varies greatly from one person to another because of the many individual factors that contribute to the situation.

Decreased caloric intake. Decreased caloric intake may be achieved by a strict diet that prescribes a specific number of calories from specific foods or by a prudent diet in which an individual maintains his customary eating patterns but selects smaller portions and avoids foods of high caloric value. Although popular literature abounds in diets designed to lead to a painless loss of weight, few have stood the test of time, and the search for the panacea continues.

One currently popular theory is that weight loss is more effective if calories are derived from fat and protein rather than carbohydrates. Experimental evidence, however, shows that weight loss is a function of caloric intake regardless of the source of calories. The distribution of total calories throughout the day can influence the relative amount of muscle and fat deposited. If a large number of calories is consumed at one time in a condition described as *nutrient overload,* some calories that might have been used in muscle growth or in tissue repair are diverted to fat depots because of the demand suddenly placed on one metabolic pathway. The same number of calories distributed in smaller, more frequent feedings leads to decreased fat and increased muscle increments. Thus some evidence appears in support of the nibbling habit in weight reduction, provided, of course, the amount of food nibbled does not exceed the needs of the individual.

In addition to a restriction in the total caloric intake, certain other considerations may be important in dieting success. Understanding guidance and support from physician or friends or family is crucial. A rigid diet may be anxiety-producing. Eating slowly, tasting food thoroughly, using a smaller than average plate, and including such carbohydrates as potatoes because of their satiety value may contribute to a successful weight-reducing program. Even more important is the necessity of developing a set of eating patterns in which the caloric intake is restricted and can be maintained to replace the eating pattern that led to the weight gain. For some persons this may involve a reeducation of their concept of serving size. Some research shows that the overweight person's concept of an average serving of food is a much larger quantity than that of a person of normal weight.

Complete starvation diets and those completely devoid of carbohydrates are effective because they lead to the accumulation of ketone bodies in the bloodstream, which in turn depress the appetite. The hazards involved in overtaxing the body's capacity to counteract excess ketones or to excrete them dictate that such regimens be employed only in extreme obesity that has been refractory to all other conventional methods and that they be undertaken with strict medical supervision. Persons on such diets are usually hospitalized and are kept in bed because of the extreme weakness accompanying the loss of sodium that occurs. The short-term effects of such programs have given dramatic results, but the long-term effects have been discouraging, with very few patients maintaining, let alone continuing, their weight loss. Part of the rapid initial weight loss can be attributed to an initial loss of sodium with the concurrent loss of water and the fact that protein has been deaminated to provide sufficient glucogenic amino acids to obtain the glucose needed to maintain the energy supply for the central nervous system and erythrocytes. This is reflected in negative nitrogen balance. Since protein is a less concentrated storage form of calories than fat tissue is, much more must be catabolized to provide the same number of calories. The extensive loss of protein in starvation diets is manifest not only by a negative nitrogen balance but also loss of body potassium. The catabolism of a pound of muscle tissue yields about one sixth as many calories as a pound of fat tissue.

Intermittent fasts of one to twelve days' duration after an initial fast of one to fifteen days have shown promising results initially, giving the patient a feeling of well-being and cheerfulness, but have proved no more satisfactory than a continuous reduction in caloric intake in the long run. Persons who have been on a fasting regimen usually eat less immediately afterwards and experience satiety with less food. This has led to the hypothesis that during fasting the satiety center in the hypothalamus may become more sensitive to satiety signals.

Criteria for evaluating diets designed for caloric restriction are discussed in Chapter 5.

Increased activity. The effectiveness of an increased level of activity in establishing caloric equilibrium has been alternately overrated and underrated. As illustrated in Chapter 5, the 3000 to 3500 kcal. represented by 1 pound of stored body fat is sufficient energy for many hours of such vigorous activity as tennis. However, a few minutes of the same activity every day for a longer period will help maintain the fine daily caloric balance necessary for weight control without undue stimulation of the appetite. Thus, while a 60 kg. (132-pound) woman will have to walk for 30 hours at an energy cost of 2 kcal. per kilogram per hour to use the energy stored in 1 pound of body fat, if she walks half a mile a day at this rate of 3 miles per hour, after 180 days she will have used the equivalent amount of energy. Such a mild degree of exercise can represent 2 pounds per year. Sometimes the initiation of a program of moderate exercise not only increases caloric expenditures sufficiently that a weight loss will occur on a diet that previously maintained weight but also improves muscle tonus, stimulates circulation, and creates a general sense of well-being. Strenuous exercise, on the other hand, may lead initially to a loss of appetite but may later stimulate the appetite to counter-balance any advantages of the regimen.

A study to determine the effectiveness of a program of nutrition education and exercise on the course of obesity in 13- to 14-year-old boys more than 30% overweight in the beginning of the program showed that obese boys in the experimental group gained 5.8 pounds during the 18-month study period, whereas those in the control group who did not receive nutrition education and who did not participate in a program of physical activity gained 13.5 pounds. These results suggest that a program of nutrition education coupled with one of prescribed physical activity can be an effective method of controlling adolescent obesity. The energy costs of activity in relation to the energy value of representative foods is shown in Table 20-3.

Dietary aids

A discussion of weight control would not be complete without some mention of the types of dietary aids, representing a $100 million business, with which the adult public is constantly confronted. The magnitude of this enterprise likely reflects the fact that many obese persons cannot adhere to a diet without supportive measures. It also represents the constant search of the overweight for some easy, painless, and quick road to weight loss. Since few of these aids stand the test of time and remain on the market for more than a brief period, this discussion will be confined to the general types of dietary aids.

Agents reducing food intake. Appetite depressants, or anorexigenic drugs, are the basis of many dietary aids. Pills containing sugar, milk solids, or gelatin taken about half an hour before meals act as an appetite depressant by raising blood glucose levels, increasing the difference between arterial and venous glucose levels, hence depressing the appetite at mealtime. These are relatively harmless but generally greatly overpriced even when the cost of minerals and vitamins that are often added to them is considered. The same effect could be achieved with caramels from the

1000 c = 1 C

Table 20-3. Energy equivalents of food calories expressed in minutes of activity*

Food	kcal.	Activity				
		Walking† (min.)	Riding bicycle‡ (min.)	Swimming§ (min.)	Running‖ (min.)	Reclining¶ (min.)
Apple, large	101	19	12	9	5	78
Bacon (2 strips)	96	18	12	9	5	74
Banana, small	88	17	11	8	4	68
Beans, green (1 cup)	27	5	3	2	1	21
Beer (1 glass)	114	22	14	10	6	88
Bread and butter	78	15	10	7	4	60
Cake (1/12, 2-layer)	356	68	43	32	18	274
Carbonated beverage (1 glass)	106	20	13	9	5	82
Carrot, raw	42	8	5	4	2	32
Cereal, dry (½ cup) with milk and sugar	200	38	24	18	10	154
Cheese, cottage (1 tablespoon)	27	5	3	2	1	21
Cheese, Cheddar (1 ounce)	111	21	14	10	6	85
Chicken, fried (½ breast)	232	45	28	21	12	178
Chicken, "TV" dinner	542	104	66	48	28	417
Cookie, plain (148/pound)	15	3	2	1	1	12
Cookie, chocolate chip	51	10	6	5	3	39
Doughnut	151	29	18	13	8	116
Egg, fried	110	21	13	10	6	85
Egg, boiled	77	15	9	7	4	59
French dressing (1 tablespoon)	59	11	7	5	3	45
Halibut steak (¼ pound)	205	39	25	18	11	158
Ham (2 slices)	167	32	20	15	9	128
Ice cream (1/6 quart)	193	37	24	17	10	148
Ice cream soda	255	49	31	23	13	196
Ice milk (1/6 quart)	144	28	18	13	7	111
Gelatin, with cream	117	23	14	10	6	90
Malted milk shake	502	97	61	45	26	386

corner grocery store if only one were taken. Fruit juices high in carbohydrate, such as grape juice or prune juice, would have a similar effect.

Stimulants. Products containing amphetamines, which are stimulants for the central nervous system, are useful in overcoming depression and its attendant nibbling. They are the basis of other products but must be used with caution, since they result in an elevated blood pressure, dryness of the mouth, and a rapid heartbeat, effects that cannot be divorced from its effect on the appetite. Dexedrine and Benzedrine, common appetite depressants, are also cardiac stimulants, as are epinephrine or ephedrine-like compounds. These anorexigenic drugs may be an essential crutch in the initial period of caloric restriction for the person who has become addicted to food and who eats compulsively but should be used only under strict medical supervision.

Tranquilizers as weight-reducing aids function by decreasing activity but at the same time reducing nibbling, which may have been the cause of weight gain.

Loss of body water. Diuretics lead to a

Table 20-3. Energy equivalents of food calories expressed in minutes of activity—cont'd

		Activity				
Food	kcal.	Walking† (min.)	Riding bicycle‡ (min.)	Swimming§ (min.)	Running‖ (min.)	Reclining¶ (min.)
Mayonnaise (1 tablespoon)	92	18	11	8	5	71
Milk (1 glass)	166	32	20	15	9	128
Milk, skim (1 glass)	81	16	10	7	4	62
Milk shake	421	81	51	38	22	324
Orange, medium	68	13	8	6	4	52
Orange juice (1 glass)	120	23	15	11	6	92
Pancake with sirup	124	24	15	11	6	95
Peach, medium	46	9	6	4	2	35
Peas, green (½ cup)	56	11	7	5	3	43
Pie, apple (1/6)	377	73	46	34	19	290
Pie, raisin (1/6)	437	84	53	39	23	336
Pizza, cheese (1/8)	180	35	22	16	9	138
Pork chop, loin	314	60	38	28	16	242
Potato chips (1 serving)	108	21	13	10	6	83
Sandwiches						
Club	590	113	72	53	30	454
Hamburger	350	67	43	31	18	269
Roast beef with gravy	430	83	52	38	22	331
Tuna fish salad	278	53	34	25	14	214
Sherbert (1/6 quart)	177	34	22	16	9	136
Shrimp, French fried	180	35	22	16	9	138
Spaghetti (1 serving)	396	76	48	35	20	305
Steak, T-bone	235	45	29	21	12	181
Strawberry shortcake	400	77	49	36	21	308

*From Konishi, F.: Food energy equivalents of various activities, J. Amer. Diet. Ass. **46**:186, 1965.
†Energy cost of walking for 70 kg. individual = 5.2 kcal. per minute at 3.5 mph.
‡Energy cost of riding bicycle = 8.2 kcal. per minute.
§Energy cost of swimming = 11.2 kcal. per minute.
‖Energy cost of running = 19.4 kcal. per minute.
¶Energy cost of reclining = 1.3 kcal. per minute.

loss of body water but no loss of body fat. If extra weight is caused by an accumulation of water in the tissues, diuretics will lead to permanent weight loss, but under normal conditions such water must be quickly replaced to maintain normal electrolyte balance. Steam baths, special plastic clothing, and bath salts—also designed to reduce weight by reduction in body water—will effect only transient weight loss.

Bulk-producing substances. Noncaloric substances such as methyl cellulose are advocated as appetite depressants because of their affinity for water and their tendency to increase in volume on the theory that bulk in the stomach will depress appetite. It has been experimentally demonstrated that the swelling of methyl cellulose takes place in the small intestine rather than in the stomach, thus limiting its supposed effectiveness.

Psychological aids. Testimony of individuals who have thought or prayed their way to slimness is evidence of the use being made of psychologically oriented devices in weight control. Other devices with strong powers of suggestion such as records played during sleep or pictures of the individual in slimming clothes are some of the current psychological gimmicks.

Transition diet

Once a desired weight adjustment is achieved, it is important that the individual be given guidance in the transition from a reducing diet to a maintenance diet. It is especially important that one recognize the level of intake that will maintain the desired weight and that is sufficiently different from the regular diet that led to the initial weight gain to prevent a recurrence. Although no clear explanation exists for the phenomenon, maintenance requirements for a person who has lost weight have often been found to be lower than those for a person of comparable weight who has not reduced. Any maintenance diet must be sufficiently individualized to conform to the cultural, environmental, and social situation in which the individual lives.

Prevention

From a public health point of view the most feasible attacks on the problem of obesity are through prevention. By learning to identify those individuals who, because of genetic makeup, personality characteristics, or environmental factors, are most likely to become obese, it should be possible to develop an educational program designed to control weight gain in the incipient stage. Such an approach could embrace a program of exercise coupled with education and training in the choice of foods and patterns of eating to minimize caloric intake. Pediatricians, with access to weight grids, which help identify deviations in growth patterns in the early stages, have an opportunity to alert parents and to encourage them to help the child acquire a set of eating patterns that will help forestall weight gain. Obstetricians and gynecologists working with women during pregnancy and menopause, two periods when weight gain is easy, are in a position to help the women to cope with such an eventuality. Similarly, physicians dealing with middle-aged males working under any form of emotional stress who have a family history of heart disease have a unique opportunity to offer preventive therapy before weight reaches the stage where it enhances the possibility of coronary or arteriosclerotic heart disease. Persons with deviant activity patterns are just as prone to caloric imbalances as are those with deviant eating habits; thus it is important to work on both sides of the energy equation, promoting a habit of moderate but consistent exercise along with moderation in food intake.

It is becoming increasingly clear as we learn more about the problems of weight control that these problems are extremely complex and that many questions are still unresolved. Indeed, it may be necessary to reevaluate some of our current concepts and possibly reject some of them.

UNDERWEIGHT

A person whose weight is more than 15% below desirable weight, although not subjected to the same social pressures to adjust as is his overweight counterpart, is more susceptible to certain health hazards. He is almost twice as likely to succumb to respiratory disease such as tuberculosis and has greater difficulty maintaining body temperature as environmental temperature drops.

Treatment

The treatment of underweight individuals involves creating a positive energy balance by increasing energy consumption beyond energy expenditure regardless of the level of the latter. Just as in obesity, it is important to recognize the cause of the undernutrition if it is to be adequately treated. If a depressed appetite is involved, various techniques can be used. Thiamin-deficiency anorexia may be reversed by the use of thiamin supplements. Handling of anorexia nervosa is considerably more complex and should involve determining the underlying cause. The use of smaller, more frequent meals of lower caloric value rather than fewer larger meals may help promote an increased energy intake. The addition to regular foods of highly concentrated sources of energy such as sugar, jellies, butter, mayonnaise, sauces, or dried milk solids

is a fairly successful way of increasing the energy value of a diet without an increase in bulk. Just as in weight reduction, the adjustment in weight needs to be made gradually, and it may be even more difficult, albeit more pleasant, for an underweight person to try to gain 1 pound per week than for an obese person to lose it.

SELECTED REFERENCES

Obesity

Ayers, W.: Changing attitudes toward overweight and reducing, J. Amer. Diet. Ass. **34**:23, 1958.

Bakwin, H.: Feeding program for infants, Fed. Proc. **23**:66, 1964.

Bortz, W. M., Wroldsen, A., Issekietz, B., and Rodahl, K.: Weight loss and frequency of feeding, New Eng. J. Med. **274**:376, 1966.

Bruch, H.: Psychiatric aspects of obesity, Metabolism **6**:461, 1957.

Darling, C. D., and Summerskill, J.: Emotional factors in obesity and weight reduction, J. Amer. Diet. Ass. **29**:1204, 1953.

Drenick, E. J., and Smith, R.: Weight reduction by prolonged starvation, Postgrad. Med. **36**:A95, 1964.

Dudleston, A. K., and Bennion, M.: Effect of diet and/or exercise on obese college women, J. Amer. Diet. Ass. **56**:126, 1970.

Fabry, P., and Tepperman, J.: Meal frequency— a possible factor in human pathology, Amer. J. Clin. Nutr. **23**:1059, 1970.

Fellner, C. H., and Levitt, H.: A new approach to overweight, Amer. J. Clin. Nutr. **15**:50, 1964.

Forbes, G.: Lean body mass and fat in obese children, Pediatrics **34**:308, 1964.

Goldberg, M., and Gordon, E. S.: Energy metabolism in human obesity, J.A.M.A. **189**:616, 1964.

Gordon, E. S.: New concepts of the biochemistry and physiology of obesity, Med. Clin. N. Amer. **48**:1285, 1964.

Halpern, S. L.: Methodology of effective weight reduction, Med. Clin. N. Amer. **48**:1335, 1964.

Hamburger, W. W.: The psychology of weight reduction, J. Amer. Diet. Ass. **34**:17, 1958.

Hashim, S. A., and Van Itallie, T. B.: Clinical and physiologic aspects of obesity, J. Amer. Diet. Ass. **46**:15, 1965.

Jacobs, D., Heald, F. P., White, P. L., and McGanity, W. J.: Obesity prevention, J.A.M.A. **186**(supp. 1):27, 1963.

MacBryde, C. M.: The diagnosis of obesity, Med. Clin. N. Amer. **48**:1307, 1964.

McCracken, B. H.: Etiological aspects of obesity, Amer. J. Med. Sci. **243**:99, 1962.

Mayer, J.: Physical activity and anthropometric measurements of obese adolescents, Fed. Proc. **25**:11, 1966.

Mayer, J.: Some aspects of the problem of the regulation of food intake and obesity, New Eng. J. Med. **274**:610, 662, 722, 1966.

Mayer, J.: Overweight causes, cost and control, Englewood Cliffs, N. J., 1968, Prentice-Hall, Inc.

Mendelson, M.: Deviant patterns of feeding behavior in man, Fed. Proc. **23**(part 1):69, 1964.

Mendelson, M.: Psychological aspects of obesity, Med. Clin. N. Amer. **48**:1373, 1964.

Moore, M. E., Stunkard, A., and Strole, L.: Obesity, social class and mental illness, J.A.M.A. **181**:962, 1962.

Pollack, H.: Prophylaxis of obesity in the adult, Bull. N. Y. Acad. Med. **36**:87, 1960.

Prugh, D. E.: Some psychological considerations concerned with the problem of overnutrition, Amer. J. Clin. Nutr. **9**:538, 1961.

Rosenberg, B. A., Bloom, W., and Spencer, H.: Obesity—treatment and hazards, J.A.M.A. **186**(supp.):43, 1963.

Ruffer, W. A.: Two simple indexes for identifying obesity compared, J. Amer. Diet. Ass. **56**: 326, 1970.

Sebrell, W. H.: Weight control through prevention of obesity, J. Amer. Diet. Ass. **34**:919, 1958.

Seltzer, C. C.: Some re-evaluations of the build and blood pressure study, 1959 as related to ponderal index, somatotype and mortality, New Eng. J. Med. **274**:254, 1966.

Seltzer, C. C., Goldman, R. F., and Mayer, J.: The triceps skinfold as a predictive measure of body density and body fat in obese adolescent girls, Pediatrics **36**:212, 1965.

Seltzer, C. C., and Mayer, J.: Body build and obesity. Who are the obese? J.A.M.A. **189**:677, 1964.

Shank, R.: Weight reduction and its significance, Nutr. Rev. **19**:289, 1961.

Shipman, W. G., and Plesset, M. R.: Predicting the outcome for obese dieters, J. Amer. Diet. Ass. **42**:383, 1963.

Swendseid, M. E., Mulcare, D. B., and Drenick, E. J.: Nitrogen and weight losses during starvation and realimentation in obesity, J. Amer. Diet. Ass. **46**:276, 1965.

Wright, F. H.: Preventing obesity in childhood, J. Amer. Diet. Ass. **40**:516, 1962.

Young, C. M.: Some comments on the obesities, J. Amer. Diet. Ass. **45**:134, 1963.

Young, C. M.: The prevention of obesity, Med. Clin. N. Amer. **48**:1317, 1964.

21 | *Food faddism and quackery*

Food faddism and quackery are aspects of nutrition that are receiving increasing attention from nutritionists because of the health, economic, and social problems they create. Nutritionists are recognizing that the food quack, with his strongly emotional appeal, his exaggerated claims, and his powers of persuasion, is commanding attention from a significant segment of the population and is rapidly undermining the teaching of the legitimate nutritionists. So far they have had little success competing with the faddist because of their unwillingness to misrepresent the knowledge in the field by making unrealistic claims. Faddism is not confined to the superstitious, the uninformed, and the poor. Although these people are easily influenced, persons with the easiest access to sound scientific information in the field are frequently attracted to faddism also. The forces that operate to keep food faddism alive are a complex of economic, sociocultural, and educational factors.

Food fads, defined as favored or popular fashions in food consumption that prevail for a period of time, are constantly changing. Although some basic beliefs of the food faddist recur and gain wide acceptance, the form in which they are manifest changes, and they can usually be destroyed if adequately and persistently attacked. A person who follows a food fad, usually with exaggerated zeal, becomes known as a food faddist, and the whole subject of fashions in food is known as food faddism. In many ways, food faddism can be considered a paradox of advancing medical and food technology. Only since nutritionists created an awareness of the importance of good food habits in maintaining a high level of health have the food faddists been able to capitalize on the public's concern that they eat well.

Some food fads, such as coffee drinking, are merely fashions that cannot be considered harmful in any way, but others, such as the use of food grown only on organically fertilized soil, may lead to bizarre eating habits at greatly inflated costs. In addition to attacking the problem of food fads, the legitimate nutritionist is constantly combatting food misinformation; this is often more difficult to fight, since it involves scientific half-truths, distortions, or misrepresentations of scientific information as well as outright fallacies and fancies. The food quack pretends to have information he does not possess, perpetrates his ideas or products on large groups of people, and is usually motivated by personal financial gain.

EXTENT OF FOOD FADDISM AND QUACKERY

The Food and Drug Administration believes that 10 million Americans are being bilked of at least half a billion dollars per year by food quacks, purveyors of nutritional supplements, and vendors of books and special devices reputed to solve the nutritional ills of the country. If a comparable amount were spent on improved food intakes, both the consumer and the food industry would benefit. Such a large expenditure of money on unnecessary supplementation or modification of the diet could occur only in an affluent society and reflects the health consciousness of the nation and our eternal quest for longer and healthier lives. Thus food quackery is confined to the technically developed countries that enjoy a high standard of living. It has been suggested that if the amount of money spent in the United States on dietary supplements is any indication of the nutritional status of the population, we must be considered the most poorly nourished nation in the world. In reality it takes more effort to be malnourished than well nourished with prevailing food patterns in the United States.

Jalso, in a study of nutritional beliefs and practices in New York state, found that food faddists had less formal education and less nutrition education than did nonfaddists and were concentrated in the older age and lower socioeconomic groups. On the basis of a personality test, food faddists were found to have more rigid personalities than did nonfaddists.

Nature of food fads

Food fads, in addition to representing mere fashions in food or the persistence of folk beliefs, follow several prescribed patterns, usually stressing a food concept rather than a nutrient concept.

Exaggeration of the virtues of a particular food. Many food fads revolve around the belief that specific foods have almost magical medicinal properties, usually in the cure of conditions over which medical science has produced no effective control or cure. Among the more common beliefs are that fruits cure cancer, carrot juice relieves leukemia, garlic reduces high blood pressure, and royal jelly extends the prime of life and leads to sexual rejuvenation. It is interesting to note that different cultures ascribe different properties to the same food. For instance, the tomato is considered poisonous by some, an aphrodisiac by others, and a cancer cure in still other situations. The folk belief that honey and vinegar are capable of curing ailments ranging from warts to hypertension to cataracts has been popularized in a book by a New England physician.

Food quacks constantly refer to the "secret formula" of a product, to which they attribute its special merits. In one case the secret formula was alfalfa, ground bones, and the germ from cereal products and in another garlic, lecithin, and wheat germ.

Omission of foods because of harmful properties. The omission of certain foods is as much a food fad as is the exaggerated use of them in the diet. The notion that any food enriched with nutrients (called "chemicals" by the faddists) is poisonous has led to the rejection of such staples in the diet as enriched white bread or milk fortified with vitamin D. The belief in a relationship between fruit and fever has led to the exclusion of fruit from the diet.

Foods high in cholesterol are avoided by many persons in the unsubstantiated fear that their use will lead to heart disease. For cholesterol-containing foods it is not unusual to find a person substituting high intakes of liquid oils, with a concurrent equally harmful increase in energy intake.

Emphasis on "natural" foods. A whole segment of the food faddist cult supports the notion that only "natural" foods are safe for human consumption. To qualify as a natural food, it must have been grown on soil fertilized with natural or organic fertilizers rather than chemical fertilizers, it must not have been subjected to herbicides or pesticides, and it must be unprocessed.

Many natural food organizations with very impressive and authoritative-sounding names propound the basic philosophy that all mental and metabolic diseases are caused by commercially processed foods. In several cases it has been established that the president of the organization or editor of its publication is the owner of a natural food store. Their propaganda war against all foods other than natural foods is continuous and knows no bounds.

Stores devoted entirely to sale of foods reportedly grown on naturally fertilized soil do a thriving business with customers who have lost all faith in the adequacy of food bought in normal food outlets and who fear the dangers of chemicals. Such persons travel long distances and pay exorbitant prices to avoid these "contaminants" in the food supply. A list of the foods available in such outlets includes carrot juice, stone-milled buckwheat flour, unsulfured fruit, wheat germ, fertile eggs, and Irish sea moss as well as more conventional food items. All these, the customer is led to believe, have been grown on soil that has not been treated with chemical fertilizers and are sold in their natural, unprocessed form. The use of such terms as "counterfeited," "prefabricated," "worthless," "national scandal," and "devitalized" to describe processed foods and "natural" and "vital" for unprocessed foods is designed to heighten the effect.

A survey of prices at a health food store revealed that unsulfured raisins cost six times the price of regular raisins; unenriched, unbleached flour four times as much as enriched all-purpose flour, canned tomatoes from "untreated" tomatoes five times as much as regular canned tomatoes; and apple butter from unsprayed apples ten times the cost of conventional apple butter. The inflated prices may be a function of a low volume of business or excessive profits. They may also reflect the fact that if crops are indeed grown without the benefit of chemical fertilizers, herbicides, and pesticides, the production will be low and the per unit price high.

Natural foods are for the most part wholesome foods that are rich in nutrients and flavor and certainly should never be condemned from a nutritional standpoint, but neither are they *essential* for health. Most processed foods have not been shown to be inferior and should not be excluded.

Special devices. Food faddists may also direct their attention to the types of equipment in which or on which food is prepared. Great merit has been attributed to devices for grating or shredding vegetables, to blenders often selling at twice the price of conventional blenders, or to cooking utensils (available only in large sets) that are said to be capable of conserving nutrients.

Dangers of food faddism

The major concern of the government and other agencies involved in protecting the consumer against the fraudulent claims and ineffectual products of the food quack stems not only from a fear that the product he sells is in itself harmful but also from a concern over the economic and ethical aspects of his operation. The government is concerned that millions of people are spending money for products that cannot possibly do what they are reported to do and more specifically that among the victims are many who can ill afford to divert their food money to nutritional supplements or overrated food products. The vitamins in many products are useless unless they have some substrate on which to act so that the supplements are useless without food. Older people in whom the fear of becoming ill or dependent is ever present are particularly susceptible. In addition to spending money on a product that is worthless for the purpose for which it was bought, people, in the belief that it may be effective, often delay the time when competent medical advice is sought until the damage is irreparable.

Mode of operation of the quack

The food quack capitalizes on people's desire for information and creates a market for his product or ideas through a variety of highly emotional appeals. He uses the overriding fear of many that they will become incapacitated through illness. For others he provides a crutch for their organic and psychic ailments. Quacks undermine the public's faith in the adequacy of the nation's food supply to provide them with the essentials for good health. Not only do quacks suggest that it may be incapable of providing the essentials, but also they claim that certain products used to increase our food production, such as chemical fertilizers, herbicides, pesticides, and the chemicals used in processing, are toxic substances undermining health and leading to all kinds of dire consequences. Competent scientists recognize that there can be hazards from the indiscriminate use of these substances and urge that their use be kept under surveillance so that we may have the benefits without the hazards.

By his contentions that all disease is caused by faulty diet, that the population suffers from widespread malnutrition, that food-processing destroys the nutritive value of foods, and that soil depletion is an underlying cause of faulty diets, the quack is able to create such a fear of sickness in his victim that he has little trouble selling his panacea. The imaginary illnesses he conjures up are often created by the use of vague, meaningless terms such as "roundness of corpuscles," "tired blood," and "vitagenic," all of which have scientific overtones to the gullible.

Food quacks frequently pose as members of legitimate-sounding professional organizations. It is virtually impossible for a lay person to recognize the names of the official organs of the profession, let alone to discriminate them from others with equally impressive names. To expect the general public to recognize that the American Institute of Nutrition, the official organization of nutritionists, is different from the American Academy of Applied Nutrition or the American Nutrition Society, both of which are nonscientific organizations, is to assume a level of interest that does not exist. In at least one case the telephone number listed on the letterhead of one of these pseudoscientific societies is answered by a health food store. Many of these organizations publish their own monthly journal with "scientific" articles by their own members, most of which support the use of the type of product sold in their outlets. Even reputable scientific groups have been temporarily deceived into accepting them as scientific. Besides mentioning specific organizations, quacks also promote themselves by the use of self-conferred titles such as "world-renowned nutritionist," "dietitian," "international authority," and other convincing accolades. Indeed, several individuals who have earned degrees that qualify them to use the title of doctor have been diverted into the lucrative food faddism business. By quoting scientific data out of context or in an incomplete form or by applying findings of animal studies to humans, they are able to create an illusion of scientific know-how.

The faddist is quick to capitalize on new developments in science by taking an observation from scientific literature and by smart and timely merchandising parlaying it into a neat profit. The promoters of safflower oil as an aid to reducing blood cholesterol levels were able for a short time to convince the public to buy it at the drugstore in 1100 mg. capsules at 6 cents each or approximately $25 per pint when the same product was available across the street in the grocery store at 80 cents a pint. Similarly, people with the unfounded belief that gelatin will improve the condition of their fingernails eagerly pay $2 per ounce for gelatin in capsule form that the grocer offers at 10 cents for the same amount. The ingredients in one widely distributed pill selling for 12 cents each were found to be the same as those in half a cent's worth of dried nonfat milk solids. The discovery of vitamin K, naturally present in alfalfa, as necessary for blood coagulation gave food supplement promoters another product in which the margin of profit was very high. Vitamin E, for which a human deficiency has seldom been demonstrated, is a favorite promotion of the quack, who attributes to the human being all the most severe deficiency symptoms ever observed in animals.

Characteristics of a quack

One can be suspicious of food quackery under any of the following conditions:

1. The promoter claims that his food has miraculous powers, usually in the cure of conditions that are still baffling medical science, such as arthritis, leukemia, and arteriosclerosis. He usually claims to have information not available through regular medical channels.

2. He claims that he is being persecuted by medical "trusts and cartels" whose livelihood is threatened by him and his product.

3. He maintains that the soil is depleted and is no longer capable of producing a food supply sufficient to meet the nutritional needs of the population. His only solutions to this are the use of food supplements or the exclusive use of the nutritious foods grown in soil fertilized with organic fertilizers.

4. He maintains that practically everyone is suffering from some degree of malnutrition that cannot possibly be corrected by foods readily available. He attributes this to the following dietary habits:

   a. Use of pasteurized rather than raw milk

   b. Use of nonfertile rather than fertile eggs

   c. Ingestion of mixed meals of a variety of foods

   d. Use of canned fruits and vegetables

   e. Use of white flour rather than freshly milled whole grains or sprouted grains

   f. Use of refined sugars

   g. Use of plant foods of all types grown on impoverished soils

   h. Use of chemically pure or synthetic vitamins

   i. Use of chemically contaminated foodstuffs resulting from pesticides, etc. (addition of fluorine to water supplies is opposed)

Methods of merchandising

Food quacks can be found in almost any aspect of the food-marketing business, but they have tended to rely on the less conventional merchandising procedures. High-pressure advertising in their own publications, Sunday supplements, and some magazines in which an introductory offer with refund privileges for dissatisfied customers is offered are common. They are sufficiently astute psychologists to realize that very few disillusioned buyers are going to bother to seek a refund.

Door-to-door salesmen or "doorbell doctors" are successful in convincing the housewife that the only way she can protect her own health and her family's health is through the use of whatever product he is promoting, be it special saucepans, a recipe book, vitamins, food supplements, or a potential cure for asthma. Usually these products are available at a "special low price" for quantity purchases on a cash basis. In many cases a victim realizes too late that to safeguard the health of her whole family she has committed an unreasonable part of the family income. In some door-to-door selling situations the parent company protects itself against responsibility for the claims of its salesmen, making it difficult to take effective legal action to stop the sales. Some states have introduced legislation that allows a person who has been a victim of high-pressure sales techniques to cancel any contract within 24 hours.

Public lectures, often "by invitation only," are used to lure people. After an initial period in which some fairly plausible nutritional information is given, the lecturer launches into a train of thought designed to lead the audience to only one conclusion—that their only hope of salvation is to rely on the product for which he will be glad to take orders. Radio and television time are also purchased and used in much the same way.

Health food stores thrive in the densely populated areas of large cities, especially when they offer food grown on organically fertilized soil. Their inventory includes several hundred items, such as carrot powder, papaya tablets, alfalfa and alfalfa concentrates, rose hips, miracle wafers, amino acid tablets, royal jelly, millet, special-formula tablets of natural vitamins and minerals, bone meal, wheat germ, brewer's yeast, dessicated liver, fish-liver oil, kelp, parsley, and iron. At the other end of the merchandising continuum are the health food farms located in a pastoral setting uncontaminated by herbicides, pesticides, and chemical fertilizers; to these the devotee may travel for the privilege of paying two to three times regular grocery prices for the same products. Practically all these outlets also offer mail order service.

The labelling on a product may also purposefully be misleading. For instance, 10 gm. capsules of gelatin bore a listing of the percentage of the total protein represented by seventeen different amino acids, the names of which would give the average consumer the impression that the product was highly nutritious. The fact that the whole capsule provided about 0.0014% of the day's protein requirement was not mentioned.

Books on nutrition have been a source of much misinformation and half-truths for the consumer and a source of tremendous income for the successful writer, especially one who can legitimately use the title M.D. Since the food quack is not limited in his claims by established findings, he is able to make a much stronger and more emotional appeal than is the legitimate scientist, who often tends to be overly cautious in his attempts to avoid violating the limits of knowledge. A perusal of the following titles of chapters in some of the more popular publications gives the reader some notion of the approach used: *"Are poisons making you old?"* *"Help for prostates,"* *"Learn to live without an ulcer,"* *"Skin problems are more than skin deep,"* and *"Arthritis can often be relieved!"* Again, much of the information is based on sound basic principles of nutrition, but in their zeal to sell books the authors frequently distort facts to achieve a strong emotional appeal. The sale of half a million copies of a book can earn the author a quarter of a million dollars and the publisher half a million, and so the motivation to appeal to a wide audience is great.

Special equipment for food preparation has been another lucrative approach of the food quack. This is often demonstrated at fairs, summer resorts, arcades, department stores, or invitational parties in private homes in all of which the promoter relies heavily on impulse buying. He attributes a wide range of merits to the equipment, such as increasing the consumption of fruits and vegetables, eliminating poisons from foods, conserving vitamins, or incorporating oxygen in food.

Types of products

"Shotgun" formula. Products characterized by "shotgun" formulas may list as many as fifty different nutrients on the label and are designed to impress the gullible consumer who is awed by the range of items included. Some of these are nutrients for which recommended daily allowances and minimum daily requirements have been established; others are those known to be essential but for which no requirements have been established; and still others are substances of no known nutritional significance but harmless. Of those known to be required, some will be present at many times the recommended level, whereas others will be present in insignificant amounts. For instance, one product in the recommended daily dose contains 400% of the minimum daily requirement of vitamins A, D, C, B_1, and B_2 and about 2% of

the daily requirement of potassium. This same product lists 10 mg. of unsaturated fatty acids, which represents about 0.1% of the 1% of the calories from linoleic acid recommended in the adult diet. The mixture is obviously irrational from a nutritional and physiological point of view but completely rational from the point of view of the uninformed consumer.

"Loaded" formula. The term *"loaded" formula* is applied to the high-potency product that competes by providing more of a nutrient than its competitor. Thus we find a spiraling in trade competition, with one company adding more of a nutrient for a very insignificant difference in price than his competitor. The average consumer does not realize that he merely excretes the excess amounts of the water-soluble vitamins and may develop toxic reactions from excessive levels of the fat-soluble vitamins.

The Food and Drug Administration has been trying since 1966 to have legislation enacted that would limit the number of nutrients that could be used in dietary supplements to those for which need in the American population has been demonstrated. In addition, it would establish upper and lower limits of nutrient content so that the consumer would be assured of an effective but not toxic dose. As yet this is still in the hearing stage in the legislative process. Their proposals are shown in Table 16-4.

Natural organic products. Natural organic foods are reportedly grown in organically fertilized soil without the addition of insecticides and herbicides or chemical fertilizers.

Miracle products. Miracle products include such products as garlic pills to relieve high blood pressure, honey and vinegar for arthritis, wheat germ for sterility, and lecithin for coronary disease.

Unnecessary supplements. The sale of protein supplements to the American population may well be questioned, especially at suggested prices. One firm created doubts about the adequacy of protein in the American diet to soften the market for its protein pills, each of which contained 728 mg. of protein. To obtain the equivalent of the 20 gm. of protein in one serving of meat, a person would need to take 28 pills at a cost of 25 cents, or 1 cent each.

Useless products. Seawater, which enterprising persons living in coastal areas were shipping all over the country, would be placed in the category of useless products. When the cost of shipping used up some of the profit, they reverted to dehydrated seawater to further enhance their earnings. Many products that may be beneficial in significant amounts are useless at the levels at which they are sold.

COMBATTING MISINFORMATION AND FOOD FADDISTS

Efforts to protect the public against unscrupulous purveyors of misinformation and nutritional supplements in the name of nutritional science and to prevent exaggerated claims of the efficiency of food products are the concern of several government and community agencies.

Better Business Bureaus in many communities attempt to police, restrict, or regulate the activities of peddlers of health foods, special cooking devices, or nutrition supplements within their regions. They also require the registration of all persons giving public lectures, and on the basis of information available from one community to another are able to deny lecture privileges to those with a reputation for abusing these privileges. They describe their efforts to combat food misinformation as preventive, corrective, and educational.

The Food and Drug Administration is constantly concerned with protecting the consumer against mislabelling and harmful, contaminated, and worthless products but are faced with an overwhelming job, considering the resources available. When personnel and funds are limited, it is frequently necessary to restrict their activities to those aspects that present immediate dangers to the population. It takes time to prove that labelling is misleading or that the product is injurious to health. After the FDA believes it has sufficient evidence to press charges, court proceedings are extremely slow and costly to both parties. In some instances by the time enforcement agencies have been prepared to take action, the defendant has already realized sufficient profit that he does not contest the action. Regulations enacted in 1963, which require that a company present evidence that the product it proposes to sell is safe for human consumption, have done much to lighten the load of this agency, which previously had to prove that a product was harmful before its sale could be restricted. A reluctance on the part of the public to initiate charges against a firm by which they have been victimized also hampers the operation of enforcement agencies. To admit that one has been "taken" is to admit a human frailty that many persons prefer not to publicize.

The FDA is responsible for formulating and enforcing regulations regarding the processing and sale of food products. On their recommendation the amount of folic acid that can be included in nutritional supplements was restricted to 0.1 mg. in a daily dose; the addition of vitamin D was limited to milk and infant formula at a level to provide no more than 400 I.U. in the recommended daily dose, and the use of the term *low-calorie* is allowed only for foods providing less than 15 kcal. in an average serving. The FDA has suggested that the quantities of vitamins and minerals in nutritional supplements be limited to amounts that are nutritionally useful to reduce the wild claims of manufacturers, that only nutrients for which a deficiency is likely to occur be allowed, that the use of cyclamates as artificial sweeteners should be banned, and that a more meaningful term than *minimum daily requirement* be used in labelling foods. It is also concerned with artificial and natural contaminants in food.

Many of the efforts of the FDA to have more effective legislation enacted have been actively opposed by natural food organizations, which have launched an organized mail campaign to the members of Congress and the Department of Health, Education, and Welfare opposing the proposed legislation.

The American Medical Association has recognized the threat that quackery and faddism poses for the health of the nation and has launched a counterattack in the form of an exposé of the tactics and claims of the quack and faddist. They have developed films for use in nutrition education programs with supporting literature; they prepare periodical statements of their stand on prevailing practices and products; and they publish a popular magazine that frequently includes articles pertaining to the use of nutritional supplements and special health foods or devices. In spite of the efforts of this professional group to promote sound information, occasionally one of their own members, under the protection and aura associated with his degree, has published books on nutrition-related topics about which he was not adequately informed or qualified to speak. The American Medical Association also maintains a Bureau of Investigation that answers inquiries about specific persons or products and promotes an active campaign against quackery.

Other professional groups such as the American Public Health Association, The American Dietetic Association, and the American Home Economics Association all have active programs designed to combat food faddism and misinformation and are constantly attempting to inform the public in an effort to help them separate the foibles from the facts.

The Federal Trade Commission is involved in the fight against food quackery in its responsibility to protect the American public against false and misleading advertising. Cases involving charges of false advertising may take several years to try and will involve hundreds of hours of testimony. Some of their cases have concerned the superiority of vitamins from natural sources over synthetic vitamins, the need for delivery of garden-fresh vitamins, the need for time-released vitamin-mineral capsules, and claims that juices prepared in special blenders have miraculous curative powers.

The Post Office Department, which regulates the use of the mails to defraud, also performs a watchdog function to protect the public against nutritional hoaxes.

On the theory that an informed public is a less gullible public, nutrition education should be one of the most effective ways of combatting food fads and quackery, especially with the potential of all the media available to disseminate sound information. When even the well-educated and scientifically enlightened are prey to the wiles of the faddist and the quack, one wonders what level of education is necessary to protect people from becoming victims of the promoter who claims his product will cure everything from corns to sterility to leukemia. To combat faddism, it is necessary to recognize the emotional and psychological influences that perpetuate it. Thus an educational campaign aimed at combatting it must be multifaceted, attacking as many of the forces that support it as possible.

Only through a constant flow of legitimate nutrition information can progress be made in combatting the high-pressure salesmanship of the quack. It appears that for every one person involved in merchandising sound nutritional information, several hundred are merchandising their own pet schemes. Several nutritionists who write regular syndicated columns for daily or weekly newspapers utilize this opportunity to fight faddism and to help enlighten the public. Dietitians in some larger cities operate a service known as Dial-a-titian in which people with questions related to nutrition may call the service and have their query referred to the person most qualified to answer it.

The difficulties in combatting misinformation in the press are much more formidable than those on labels or ads for products. Only when a book containing untenable claims for a certain food or product is displayed in a store along with the product it recommends can the book be confiscated along with the product on the grounds that it constitutes labelling. Even then it must involve interstate trade.

The final chapter in the saga of food faddism is far from written. One can only hope that it can be brought under reasonable control before the health of too many persons is jeopardized by the use of products promoted by unscrupulous salesmen. On the other hand, one should not overlook the fact that the faddists have done much to dramatize the importance of nutrition and have created a nutrition consciousness in a larger segment of the population. The challenge to nutritionists is to tap this interest and divert the attention of the concerned to more reasonable and appropriate solutions.

SELECTED REFERENCES

Beeuwkes, A. M.: Food faddism and consumer, Fed. Proc. **13**:785, 1954.

Bernard, V. W.: Why people become the victims of medical quackery, Amer. J. Public Health **55**:1142, 1965.

Bruch, H.: The allure of food cults and nutrition quackery, J. Amer. Diet. Ass. **57**:316, 1970.

Council on Foods and Nutrition: Problems of antibiotics in food, J.A.M.A. **170**:139, 1959.

Council on Foods and Nutrition: Vitamin preparations as dietary supplements and as therapeutic agents, J.A.M.A. **169**:41, 1959.

Council on Foods and Nutrition: General policy on addition of specific nutrients to foods, J.A.M.A. **178**:1024, 1961.

Council on Foods and Nutrition: Safe use of chemicals in food, J.A.M.A. **178**:749, 1961.

Darby, W. J.: The rational use of vitamins in medical practice, Med. Clin. N. Amer. **48**:1203, 1964.

422 *Applied nutrition*

Deutsch, R.: Nuts among the berries, New York, 1961, Ballantine Books, Inc.

Food facts talk back, Chicago, 1967, The American Dietetic Association.

Larrick, G. P.: The nutritive adequacy of our food supply, J. Amer. Diet. Ass. 39:117, 1961.

Let's talk about food, Chicago, 1967, American Medical Association.

Jalso, S. B., Burns, M. M., and Rivers, J. M.: Nutritional beliefs and practices, J. Amer. Diet. Ass. 47:263, 1965.

Kulp, K., Golosinec, O. C., Shank, C. W., and Bradley, W. B.: Current practices in bread enrichment, J. Amer. Diet. Ass. 32:331, 1956.

Milstead, K. L.: Science works through law to protect consumers, J. Amer. Diet. Ass. 48:187, 1966.

Mitchell, H. S.: Food fads—what protection have we? J. Home Economics 53:100, 1961.

Mott, M. A.: Better business bureaus fight food faddism, J. Amer. Diet. Ass. 39:122, 1961.

Olson, R. E.: Food faddism—why? Nutr. Rev. 16:97, 1958.

Roe, D. A.: Nutrient toxicity with excessive intake, New York J. Med. 66:1233, 1966.

The role of nutrition education in combating food fads, New York, 1959, The Nutrition Foundation.

Sherlock, P., and Rothschild, E. O.: Scurvy produced by a Zen macrobiotic diet, J.A.M.A. 199:794, 1967.

Sipple, H. L.: Opportunities in nutrition education, J. Amer. Diet. Ass. 42:140, 1963.

Stare, F. J.: Your food and your health, Garden City, N. Y., 1969, Doubleday & Co., Inc.

Todhunter, E. N.: The foods we eat, J. Home Economics 50:510, 1958.

Wagner, M.: The irony of affluence, J. Amer. Diet. Ass. 57:311, 1970.

Walker, A. R. P.: Problems in nutritional supplementation and enrichment, Amer. J. Clin. Nutr. 12:157, 1963.

Williams, R. J.: Nutrition in a nutshell, Garden City, N. Y., 1962, Doubleday & Co., Inc.

22

Nutrition—a national and an international concern

Interest in nutrition as a national and an international concern has come into focus only in the last one or two decades. At the international level, concern stems from an analysis of the increase in world population relative to the capacity of the world to provide adequate amounts of food for an expanding population. Since 60% of the current population and 70% of its children are judged to be undernourished, the problem is one not only of improving the level of nutrition but also of providing this more desirable level for a large population increase. The magnitude of the problem became evident with the recognition in 1950 that a protein deficiency resulted in kwashiorkor, a major cause of infant mortality in developing countries. The effects include permanently retarded physical growth, increased susceptibility to infection, and if it occurs early enough in life, depressed development of the central nervous system. High-quality protein is an expensive nutrient in terms of the productivity of the land, since 1 acre will yield twenty-five times as much protein from soybeans and ten times as much from rice as from beef. Under conditions of high land pressures it is evident that other protein sources such as vegetable protein mixtures and legumes rather than animal proteins must be developed and exploited to narrow the protein gap.

Recognition of malnutrition as a national concern for developed countries is an even more recent phenomenon. In the United States the publication *Hunger USA* by the Citizens Board of Inquiry into Hunger and Malnutrition in 1968 and the CBS television program *Hunger in America,* both charging that hunger in the midst of plenty was a national disgrace, shocked the nation. This was followed by the senate hearings on Nutrition and Human Needs from 1968 to 1970 and the White House Conference on Food, Nutrition, and Health in December, 1969. Both presented evidence not only that malnutrition was much more prevalent than previously suspected but that relatively little information on the nutritional status of the American population has been compiled.

Thus we now find that nutrition has become both a national and international concern, with many agencies dedicated to alleviating it. It is the subject of much research effort not only by nutritionists, agronomists, and biochemists but also by social scientists—economists, sociologists, psychologists, and anthropologists. The following discussion will focus on our current knowledge of some of the factors that are contributing to the problem. Although the foregoing chapters have been concerned primarily with the physiological and biochemical aspects of nutritional inadequacies, this chapter will concentrate on the social, economic, and psychological aspects of nutritional disease as they pertain to causes and solutions of the problem.

A NATIONAL CONCERN

Until 1968 attempts to evaluate the nutritional status of the American population had been confined to small geographically isolated groups selected to meet the criterion of individual investigators. The findings of many of these were summarized in *Nutritional Status USA,* a compilation of studies supported by the U. S. Department of Agriculture, published in 1960. A subsequent compendium of similar studies appeared in 1969. These studies showed that the quality of nutrition was generally related to economic status and level of education. Infants and children from families of lower socioeconomic levels tended to be below average in height and weight. From 15% to 20% of adolescents were found to be obese, and older people tended to be overweight. Iron deficiency was common in pregnant women and infants but not among adolescents. Ascorbic acid, vitamin A, calcium, and iron were the nutrients most commonly consumed at levels below the recommended dietary allowances, but biochemical evidence of vitamin deficiencies was rare.

The United States Department of Agriculture has regularly assessed food consumption of households every ten years and is now planning to repeat the study every five years.

The most recent survey in the spring of 1965 included 7500 households drawn to be representative of all housekeeping households in the United States. Dietary intakes were assessed on the basis of a 7-day dietary recall by the homemaker of food available for consumption by the household, with adjustments for meals eaten away from home. This study showed that half the households had diets rated good on the basis that they provided the recommended levels of all nutrients. One fifth of the families had diets rated poor, since they provided less than two thirds of the recommended levels for one or more nutrients. Diets were most often inadequate in calcium, vitamin A, and ascorbic acid. Intakes of protein, iron, thiamin, and riboflavin met the recommended standards for 90% of the families. Dietary adequacy improved as income increased, although an adequate income provided no assurance of

a good diet, since 9% of households with incomes over $10,000 had poor diets.

Analysis of 24-hour dietary recall records of food eaten at home and away from home for 14,500 individual members of the household as reported by the homemaker showed that calcium and iron were the nutrients most often taken at levels below recommended allowances. Individuals in families with incomes below $3000 also had diets with less than recommended amounts of ascorbic acid and vitamin A.

The first comprehensive attempt to assess the nutritional status of the American people was launched in 1968 and has been identified as the *National Nutrition Survey.* This study was designed to examine the dietary practices and nutritional status of a representative sample of persons identified by the 1960 census data in the lower quartile on the basis of income. Most families had incomes below $3000 per year. Ten states—Louisiana, North Carolina, Washington, New York, California, Texas, Kentucky, Michigan, West Virginia, and Massachusetts—were chosen to provide representation of the various ethnic and social groups within the population. Nutritional status is assessed on the basis of physical and anthropological measurements, biochemical determinations on blood and urine, and a dental examination. Dietary intake is evaluated on the basis of a 24-hour dietary recall by the homemaker and selected nutritionally vulnerable members of the household. A preliminary evaluation of the data indicates regional differences, but in all areas vitamin A, ascorbic acid, and iron are the nutrients most often taken in less than recommended amounts. Low hemoglobin levels were encountered in a significant portion of the population, low vitamin A levels in the serum of children, low vitamin C levels in that of mothers, and some evidence of growth retardation in children. Rickets was observed in 2% of children and goiter in 5% of adults. Complete analysis of the data should yield information on the extent of nutritional inadequacies and their relation to dietary intake.

Another federally sponsored nationwide study of the dietary practices and nutritional status of preschool children in all socioeconomic strata of the American population is also underway. This age group has been singled out for attention because it represents a nutritionally vulnerable group. In 1970 the Department of Health, Education, and Welfare announced plans for continuing surveillance of the nutritional status of the population through an examination of 30,000 individuals every two years.

Although undernutrition and malnutrition are not confined to any one social, economic, cultural, or ethnic group, available studies show several groups within the United States for whom they are special problems. These include the Indians, migrant workers, Eskimos, the poor, and the elderly. In many respects these groups are difficult to reach, since they neither belong to organized groups nor tend to seek help. In general, it has been suggested that their nutritional status may be a function of their cultural backgrounds, their inadequate knowledge of the nutritive value of foods, the economic problems resulting from low and often irregular incomes, the pressures of large families, and the trauma of high morbidity rates. Some of the specific factors involved for each particular group will be considered briefly.

American Indians, numbering less than half a million, live on 53 million acres of barren, dry, unproductive land, and are restricted in terms of freedom to earn and to roam for food. The animals and fruit on which they formerly depended for food are vanishing. Meat is less available at higher prices, which leads Indians whose incomes average less than $1000 per year to consume a less expensive high-carbohydrate diet. Infant mortality rates of 140 per 1000 live births compared to a national average of 21.4, and a tuberculosis rate eight times

the national average are evidence of poor health conditions. Studies of dietary adequacy among Indians indicate that low intakes of ascorbic acid and vitamin A are the most prevalent nutritional inadequacies.

Migrant workers, dependent on agriculture for a living, have virtually no financial security. Because of the mobile nature of their existence, they have limited and irregular opportunities for education and their housing is marginal, often lacking facilities for the preparation and storage of food and for adequate sanitation. The latter increases the possibility of infection to which resistance is low because of poor nutrition and possible intestinal parasitism. In many cases the mother who must work in the field all day is home to cook at most two meals a day. Older children care for younger ones and thus cannot attend school. Dietary studies indicate that diets of migrant families are low in vitamins C and A, calcium, and riboflavin, reflecting limited use of fruit and vegetables and milk.

Eskimos traditionally consumed a diet obtained largely by hunting and fishing, high in fat and protein, and low in carbohydrate. They have migrated to the city in search of a fixed income. At the same time, they have lost their food-gathering skills and resources. The result has been a shift to a high-carbohydrate diet, with a concurrent increase in dental caries.

The poor have been identified in many nutritional surveys as a group with generally less than adequate diets. This is attributed in part to their limited resources for all necessities of life, including food, and in part to the fact that low-income families in general have less education and less sound nutritional knowledge on which to base their food choices.

The nutritional practices of the elderly have been discussed in Chapter 19, in which it was pointed out that physiological as well as social factors such as low income, long-standing food habits, loneliness, poor housing, lack of adequate storage and preparation facilities, lack of transportation to stores, and indifference to or ignorance of adequate food habits are involved. Physiologically they suffer from decreased ability to absorb and transport nutrients, increased excretion of nutrients, and thus relatively increased need.

Nutritional problems are by no means confined to these groups. Many others, such as adolescent girls and pregnant women, are often underfed. Another significant group, the overfed, suffer from obesity and may represent up to 20% of some population groups. Although the causes may be multiple, nutrition is one factor in the etiology of atherosclerosis, responsible for premature death of a large number of middle-aged men.

Improvement of nutritive intake in the United States

National programs to improve nutrient intake and to alleviate malnutrition in the United States have included the National School Lunch Program (Chapter 18), the Special Milk Program, and the School Breakfast Program, the Expanded Nutrition Program, Head Start, the Commodity Distribution Program, and the Food Stamp Program.

The National School Lunch Program, discussed in detail in Chapter 18, makes lunches available free or at reduced prices for 4.8 million of the 25 million children participating. With more federal funds being allocated to the School Lunch Program, participation is expected to increase. In addition, several states are making nutrition education an integral part of the School Lunch Program and are urging that it be incorporated into other academic programs.

The School Lunch Act also provides support for the Special Milk Program. Under this plan the United States Department of Agriculture reimburses schools and child care institutions for part of the cost of providing a special milk service as snacks or at mealtime to children not participating in the lunch program.

The Child Nutrition Act passed in 1966 provided funds for the purchase of equipment for schools in districts wishing to establish, maintain, and expand school food service programs to participate in the School Lunch Program. In addition, it provided for a pilot study of a School Breakfast Program to initiate, maintain, and expand nonprofit breakfast programs in schools and authorized the use of federal school feeding funds for feeding preschool children. The pilot School Breakfast Program has been extended until 1971. In 1969 over 3600 schools, 90% of which also had a School Lunch Program, participated. Only 5% of the schools with a lunch program also have a breakfast program, however.

In 1969 funds for the Expanded Nutrition Program were allocated by the United States Department of Agriculture. The Extension Service supervises the training of nutrition aides with the responsibility of working on a one-to-one basis with low-income homemakers to help them with homemaking skills and to provide nutrition education. Most of the aides are recruited from the same socioeconomic group as the people with whom they will be working. In 1970 the funds were increased, with a provision that 25% of available resources must be allocated for work by youth professionals in the inner city. These people are to integrate nutrition education in other programs for the young.

Head Start has provided a feeding program along with medical, psychological, educational, and social services for children enrolled in their program. By 1969 this included 2 million children. Little information has been collected on the nature and extent of hunger and malnutrition among this group.

The Commodity Distribution Program was introduced with a dual purpose of improving the nutrient intake of families with limited incomes and at the same time providing an outlet for domestically produced agricultural products. Originally it involved making foods purchased by the government under agricultural price-support programs available to people with limited incomes. Local governments wishing to participate must bear the costs of administering the program and must apply to the United States Department of Agriculture. Participation is limited by the funds available, and priority is based on the per capita income of the county or administrative unit. In 1960 when the primary emphasis was on providing a few surplus foods, only lard, rice, dried milk, flour, and cornmeal were available. With a change in emphasis toward providing a more adequately balanced diet, up to fifty-nine foods, many nutritionally improved, are available. The choice within any one district is the choice of local officials and is determined in part by availability in relation to demand. The fact that food is usually distributed only once a month and often at a center remote from the recipient's home, coupled with problems of transporting and storing large quantities of food, is a deterrent to the success of the program. In 1970, although 4 million people received food commodities, only one third of the eligible families were participating in the program. Eligibility of individual households, which must be certified every three months, is based on income relative to number in the family and total cash assets. In addition to providing food for individual families, the Commodity Distribution Program made food available to schools, nonprofit institutions, and nonprofit summer camps for children. In 1970 donated foods amounted to about 2000 million pounds, over half of which went to needy families. Additional commodities are also available through maternal and child health centers to expectant and nursing mothers and young infants in an attempt to decrease the risk to these nutritionally vulnerable groups.

The Food Stamp Program, begun as a pilot program in 1961 and initiated under the Food Stamp Act of 1964, has been rapidly replacing the Commodity Distribution Program. In 1970, 3050 of the 3129 eligible counties in the United States were participating in either program, and 69 counties were planning to operate a program. Over half had elected the Food Stamp Program, which was used by 7.2 million people. This program is designed to improve the diets of low-income households and at the same time to expand the market for domestically produced food. Basically the program increases the purchasing power of the eligible family by allowing the purchase of sufficient food stamps to provide sufficient food for an adequate diet for the family. The cost of the stamps varies on the basis of income and represents a reasonable amount to spend for food. Thus a family of 5 with an income of $120 per month is able to purchase $126 worth of food stamps for $33, whereas a similar family with an income of $300 pays $84 for the same value in stamps. Stamps that can be purchased twice a month at the bank are used as cash at participating and approved grocery stores. This program is currently being expanded and modified to provide for more equitable use of funds. The program is directed by the state agency responsible for administering other federally aided assistance program.

Many other innovative programs are being introduced to improve food habits, especially among low-income groups for whom nutritional intakes are least adequate. For instance, a housing authority is providing after-school snacks for 1500 children in the city housing developments. Another community is sponsoring a summer recreational feeding program in a low-income area to provide lunches for children. Feeding programs in migrant camps are increasing in number. Several cities have introduced noon feeding programs for older people. All these programs are utilizing donated commodities, and, in many cases, labor and equipment costs are borne by the federal government.

Enrichment. Enrichment or fortification of food products has been an effective way of correcting some aspects of undernutrition. Compulsory enrichment of bread and flour introduced in 1940 remained in effect during the national emergency of World War II. At the end of that period, jurisdiction for enrichment policies reverted to the individual states. Currently thirty states require the enrichment of bread and flour, with thiamin, riboflavin, niacin, and iron mandatory and calcium and vitamin D optional within prescribed limits. Since most wheat is milled in three or four large milling centers, 90% of the bread and cereal sold in the United States is enriched. Some states require the addition of these same nutrients to cornmeal, corn grits, farina, and macaroni and noodles and the addition of thiamin, niacin, and iron to rice.

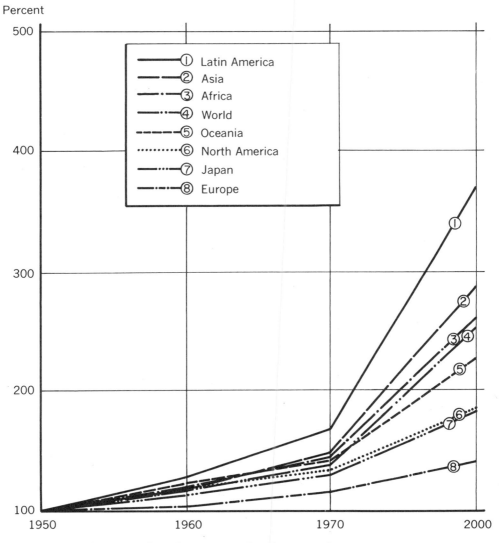

Fig. 22-1. Population trends and projections based on population in selected areas of the world, 1950. (Adapted from Freedom From Hunger Campaign: Basic Study No. 7, Population and food supply, Rome, 1963, Food and Agricultural Organization.)

Iodization of salt, although not compulsory, has contributed to a reduction in the incidence of goiter in the United States. Fortification of fresh whole and evaporated milk with vitamin D, nonfat milk with both vitamins A and D, and margarine with vitamin A are general practices. Iron enrichment of infant cereals is not governed by any state or federal regulation other than that it be adequately labelled but has contributed to the control of iron-deficiency anemia in infants. Although many other forms of enrichment are used by the food industry, they have not received the endorsement of nutritionists for several reasons. They may not be used in foods that are effective carriers. Demonstrable deficiency of the nutrient may not have been found in the population consuming the product, or the nutrient may be unstable under normal conditions of preparation. With the possibility of toxicity from the excessive intake of fat-soluble vitamin D, there is concern about the indiscriminate practice of food enrichment and fortification.

Because of the confusion resulting from the terms *enrichment,* generally used to refer to the addition of nutrients to cereals, and *fortification,* generally used to refer to the addition of nutrients to other foods, it has been suggested that the term *nutritionally improved* be used to identify all foods that have been modified in an attempt to increase their nutritive value.

AN INTERNATIONAL CONCERN

At the global level, efforts toward improving the nutritional status of the world's population have centered on the possibility of balancing the increase in population with an increase in food production. At the present rate of increase of 2.5% to 3% per year, world population will double in twenty-four years. Unfortunately, this increase is not occurring evenly in all areas of the world. The largest increases are occurring in the poor, ill-fed areas with the most limited potential for food production.

At present the food-deficit areas of Asia, Africa, and Latin America have 50% of the world's population, 25% of the world's food supply, 12.5% of the income, and 50% of the arable land. On the other hand, Europe, Oceania, and North America, with 20% of the population, have 59% of the food and 80% of the income. Fig. 22-1 shows recent and predicted changes in population for various parts of the world. If these predicted population trends materialize, it is estimated that to maintain present nutrient intake, food supplies must increase 36% by 1975 and 123% by 2000 over levels for 1965. This calls for an increase of 3.9% annually compared to the current rate of 2.7%. To improve nutritional status, the Food and Agricultural Organization estimates comparable needs would be 151% and 274% for the world and 179% and 393% for the less developed countries. Current trends in population relative to food production are shown in Fig. 22-2. The Indicative World Plan (IWP) for Agricultural Production forecasts a food demand in developing countries in 1985 two and a half times current production. Since even the most optimistic view of the potential for increased food production does not foresee an increase of this magnitude, it is obvious that efforts must be made simultaneously to reverse or to slow down the population trend. Should this not be accomplished, the possibility of the malthusian correctives of famine, pestilence, and war are ever present.

Efforts to increase world food production must include increasing the yield of land currently under cultivation, increasing the amount of land under cultivation, making maximum use of land not suitable for agriculture for the grazing of animals, exploiting the sea as a potential source of food, and capitalizing on the capability of advancing food technology to provide nonconventional food sources. The success of these efforts will depend to a certain extent on the application of agricultural technology in the form of improved plant and ani-

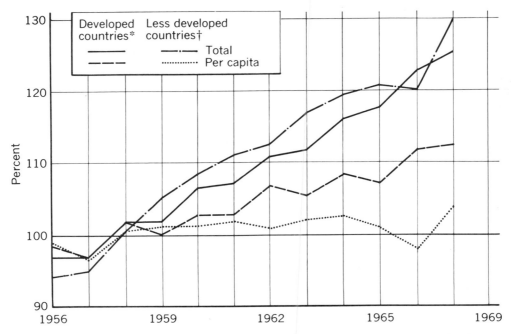

Fig. 22-2. Trends in total and per capita agricultural production in developed and developing countries. *United States, Canada, U.S.S.R., Japan, Europe, Australia, New Zealand, and South Africa. †Latin America, south Asia, east Asia, west Asia, and Africa. (From Editorial: A year of action, War on Hunger No. 2, p. 3, Feb., 1969.)

mal breeding; the use of herbicides, pesticides, fertilizers and irrigation; and social changes in the form of an available market and credit and efficient transportation and distribution systems. These approaches will be effective, however, only when introduced with an understanding of the social and cultural framework of society. Such influences as traditional value systems, social organization, land ownership and tenure relationships, and political climate are equally as important as technology in the success of innovations in agricultural production and marketing. For a more complete understanding of the complexity of the problem a consideration of the ecology of nutritional disease is in order.

Ecology of nutritional disease

Epidemiologists have traditionally considered disease to be the result of a complex interaction between *host, environmental factors,* and *agent,* as depicted in Fig.

22-3. The use of this model provides a meaningful basis for a discussion of factors contributing to nutritional disease. Such considerations help explain the varying incidence of nutritional disease under seemingly similar patterns of food consumption—differences that may be a function of time, place, or person.

Host. The nature of the nutritional needs and the extent to which the available nutrients are utilized are known to vary from one individual to another. The factors affecting needs include age, sex, prior nutritional state, health, rate of growth, stage of maturity, and genetic background. In general, the needs for nutrients are relatively high during periods of rapid growth and decline gradually with age after maturity. Differences attributed to sex are due not only to variations in body composition and in rate of growth, as well as the effect of different endocrine secretions, but also to different patterns of activity. That the

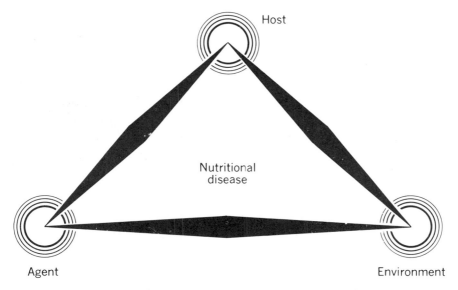

Fig. 22-3. Epidemiological triad depicting relationship among agent, host, and environment as factors in nutritional disease.

needs and utilization of nutrients vary as a result of genetically determined characteristics has been well established. In his discussion on biochemical individuality, Williams demonstrates evidence for a wide range of normal requirements of specific nutrients—a consideration that has been recognized in formulating dietary allowances for healthy individuals.

Whether or not a certain dietary intake will be nutritionally inadequate is influenced by the extent to which the individual is able to adapt to, or to compensate for, suboptimal intakes. For instance, people accustomed to low-calcium diets are able to use the calcium more effectively than are those accustomed to higher intakes. Similarly, when sodium intake is restricted or sodium needs are increased, a series of hormonal changes occur that lead to increased retention and decreased excretion of the nutrient. The lethargy so common in undernourished people may represent a conservation of energy to compensate for the energy deficit.

The physiological state of the person—pregnancy, lactation, or growth—will ac-

count for varying nutritional needs. Such stress factors normally result in an increased need for nutrients, but at the same time, physiological adjustments increase the efficiency with which a nutrient can be utilized. Similarly, the stress of infections, such as tonsillitis, measles, tuberculosis, or pneumonia, and of parasitic infestations increases the nutrient need and in cases of marginal intake are often regarded as responsible for precipitating a nutrient inadequacy. Such a synergism between malnutrition and infection is considered a major cause of the high mortality and morbidity, or sickness, rates among preschool children in developing countries.

Environmental factors. The role of environmental factors in nutritional disease is the result of their effect on the availability of nutrients, the nutritional requirements of the host, and the intake of nutrients. The environment includes not only the important physical and biological environment but also the social or cultural environment.

The availability of nutrients for both a population and an individual will vary with the season. The phenomenon of seasonal hunger in which food intakes hit a low point just before harvest season and a peak after harvest is well known in developing countries. For persons dependent on sunshine as a source of vitamin D, the rainy season will lead to a marked reduction in the amount of the nutrient available. Similarly, the practice in many cultures of protecting infants from exposure to sunlight deprives the child of a supply of the nutrient at a time of maximum need. Seasonal fluctuations in employment, such as those experienced by migrant workers, with the resultant fluctuations in income account for seasonal variations in availability of nutrients.

Agricultural productivity, especially in economically underdeveloped areas with poorly developed transportation and storage facilities, is an obvious determinant of availability of food. This in turn is dependent on the nature and fertility of the soil, the climate, the topography of the land, and the prevalence of natural disasters, such as floods, droughts, and storms. These determine the type of plant or animal that can be raised in the area and the nutritive value of the food produced. For instance, cassava and soybeans can be grown on marginal land, whereas rice and wheat require more productive soil. The trace mineral content of the soil determines the mineral content of the plants produced, and this in turn influences the growth of animals feeding on the crops or the nutrient intake of people eating plant foods directly.

Even where the physical and biological environment would be conducive to agricultural productivity, social factors may act as a deterrent. Education of the farmer in effective agricultural practices and the provision of adequate incentives to increase production are of prime importance. These in turn may be a function of the effectiveness of mass communication or the availability of a resource person who can inspire the confidence of the farmers. Adequate irrigation systems, terracing of hillsides, land tenure policies, availability of credit for seed at planting time and for herbicides and pesticides during cultivation, adequate food storage and distribution systems, and price-support policies are all socially and often politically determined factors that can influence agricultural practices and hence productivity.

The capacity of the farmer to produce food is influenced by the condition of his health. A malaria or a tuberculosis victim has reduced work capacity. A farmer suffering with intestinal parasites experiences a blood loss, with a resultant decrease in hemoglobin level and a concomitant apathy. The reduced work capacity reduces his food production and income, which in turn reduce his food intake and his ability to resist intestinal parasites and infectious agents. Thus he finds himself caught in a vicious circle that must be broken if his situation is to improve.

Nutrient requirements also fall under the influence of environmental variables. Climate as it affects heat and water and hence electrolyte losses accounts for variations in nutrient requirements. Loss of nutrients through perspiration in a hot climate may be a precipitating factor in nutritional deficiency diseases. In highly developed countries the ubiquitous nature of laborsaving devices, such as push-button ranges, electric typewriters, and automatic transmission, reduce the requirements for calories and concomitantly for nutrients involved in energy metabolism. Dietary practices, themselves an element in the environment, can influence nutrient requirements. For instance, a high-carbohydrate diet calls for an increase in thiamin; a diet high in polyunsaturates, more vitamin E; a goitrogenic diet, more iodine; and a vegetarian diet, a supplementary source of cobalamin.

The intake of nutrients is determined to a large extent by both the physical and social environment. In the cold arctic climate only 20% of dietary calories are derived from carbohydrate, whereas in the tropical regions about 80% are from the carbohydrate sources, which grow well there at a high yield per acre. Long-standing food habits are a function of the availability of food. To a certain degree they are also culturally determined. Food taboos, such as the Hindus' avoidance of meat and the Jews' avoidance of pork, are religious in origin. Superstitions, such as fish causing worms, eggplant causing the skin to be dark, eggs causing sterility, and a combination of cherries and milk causing illness, have their origins in folk beliefs. The association of milk intake and diarrhea originally attributed to inadequate sanitation has been found to have a sound physiological basis for those persons who fail to produce the enzyme lactase necessary to digest milk sugar.

Lack of income has been identified as a significant factor in undernutrition. It has led older people to adopt a high-carbohydrate diet, mothers to feed diluted milk to their children, the poor to exist on a monotonous and inadequate diet of rice and beans, and people in developing countries to use insignificant amounts of relatively expensive animal protein of high biological value. Although availability of money is no guarantee of an adequate diet, when income falls below a certain point, the chances of obtaining an adequate nutrient intake decrease as income decreases.

Food intake is influenced by many physiological factors. The inability to chew, the loss of neuromuscular coordination, or the inability to tolerate certain foods because of allergy, gastric distress, or heartburn lead to marked changes in the character of the diet, often with resulting nutritional inadequacies. Recently the Chinese restaurant syndrome, in which the consumption of monosodium glutamate has been implicated in a series of adverse physical symptoms, has provided further evidence of an environmental factor influencing food consumption. Loss of appetite may accompany emotional states such as fear or anxiety,

whereas overeating may be a compensatory mechanism to combat unhappiness or loneliness.

In developed countries particularly, one of the major determinants of food intake may be food faddism. Practices advocated by faddists often result in diets completely devoid of a particular nutrient. Scurvy has occurred among adherents to the Zen macrobiotic diet, which is based solely on brown rice. Vegetarians put themselves on a vitamin B_{12}–deficient diet, with the possibility of precipitating pernicious anemia. Any diet that restricts consumption to one or two food groups increases the likelihood of a nutrient deficiency.

Agent. The third member of the epidemiological triad, the agent, is a relative lack of a nutrient. As has been discussed, the need for a nutrient varies with host and environmental variables. Diets also vary in their nutritive content. In addition, many factors, such as method of food processing and storage, cooking procedures, and distribution of nutrients in a day's meals, affect the amount actually available. When nutrient stores have been depleted or cannot be mobilized and when the amount of the available nutrient is inadequate relative to the need, a nutrient deficiency develops. The nature and severity of the symptoms vary with the specific nutrient, as does the speed with which deficiency symptoms manifest themselves. The detection of the biochemical changes in the blood and urine that usually precede physical symptoms is of prime importance in prevention.

Increasing the world food supply

As just pointed out, the causes of malnutrition may be multiple and interrelated. By the same token, the cure or prevention of malnutrition involves the identification of the basic cause or causes and their interrelationship. Thus an increase in availability and utilization of food for the prevention of malnutrition may necessitate a modification of the social, physical, or biological environment, rather than a mere increase in food production. In this discussion we will consider some of the approaches that are being used to increase food production with a goal of increasing nutrient intake and improving nutritional status.

Increased agricultural productivity has resulted from more extensive use of pesticides and herbicides. Although safe and effective when used properly, they are not without hazards, however, since their indiscriminate use may result in environmental contamination that adversely affects the life of animals, themselves an important source of foods. Similarly, animal food production has been increased through the use of antibiotics and some hormones. Again, controls are necessary to prevent misuse so that levels in animal tissues as used for human consumption do not exceed established standards.

Selective breeding of plants has resulted in high-yielding crops particularly suited to the area. The Maize and Wheat Improvement Center in Mexico has produced a strain of wheat especially suited to the climatic and soil conditions of Central and South America. The International Rice Institute in the Philippines was responsible for so-called miracle rice (1R8) that is high yielding, responds well to fertilizer and irrigation, and has a shorter maturation period that makes it possible to produce more crops each year. This product has been responsible for a large increase in rice production throughout southeast Asia—a development that has been characterized as a Green Revolution. The newly built (1970) Institute for Tropical Agriculture in Nigeria is expected to stimulate similar advances for Africa for stable crops, such as sorghum, millet, and corn. Purdue University plant geneticists have perfected a high-yielding corn with high disease resistance and a content of the amino acid lysine sufficient to raise the normally low biological value of corn protein from 1.3 to 2.3, a level approaching that of casein. Similar advances will undoubtedly follow for other staple crops.

Animal breeders have also contributed. The International Center for Tropical Agriculture in Colombia will concentrate on improving tropical livestock production. By developing a cow that thrives in the tropics, is resistant to tropical diseases, and can range on rough marginal land, the potential supply of animal protein in such areas where only 20% to 30% of the animal protein is now produced has been increased. The nonprotein nitrogen sources such as urea, which can be manufactured from carbon dioxide and ammonia, can be used as at least a partial source of nitrogen in feeding some animals. The development of a rapidly maturing chicken with a high-protein efficiency ratio in converting food into protein and an early maturing pig with an increased proportion of its body weight as protein are other examples of the potential of animal breeding techniques. The raising of rapid-turnover species such as poultry and hogs is also encouraged. In addition, the "farming" of animals not now extensively used for food, such as the elephant, antelope, or hippopotamus, is being investigated for countries with large game lands, for example, those in Africa. The use of these animals by cultures that prohibit the use of more conventional domestic animals, such as the cow, for human food has great potential.

The addition of fertilizer in areas of food deficiency could result in a marked increase in food supply from current acreage. At the present time only 15% of the fertilizer is used in the areas of the world that feed 50% of the world's population. To increase the use of fertilizer, it will be necessary not only to develop fertilizer manufacturing plants close to the areas where it is needed and to make credit readily available at the time of planting but also to make available information on its proper and effective use. Since a sizeable financial outlay is involved, subsistence farmers who operate on a small margin with virtually no cash reserves need to be convinced that the returns will justify the risk. Demonstrations of its effectiveness, especially by farmers identified as more progressive, have been feasible methods of increasing its acceptance.

Adequate irrigation systems have increased the productivity of land and have made it possible to convert much unproductive land to productive land. The use of either atomic or solar energy to run plants to desalinate ocean water is being explored as a means of using salt water for land irrigation. Recognition of the importance of a water supply is evident in the inheritance patterns of many primitive societies in which the water rights to land are considered as important as the land itself.

Scientific animal feeding techniques that include the use of cut forage crops, urea, oilseed cakes, by-products of the sugar industry, and other foods not used by humans are being promoted. Since the energy value of food from animal sources is only one third that of the vegetable crops fed, the use of animal foods is economically unsound under conditions of land pressures unless animals eat foods that could not otherwise be used for human consumption or graze on lands that are suitable for grazing only. Control of animal diseases, such as hoof-and-mouth disease, rinderpest, hog cholera, and tuberculosis, is now possible, but losses from these causes still account for 15% to 20% of annual animal food production.

The potential of the sea, which now provides 1% of calories and 3% of protein in the world food supply, as a source of food has been considered, but opinions as to its feasibility are controversial. Those who maintain that it represents an untapped resource point to the fact the sea is capable of yielding over 140 million tons of fish per year compared to the current production of 61 million tons and a projected need of 107 million tons in 1985. They also point to the feasibility of harvesting small fish otherwise unfit for human food that can be utilized in the production of fish protein concentrate (FPC). Experimental floating factories are harvesting such fish in the Atlantic, converting them into a powder containing 90% protein. This product, now deodorized and defatted, has been suggested as an addition to basic cereal products, such as noodles, breads, and pasta, in which the FPC is incorporated with the basic cereal to provide a product with protein of enhanced biological value. Those less optimistic about the potential of the sea as a source of protein point to the role of small fish in the food chain and suggest that by removing the small fish, we will eventually decrease the size of the herd of large fish—a more acceptable source of protein. They also point to the restrictions that have already been placed on the size of the catch of big fish to preserve the larger species. In addition, they also indicate the need for considerable advances in food technology if we are to utilize the potential of the sea. Aquaculture is now recognized as a separate field of agriculture, and this discipline is concentrating on the development of new species and methods that can be employed to maximize the potential of the sea as a source of food. The Food and Agricultural Organization has promoted the development of fish ponds in which either brackish water or freshwater can be used for the cultivation of freshwater fish. Yields as high as 5 tons per acre have been reported from properly fertilized ponds. Even higher yields are obtained if flowing water prevents the buildup of wastes and oxygen depletion.

Supplementation of food either with synthetically produced nutrients or with concentrates of natural foods holds promise. The enrichment of rice with thiamin, riboflavin, niacin, and iron; the iodization of salt; the enrichment of wheat and rice with the amino acid lysine; the addition of FPC to cereal products; and the addition of soybean hydrolysates to infant foods are examples. The effectiveness of an enrichment program depends on its use with a staple food product that is bought from major production sources, rather than produced in many small places, and that can be purchased by all economic segments of the population. Decentralization of rice milling and an unfavorable taxation system have been a deterrent to the success of rice enrichment in the Philippines. Similarly, in India the value of adding lysine to milled wheat has been minimal because it has been impossible to provide the machinery and control necessary in a multitude of small mills. Indian authorities are investigating the possibility of employing salt, a universally used product that even the very poor must buy, as a carrier for enrichment nutrients.

Incentives for increased food production must be present. These must be great enough to overcome the old habits, customs, and traditions on which existing food production is based. In some cases marked changes in the social structure may be involved—changes that have profound implications. In any case, increases in food production must be accompanied by comparable advances in facilities for the storage and distribution of crops.

Activities of international organizations

The World Health Organization (WHO) is primarily concerned with combatting disease and other health problems and strengthening national health services. Since nutrition plays a significant role in combatting infection and reducing infant mortality and morbidity, WHO has cooperated with other agencies in seeking means of improving nutritional intakes. Much of their effort has been focussed on improvement of infant and maternal nutrition, and this is undertaken primarily through the medical profession, rather than on a direct contact basis.

The Food and Agricultural Organization (FAO), first organized under the auspices of the United Nations, has been charged with the responsibility to increase food production, to encourage agricultural practices that will increase food production and will result in a more equitable distribution of food for the world population, and to improve the nutritional status of rural population in underdeveloped areas of the world. Working in conjunction with WHO, they have formulated practical dietary standards for energy, protein, calcium, iron, vitamin A, thiamin, riboflavin, niacin, folacin, and cobalamin. They believe that these standards are compatible with a high level of health and that it is within the potential of the world to produce this level of intake.

The United Nation's Children's Emergency Fund (UNICEF), another organization within the United Nations, has focussed its attention on the nutritional needs of children. They were responsible for the distribution of surplus dried milk solids in infant- and child-feeding projects throughout food-deficit areas of the world. They have also promoted school gardens through the provision of seeds and tools.

Many other agencies sponsored by both private and government groups have contributed to the solution of the nutritional concerns of developing nations.

• • •

In summary one can say that in 1971 we find ourselves at both a national and an international level with a vast fund of nutritional knowledge but with stark evidence that much of this is not being used for the betterment of human health. Many questions at the level of basic nutritional knowledge are still unanswered, but the gap between the knowledge we have and the application of this knowledge is even more disconcerting. Correction of this situation is going to call for a united effort on the part of nutritionists working with anthropologists, sociologists, and agriculturists as well as biological and physical scientists. The challenge in terms of the alleviation of human suffering is ever present.

SELECTED REFERENCES

Altschul, A. M.: Food proteins: new sources from seeds, Science **158**:221, 1967.

Bardach, J. E.: Aquaculture, Science **161**:1098, 1968.

Bradfield, R. B., and Brun, T.: Nutritional status of California Mexican-Americans, Amer. J. Clin. Nutr. **23**:798, 1970.

Coffey, J. D.: World food supply and population explosion, J. Amer. Diet. Ass. **52**:43, 1968.

deGarine, I.: The social and cultural background of food habits in developing countries, FAO Nutr. Newsletter **8**(1):9, 1970.

Emery, K. O., and Iselin, C. O. D.: Human food from ocean and land, Science **157**:1279, 1967.

Feeley, R. M., and Watt, B. K.: Nutritive values of foods available in USDA Food Assistance Programs, J. Amer. Diet. Ass. **57**:528, 1970.

Freedom From Hunger Campaign: Basic Study No. 7, Population and food supply, 1963; No. 10, Possibilities of increasing world food production, 1963; No. 11, Third World Food Survey, 1963; No. 12, Malnutrition and disease, 1963; No. 14, Hunger and social policy, 1963; No. 15, Education and agricultural development, 1964; and No. 22, Manual on food and nutrition policy, Rome, 1969, Food and Agricultural Organization.

Guthrie, H. A.: Nutrition in a fishing community, Institute of Philippine Culture Papers, No. 6, p. 129, 1969.

Guthrie, H. A.: Infant and maternal nutrition in four Tagalog communities, Institute of Philippine Culture Papers, No. 7, p. 60, 1969.

Indicative World Plan for Agricultural Development, vols. 1 to 3, Rome, 1969, Food and Agricultural Organization.

Kallen, D.: Nutrition and society, J.A.M.A. **215**: 94, 1971.

Kelsay, J. L.: A compendium of nutritional status studies and dietary evaluation studies conducted in the United States, 1957-1967, J. Nutr. **99**:119, 1969.

Mayer, J.: White House Conference on Food, Nutrition and Health, J. Amer. Diet. Ass. **55**:553, 1969.

Morgan, A. F.: Nutritional status USA, Interregional Research Pub., California Agricultural Experiment Station Bull. 769, University of California, Berkeley, Calif., 1959.

Rasmussen, C. L.: Man and his food: 2000 A.D., Food Techn. **23**:57, 1969.

Schaefer, A.: Are we well fed? The search for the answer, Nutr. Today **4**:2, 1969.

Schrimshaw, N. S.: Ecological factors in nutritional disease, Amer. J. Clin. Nutr. **14**:112, 1964.

Schrimshaw, N. S.: Meeting tomorrow's protein needs, J. Amer. Diet. Ass. **54**:94, 1969.

Stare, F. J.: Nutritional improvement and world health potential, J. Amer. Diet. Ass. **57**:107, 1970.

Tauber, C.: Population and food supply, Ann. Amer. Acad. Polit. Social Sci. **369**:73, 1967.

APPENDICES

Appendix A | *Glossary*

absorption Process by which the products of digestion are transferred from the intestinal tract into the blood and lymph or by which substances in the interstitial fluid are taken up by the cells.

acid-base balance Relationship of the acid-forming and base-forming elements in the body.

aerobic Living or functioning in air or free oxygen. Opposite of anaerobic.

active transport Energy-requiring process by which a substance crosses a biological membrane.

alopecia Loss of hair.

amino acid Organic compounds of carbon, hydrogen, oxygen, and nitrogen. Each amino acid molecule contains one or more amino groups ($-NH_2$) and at least one carboxyl group ($-COOH$). In addition, some amino acids (cystine and methionine) contain sulfur. Many amino acids are linked together in some definite pattern to form a molecule of protein.

anabolism Process by which substances are formed or built up. It includes all the chemical reactions that nutrients undergo in the construction of body compounds, such as blood, enzymes, muscle tissue, and fat. Opposite of catabolism.

anaerobic Living or functioning in the absence of air or free oxygen. Opposite of aerobic.

antibody One of many specific substances produced in the body to react against disease-producing or other foreign materials in the bloodstream. Some antibodies remain available for many years and help to give a person permanent immunity.

antioxidant Substance capable of chemically protecting other substances against oxidation.

antivitamin, or vitamin antagonist Substance chemically similar to a vitamin that is able to replace the vitamin in an essential compound but is not capable of performing its role.

anorexia Pathological absence of appetite or hunger in spite of a need for food.

apatite Crystals of calcium phosphate that give strength to bone or tooth matrix.

appetite Complex sensations by which an organism is aware of desire for and anticipation of ingestion of palatable food.

atrophy Wasting away or degeneration.

basal metabolism Irreducible minimum of energy needed to carry on the body processes vital to life.

biosynthesis The coming together of chemical building units to form new materials in the living plant or animal.

blood serum Whole blood from which the cells and the clotting factor have been removed. It is the colorless fluid portion of the blood that separates when blood clots.

buffer Substance that can help a solution resist or counteract changes in free acid or alkali concentration. Many buffers in the body help maintain the acid-base balance compatible with life.

calcification Process by which organic tissue becomes hardened by a deposit of calcium salts.

calorimeter Instrument for measuring heat changes in any system.

calorimetry Science of measuring heat.

carbon Chemical element present in all substances designated as organic. These include proteins, carbohydrates, and fats. When a compound containing carbon combines with oxygen in the body, energy is liberated and carbon dioxide is formed. Compounds that do not contain carbon are classed as inorganic.

carbon dioxide Compound that is formed when carbon combines with oxygen. It leaves the body chiefly when air is exhaled from the lungs.

cartilage Special form of white connective tissue attached to the ends of bones that are either divided into joints or united by joints. It is more flexible than but not as strong as bone. Cartilage is the first substance to form in growing bone; then calcium and phosphorus are deposited in the cartilage to change it to bone.

catabolism The breaking down in the body of chemical compounds into simpler ones, usually accompanied by the production of heat. Opposite of anabolism.

catalyst Substance that speeds up the rate of a chemical reaction but is not itself used up in the reaction.

cell Smallest structural unit of living material.

cheilosis Condition characterized by lesions of the lips and corners of the mouth.

chlorophyll Magnesium-containing green coloring matter present in growing plants, which under stimulus of light is active in the manufacture of carbohydrates from carbon dioxide and water in a process known as photosynthesis.

chylomicrons Very small (micro-) globules of fat of varying sizes in transport in the blood.

coenzymes Enzyme usually containing a vitamin that activates or combines with another enzyme to give a substance with enzyme activity.

collagen Protein that forms the chief constituent of connective tissue, cartilage, tendon, bone, and skin. Collagen is changed to gelatin by the action of water and heat.

colostrum Thin watery yellowish fluid secreted during the first few days of lactation.

combustion Combination of substances with oxygen, accompanied by the liberation of energy.

decalcification Withdrawal of calcium from the bones on teeth, where it has been deposited.

edema Swelling of a part of or the entire body caused by the accumulation of excess water.

element Any one of the fundamental atoms of which all matter is composed.

endemic Occurring infrequently but more or less constantly in a particular region or population.

endocrine Secreting internally or into the bloodstream, as in endocrine glands, or glands of internal secretion.

endogenous Originating within or inside the cells or tissues.

enrichment Addition of nutrients to cereals to replace those lost during processing.

enzymatic Related to that class of complex organic substances called enzymes, such as amylase and pepsin, that accelerate (catalyze) specific chemical reactions in plants and animals, as in digestion of foods.

epithelial Those cells that form the outer layer of the skin or those that line all the portions of the body that have contact with the external air, such as the eyes, ears, nose, throat, and lungs.

erythropoiesis Process by which red blood cells are produced.

etiology Theory or study of the causes of a disease or a disorder.

exudation Abnormal outpouring of a substance that becomes deposited in or on tissues.

fetus Unborn young or embryo of animals in the later stages of their development before birth (adj., fetal).

flora (intestinal) Bacteria and other small organisms that are found in the intestinal contents.

Food and Agriculture Organization (FAO), Branch of the United Nations concerned with problems of food supply and distribution on a worldwide basis to help provide an adequate level of nutrition for all people.

Food and Nutrition Board Group of scientists in foods and nutrition or related fields who act in an advisory capacity to the National Research Council of the National Academy of Sciences.

fortification Addition of nutrients to foods other than cereals to replace those lost during processing.

gluconeogenesis Formation of glucose from noncarbohydrate substances, such as amino acids or glycerol.

homeostasis Steady biochemical states in the body maintained by physiological processes.

hormone Chemical substance that is produced in an organ called an endocrine gland and is transported by the blood or other body fluids to other cells. A hormone greatly influences the functions of some specific organs and of the body as a whole.

hunger Complex of unpleasant sensations felt after prolonged food deprivation that will impel an animal or man to seek, work for, or fight for immediate relief by ingestion of food.

hydrogenation Addition of hydrogen to any unsaturated compounds. Oils are changed to solid fats by hydrogenation.

hydrolysis Splitting of a substance into the smaller units of which it is composed by the addition of the elements of water. For example, when starch is heated in water containing a small amount of acid or is subjected to the action of digestive enzymes, the simpler sugar glucose is released.

hypervitaminosis Condition in which the level of a vitamin in the blood or tissues is high enough to cause undesirable symptoms.

ingest To eat or take in through the mouth.

isocaloric Having the same energy value.

labile Unstable; easily decomposed.

lactation Secretion of milk or the period during which milk is formed.

lipids Broad term for fats and fatlike substances; characterized by the presence of one or more fatty acids. Lipids include fats, cholesterol, lecithins, phospholipids, and similar substances that do not mix readily with water.

lysosome (perinuclear dense body) Organelle of the cell that contains enzymes capable of destroying the cell.

matrix Intercellular framework of a tissue.

metabolism All the chemical changes that occur from the time nutrients are absorbed until they are built into body substances or are excreted. This term includes both anabolism and catabolism.

microorganisms Very small living cells, such as bacteria, yeasts, and molds.

mitochondrion Organelle of the cell in which most of the transformation of energy occurs.

mucosa Mucous membrane in an epithelial tissue that lines the passages and cavities of the body, such as the gastrointestinal tract and the respiratory tract. It usually has the ability to secrete.

National Research Council (NRC) Group of leading scientists appointed by the National Academy of Sciences to coordinate the efforts of major scientific and technical societies of this country to serve science and government.

organelle Part or division of a cell that has a definite structure and function within the cell.

organic acids Acids containing only carbon, hydrogen, and oxygen. Among the best known are citric acid (in citrus fruits) and acetic acid (in vinegar).

osmosis Transfer of materials that takes place through a semipermeable membrane that separates two solutions or between a solvent and a solution, tending to equalize their concentrations. The walls of living cells are semipermeable membranes, and much of the activity of the cells depends on osmosis.

ossification Process of forming bone. Cartilage is made into bone by the process of ossification. The minerals calcium and phosphorus are deposited in the cartilage, changing it into bone.

oxidation Removal of electrons in the most general sense; it may also mean the combining with oxygen or the removal of hydrogen.

phagocyte Cell that can engulf particles or cells that are foreign or harmful to the body. Phagocytes are present in the blood and lymph and also in the lungs, liver, and spleen.

phosphorylate Chemical term that applies to the introduction of a phosphorus and oxygen group into a complex chemical compound.

physiological Refers to the science of physiology, which deals with functions of living organisms or their parts.

placenta Organ on the wall of the uterus (womb), to which the developing young animal is attached by means of the umbilical cord. Nourishment is transferred from the maternal organism to the fetus and fetal waste products are returned to the maternal circulation through it.

plasma Colorless fluid portion of the blood from which the cells have been removed.

protoplasm Living matter possessing capability for growth, repair, and reproduction. It is composed of water, inorganic salts, and organic compounds.

passive transport Process by which a substance crosses a biological membrane by diffusion or without the use of energy.

pituitary gland Gland in the lower part of the brain that produces a number of hormones that regulate the growth of all body tissues and regulate the development and action of other endocrine glands, such as the thyroid, pancreas, and adrenal glands.

portal vein Blood vessel leading from the wall of the intestine to the liver.

radical In chemistry, a group of elements joined in a set formation, which appears as a unit in a series of compounds or behaves as one piece without decomposition in chemical reactions. Examples are the glycerol radical in fats, the carboxyl group in organic acids, and the phenol radical (benzene ring) in certain amino acids. Amino acids themselves act as larger radicals in making up proteins.

reticuloendothelial system Liver, spleen, and bone marrow.

ribosome Organelle of a cell responsible for protein synthesis. It frequently occurs in groupings known as polyribosomes, polysomes, or ergosomes.

satiety Cessation of desire for further nourishment at the end of the meal.

syndrome Medical term meaning a group of symptoms that occur together.

synthesis Process by which a new substance is formed from its individual parts.

toxicity Quality of a substance that makes it poisonous, or toxic; it sometimes refers to the degree of severity of the poison or the possibility of being poisonous.

trimester Three months or one third of the nine months of pregnancy. The nine months of pregnancy are divided into the first, second, and third trimesters.

urinary Occurring in the urine.

Appendix B | *Meaning of prefixes and suffixes used in nutrition terms*

Prefix	Meaning	Example
a-	lack of	avitaminosis
ab-	away from	abnormal
ad-	toward	addiction
amyl-	starch	amylose
an-	negative, lack of	anemia
ante-	before, preceding	antenatal
anti-	against	antibiotic
bi-	two, double	bilateral
calori-	heat	calorimetry
co-	with	coenzymes
di-	in two parts	disaccharides
dys-	bad	dysentery
endo-	within	endogenous
epi-	upon, on, over, above	epithelium
ex-	out	exogenous
hepato-	pertaining to the liver	hepatitis
hyper-	excessive, above	hyperactive
hypo-	under	hypothyroidism
iso-	the same	isocaloric
lacto-	pertaining to milk	lactose
lip-	fat	lipid
leuko-	white	leukocyte
mono-	one	monosaccharide
neo-	new	neonatal
os-	bone	osteoblast
pan-	all, entire	panacea
peri-	around, on all sides	pericardium
poly-	many	polyneuritis
post-	after, behind	postnatal
ren-	kidney	renal
syn-	with, together	synthesis
tachy-	rapid	tachycardia
thio-	containing sulfur	thiamin
tox-	poison	toxemia

Suffix	Meaning	Example
-algia	suffering, pain	neuralgia
-ase	enzyme	protease
-blast	cell that builds	osteoblast
-cide	causing death	pesticide
-clast	cell that destroys	osteoclast
-cyte	mature cell	erythrocyte
-ectomy	removal	thyroidectomy
-emia	blood	anemia

Suffix	Meaning	Example
-gen	get or produce	antigen
-genesis	produce	glucogenesis
-gram	tracing or mark	cardiogram
-graph	instrument	cardiograph
-heme	iron-containing	hemoglobin
-ia, iasis	disease of	cholelithiasis
-itis	inflammation of	hepatitis
-logy	study of	biology
-lysis	solution, breakdown	hydrolysis
-meter	instrument for measuring	calorimeter
-oid	like	lipoid
-oma	tumor, swelling	adenoma
-osis	disease of, state or condition	fluorosis
-pathy	suffering, disease	osteopathy
-phagia	swallowing, eating	hyperphagia
-phobia	fear of, antagonism	hydrophobia
-plasty	repair of	rhinoplasty
-rhea	flow, discharge	steatorrhea
-tomy	cut into	appendectomy

443

Appendix C | *National Research Council recommended allowances*

National Research Council recommended allowances°

Recommended daily dietary allowances,† designed for the maintenance of good nutrition of practically all healthy people in the United States

	Age‡ (years) From Up to	Weight (kg.)	Weight (lbs.)	Height (cm.)	Height (in.)	kcal.	Protein (gm.)	Fat-soluble vitamins Vitamin A activity (I.U.)	Vitamin D (I.U.)	Vitamin E activity (I.U.)
Infants	0 - 1/6	4	9	55	22	kg. × 120	kg. × 2.2¶	1500	400	5
	1/6 - 1/2	7	15	63	25	kg. × 110	kg. × 2.0¶	1500	400	5
	1/2 - 1	9	20	72	28	kg. × 100	kg. × 1.8¶	1500	400	5
Children	1 - 2	12	26	81	32	1,100	25	2000	400	10
	2 - 3	14	31	91	36	1,250	25	2000	400	10
	3 - 4	16	35	100	39	1,400	30	2500	400	10
	4 - 6	19	42	110	43	1,600	30	2500	400	10
	6 - 8	23	51	121	48	2,000	35	3500	400	15
	8 - 10	28	62	131	52	2,200	40	3500	400	15
Males	10 - 12	35	77	140	55	2,500	45	4500	400	20
	12 - 14	43	95	151	59	2,700	50	5000	400	20
	14 - 18	59	130	170	67	3,000	60	5000	400	25
	18 - 22	67	147	175	69	2,800	60	5000	400	30
	22 - 35	70	154	175	69	2,800	65	5000	—	30
	35 - 55	70	154	173	68	2,600	65	5000	—	30
	55 - 75+	70	154	171	67	2,400	65	5000	—	30
Females	10 - 12	35	77	142	56	2,250	50	4500	400	20
	12 - 14	44	97	154	61	2,300	50	5000	400	20
	14 - 16	52	114	157	62	2,400	55	5000	400	25
	16 - 18	54	119	160	63	2,300	55	5000	400	25
	18 - 22	58	128	163	64	2,000	55	5000	400	25
	22 - 35	58	128	163	64	2,000	55	5000	—	25
	35 - 55	58	128	160	63	1,850	55	5000	—	25
	55 - 75+	58	128	157	62	1,700	55	5000	—	25
Pregnancy						+200	65	6000	400	30
Lactation						+1,000	75	8000	400	30

*Food and Nutrition Board: Recommended dietary allowances, ed. 7, Publication No. 1694, Washington, D. C., revised 1968, National Academy of Sciences–National Research Council.

†The allowance levels are intended to cover individual variations among most normal persons as they live in the United States under usual environmental stresses. The recommended allowances can be attained with a variety of common foods, providing other nutrients for which human requirements have been less well defined. See text for more detailed discussion of allowances and of nutrients not tabulated.

‡Entries on lines for age range 22-35 years represent the reference man and woman at 22 years of age. All other entries represent allowances for the midpoint of the specified age range.

Water-soluble vitamins							Minerals				
Ascorbic acid (mg.)	Folacin§ (mg.)	Niacin (mg. equiv.)||	Riboflavin (mg.)	Thiamin (mg.)	Vitamin B_6 (mg.)	Vitamin B_{12} (µg.)	Calcium (gm.)	Phosphorus (gm.)	Iodine (µg.)	Iron (mg.)	Magnesium (mg.)
35	0.05	5	0.4	0.2	0.2	1.0	0.4	0.2	25	6	40
35	0.05	7	0.5	0.4	0.3	1.5	0.5	0.4	40	10	60
35	0.1	8	0.6	0.5	0.4	2.0	0.6	0.5	45	15	70
40	0.1	8	0.6	0.6	0.5	2.0	0.7	0.7	55	15	100
40	0.2	8	0.7	0.6	0.6	2.5	0.8	0.8	60	15	150
40	0.2	9	0.8	0.7	0.7	3	0.8	0.8	70	10	200
40	0.2	11	0.9	0.8	0.9	4	0.8	0.8	80	10	200
40	0.2	13	1.1	1.0	1.0	4	0.9	0.9	100	10	250
40	0.3	15	1.2	1.1	1.2	5	1.0	1.0	110	10	250
40	0.4	17	1.3	1.3	1.4	5	1.2	1.2	125	10	300
45	0.4	18	1.4	1.4	1.6	5	1.4	1.4	135	18	350
55	0.4	20	1.5	1.5	1.8	5	1.4	1.4	150	18	400
60	0.4	18	1.6	1.4	2.0	5	0.8	0.8	140	10	400
60	0.4	18	1.7	1.4	2.0	5	0.8	0.8	140	10	350
60	0.4	17	1.7	1.3	2.0	5	0.8	0.8	125	10	350
60	0.4	14	1.7	1.2	2.0	6	0.8	0.8	110	10	350
40	0.4	15	1.3	1.1	1.4	5	1.2	1.2	110	18	300
45	0.4	15	1.4	1.2	1.6	5	1.3	1.3	115	18	350
50	0.4	16	1.4	1.2	1.8	5	1.3	1.3	120	18	350
50	0.4	15	1.5	1.2	2.0	5	1.3	1.3	115	18	350
55	0.4	13	1.5	1.0	2.0	5	0.8	0.8	100	18	350
55	0.4	13	1.5	1.0	2.0	5	0.8	0.8	100	18	300
55	0.4	13	1.5	1.0	2.0	5	0.8	0.8	90	18	300
55	0.4	13	1.5	1.0	2.0	6	0.8	0.8	80	10	300
60	0.8	15	1.8	+0.1	2.5	8	+0.4	+0.4	125	18	450
60	0.5	20	2.0	+0.5	2.5	6	+0.5	+0.5	150	18	450

§The folacin allowances refer to dietary sources as determined by *Lactobacillus casei* assay. Pure forms of folacin may be effective in doses less than one fourth of the RDA.

||Niacin equivalents include dietary sources of the vitamin itself, plus 1 mg. equivalent for each 60 mg. of dietary tryptophan.

¶Assumes protein equivalent to human milk. For proteins not 100% utilized, factors should be increased proportionately.

$\mathcal{A}ppendix$ D | $\mathit{Growth\ standards}$ $\mathit{for\ children}$

Height and weight of children 4-18 years of age*

Ages (years)	Boys					
	Height (inches)			Weight (pounds)		
	5th P†	50th P	95th P	5th P	50th P	95th P
4	38.3	40.8	43.3	30.0	36.1	42.2
5	40.3	43.4	46.4	33.0	40.3	47.6
6	42.8	45.9	49.0	36.0	44.7	53.4
7	44.8	48.1	51.4	40.3	50.9	61.5
8	46.9	50.5	54.1	44.4	57.4	70.4
9	48.8	52.8	56.8	48.0	64.4	80.4
10	50.6	54.9	59.2	51.4	71.4	91.4
11	51.9	56.4	60.9	53.3	78.9	102.5
12	53.5	58.6	63.7	60.0	86.0	113.5
13	55.2	61.3	67.4	65.3	98.6	131.9
14	57.5	64.1	70.7	75.5	111.8	148.1
15	61.0	66.9	72.8	88.0	124.3	160.6
16	63.8	68.9	74.0	97.8	133.8	169.8
17	65.2	69.8	74.4	106.5	139.8	174.0
18	65.9	70.2	74.5	110.3	144.8	179.3

*From Falkner, F.: Some physical growth standards for white North American children, Pediatrics **29:**448, 1962.
†P = percentile.

446

Height and weight of children 4-18 years of age—cont'd

				Girls			

Ages (years)	Height (inches)			Weight (pounds)		
	5th P	50th P	95th P	5th P	50th P	95th P
4	38.1	40.7	43.3	28.8	36.1	43.4
5	40.6	43.4	46.2	32.2	40.9	49.6
6	42.8	45.9	49.0	35.5	45.7	55.9
7	44.5	47.8	51.1	38.3	51.0	63.7
8	46.4	50.0	53 6	42.0	57.2	72.4
9	48.2	52.2	56.2	45.1	63.6	82.1
10	49.9	54.5	59.1	48.2	71.0	95.0
11	51.9	57.0	62.1	55.4	82.0	108.6
12	54.1	59.5	64.9	63.9	94.4	124.9
13	57.1	62.2	66.8	72.8	105.5	138.2
14	58.5	63.1	67.7	83.0	113.0	144.0
15	59.5	63.8	68.1	89.5	120.0	150.5
16	59.8	64.1	68.4	95.1	123.0	150.1
17	60.1	64.2	68.3	97.9	125.8	153.7
18	60.1	64.4	68.7	96.0	126.2	156.4

Annual height gains (inches)			*Annual weight gains (pounds)*		
Boys	Age (years)	Girls	Boys	Age (years)	Girls
2.8	4	2.8	4.4	4	4.4
2.6	5	2.7	4.5	5	4.4
2.5	6	2.5	4.8	6	4.4
2.4	7	2.25	5.5	7	5.3
2.4	8	2.3	6.4	8	6.4
2.3	9	2.3	7.0	9	7.6
2.1	10	2.4	7.0	10	9.4
1.7	11	2.5	6.8	11	10.6
1.6	11½	—	7.4	11½	—
1.9	12	3.1	8.4	12	12.6
2.6	13	2.3	—	12½	13.3
3.0	13½	—	11.8	13	13.2
3.2	14	1.4	—	13½	—
3.4	14½	—	15.0	14	8.6
3.1	15	0.6	15.4	14½	—
2.0	16	0.3	10.8	15	4.4
0.9	17	0.1	8.8	16	2.8
0.4	18	0.0	6.6	17	0.7
			4.4	18	0.0

Appendix E | *Desirable weights for height for adults*

Desirable weights for men 25 years of age and over[*][†]

Height with shoes on (1-inch heels)		Small frame	Medium frame	Large frame
(Feet)	*(Inches)*			
5	2	112-120	118-129	126-141
5	3	115-123	121-133	129-144
5	4	118-126	124-136	132-148
5	5	121-129	127-139	135-152
5	6	124-133	130-143	138-156
5	7	128-137	134-147	142-161
5	8	132-141	138-152	147-166
5	9	136-145	142-156	151-170
5	10	140-150	146-160	155-174
5	11	144-154	150-165	159-179
6	0	148-158	154-170	164-184
6	1	152-162	158-175	168-189
6	2	156-167	162-180	173-194
6	3	160-171	167-185	178-199
6	4	164-175	172-190	182-204

*Courtesy Metropolitan Life Insurance Co., How to control your weight, New York, 1960 supplement. Based on 1959 Build and blood pressure study.
†Weight in pounds, according to frame (in indoor clothing).

Desirable weights for women 25 years of age and over°†

Height with shoes on (2-inch heels) (Feet)	(Inches)	Small frame	Medium frame	Large frame
4	10	92-98	96-107	104-119
4	11	94-101	98-110	106-122
5	0	96-104	101-113	109-125
5	1	99-107	104-116	112-128
5	2	102-110	107-119	115-131
5	3	105-113	110-122	118-134
5	4	108-116	113-126	121-138
5	5	111-119	116-130	125-142
5	6	114-123	120-135	129-146
5	7	118-127	124-139	133-150
5	8	122-131	128-143	137-154
5	9	126-135	132-147	141-158
5	10	130-140	136-151	145-163
5	11	134-144	140-155	149-168
6	0	138-148	144-159	153-173

*Courtesy Metropolitan Life Insurance Co., How to control your weight, New York, 1960 supplement. Based on 1959 Build and blood pressure study.
Weight in pounds, according to frame (in indoor clothing).

Appendix **F** | *Table of food composition*

Table of food composition*†

Milk, cheese, cream, imitation cream; related products

Food, approximate measure, and weight (in grams)		Water (%)	Food energy (kcal.)	Protein (gm.)	Fat (gm.)	Fatty acids			Carbohydrate (gm.)	Calcium (mg.)	Iron (mg.)	Vitamin A value (I.U.)	Thiamin (mg.)	Riboflavin (mg.)	Niacin (mg.)	Ascorbic acid (mg.)
						Saturated (total) (gm.)	Unsaturated									
							Oleic (gm.)	Linoleic (gm.)								
Milk:																
Fluid:																
Whole, 3.5% fat	1 cup	244	87	160	9	9	5	3	Trace	12	288	0.1	350	0.07	0.41	0.2	2
Nonfat (skim)	1 cup	245	90	90	9	Trace	—	—	—	12	296	0.1	10	0.09	0.44	0.2	2
Partly skimmed, 2% nonfat milk solids added.	1 cup	246	87	145	10	5	3	2	Trace	15	352	0.1	200	0.10	0.52	0.2	2
Canned, concentrated, undiluted:																
Evaporated, un-sweetened.	1 cup	252	74	345	18	20	11	7	1	24	635	0.3	810	0.10	0.86	0.5	3
Condensed, sweetened.	1 cup	306	27	980	25	27	15	9	1	166	802	0.3	1,100	0.24	1.16	0.6	3
Dry, nonfat instant:																
Low-density (1⅓ cups needed for reconstitution to 1 quart).	1 cup	68	4	245	24	Trace	—	—	—	35	879	0.4	20‡	0.24	1.21	0.6	5
High-density (⅞ cup needed for reconstitution to 1 quart).	1 cup	104	4	375	37	1	—	—	—	54	1,345	0.6	30‡	0.36	1.85	0.9	7
Buttermilk:																
Fluid, cultured, made from skim milk.	1 cup	245	90	90	9	Trace	—	—	—	12	296	0.1	10	0.10	0.44	0.2	2
Dried, packaged	1 cup	120	3	465	41	6	3	2	Trace	60	1,498	0.7	260	0.31	2.06	1.1	—
Cheese:																
Natural:																
Blue or Roquefort type:																
Ounce	1 ounce	28	40	105	6	9	5	3	Trace	1	89	0.1	350	0.01	0.17	0.3	0
Cubic inch	1 cubic inch	17	40	65	4	5	3	2	Trace	Trace	54	0.1	210	0.01	0.11	0.2	0
Camembert, packaged in 4-ounce package with 3 wedges per package	1 wedge	38	52	115	7	9	5	3	Trace	1	40	0.2	380	0.02	0.29	0.3	0

*From Nutritive values of the edible part of foods, Home and Garden Bulletin No. 72, Washington, D.C., 1970, U.S. Department of Agriculture.

†Dashes in the columns for nutrients show that no suitable value could be found, although there is reason to believe that a measurable amount of the nutrient may be present.

‡Value applies to unfortified product; value for fortified low-density product would be 1,500 I.U., and the fortified high-density product would be 2,290 I.U.

Table of food composition—cont'd

Food, approximate measure, and weight (in grams)	Water (%)	Food energy (kcal.)	Protein (gm.)	Fat (gm.)	Fatty acids Saturated (total) (gm.)	Fatty acids Unsaturated Oleic (gm.)	Fatty acids Unsaturated Linoleic (gm.)	Carbohydrate (gm.)	Calcium (mg.)	Iron (mg.)	Vitamin A value (I.U.)	Thiamin (mg.)	Riboflavin (mg.)	Niacin (mg.)	Ascorbic acid (mg.)
Cheddar:															
Ounce 1 ounce 28	37	115	7	9	5	3	Trace	1	213	0.3	370	0.01	0.13	Trace	0
Cubic inch 1 cubic inch 17	37	70	4	6	3	2	Trace	Trace	129	0.2	230	0.01	0.08	Trace	0
Cottage, large or small curd:															
Creamed:															
Package of 12 ounces, net weight 1 package 340	78	360	46	14	8	5	Trace	10	320	1.0	580	0.10	0.85	0.3	0
Cup, curd pressed down 1 cup 245	78	260	33	10	6	3	Trace	7	230	0.7	420	0.07	0.61	0.2	0
Uncreamed:															
Package of 12 ounces, net weight 1 package 340	79	290	58	1	1	Trace	Trace	9	306	1.4	30	0.10	0.95	0.3	0
Cup, curd pressed down 1 cup 200	79	170	34	1	Trace	Trace	Trace	5	180	0.8	20	0.06	0.56	0.2	0
Cream:															
Package of 8 ounces, net weight 1 package 227	51	850	18	86	48	28	3	5	141	0.5	3,500	0.05	0.54	0.2	0
Package of 3 ounces, net weight 1 package 85	51	320	7	32	18	11	1	2	53	0.2	1,310	0.02	0.20	0.1	0
Cubic inch 1 cubic inch 16	51	60	1	6	3	2	Trace	Trace	10	Trace	250	Trace	0.04	Trace	0
Parmesan, grated:															
Cup, pressed down 1 cup 140	17	655	60	43	24	14	1	5	1,893	0.7	1,760	0.03	1.22	0.3	0
Tablespoon 1 tablespoon 5	17	25	2	2	1	Trace	Trace	Trace	68	Trace	60	Trace	0.04	Trace	0
Ounce 1 ounce 28	17	130	12	9	5	3	Trace	1	383	0.1	360	0.01	0.25	0.1	0
Swiss:															
Ounce 1 ounce 28	39	105	8	8	4	3	Trace	1	262	0.3	320	Trace	0.11	Trace	0
Cubic inch 1 cubic inch 15	39	55	4	4	2	1	Trace	Trace	139	0.1	170	Trace	0.06	Trace	0
Pasteurized process cheese:															
American:															
Ounce 1 ounce 28	40	105	7	9	5	3	Trace	1	198	0.3	350	0.01	0.12	Trace	0
Cubic inch 1 cubic inch 18	40	65	4	5	3	2	Trace	Trace	122	0.2	210	Trace	0.07	Trace	0
Swiss:															
Ounce 1 ounce 28	40	100	8	8	4	3	Trace	1	251	0.3	310	Trace	0.11	Trace	0
Cubic inch 1 cubic inch 18	40	65	5	5	3	2	Trace	Trace	159	0.2	200	Trace	0.07	Trace	0
Pasteurized process cheese food, American:															
Tablespoon 1 tablespoon 14	43	45	3	3	2	1	Trace	1	80	0.1	140	Trace	0.08	Trace	0
Cubic inch 1 cubic inch 18	43	60	4	4	2	1	Trace	1	100	0.1	170	Trace	0.10	Trace	0

Pasteurized process cheese spread, American.	1 ounce	28	49	80	5	6	3	2	Trace	2	160	0.2	250	Trace	0.15	Trace	0
Cream:																	
Half-and-half (cream and milk).	1 cup	242	80	325	8	28	15	9	1	11	261	0.1	1,160	0.07	0.39	0.1	2
	1 tablespoon	15	80	20	1	2	1	1	Trace	1	16	Trace	70	Trace	0.02	Trace	Trace
Light, coffee or table	1 cup	240	72	505	7	49	27	16	1	10	245	0.1	2,020	0.07	0.36	0.1	Trace
	1 tablespoon	15	72	30	1	3	2	1	Trace	1	15	Trace	130	Trace	0.02	Trace	Trace
Sour	1 cup	230	72	485	7	47	26	16	1	10	235	0.1	1,930	0.07	0.35	0.1	2
	1 tablespoon	12	72	25	Trace	2	1	1	Trace	1	12	Trace	100	Trace	0.02	Trace	Trace
Whipped topping (pressurized).	1 cup	60	62	155	2	14	8	5	Trace	6	67	—	570	—	0.04	—	—
	1 tablespoon	3	62	10	Trace	1	Trace	Trace	Trace	Trace	3	—	30	—	Trace	—	—
Whipping, unwhipped (volume about double when whipped):																	
Light	1 cup	239	62	715	6	75	41	25	2	9	203	0.1	3,060	0.05	0.29	0.1	2
	1 tablespoon	15	62	45	Trace	5	3	2	Trace	1	13	Trace	190	Trace	0.02	Trace	Trace
Heavy	1 cup	238	57	840	5	90	50	30	3	7	179	0.1	3,670	0.05	0.26	0.1	2
	1 tablespoon	15	57	55	Trace	6	3	2	Trace	1	11	Trace	230	Trace	0.02	Trace	Trace
Imitation cream products (made with vegetable fat):																	
Creamers:																	
Powdered	1 cup	94	2	505	4	33	31	1	0	52	21	0.6	200*	—	—	Trace	—
	1 teaspoon	2	2	10	Trace	1	Trace	Trace	0	1	1	Trace	Trace*	—	—	—	—
Liquid (frozen)	1 cup	245	77	345	3	27	25	1	0	25	29	—	100*	0	0	—	—
	1 tablespoon	15	77	20	Trace	2	1	Trace	0	2	2	—	10*	0	0	—	—
Sour dressing (imitation sour cream) made with nonfat dry milk.	1 cup	235	72	440	9	38	35	1	Trace	17	277	0.1	10	0.07	0.38	0.2	1
	1 tablespoon	12	72	20	Trace	2	2	Trace	Trace	1	14	Trace	Trace	Trace	Trace	Trace	Trace
Whipped topping:																	
Pressurized	1 cup	70	61	190	1	17	15	1	0	9	5	—	340*	0	0	—	—
	1 tablespoon	4	61	10	Trace	1	1	Trace	0	Trace	Trace	—	20*	0	0	—	—
Frozen	1 cup	75	52	230	1	20	18	Trace	0	15	5	—	560*	0	0	—	—
	1 tablespoon	4	52	10	Trace	1	1	Trace	0	1	Trace	—	30*	0	0	—	—
Powdered, made with whole milk.	1 cup	75	58	175	3	12	10	1	Trace	15	62	Trace	330*	0.02	0.08	0.1	Trace
	1 tablespoon	4	58	10	Trace	1	1	Trace	Trace	1	3	Trace	20*	Trace	Trace	Trace	Trace
Milk beverages:																	
Cocoa, homemade	1 cup	250	79	245	10	12	7	4	Trace	27	295	1.0	400	0.10	0.45	0.5	3
Chocolate-flavored drink made with skim milk and 2% added butterfat.	1 cup	250	83	190	8	6	3	2	Trace	27	270	0.5	210	0.10	0.40	0.3	3
Malted milk:																	
Dry powder, approx. 3 heaping teaspoons per ounce.	1 ounce	28	3	115	4	2	—	—	—	20	82	0.6	290	0.09	0.15	0.1	0
Beverage	1 cup	235	78	245	11	10	—	—	—	28	317	0.7	590	0.14	0.49	0.2	2

*Contributed largely from beta-carotene used for coloring.

Table of food composition—cont'd

Food, approximate measure, and weight (in grams)	Weight (in grams)	Water (%)	Food energy (kcal.)	Protein (gm.)	Fat (gm.)	Fatty acids Saturated (total) (gm.)	Unsaturated Oleic (gm.)	Unsaturated Linoleic (gm.)	Carbohydrate (gm.)	Calcium (mg.)	Iron (mg.)	Vitamin A value (I.U.)	Thiamin (mg.)	Riboflavin (mg.)	Niacin (mg.)	Ascorbic acid (mg.)
Milk desserts:																
Custard, baked ... 1 cup	265	77	305	14	15	7	5	1	29	297	1.1	930	0.11	0.50	0.3	1
Ice cream:																
Regular (approx. 10% fat) ... ½ gallon	1,064	63	2,055	48	113	62	37	3	221	1,553	0.5	4,680	0.43	2.23	1.1	11
1 cup	133	63	255	6	14	8	5	Trace	28	194	0.1	590	0.05	0.28	0.1	1
3 fluid ounces cup	50	63	95	2	5	3	2	Trace	10	73	Trace	220	0.02	0.11	0.1	1
Rich (approx. 16% fat) ... ½ gallon	1,188	63	2,635	31	191	105	63	6	214	927	0.2	7,840	0.24	1.31	1.2	12
1 cup	148	63	330	4	24	13	8	1	27	115	Trace	980	0.03	0.16	0.1	1
Ice milk:																
Hardened ... ½ gallon	1,048	67	1,595	50	53	29	17	2	235	1,635	1.0	2,200	0.52	2.31	1.0	10
1 cup	131	67	200	6	7	4	2	Trace	29	204	0.1	280	0.07	0.29	0.1	1
Soft-serve ... 1 cup	175	67	265	8	9	5	3	Trace	39	273	0.2	370	0.09	0.39	0.2	2
Yoghurt:																
Made from partially skimmed milk ... 1 cup	245	89	125	8	4	2	1	Trace	13	294	0.1	170	0.10	0.44	0.2	2
Made from whole milk ... 1 cup	245	88	150	7	8	5	3	Trace	12	272	0.1	340	0.07	0.39	0.2	2
Eggs																
Eggs, large, 24 ounces per dozen:																
Raw or cooked in shell with nothing added:																
Whole, without shell ... 1 egg	50	74	80	6	6	2	3	Trace	Trace	27	1.1	590	0.05	0.15	Trace	0
White of egg ... 1 white	33	88	15	4	Trace	—	—	—	Trace	3	Trace	0	Trace	0.09	Trace	0
Yolk of egg ... 1 yolk	17	51	60	3	5	2	2	Trace	Trace	24	0.9	580	0.04	0.07	Trace	0
Scrambled, with milk and fat ... 1 egg	64	72	110	7	8	3	3	Trace	1	51	1.1	690	0.05	0.18	Trace	0
Meat, poultry, fish, shellfish; related products																
Bacon, (20 slices per pound raw), broiled or fried, crisp ... 2 slices	15	8	90	5	8	3	4	1	1	2	0.5	0	0.08	0.05	0.8	—
Beef,* cooked:																
Cuts braised, simmered, or pot-roasted:																
Lean and fat ... 3 ounces	85	53	245	23	16	8	7	Trace	0	10	2.9	30	0.04	0.18	3.5	—
Lean only ... 2.5 ounces	72	62	140	22	5	2	2	Trace	0	10	2.7	10	0.04	0.16	3.3	—
Hamburger (ground beef), broiled:																
Lean ... 3 ounces	85	60	185	23	10	5	4	Trace	0	10	3.0	20	0.08	0.20	5.1	—
Regular ... 3 ounces	85	54	245	21	17	8	8	Trace	0	9	2.7	30	0.07	0.18	4.6	—

Food	Measure																
Roast, oven-cooked, no liquid added:																	
Relatively fat, such as rib:																	
Lean and fat	3 ounces	85	40	375	17	34	16	15	1	0	8	2.2	70	0.05	0.13	3.1	—
Lean only	1.8 ounces	51	57	125	14	7	3	3	Trace	0	6	1.8	10	0.04	0.11	2.6	—
Relatively lean, such as heel of round:																	
Lean and fat	3 ounces	85	62	165	25	7	3	3	Trace	0	11	3.2	10	0.06	0.19	4.5	—
Lean only	2.7 ounces	78	65	125	24	3	1	1	Trace	0	10	3.0	Trace	0.06	0.18	4.3	—
Steak, broiled:																	
Relatively fat, such as sirloin:																	
Lean and fat	3 ounces	85	44	330	20	27	13	12	1	0	9	2.5	50	0.05	0.16	4.0	—
Lean only	2 ounces	56	59	115	18	4	2	2	Trace	0	7	2.2	10	0.05	0.14	3.6	—
Relatively lean, such as round:																	
Lean and fat	3 ounces	85	55	220	24	13	6	6	Trace	0	10	3.0	20	0.07	0.19	4.8	—
Lean only	2.4 ounces	68	61	130	21	4	2	2	Trace	0	9	2.5	10	0.06	0.16	4.1	—
Beef, canned:																	
Corned beef	3 ounces	85	59	185	22	10	5	4	Trace	0	17	3.7	20	0.01	0.20	2.9	—
Corned beef hash	3 ounces	85	67	155	7	10	5	4	Trace	9	11	1.7	—	0.01	0.08	1.8	—
Beef, dried or chipped	2 ounces	57	48	115	19	4	2	2	Trace	0	11	2.9	—	0.04	0.18	2.2	—
Beef and vegetable stew	1 cup	235	82	210	15	10	5	4	Trace	15	28	2.8	2,310	0.13	0.17	4.4	15
Beef potpie, baked, 4¼-inch diameter, weight before baking about 8 ounces.	1 pie	227	55	560	23	33	9	20	2	43	32	4.1	1,860	0.25	0.27	4.5	7
Chicken, cooked:																	
Flesh only, broiled	3 ounces	85	71	115	20	3	1	1	1	0	8	1.4	80	0.05	0.16	7.4	—
Breast, fried, ½ breast:																	
With bone	3.3 ounces	94	58	155	25	5	1	2	1	1	9	1.3	70	0.04	0.17	11.2	—
Flesh and skin only	2.7 ounces	76	58	155	25	5	1	2	1	1	9	1.3	70	0.04	0.17	11.2	—
Drumstick, fried:																	
With bone	2.1 ounces	59	55	90	12	4	1	2	1	Trace	6	0.9	50	0.03	0.15	2.7	—
Flesh and skin only	1.3 ounces	38	55	90	12	4	1	2	1	Trace	6	0.9	50	0.03	0.15	2.7	—
Chicken, canned, boneless	3 ounces	85	65	170	18	10	3	4	2	0	18	1.3	200	0.03	0.11	3.7	3
Chicken potpie, baked, 4¼-inch diameter, weight before baking about 8 ounces.	1 pie	227	57	535	23	31	10	15	3	42	68	3.0	3,020	0.25	0.26	4.1	5
Chile con carne, canned:																	
With beans	1 cup	250	72	335	19	15	7	7	Trace	30	80	4.2	150	0.08	0.18	3.2	—
Without beans	1 cup	255	67	510	26	38	18	17	1	15	97	3.6	380	0.05	0.31	5.6	—
Heart, beef, lean, braised	3 ounces	85	61	160	27	5	—	—	—	1	5	5.0	20	0.21	1.04	6.5	1
Lamb,* cooked:																	
Chop, thick, with bone, broiled.	1 chop, 4.8 ounces	137	47	400	25	33	18	12	1	0	10	1.5	—	0.14	0.25	5.6	—
Lean and fat	4.0 ounces	112	47	400	25	33	18	12	1	0	10	1.5	—	0.14	0.25	5.6	—
Lean only	2.6 ounces	74	62	140	21	6	3	—	Trace	0	9	1.5	—	0.11	0.20	4.5	—

*Outer layer of fat on the cut was removed to within approximately ½ inch of the lean. Deposits of fat within the cut were not removed.

Table of food composition—cont'd

Food, approximate measure, and weight (in grams)		Water (%)	Food energy (kcal.)	Protein (gm.)	Fat (gm.)	Fatty acids			Carbohydrate (gm.)	Calcium (mg.)	Iron (mg.)	Vitamin A value (I.U.)	Thiamin (mg.)	Riboflavin (mg.)	Niacin (mg.)	Ascorbic acid (mg.)
						Saturated (total) (gm.)	Unsaturated									
							Oleic (gm.)	Linoleic (gm.)								
Leg, roasted:																
Lean and fat	3 ounces	85	54	235	22	16	9	6	Trace	0	9	1.4	—	0.13	0.23	4.7	—
Lean only	2.5 ounces	71	62	130	20	5	3	2	Trace	0	9	1.4	—	0.12	0.21	4.4	—
Shoulder, roasted:																
Lean and fat	3 ounces	85	50	285	18	23	13	8	1	0	9	1.0	—	0.11	0.20	4.0	—
Lean only	2.3 ounces	64	61	130	17	6	3	2	Trace	0	8	1.0	—	0.10	0.18	3.7	—
Liver, beef, fried	2 ounces	57	57	130	15	6	—	—	—	3	6	5.0	30,280	0.15	2.37	9.4	15
Pork, cured, cooked:																
Ham, light cure, lean and fat, roasted.	3 ounces	85	54	245	18	19	7	8	2	0	8	2.2	0	0.40	0.16	3.1	—
Luncheon meat:																
Boiled ham, sliced	2 ounces	57	59	135	11	10	4	4	1	0	6	1.6	0	0.25	0.09	1.5	—
Canned, spiced or unspiced	2 ounces	57	55	165	8	14	5	6	1	1	5	1.2	0	0.18	0.12	1.6	—
Pork, fresh,* cooked:																
Chop, thick, with bone	1 chop, 3.5 ounces	98	42	260	16	21	8	9	2	0	8	2.2	0	0.63	0.18	3.8	—
Lean and fat	2.3 ounces	66	42	260	16	21	8	9	2	0	8	2.2	0	0.63	0.18	3.8	—
Lean only	1.7 ounces	48	53	130	15	7	2	3	1	0	7	1.9	0	0.54	0.16	3.3	—
Roast, oven-cooked, no liquid added:																
Lean and fat	3 ounces	85	46	310	21	24	9	10	2	0	9	2.7	0	0.78	0.22	4.7	—
Lean only	2.4 ounces	68	55	175	20	10	3	4	1	0	9	2.6	0	0.73	0.21	4.4	—
Cuts, simmered:																
Lean and fat	3 ounces	85	46	320	20	26	9	11	2	0	8	2.5	0	0.46	0.21	4.1	—
Lean only	2.2 ounces	63	60	135	18	6	2	3	1	0	8	2.3	0	0.42	0.19	3.7	—
Sausage:																
Bologna, slice, 3-inch diameter by 1/8 inch.	2 slices	26	56	80	3	7	—	—	—	Trace	2	0.5	—	0.04	0.06	0.7	—
Braunschweiger, slice 2-inch diameter by 1/4 inch.	2 slices	20	53	65	3	5	—	—	—	Trace	2	1.2	1,310	0.03	0.29	1.6	—
Deviled ham, canned	1 tablespoon	13	51	45	2	4	2	2	Trace	0	1	0.3	—	0.02	0.01	0.2	—
Frankfurter, heated (8 per pound purchased package).	1 frank	56	57	170	7	15	—	—	—	1	3	0.8	—	0.08	0.11	1.4	—
Pork links, cooked (16 links per pound raw).	2 links	26	35	125	5	11	4	5	1	Trace	2	0.6	0	0.21	0.09	1.0	—

Food	Measure																
Salami, dry type	1 ounce	28	30	130	7	11	—	—	—	Trace	4	1.0	—	0.10	0.07	1.5	—
Salami, cooked	1 ounce	28	51	90	5	7	—	—	—	Trace	3	0.7	—	0.07	0.07	1.2	—
Vienna, canned (7 sausages per 5-ounce can).	1 sausage	16	63	40	2	3	—	—	—	Trace	1	0.3	—	0.01	0.02	0.4	—
Veal, medium fat, cooked, bone removed:																	
Cutlet	3 ounces	85	60	185	23	9	5	4	Trace	—	9	2.7	—	0.06	0.21	4.6	—
Roast	3 ounces	85	55	230	23	14	7	6	Trace	0	10	2.9	—	0.11	0.26	6.6	—
Fish and shellfish:																	
Bluefish, baked with table fat	3 ounces	85	68	135	22	4	—	—	—	0	25	0.6	40	0.09	0.08	1.6	—
Clams:																	
Raw, meat only	3 ounces	85	82	65	11	1	—	—	—	2	59	5.2	90	0.08	0.15	1.1	8
Canned, solids and liquid.	3 ounces	85	86	45	7	1	—	—	—	2	47	3.5	—	0.01	0.09	0.9	—
Crabmeat, canned	3 ounces	85	77	85	15	2	—	—	—	1	38	0.7	—	0.07	0.07	1.6	—
Fish sticks, breaded, cooked, frozen; stick, 3¾ by 1 by ½ inch	10 sticks or 8-ounce package	227	66	400	38	20	5	4	10	15	25	0.9	—	0.09	0.16	3.6	—
Haddock, breaded, fried	3 ounces	85	66	140	17	5	1	3	Trace	5	34	1.0	—	0.03	0.06	2.7	2
Ocean perch, breaded, fried.	3 ounces	85	59	195	16	11	—	—	—	6	28	1.1	—	0.08	0.09	1.5	—
Oysters, raw, meat only (13-19 medium selects).	1 cup	240	85	160	20	4	—	—	—	8	226	13.2	740	0.33	0.43	6.0	—
Salmon, pink, canned	3 ounces	85	71	120	17	5	1	1	Trace	0	167†	0.7	60	0.03	0.16	6.8	—
Sardines, Atlantic, canned in oil, drained solids.	3 ounces	85	62	175	20	9	—	—	—	0	372	2.5	190	0.02	0.17	4.6	—
Shad, baked with table fat and bacon	3 ounces	85	64	170	20	10	—	—	—	0	20	0.5	20	0.11	0.22	7.3	—
Shrimp, canned, meat	3 ounces	85	70	100	21	1	—	—	—	1	98	2.6	50	0.01	0.03	1.5	—
Swordfish, broiled with butter or margarine.	3 ounces	85	65	150	24	5	—	—	—	0	23	1.1	1,750	0.03	0.04	9.3	—
Tuna, canned in oil, drained solids.	3 ounces	85	61	170	24	7	2	1	1	0	7	1.6	70	0.04	0.10	10.1	—
Mature dry beans and peas, nuts, peanuts; related products																	
Almonds, shelled, whole kernels.	1 cup	142	5	850	26	77	6	52	15	28	332	6.7	0	0.34	1.31	5.0	Trace
Beans, dry:																	
Common varieties as Great Northern, navy, and others:																	
Cooked, drained:																	
Great Northern	1 cup	180	69	210	14	1	—	—	—	38	90	4.9	0	0.25	0.13	1.3	0
Navy (pea)	1 cup	190	69	225	15	1	—	—	—	40	95	5.1	0	0.27	0.13	1.3	0

*Outer layer of fat on the cut was removed to within approximately ½ inch of the lean. Deposits of fat within the cut were not removed.
†If bones are discarded, value will be greatly reduced.

Table of food composition—cont'd

Food, approximate measure, and weight (in grams)		Water (%)	Food energy (kcal.)	Protein (gm.)	Fat (gm.)	Saturated (total) (gm.)	Oleic (gm.)	Linoleic (gm.)	Carbohydrate (gm.)	Calcium (mg.)	Iron (mg.)	Vitamin A value (I.U.)	Thiamin (mg.)	Riboflavin (mg.)	Niacin (mg.)	Ascorbic acid (mg.)
Canned, solids and liquid:																
White with—																
Frankfurters (sliced).	1 cup 255	71	365	19	18	—	—	—	32	94	4.8	330	0.18	0.15	3.3	Trace
Pork and tomato sauce.	1 cup 255	71	310	16	7	2	3	1	49	138	4.6	330	0.20	0.08	1.5	5
Pork and sweet sauce.	1 cup 255	66	385	16	12	4	5	1	54	161	5.9	—	0.15	0.10	1.3	—
Red kidney	1 cup 255	76	230	15	1	—	—	—	42	74	4.6	10	0.13	0.10	1.5	—
Lima, cooked, drained.	1 cup 190	64	260	16	1	—	—	—	49	55	5.9	—	0.25	0.11	1.3	—
Cashew nuts, roasted	1 cup 140	5	785	24	64	11	45	4	41	53	5.3	140	0.60	0.35	2.5	—
Coconut, fresh, meat only:																
Pieces, approx. 2 by 2 by ½ inch.	1 piece 45	51	155	2	16	14	1	Trace	4	6	0.8	0	0.02	0.01	0.2	1
Shredded or grated, firmly packed.	1 cup 130	51	450	5	46	39	3	Trace	12	17	2.2	0	0.07	0.03	0.7	4
Cowpeas or blackeye peas, dry, cooked.	1 cup 248	80	190	13	1	—	—	—	34	42	3.2	20	0.41	0.11	1.1	Trace
Peanuts, roasted, salted, halves.	1 cup 144	2	840	37	72	16	31	21	27	107	3.0	—	0.46	0.19	24.7	0
Peanut butter	1 tablespoon 16	2	95	4	8	2	4	2	3	9	0.3	—	0.02	0.02	2.4	0
Peas, split, dry, cooked	1 cup 250	70	290	20	1	—	—	—	52	28	4.2	100	0.37	0.22	2.2	—
Pecans, halves	1 cup 108	3	740	10	77	5	48	15	16	79	2.6	140	0.93	0.14	1.0	2
Walnuts, black or native, chopped.	1 cup 126	3	790	26	75	4	26	36	19	Trace	7.6	380	0.28	0.14	0.9	—
Vegetables and vegetable products																
Asparagus, green:																
Cooked, drained:																
Spears, ½-inch diameter at base.	4 spears 60	94	10	1	Trace	—	—	—	2	13	0.4	540	0.10	0.11	0.8	16
Pieces, 1½- to 2-inch lengths.	1 cup 145	94	30	3	Trace	—	—	—	5	30	0.9	1,310	0.23	0.26	2.0	38
Canned, solids and liquid.	1 cup 244	94	45	5	1	—	—	—	7	44	4.1	1,240	0.15	0.22	2.0	37
Beans:																
Lima, immature seeds, cooked, drained.	1 cup 170	71	190	13	1	—	—	—	34	80	4.3	480	0.31	0.17	2.2	29

Food	Measure																
Snap:																	
Green:																	
Cooked, drained	1 cup	125	92	30	2	Trace	—	—	—	7	63	0.8	680	0.09	0.11	0.6	15
Canned, solids and liquid.	1 cup	239	94	45	2	Trace	—	—	—	10	81	2.9	690	0.07	0.10	0.7	10
Yellow or wax:																	
Cooked, drained	1 cup	125	93	30	2	Trace	—	—	—	6	63	0.8	290	0.09	0.11	0.6	16
Canned, solids and liquid.	1 cup	239	94	45	2	1	—	—	—	10	81	2.9	140	0.07	0.10	0.7	12
Sprouted mung beans, cooked, drained.	1 cup	125	91	35	4	Trace	—	—	—	7	21	1.1	30	0.11	0.13	0.9	8
Beets:																	
Cooked, drained, peeled:																	
Whole beets, 2-inch diameter.	2 beets	100	91	30	1	Trace	—	—	—	7	14	0.5	20	0.03	0.04	0.3	6
Diced or sliced	1 cup	170	91	55	2	Trace	—	—	—	12	24	0.9	30	0.05	0.07	0.5	10
Canned, solids and liquid.	1 cup	246	90	85	2	Trace	—	—	—	19	34	1.5	20	0.02	0.05	0.2	7
Beet greens, leaves and stems, cooked, drained.	1 cup	145	94	25	3	Trace	—	—	—	5	144	2.8	7,400	0.10	0.22	0.4	22
Blackeye peas. See Cowpeas.																	
Broccoli, cooked, drained:																	
Whole stalks, medium size.	1 stalk	180	91	45	6	1	—	—	—	8	158	1.4	4,500	0.16	0.36	1.4	162
Stalks cut into ½-inch pieces.	1 cup	155	91	40	5	1	—	—	—	7	136	1.2	3,880	0.14	0.31	1.2	140
Chopped, yield from 10-ounce frozen package.	1⅜ cups	250	92	65	7	1	—	—	—	12	135	1.8	6,500	0.15	0.30	1.3	143
Brussels sprouts, 7-8 sprouts (1¼- to 1½-inches diameter) per cup, cooked.	1 cup	155	88	55	7	1	—	—	—	10	50	1.7	810	0.12	0.22	1.2	135
Cabbage:																	
Common varieties:																	
Raw:																	
Coarsely shredded or sliced.	1 cup	70	92	15	1	Trace	—	—	—	4	34	0.3	90	0.04	0.04	0.2	33
Finely shredded or chopped.	1 cup	90	92	20	1	Trace	—	—	—	5	44	0.4	120	0.05	0.05	0.3	42
Cooked	1 cup	145	94	30	2	Trace	—	—	—	6	64	0.4	190	0.06	0.06	0.4	48
Red, raw, coarsely shredded.	1 cup	70	90	20	1	Trace	—	—	—	5	29	0.6	30	0.06	0.04	0.3	43
Savoy, raw, coarsely shredded.	1 cup	70	92	15	2	Trace	—	—	—	3	47	0.6	140	0.04	0.06	0.2	39
Cabbage, celery or Chinese, raw, cut in 1-inch pieces.	1 cup	75	95	10	1	Trace	—	—	—	2	32	0.5	110	0.04	0.03	0.5	19
Cabbage, spoon (or pakchoy), cooked.	1 cup	170	95	25	2	Trace	—	—	—	4	252	1.0	5,270	0.07	0.14	1.2	26

Table of food composition—cont'd

Food, approximate measure, and weight (in grams)	Water (%)	Food energy (kcal.)	Protein (gm.)	Fat (gm.)	Fatty acids Saturated (total) (gm.)	Fatty acids Unsaturated Oleic (gm.)	Fatty acids Unsaturated Linoleic (gm.)	Carbohydrate (gm.)	Calcium (mg.)	Iron (mg.)	Vitamin A value (I.U.)	Thiamin (mg.)	Riboflavin (mg.)	Niacin (mg.)	Ascorbic acid (mg.)
Carrots:															
Raw:															
Whole, 5½ by 1 inch, (25 thin strips).	1 carrot	50	88	20	1	Trace	—	—	—	5	18	0.4	5,500	0.03	0.03	0.3	4
Grated	1 cup	110	88	45	1	Trace	—	—	—	11	41	0.8	12,100	0.06	0.06	0.7	9
Cooked, diced	1 cup	145	91	45	1	Trace	—	—	—	10	48	0.9	15,220	0.08	0.07	0.7	9
Canned, strained or chopped (baby food).	1 ounce	28	92	10	Trace	Trace	—	—	—	2	7	0.1	3,690	0.01	0.01	0.1	1
Cauliflower, cooked, flowerbuds.	1 cup	120	93	25	3	Trace	—	—	—	5	25	0.8	70	0.11	0.10	0.7	66
Celery, raw:															
Stalk, large outer, 8 by about 1½ inches at root end.	1 stalk	40	94	5	Trace	Trace	—	—	—	2	16	0.1	100	0.01	0.01	0.1	4
Pieces, diced	1 cup	100	94	15	1	Trace	—	—	—	4	39	0.3	240	0.03	0.03	0.3	9
Collards, cooked	1 cup	190	91	55	5	1	—	—	—	9	289	1.1	10,260	0.27	0.37	2.4	87
Corn, sweet:															
Cooked, ear 5 by 1¾ inches.*	1 ear	140	74	70	3	1	—	—	—	16	2	0.5	310†	0.09	0.08	1.0	7
Canned, solids and liquid.	1 cup	256	81	170	5	2	—	—	—	40	10	1.0	690†	0.07	0.12	2.3	13
Cowpeas, cooked, immature seeds.	1 cup	160	72	175	13	1	—	—	—	29	38	3.4	560	0.49	0.18	2.3	28
Cucumbers, 10-ounce; 7½ by about 2 inches:															
Raw, pared	1 cucumber	207	96	30	1	Trace	—	—	—	7	35	0.6	Trace	0.07	0.09	0.4	23
Raw, pared, center slice ⅛-inch thick.	6 slices	50	96	5	Trace	Trace	—	—	—	2	8	0.2	Trace	0.02	0.02	0.1	6
Dandelion greens, cooked	1 cup	180	90	60	4	1	—	—	—	12	252	3.2	21,060	0.24	0.29	—	32
Endive, curly (including escarole).	2 ounces	57	93	10	1	Trace	—	—	—	2	46	1.0	1,870	0.04	0.08	0.3	6
Kale, leaves including stems, cooked.	1 cup	110	91	30	4	1	—	—	—	4	147	1.3	8,140	—	—	—	68
Lettuce, raw:															
Butterhead, as Boston types; head, 4-inch diameter.	1 head	220	95	30	3	Trace	—	—	—	6	77	4.4	2,130	0.14	0.13	0.6	18

Food	Measure																
Crisphead, as iceberg; head, 4¾-inch diameter.	1 head	454	96	60	4	Trace	—	—	—	13	91	2.3	1,500	0.29	0.27	1.3	29
Looseleaf, or bunching varieties, leaves.	2 large	50	94	10	1	Trace	—	—	—	2	34	0.7	950	0.03	0.04	0.2	9
Mushrooms, canned, solids and liquid.	1 cup	244	93	40	5	Trace	—	—	—	6	15	1.2	Trace	0.04	0.60	4.8	4
Mustard greens, cooked	1 cup	140	93	35	3	1	—	—	—	6	193	2.5	8,120	0.11	0.19	0.9	68
Okra, cooked, pod 3 by ⅝ inch.	8 pods	85	91	25	2	Trace	—	—	—	5	78	0.4	420	0.11	0.15	0.8	17
Onions: Mature: Raw, onion 2½-inch diameter.	1 onion	110	89	40	2	Trace	—	—	—	10	30	0.6	40	0.04	0.04	0.2	11
Cooked	1 cup	210	92	60	3	Trace	—	—	—	14	50	0.8	80	0.06	0.06	0.4	14
Young green, small, without tops.	6 onions	50	88	20	1	Trace	—	—	—	5	20	0.3	Trace	0.02	0.02	0.2	12
Parsley, raw, chopped	1 tablespoon	4	85	Trace	Trace	Trace	—	—	—	Trace	8	0.2	340	Trace	0.01	Trace	7
Parsnips, cooked	1 cup	155	82	100	2	1	—	—	—	23	70	0.9	50	0.11	0.12	0.2	16
Peas, green: Cooked	1 cup	160	82	115	9	1	—	—	—	19	37	2.9	860	0.44	0.17	3.7	33
Canned, solids and liquid	1 cup	249	83	165	9	1	—	—	—	31	50	4.2	1,120	0.23	0.13	2.2	22
Canned, strained (baby food).	1 ounce	28	86	15	1	Trace	—	—	—	3	3	0.4	140	0.02	0.02	0.4	3
Peppers, hot, red, without seeds, dried (ground chili powder, added seasonings).	1 tablespoon	15	8	50	2	2	—	—	—	8	40	2.3	9,750	0.03	0.17	1.3	2
Peppers, sweet: Raw, about 5 per pound: Green pod without stem and seeds.	1 pod	74	93	15	1	Trace	—	—	—	4	7	0.5	310	0.06	0.06	0.4	94
Cooked, boiled, drained	1 pod	73	95	15	1	Trace	—	—	—	3	7	0.4	310	0.05	0.05	0.4	70
Potatoes, medium (about 3 per pound raw): Baked, peeled after baking.	1 potato	99	75	90	3	Trace	—	—	—	21	9	0.7	Trace	0.10	0.04	1.7	20
Boiled: Peeled after boiling	1 potato	136	80	105	3	Trace	—	—	—	23	10	0.8	Trace	0.13	0.05	2.0	22
Peeled before boiling	1 potato	122	83	80	2	Trace	—	—	—	18	7	0.6	Trace	0.11	0.04	1.4	20
French-fried, piece 2 by ½ by ½ inch: Cooked in deep fat	10 pieces	57	45	155	2	7	2	2	4	20	9	0.7	Trace	0.07	0.04	1.8	12
Frozen, heated	10 pieces	57	53	125	2	5	1	1	2	19	5	1.0	Trace	0.08	0.01	1.5	12
Mashed: Milk added	1 cup	195	83	125	4	1	—	—	—	25	47	0.8	50	0.16	0.10	2.0	19
Milk and butter added	1 cup	195	80	185	4	8	4	3	Trace	24	47	0.8	330	0.16	0.10	1.9	18

*Measure and weight apply to entire vegetable or fruit, including parts not usually eaten.

†Based on yellow varieties; white varieties contain only a trace of cryptoxanthin and carotenes, the pigments in corn that have biological activity.

Table of food composition—cont'd

Food, approximate measure, and weight (in grams)		Water (%)	Food energy (kcal.)	Protein (gm.)	Fat (gm.)	Fatty acids Saturated (total) (gm.)	Fatty acids Unsaturated Oleic (gm.)	Fatty acids Unsaturated Linoleic (gm.)	Carbohydrate (gm.)	Calcium (mg.)	Iron (mg.)	Vitamin A value (I.U.)	Thiamin (mg.)	Riboflavin (mg.)	Niacin (mg.)	Ascorbic acid (mg.)
Potato chips, medium, 2-inch diameter	10 chips	2	115	1	8	2	2	4	10	8	0.4	Trace	0.04	0.01	1.0	3
Pumpkin, canned	1 cup	90	75	2	1	—	—	—	18	57	0.9	14,590	0.07	0.12	1.3	12
Radishes, raw, small, without tops.	4 radishes	94	5	Trace	Trace	—	—	—	1	12	0.4	Trace	0.01	0.01	0.1	10
Sauerkraut, canned, solids and liquid.	1 cup	93	45	2	Trace	—	—	—	9	85	1.2	120	0.07	0.09	0.4	33
Spinach:																
Cooked	1 cup	92	40	5	1	—	—	—	6	167	4.0	14,580	0.13	0.25	1.0	50
Canned, drained solids	1 cup	91	45	5	1	—	—	—	6	212	4.7	14,400	0.03	0.21	0.6	24
Squash:																
Cooked:																
Summer, diced	1 cup	96	30	2	Trace	—	—	—	7	52	0.8	820	0.10	0.16	1.6	21
Winter, baked, mashed	1 cup	81	130	4	1	—	—	—	32	57	1.6	8,610	0.10	0.27	1.4	27
Sweet potatoes:																
Cooked, medium, 5 by 2 inches, weight raw about 6 ounces:																
Baked, peeled after baking.	1 sweet potato	64	155	2	1	—	—	—	36	44	1.0	8,910	0.10	0.07	0.7	24
Boiled, peeled after boiling.	1 sweet potato	71	170	2	1	—	—	—	39	47	1.0	11,610	0.13	0.09	0.9	25
Candied, 3½ by 2¼ inches.	1 sweet potato	60	295	2	6	2	3	1	60	65	1.6	11,030	0.10	0.08	0.8	17
Canned, vacuum or solid pack.	1 cup	72	235	4	Trace	—	—	—	54	54	1.7	17,000	0.10	0.10	1.4	30
Tomatoes:																
Raw, approx. 3-inch diameter, 2⅛ inches high; weight, 7 ounces.	1 tomato	94	40	2	Trace	—	—	—	9	24	0.9	1,640	0.11	0.07	1.3	42*
Canned, solids and liquid.	1 cup	94	50	2	1	—	—	—	10	14	1.2	2,170	0.12	0.07	1.7	41
Tomato catsup:																
Cup	1 cup	69	290	6	1	—	—	—	69	60	2.2	3,820	0.25	0.19	4.4	41
Tablespoon	1 tablespoon	69	15	Trace	Trace	—	—	—	4	3	0.1	210	0.01	0.01	0.2	2
Tomato juice, canned:																
Cup	1 cup	94	45	2	Trace	—	—	—	10	17	2.2	1,940	0.12	0.07	1.9	39
Glass (6 fluid ounces)	1 glass	94	35	2	Trace	—	—	—	8	13	1.6	1,460	0.09	0.05	1.5	29

Food	Measure	Grams	Water (%)	Food energy	Protein	Fat	Sat.	Oleic	Linoleic	Carbohydrate	Calcium	Iron	Vitamin A	Thiamine	Riboflavin	Niacin	Ascorbic acid
Turnips, cooked, diced	1 cup	155	94	35	1	Trace	—	—	—	8	54	0.6	Trace	0.06	0.08	0.5	34
Turnip greens, cooked	1 cup	145	94	30	3	Trace	—	—	—	5	252	1.5	8,270	0.15	0.33	0.7	68

Fruits and fruit products

Food	Measure	Grams	Water (%)	Food energy	Protein	Fat	Sat.	Oleic	Linoleic	Carbohydrate	Calcium	Iron	Vitamin A	Thiamine	Riboflavin	Niacin	Ascorbic acid
Apples, raw, about 3 per pound.†	1 apple	150	85	70	Trace	Trace	—	—	—	18	8	0.4	50	0.04	0.02	0.1	3
Apple juice, bottled or canned.	1 cup	248	88	120	Trace	Trace	—	—	—	30	15	1.5	—	0.02	0.05	0.2	2‡
Applesauce, canned: Sweetened	1 cup	255	76	230	1	Trace	—	—	—	61	10	1.3	100	0.05	0.03	0.1	3‡
Unsweetened or artificially sweetened.	1 cup	244	88	100	1	Trace	—	—	—	26	10	1.2	100	0.05	0.02	0.1	2‡
Apricots: Raw (about 12 per pound).†	3 apricots	114	85	55	1	Trace	—	—	—	14	18	0.5	2,890	0.03	0.04	0.7	10
Canned in heavy syrup	1 cup	259	77	220	2	Trace	—	—	—	57	28	0.8	4,510	0.05	0.06	0.9	10
Dried, uncooked (40 halves per cup).	1 cup	150	25	390	8	1	—	—	—	100	100	8.2	16,350	0.02	0.23	4.9	19
Cooked, unsweetened, fruit and liquid.	1 cup	285	76	240	5	1	—	—	—	62	63	5.1	8,550	0.01	0.13	2.8	8
Apricot nectar, canned	1 cup	251	85	140	1	Trace	—	—	—	37	23	0.5	2,380	0.03	0.03	0.5	8‡
Avocados, whole fruit, raw‡: California (mid- and late-winter; diameter 3⅛ inches).	1 avocado	284	74	370	5	37	7	17	5	13	22	1.3	630	0.24	0.43	3.5	30
Florida (late summer, fall; diameter 3⅝ inches).	1 avocado	454	78	390	4	33	7	15	4	27	30	1.8	880	0.33	0.61	4.9	43
Bananas, raw, medium size.†	1 banana	175	76	100	1	Trace	—	—	—	26	10	0.8	230	0.06	0.07	0.8	12
Banana flakes	1 cup	100	3	340	4	1	—	—	—	89	32	2.8	760	0.18	0.24	2.8	7
Blackberries, raw	1 cup	144	84	85	2	1	—	—	—	19	46	1.3	290	0.05	0.06	0.5	30
Blueberries, raw	1 cup	140	83	85	1	1	—	—	—	21	21	1.4	140	0.04	0.08	0.6	20
Cantaloupes, raw; medium, 5-inch diameter, about 1⅔ pounds.†	½ melon	385	91	60	1	Trace	—	—	—	14	27	0.8	6,540§	0.08	0.06	1.2	63
Cherries, canned, red, sour, pitted, water pack.	1 cup	244	88	105	2	Trace	—	—	—	26	37	0.7	1,660	0.07	0.05	0.5	12
Cranberry juice cocktail, canned.	1 cup	250	83	165	Trace	Trace	—	—	—	42	13	0.8	Trace	0.03	0.03	0.1	40‖
Cranberry sauce, sweetened, canned, strained.	1 cup	277	62	405	Trace	1	—	—	—	104	17	0.6	60	0.03	0.03	0.1	6
Dates, pitted, cut.	1 cup	178	22	490	4	1	—	—	—	130	105	5.3	90	0.16	0.17	3.9	0

*Year-round average. Samples marketed from November through May average around 20 mg. per 200-gram tomato; from June through October, around 52 mg.

†Measure and weight apply to entire vegetable or fruit, including parts not usually eaten.

‡This is the amount from the fruit. Additional ascorbic acid may be added by the manufacturer. Refer to the label for this information.

§Value for varieties with orange-colored flesh; value for varieties with green flesh would be about 540 I.U.

‖Value listed is based on product with label stating 30 mg. per 6 fluid ounce serving.

Table of food composition—cont'd

Food, approximate measure, and weight (in grams)			Water (%)	Food energy (kcal.)	Protein (gm.)	Fat (gm.)	Fatty acids Saturated (total) (gm.)	Unsaturated Oleic (gm.)	Unsaturated Linoleic (gm.)	Carbohydrate (gm.)	Calcium (mg.)	Iron (mg.)	Vitamin A value (I.U.)	Thiamin (mg.)	Riboflavin (mg.)	Niacin (mg.)	Ascorbic acid (mg.)
Figs, dried, large, 2 by 1 inch	1 fig	21	23	60	1	Trace	—	—	—	15	26	0.6	20	0.02	0.02	0.1	0
Fruit cocktail, canned, in heavy syrup.	1 cup	256	80	195	1	Trace	—	—	—	50	23	1.0	360	0.05	0.03	1.3	5
Grapefruit:																	
Raw, medium, 3¾-inch diameter*:																	
White	½ grapefruit	241	89	45	1	Trace	—	—	—	12	19	0.5	10	0.05	0.02	0.2	44
Pink or red	½ grapefruit	241	89	50	1	Trace	—	—	—	13	20	0.5	540	0.05	0.02	0.2	44
Canned, syrup pack	1 cup	254	81	180	2	Trace	—	—	—	45	33	0.8	30	0.08	0.05	0.5	76
Grapefruit juice:																	
Fresh	1 cup	246	90	95	1	Trace	—	—	—	23	22	0.5	†	0.09	0.04	0.4	92
Canned, white:																	
Unsweetened	1 cup	247	89	100	1	Trace	—	—	—	24	20	1.0	20	0.07	0.04	0.4	84
Sweetened	1 cup	250	86	130	1	Trace	—	—	—	32	20	1.0	20	0.07	0.04	0.4	78
Frozen, concentrate, unsweetened:																	
Undiluted, can, 6 fluid ounces.	1 can	207	62	300	4	1	—	—	—	72	70	0.8	60	0.29	0.12	1.4	286
Diluted with 3 parts water, by volume.	1 cup	247	89	100	1	Trace	—	—	—	24	25	0.2	20	0.10	0.04	0.5	96
Dehydrated crystals	4 ounces	113	1	410	6	1	—	—	—	102	100	1.2	80	0.40	0.20	2.0	396
Prepared with water (1 pound yields about 1 gallon).	1 cup	247	90	100	1	Trace	—	—	—	24	22	0.2	20	0.10	0.05	0.5	91
Grapes, raw*:																	
American type (slip skin)	1 cup	153	82	65	1	1	—	—	—	15	15	0.4	100	0.05	0.03	0.2	3
European type (adherent skin).	1 cup	160	81	95	1	Trace	—	—	—	25	17	0.6	140	0.07	0.04	0.4	6
Grape juice:																	
Canned or bottled.	1 cup	253	83	165	1	Trace	—	—	—	42	28	0.8	—	0.10	0.05	0.5	Trace
Frozen concentrate, sweetened:																	
Undiluted, can, 6 fluid ounces.	1 can	216	53	395	1	Trace	—	—	—	100	22	0.9	40	0.13	0.22	1.5	‡
Diluted with 3 parts water by volume.	1 cup	250	86	135	1	Trace	—	—	—	33	8	0.3	10	0.05	0.08	0.5	‡
Grape juice drink, canned.	1 cup	250	86	135	Trace	Trace	—	—	—	35	8	0.3	—	0.03	0.03	0.3	‡
Lemons, raw, 2⅛-inch diameter, size 165.* Used for juice.	1 lemon	110	90	20	1	Trace	—	—	—	6	19	0.4	10	0.03	0.01	0.1	39
Lemon juice, raw	1 cup	244	91	60	1	Trace	—	—	—	20	17	0.5	50	0.07	0.02	0.2	112

Food	Measure	Weight (g)	Water (%)	Food energy	Protein	Fat				Carbohydrate	Calcium	Iron	Vitamin A (I.U.)	Thiamine	Riboflavin	Niacin	Ascorbic acid
Lemonade concentrate:																	
Frozen, 6 fluid ounces per can.	1 can	219	48	430	Trace	Trace	—	—	—	112	9	0.4	40	0.04	0.07	0.7	66
Diluted with 4⅓ parts water, by volume.	1 cup	248	88	110	Trace	Trace	—	—	—	28	2	Trace	Trace	Trace	0.02	0.2	17
Lime juice:																	
Fresh	1 cup	246	90	65	1	Trace	—	—	—	22	22	0.5	20	0.05	0.02	0.2	79
Canned, unsweetened	1 cup	246	90	65	1	Trace	—	—	—	22	22	0.5	20	0.05	0.02	0.2	52
Limeade concentrate, frozen:																	
Undiluted, can, 6 fluid ounces.	1 can	218	50	410	Trace	Trace	—	—	—	108	11	0.2	Trace	0.02	0.02	0.2	26
Diluted with 4⅓ parts water, by volume.	1 cup	247	90	100	Trace	Trace	—	—	—	27	2	Trace	Trace	Trace	Trace	Trace	5
Oranges, raw, 2⅝-inch diameter, all commercial varieties.*	1 orange	180	86	65	1	Trace	—	—	—	16	54	0.5	260	0.13	0.05	0.5	66
Orange juice, fresh, all varieties.	1 cup	248	88	110	2	1	—	—	—	26	27	0.5	500	0.22	0.07	1.0	124
Canned, unsweetened	1 cup	249	87	120	2	Trace	—	—	—	28	25	1.0	500	0.17	0.05	0.7	100
Frozen concentrate:																	
Undiluted, can, 6 fluid ounces.	1 can	213	55	360	5	Trace	—	—	—	87	75	0.9	1,620	0.68	0.11	2.8	360
Diluted with 3 parts water, by volume.	1 cup	249	87	120	2	Trace	—	—	—	29	25	0.2	550	0.22	0.02	1.0	120
Dehydrated crystals	4 ounces	113	1	430	6	2	—	—	—	100	95	1.9	1,900	0.76	0.24	3.3	408
Prepared with water, 1 pound yields about 1 gallon.	1 cup	248	88	115	2	1	—	—	—	27	25	0.5	500	0.20	0.07	1.0	109
Orange-apricot juice drink	1 cup	249	87	125	1	Trace	—	—	—	32	12	0.2	1,440	0.05	0.02	0.5	40§
Orange and grapefruit juice:																	
Frozen concentrate:																	
Undiluted, can, 6 fluid ounces.	1 can	210	59	330	4	1	—	—	—	78	61	0.8	800	0.48	0.06	2.3	302
Diluted with 3 parts Water, by volume.	1 cup	248	88	110	1	Trace	—	—	—	26	20	0.2	270	0.16	0.02	0.8	102
Papayas, raw, ½-inch cubes	1 cup	182	89	70	1	Trace	—	—	—	18	36	0.5	3,190	0.07	0.08	0.5	102
Peaches:																	
Raw																	
Whole, medium, 2-inch diameter, about 4 per pound.*	1 peach	114	89	35	1	Trace	—	—	—	10	9	0.5	1,320‖	0.02	0.05	1.0	7
Sliced	1 cup	168	89	65	1	Trace	—	—	—	16	15	0.8	2,230‖	0.03	0.08	1.6	12

*Measure and weight apply to entire vegetable or fruit including parts not usually eaten.

†For white-fleshed varieties value is about 20 I.U. per cup; for red-fleshed varieties, 1,080 I.U. per cup.

‡Present only if added by the manufacturer. Refer to the label for this information.

§Value listed is based on product with label stating 30 mg. per 6 fluid ounce serving.

‖Based on yellow-fleshed varieties; for white-fleshed varieties value is about 50 I.U. per 114-gram peach and 80 I.U. per cup of sliced peaches.

Table of food composition—cont'd

Food, approximate measure, and weight (in grams)		Water (%)	Food energy (kcal.)	Protein (gm.)	Fat (gm.)	Fatty acids			Carbohydrate (gm.)	Calcium (mg.)	Iron (mg.)	Vitamin A value (I.U.)	Thiamin (mg.)	Riboflavin (mg.)	Niacin (mg.)	Ascorbic acid (mg.)
						Saturated (total) (gm.)	Unsaturated Oleic (gm.)	Linoleic (gm.)								
Canned, yellow-fleshed, solids and liquid:																
Syrup pack, heavy:																
Halves or slices	1 cup	257	79	200	1	Trace	—	—	—	52	10	0.8	1,100	0.02	0.06	1.4	7
Water pack	1 cup	245	91	75	1	Trace	—	—	—	20	10	0.7	1,100	0.02	0.06	1.4	7
Dried, uncooked	1 cup	160	25	420	5	1	—	—	—	109	77	9.6	6,240	0.02	0.31	8.5	28
Cooked, unsweetened, 10-12 halves and juice.	1 cup	270	77	220	3	1	—	—	—	58	41	5.1	3,290	0.01	0.15	4.2	6
Frozen:																
Carton, 12 ounces, not thawed.	1 carton	340	76	300	1	Trace	—	—	—	77	14	1.7	2,210	0.03	0.14	2.4	135†
Pears:																
Raw, 3 by 2½-inch diameter.*	1 pear	182	83	100	1	1	—	—	—	25	13	0.5	30	0.04	0.07	0.2	7
Canned, solids and liquid:																
Syrup pack, heavy:																
Halves or slices:	1 cup	255	80	195	1	1	—	—	—	50	13	0.5	Trace	0.03	0.05	0.3	4
Pineapple:																
Raw, diced	1 cup	140	85	75	1	Trace	—	—	—	19	24	0.7	100	0.12	0.04	0.3	24
Canned, heavy syrup pack, solids and liquid:																
Crushed	1 cup	260	80	195	1	Trace	—	—	—	50	29	0.8	120	0.20	0.06	0.5	17
Sliced, slices and juice.	2 small or 1 large	122	80	90	Trace	Trace	—	—	—	24	13	0.4	50	0.09	0.03	0.2	8
Pineapple juice, canned	1 cup	249	86	135	1	Trace	—	—	—	34	37	0.7	120	0.12	0.04	0.5	22‡
Plums, all except prunes:																
Raw, 2-inch diameter, about 2 ounces.*	1 plum	60	87	25	Trace	Trace	—	—	—	7	7	0.3	140	0.02	0.02	0.3	3
Canned, syrup pack (Italian prunes):																
Plums (with pits) and juice.*	1 cup	256	77	205	1	Trace	—	—	—	53	22	2.2	2,970	0.05	0.05	0.9	4
Prunes, dried, "softenized," medium:																
Uncooked*	4 prunes	32	28	70	1	Trace	—	—	—	18	14	1.1	440	0.02	0.04	0.4	1
Cooked, unsweetened, 17-18 prunes and ⅓ cup liquid.*	1 cup	270	66	295	2	1	—	—	—	78	60	4.5	1,860	0.08	0.18	1.7	2
Prune juice, canned or bottled.	1 cup	256	80	200	1	Trace	—	—	—	49	36	10.5	—	0.03	0.03	1.0	5‡

Raisins, seedless:																	
Packaged, ½ ounce or 1½ tablespoons per package.	1 package	14	18	40	Trace	Trace	—	—	—	11	9	0.5	Trace	0.02	0.01	0.1	Trace
Cup, pressed down	1 cup	165	18	480	4	Trace	—	—	—	128	102	5.8	30	0.18	0.13	0.8	2
Raspberries, red:																	
Raw	1 cup	123	84	70	1	1	—	—	—	17	27	1.1	160	0.04	0.11	1.1	31
Frozen, 10-ounce carton, not thawed.	1 carton	284	74	275	2	1	—	—	—	70	37	1.7	200	0.06	0.17	1.7	59
Rhubarb, cooked, sugar added.	1 cup	272	63	385	1	Trace	—	—	—	98	212	1.6	220	0.06	0.15	0.7	17
Strawberries:																	
Raw, capped	1 cup	149	90	55	1	1	—	—	—	13	31	1.5	90	0.04	0.10	1.0	88
Frozen, 10-ounce carton, not thawed.	1 carton	284	71	310	1	1	—	—	—	79	40	2.0	90	0.06	0.17	1.5	150
Tangerines, raw, medium, 2⅜-inch diameter, size 176.*	1 tangerine	116	87	40	1	Trace	—	—	—	10	34	0.3	360	0.05	0.02	0.1	27
Tangerine juice, canned sweetened	1 cup	240	87	125	1	1	—	—	—	30	45	0.5	1,050	0.15	0.05	0.2	55
Watermelon, raw, wedge, 4 by 8 inches (1/16 of 10 by 16-inch melon, about 2 pounds with rind).*	1 wedge	925	93	115	2	1	—	—	—	27	30	2.1	2,510	0.13	0.13	0.7	30
Grain products																	
Bagel, 3-inch diameter:																	
Egg	1 bagel	55	32	165	6	2	—	—	—	28	9	1.2	30	0.14	0.10	1.2	0
Water	1 bagel	55	29	165	6	2	—	—	Trace	30	8	1.2	0	0.15	0.11	1.4	0
Barley, pearled, light, uncooked.	1 cup	200	11	700	16	2	Trace	1	1	158	32	4.0	0	0.24	0.10	6.2	0
Biscuits, baking powder from home recipe with enriched flour, 2-inch diameter.	1 biscuit	28	27	105	2	5	1	2	1	13	34	0.4	Trace	0.06	0.06	0.1	Trace
Biscuits, baking powder from mix, 2-inch diameter.	1 biscuit	28	28	90	2	3	1	1	1	15	19	0.6	Trace	0.08	0.07	0.6	Trace
Bran flakes (40% bran), added thiamin and iron.	1 cup	35	3	105	4	1	—	—	—	28	25	12.3	0	0.14	0.06	2.2	0
Bran flakes with raisins, added thiamin and iron.	1 cup	50	7	145	4	1	—	—	—	40	28	13.5	Trace	0.16	0.07	2.7	0

*Measure and weight apply to entire vegetable or fruit including parts not usually eaten.

†This value includes ascorbic acid added by the manufacturer.

‡This is the amount from the fruit. Additional ascorbic acid may be added by the manufacturer. Refer to the label for this information.

Table of food composition—cont'd

Food, approximate measure, and weight (in grams)		Water (%)	Food energy (kcal.)	Protein (gm.)	Fat (gm.)	Fatty acids			Carbohydrate (gm.)	Calcium (mg.)	Iron (mg.)	Vitamin A value (I.U.)	Thiamin (mg.)	Riboflavin (mg.)	Niacin (mg.)	Ascorbic acid (mg.)
						Saturated (total) (gm.)	Unsaturated									
							Oleic (gm.)	Linoleic (gm.)								
Breads:																
Boston brown bread, slice, 3 by ¾ inch.	1 slice	48	45	100	3	1	—	—	—	22	43	0.9	0	0.05	0.03	0.6	0
Cracked-wheat bread:																	
Loaf, 1-pound	1 loaf	454	35	1,190	40	10	2	5	2	236	399	5.0	Trace	0.53	0.41	5.9	Trace
Slice, 18 slices per loaf	1 slice	25	35	65	2	1	—	—	—	13	22	0.3	Trace	0.03	0.02	0.3	Trace
French or vienna bread:																	
Enriched, 1-pound loaf	1 loaf	454	31	1,315	41	14	3	8	2	251	195	10.0	Trace	1.27	1.00	11.3	Trace
Unenriched, 1-pound loaf.	1 loaf	454	31	1,315	41	14	3	8	2	251	195	3.2	Trace	0.36	0.36	3.6	Trace
Italian bread:																	
Enriched, 1-pound loaf	1 loaf	454	32	1,250	41	4	Trace	1	2	256	77	10.0	0	1.32	0.91	11.8	0
Unenriched, 1-pound loaf.	1 loaf	454	32	1,250	41	4	Trace	1	2	256	77	3.2	0	0.41	0.27	3.6	0
Raisin bread:																	
Loaf, 1-pound	1 loaf	454	35	1,190	30	13	3	8	2	243	322	5.9	Trace	0.23	0.41	3.2	Trace
Slice, 18 slices per loaf	1 slice	25	35	65	2	1	—	—	—	13	18	0.3	Trace	0.01	0.02	0.2	Trace
Rye bread:																	
American, light (⅓ rye, ⅔ wheat):																	
Loaf, 1-pound	1 loaf	454	36	1,100	41	5	—	—	—	236	340	7.3	0	0.82	0.32	6.4	0
Slice, 18 slices per loaf	1 slice	25	36	60	2	Trace	—	—	—	13	19	0.4	0	0.05	0.02	0.4	0
Pumpernickel, loaf, 1-pound.	1 loaf	454	34	1,115	41	5	—	—	—	241	381	10.9	0	1.04	0.64	5.4	0
White bread, enriched*:																	
Soft-crumb type:																	
Loaf, 1-pound	1 loaf	454	36	1,225	39	15	3	8	2	229	381	11.3	Trace	1.13	0.95	10.9	Trace
Slice, 18 slices per loaf.	1 slice	25	36	70	2	1	—	—	—	13	21	0.6	Trace	0.06	0.05	0.6	Trace
Slice, toasted	1 slice	22	25	70	2	1	—	—	—	13	21	0.6	Trace	0.06	0.05	0.6	Trace
Slice, 22 slices per loaf.	1 slice	20	36	55	2	1	—	—	—	10	17	0.5	Trace	0.05	0.04	0.5	Trace
Slice, toasted	1 slice	17	25	55	2	1	—	—	—	10	17	0.5	Trace	0.05	0.04	0.5	Trace
Loaf, 1½ pounds	1 loaf	680	36	1,835	59	22	5	12	3	343	571	17.0	Trace	1.70	1.43	16.3	Trace
Slice, 24 slices per loaf.	1 slice	28	36	75	2	1	—	—	—	14	24	0.7	Trace	0.07	0.06	0.7	Trace
Slice, toasted	1 slice	24	25	75	2	1	—	—	—	14	24	0.7	Trace	0.07	0.06	0.7	Trace

Slice, 28 slices per loaf.	1 slice	24	36	65	2	1	—	—	—	12	20	0.6	Trace	0.06	0.05	0.6	Trace
Slice, toasted	1 slice	21	25	65	2	1	—	—	—	12	20	0.6	Trace	0.06	0.05	0.6	Trace
Firm-crumb type:																	
Loaf, 1-pound	1 loaf	454	35	1,245	41	17	4	10	2	228	435	11.3	Trace	1.22	0.91	10.9	Trace
Slice, 20 slices per loaf.	1 slice	23	35	65	2	1	—	—	—	12	22	0.6	Trace	0.06	0.05	0.6	Trace
Slice, toasted	1 slice	20	24	65	2	1	—	—	—	12	22	0.6	Trace	0.06	0.05	0.6	Trace
Loaf, 2 pounds	1 loaf	907	35	2,495	82	34	8	20	4	455	871	22.7	Trace	2.45	1.81	21.8	Trace
Slice, 34 slices per loaf.	1 slice	27	35	75	2	1	—	—	—	14	26	0.7	Trace	0.07	0.05	0.6	Trace
Slice, toasted	1 slice	23	35	75	2	1	—	—	—	14	26	0.7	Trace	0.07	0.05	0.6	Trace
Whole-wheat bread, soft-crumb type:																	
Loaf, 1 pound	1 loaf	454	36	1,095	41	12	2	6	2	224	381	13.6	Trace	1.36	0.45	12.7	Trace
Slice, 16 slices per loaf	1 slice	28	36	65	3	1	—	—	—	14	24	0.8	Trace	0.09	0.03	0.8	Trace
Slice, toasted	1 slice	24	24	65	3	1	—	—	—	14	24	0.8	Trace	0.09	0.03	0.8	Trace
Loaf, 1 pound	1 loaf	454	36	1,100	48	14	3	6	3	216	449	13.6	Trace	1.18	0.54	12.7	Trace
Slice, 18 slices per loaf	1 slice	25	36	60	3	1	—	—	—	12	25	0.8	Trace	0.06	0.03	0.7	Trace
Slice, toasted	1 slice	21	24	60	3	1	—	—	—	12	25	0.8	Trace	0.06	0.03	0.7	Trace
Breadcrumbs, dry, grated	1 cup	100	6	390	13	5	1	2	1	73	122	3.6	Trace	0.22	0.30	3.5	Trace
Buckwheat flour, light, sifted	1 cup	98	12	340	6	1	—	—	—	78	11	1.0	0	0.08	0.04	0.4	0
Bulgur, canned, seasoned	1 cup	135	56	245	8	4	—	—	—	44	27	1.9	0	0.08	0.05	4.1	0
Cakes made from cake mixes:																	
Angelfood:																	
Whole cake	1 cake	635	34	1,645	36	1	—	—	—	377	603	1.9	0	0.03	0.70	0.6	0
Piece, 1/12 of 10-inch-diameter cake.	1 piece	53	34	135	3	Trace	—	—	—	32	50	0.2	0	Trace	0.06	0.1	0
Cupcakes, small, 2½-inch diameter:																	
Without icing	1 cupcake	25	26	90	1	3	1	1	1	14	40	0.1	40	0.01	0.03	0.1	Trace
With chocolate icing	1 cupcake	36	22	130	2	5	2	2	1	21	47	0.3	60	0.01	0.04	0.1	Trace
Devil's food, 2-layer, with chocolate icing:																	
Whole cake	1 cake	1,107	24	3,755	49	136	54	58	16	645	653	8.9	1,660	0.33	0.89	3.3	1
Piece, 1/16 of 9-inch-diameter cake.	1 piece	69	24	235	3	9	3	4	1	40	41	0.6	100	0.02	0.06	0.2	Trace
Cupcake, small, 2½-inch diameter.	1 cupcake	35	24	120	2	4	1	2	Trace	20	21	0.3	50	0.01	0.03	0.1	Trace

*Values for iron, thiamin, riboflavin, and niacin per pound of unenriched white bread would be as follows:

	Iron (mg.)	Thiamin (mg.)	Riboflavin (mg.)	Niacin (mg.)
Soft crumb	3.2	0.31	0.39	5.0
Firm crumb	3.2	0.32	0.59	4.1

Table of food composition—cont'd

Food, approximate measure, and weight (in grams)			Water (%)	Food energy (kcal.)	Protein (gm.)	Fat (gm.)	Fatty acids			Carbo-hydrate (gm.)	Cal-cium (mg.)	Iron (mg.)	Vita-min A value (I.U.)	Thia-min (mg.)	Ribo-flavin (mg.)	Niacin (mg.)	Ascor-bic acid (mg.)
							Satu-rated (total) (gm.)	Unsaturated									
								Oleic (gm.)	Linoleic (gm.)								
Gingerbread:																	
Whole cake	1 cake	570	37	1,575	18	39	10	19	9	291	513	9.1	Trace	0.17	0.51	4.6	2
Piece, 1/9 of 8-inch square cake.	1 piece	63	37	175	2	4	1	2	1	32	57	1.0	Trace	0.02	0.06	0.5	Trace
White, 2-layer, with chocolate icing:																	
Whole cake	1 cake	1,140	21	4,000	45	122	45	54	17	716	1,129	5.7	680	0.23	0.91	2.3	2
Piece, 1/16 of 9-inch-diameter cake.	1 piece	71	21	250	3	8	3	3	1	45	70	0.4	40	0.01	0.06	0.1	Trace
Cakes made from home recipes*:																	
Boston cream pie; piece 1/12 of 8-inch diameter.	1 piece	69	35	210	4	6	2	3	1	34	46	0.3	140	0.02	0.08	0.1	Trace
Fruitcake, dark, made with enriched flour:																	
Loaf, 1-pound	1 loaf	454	18	1,720	22	69	15	37	13	271	327	11.8	540	0.59	0.64	3.6	2
Slice, 1/30 of 8-inch loaf	1 slice	15	18	55	1	2	Trace	1	Trace	9	11	0.4	20	0.02	0.02	0.1	Trace
Plain sheet cake:																	
Without icing:																	
Whole cake	1 cake	777	25	2,830	35	108	30	52	21	434	497	3.1	1,320	0.16	0.70	1.6	2
Piece, 1/9 of 9-inch square cake.	1 piece	86	25	315	4	12	3	6	2	48	55	0.3	150	0.02	0.08	0.2	Trace
With boiled white icing, piece 1/9 of 9-inch square cake.	1 piece	114	23	400	4	12	3	6	2	71	56	0.3	150	0.02	0.08	0.2	Trace
Pound:																	
Loaf, 8½ by 3½ by 3 inches.	1 loaf	514	17	2,430	29	152	34	68	17	242	108	4.1	1,440	0.15	0.46	1.0	0
Slice, ½-inch thick	1 slice	30	17	140	2	9	2	4	1	14	6	0.2	80	0.01	0.03	0.1	0
Sponge:																	
Whole cake	1 cake	790	32	2,345	60	45	14	20	4	427	237	9.5	3,560	0.40	1.11	1.6	Trace
Piece, 1/12 of 10-inch-diameter cake.	1 piece	66	32	195	5	4	1	2	Trace	36	20	0.8	300	0.03	0.09	0.1	Trace
Yellow, 2-layer, without icing:																	
Whole cake	1 cake	870	24	3,160	39	111	31	53	22	506	618	3.5	1,310	0.17	0.70	1.7	2
Piece, 1/16 of 9-inch-diameter cake.	1 piece	54	24	200	2	7	2	3	1	32	39	0.2	80	0.01	0.04	0.1	Trace
Yellow, 2-layer, with chocolate icing:																	
Whole cake	1 cake	1,203	21	4,390	51	156	55	69	23	727	818	7.2	1,920	0.24	0.96	2.4	2
Piece, 1/16 of 9-inch-diameter cake.	1 piece	75	21	275	3	10	3	4	1	45	51	0.5	120	0.02	0.06	0.2	Trace

Cake icings. See Sugars, Sweets.
Cookies:
Brownies with nuts:

Food	Measure	Grams	Water (%)	Food energy	Protein (g)	Fat (g)	Saturated (g)	Oleic (g)	Linoleic (g)	Carbohydrate (g)	Calcium (mg)	Iron (mg)	Vitamin A	Thiamine (mg)	Riboflavin (mg)	Niacin (mg)	Ascorbic acid (mg)
Made from home recipe with enriched flour.	1 brownie	20	10	95	1	6	1	3	1	10	8	0.4	40	0.04	0.02	0.1	Trace
Made from mix	1 brownie	20	11	85	1	4	1	2	1	13	9	0.4	20	0.03	0.02	0.1	Trace
Chocolate chip: Made from home recipe with enriched flour.	1 cookie	10	3	50	1	3	1	1	1	6	4	0.2	10	0.01	0.01	0.1	Trace
Commercial	1 cookie	10	3	50	1	2	1	1	Trace	7	4	0.2	10	Trace	Trace	Trace	Trace
Fig bars, commercial	1 cookie	14	14	50	1	1	—	—	—	11	11	0.2	20	Trace	0.01	0.1	Trace
Sandwich, chocolate or vanilla, commercial.	1 cookie	10	2	50	1	2	1	1	Trace	7	2	0.1	0	Trace	Trace	0.1	0
Corn flakes, added nutrients: Plain	1 cup	25	4	100	2	Trace	—	—	—	21	4	0.4	0	0.11	0.02	0.5	0
Sugar-covered	1 cup	40	2	155	2	Trace	—	—	—	36	5	0.4	0	0.16	0.02	0.8	0
Corn (hominy) grits, degermed, cooked: Enriched	1 cup	245	87	125	3	Trace	—	—	—	27	2	0.7	150†	0.10	0.07	1.0	0
Unenriched	1 cup	245	87	125	3	Trace	—	—	—	27	2	0.2	150†	0.05	0.02	0.5	0
Cornmeal: Whole-ground, unbolted, dry.	1 cup	122	12	435	11	5	1	2	2	90	24	2.9	620†	0.46	0.13	2.4	0
Bolted (nearly whole-grain) dry.	1 cup	122	12	440	11	4	Trace	1	2	91	21	2.2	590†	0.37	0.10	2.3	0
Degermed, enriched: Dry form	1 cup	138	12	500	11	2	—	—	—	108	8	4.0	610†	0.61	0.36	4.8	0
Cooked	1 cup	240	88	120	3	1	—	—	—	26	2	1.0	140†	0.14	0.10	1.2	0
Degermed, unenriched: Dry form	1 cup	138	12	500	11	2	—	—	—	108	8	1.5	610†	0.19	0.07	1.4	0
Cooked	1 cup	240	88	120	3	1	—	—	—	26	2	0.5	140†	0.05	0.02	0.2	0
Corn muffins, made with with enriched degermed cornmeal and enriched flour; muffin 2⅜-inch diameter	1 muffin	40	33	125	3	4	2	2	Trace	19	42	0.7	120†	0.08	0.09	0.6	Trace
Corn muffins, made with mix, egg, and milk; muffin 2⅜-inch diameter	1 muffin	40	30	130	3	4	1	2	1	20	96	0.07	100	0.07	0.08	0.6	Trace
Corn, puffed, presweetened, added nutrients.	1 cup	30	2	115	1	Trace	—	—	—	27	3	0.5	0	0.13	0.05	0.6	0
Corn, shredded, added nutrients.	1 cup	25	3	100	2	Trace	—	—	—	22	1	0.6	0	0.11	0.05	0.5	0

*Unenriched cake flour used unless otherwise specified.
†This value is based on product made from yellow varieties of corn; white varieties contain only a trace.

Table of food composition—cont'd

Food, approximate measure, and weight (in grams)		Water (%)	Food energy (kcal.)	Protein (gm.)	Fat (gm.)	Fatty acids — Saturated (total) (gm.)	Unsaturated Oleic (gm.)	Unsaturated Linoleic (gm.)	Carbohydrate (gm.)	Calcium (mg.)	Iron (mg.)	Vitamin A value (I.U.)	Thiamin (mg.)	Riboflavin (mg.)	Niacin (mg.)	Ascorbic acid (mg.)
Crackers:																
Graham, 2½-inch square	4 crackers	28	6	110	2	3	—	—	—	21	11	0.4	0	0.01	0.06	0.4	0
Saltines	4 crackers	11	4	50	1	1	—	1	—	8	2	0.1	0	Trace	Trace	0.1	0
Danish pastry, plain (without fruit or nuts):																
Packaged ring, 12 ounces	1 ring	340	22	1,435	25	80	24	37	15	155	170	3.1	1,050	0.24	0.51	2.7	Trace
Round piece, approx. 4¼-inch diameter by 1 inch	1 pastry	65	22	275	5	15	5	7	3	30	33	0.6	200	0.05	0.10	0.5	Trace
Ounce	1 ounce	28	22	120	2	7	2	3	1	13	14	0.3	90	0.02	0.04	0.2	Trace
Doughnuts, cake type	1 doughnut	32	24	125	1	6	1	4	Trace	16	13	0.4†	30	0.05†	0.05†	0.4†	Trace
Farina, quick-cooking, enriched, cooked.	1 cup	245	89	105	3	Trace	—	—	—	22	147	0.7‡	0	0.12‡	0.07‡	1.0‡	0
Macaroni, cooked:																
Enriched:																
Cooked, firm stage (undergoes additional cooking in a food mixture).	1 cup	130	64	190	6	1	—	—	—	39	14	1.4‡	0	0.23‡	0.14‡	1.8‡	0
Cooked until tender	1 cup	140	72	155	5	1	—	—	—	32	8	1.3‡	0	0.20‡	0.11‡	1.5‡	0
Unenriched:																
Cooked, firm stage (undergoes additional cooking in a food mixture).	1 cup	130	64	190	6	1	—	—	—	39	14	0.7	0	0.03	0.03	0.5	0
Cooked until tender	1 cup	140	72	155	5	1	—	—	—	32	11	0.6	0	0.01	0.01	0.4	0
Macaroni (enriched) and cheese, baked.	1 cup	200	58	430	17	22	10	9	2	40	362	1.8	860	0.20	0.40	1.8	Trace
Canned	1 cup	240	80	230	9	10	4	3	1	26	199	1.0	260	0.12	0.24	1.0	Trace
Muffins, with enriched white flour; muffin, 3-inch diameter.	1 muffin	40	38	120	3	4	1	2	1	17	42	0.6	40	0.07	0.09	0.6	Trace
Noodles (egg noodles), cooked:																
Enriched	1 cup	160	70	200	7	2	1	1	Trace	37	16	1.4†	110	0.22‡	0.13‡	1.9‡	0
Unenriched	1 cup	160	70	200	7	2	1	1	Trace	37	16	1.0	110	0.05	0.03	0.6	0
Oats (with or without corn) puffed, added nutrients.	1 cup	25	3	100	3	1	—	—	—	19	44	1.2	0	0.24	0.04	0.5	0
Oatmeal or rolled oats, cooked.	1 cup	240	87	130	5	2	—	—	1	23	22	1.4	0	0.19	0.05	0.2	0
Pancakes, 4-inch diameter:																
Wheat, enriched flour	1 cake	27	50	60	2	2	Trace	1	Trace	9	27	0.4	30	0.05	0.06	0.4	Trace

mix with egg and milk.

(Column headings are printed on the facing page. The implied columns, left to right, are: Measure, Weight (grams), Water (%), Food energy (calories), Protein (g), Fat (g), Saturated fatty acids (g), Oleic (g), Linoleic (g), Carbohydrate (g), Calcium (mg), Iron (mg), Vitamin A (I.U.), Thiamin (mg), Riboflavin (mg), Niacin (mg), Ascorbic acid (mg).)

Food	Measure	Wt.	Water	Cal.	Prot.	Fat	Sat.	Oleic	Lino.	Carb.	Ca	Fe	Vit. A	Thi.	Rib.	Nia.	Asc.
Plain or buttermilk (made from mix with egg and milk).	1 cake	27	51	60	2	2	1	1	Trace	9	58	0.3	70	0.04	0.06	0.2	Trace
Pie (piecrust made with unenriched flour):																	
Sector, 4-inch, 1/7 of 9-inch-diameter pie:																	
Apple (2-crust)	1 sector	135	48	350	3	15	4	7	3	51	11	0.4	40	0.03	0.03	0.5	1
Butterscotch (1-crust)	1 sector	130	45	350	6	14	5	6	2	50	98	1.2	340	0.04	0.13	0.3	Trace
Cherry (2-crust)	1 sector	135	47	350	4	15	4	7	3	52	19	0.4	590	0.03	0.03	0.7	Trace
Custard (1-crust)	1 sector	130	58	285	8	14	5	6	2	30	125	0.8	300	0.07	0.21	0.4	0
Lemon meringue (1-crust)	1 sector	120	47	305	4	12	4	6	2	45	17	0.6	200	0.04	0.10	0.2	4
Mince (2-crust)	1 sector	135	43	365	3	16	4	8	3	56	38	1.4	Trace	0.09	0.05	0.5	1
Pecan (1-crust)	1 sector	118	20	490	6	27	4	16	5	60	55	3.3	190	0.19	0.08	0.4	Trace
Pineapple chiffon (1-crust)	1 sector	93	41	265	6	11	3	5	2	36	22	0.8	320	0.04	0.08	0.4	1
Pumpkin (1-crust)	1 sector	130	59	275	5	15	5	6	2	32	66	0.7	3,210	0.04	0.13	0.7	Trace
Piecrust, baked shell for pie made with:																	
Enriched flour	1 shell	180	15	900	11	60	16	28	12	79	25	3.1	0	0.36	0.25	3.2	0
Unenriched flour	1 shell	180	15	900	11	60	16	28	12	79	25	0.9	0	0.05	0.05	0.9	0
Piecrust mix including stick form:																	
Package, 10-ounce, for double crust.	1 package	284	9	1,480	20	93	23	46	21	141	131	1.4	0	0.11	0.11	2.0	0
Pizza (cheese) 5½-inch sector; ⅛ of 14-inch-diameter pie.	1 sector	75	45	185	7	6	2	3	Trace	27	107	0.7	290	0.04	0.12	0.7	4
Popcorn, popped:																	
Plain, large kernel	1 cup	6	4	25	1	Trace	—	—	—	5	1	0.2	—	—	0.01	0.1	0
With oil and salt	1 cup	9	3	40	1	2	1	Trace	1	5	1	0.2	—	—	0.01	0.2	0
Sugar coated	1 cup	35	4	135	2	1	—	—	—	30	2	0.5	—	—	0.02	0.4	0
Pretzels:																	
Dutch, twisted	1 pretzel	16	5	60	2	1	—	—	—	12	4	0.2	0	Trace	Trace	0.1	0
Thin, twisted	1 pretzel	6	5	25	1	Trace	—	—	—	5	1	0.1	0	Trace	Trace	Trace	0
Stick, small, 2¼ inches	10 sticks	3	5	10	Trace	Trace	—	—	—	2	1	Trace	0	Trace	Trace	Trace	0
Stick, regular, 3⅛ inches	5 sticks	3	5	10	Trace	Trace	—	—	—	2	1	Trace	0	Trace	Trace	Trace	0
Rice, white:																	
Enriched:																	
Raw	1 cup	185	12	670	12	1	—	—	—	149	44	5.4§	0	0.81§	0.06§	6.5§	0
Cooked	1 cup	205	73	225	4	Trace	—	—	—	50	21	1.8§	0	0.23§	0.02§	2.1§	0
Instant, ready-to-serve	1 cup	165	73	180	4	Trace	—	—	—	40	5	1.3§	0	0.21§	—§	1.7§	0
Unenriched, cooked	1 cup	205	73	225	4	Trace	—	—	—	50	21	0.4	0	0.04	0.02	0.8	0
Parboiled, cooked	1 cup	175	73	185	4	Trace	—	—	—	41	33	1.4§	0	0.19§	—§	2.1§	0
Rice, puffed, added nutrients.	1 cup	15	4	60	1	Trace	—	—	—	13	3	0.3	0	0.07	0.01	0.7	0

†Based on product made with enriched flour. With unenriched flour, approximate values per doughnut are iron, 0.2 mg.; thiamin, 0.01 mg.; riboflavin, 0.03 mg.; niacin, 0.2 mg.

‡Iron, thiamin, riboflavin, and niacin are based on the minimum levels of enrichment specified in standards of identity promulgated under the Federal Food, Drug, and Cosmetic Act.

§Iron, thiamin, riboflavin, and niacin are based on the minimum levels of enrichment specified in standards of identity promulgated under the Federal Food, Drug, and Cosmetic Act. Riboflavin is based on unenriched rice. When the minimum level of enrichment for riboflavin specified in the standards of identity becomes effective, the value will be 0.12 mg. per cup of parboiled rice and of white rice.

Table of food composition—cont'd

Food, approximate measure, and weight (in grams)			Water (%)	Food energy (kcal.)	Protein (gm.)	Fat (gm.)	Fatty acids: Saturated (total) (gm.)	Fatty acids: Unsaturated: Oleic (gm.)	Fatty acids: Unsaturated: Linoleic (gm.)	Carbohydrate (gm.)	Calcium (mg.)	Iron (mg.)	Vitamin A value (I.U.)	Thiamin (mg.)	Riboflavin (mg.)	Niacin (mg.)	Ascorbic acid (mg.)
Rolls, enriched:																	
Cloverleaf or pan:																	
Home recipe	1 roll	35	26	120	3	3	1	1	1	20	16	0.7	30	0.09	0.09	0.8	Trace
Commercial	1 roll	28	31	85	2	2	Trace	1	Trace	15	21	0.5	Trace	0.08	0.05	0.6	Trace
Frankfurter or hamburger	1 roll	40	31	120	3	2	1	1	1	21	30	0.8	Trace	0.11	0.07	0.9	Trace
Hard, round or rectangular	1 roll	50	25	155	5	2	Trace	1	Trace	30	24	1.2	Trace	0.13	0.12	1.4	Trace
Rye wafers, whole-grain, 1⅞ by 3½ inches.	2 wafers	13	6	45	2	Trace	—	—	—	10	7	0.5	0	0.04	0.03	0.2	0
Spaghetti, cooked, tender stage, enriched	1 cup	140	72	155	5	1	—	—	—	32	11	1.3*	0	0.20*	0.11*	1.5*	0
Spaghetti with meat balls and tomato sauce:																	
Home recipe	1 cup	248	70	330	19	12	4	6	1	39	124	3.7	1,590	0.25	0.30	4.0	22
Canned	1 cup	250	78	260	12	10	2	3	4	28	53	3.3	1,000	0.15	0.18	2.3	5
Spaghetti in tomato sauce with cheese:																	
Home recipe	1 cup	250	77	260	9	9	2	5	1	37	80	2.3	1,080	0.25	0.18	2.3	13
Canned	1 cup	250	80	190	6	2	1	1	1	38	40	2.8	930	0.35	0.28	4.5	10
Waffles, with enriched flour, 7-inch diameter.	1 waffle	75	41	210	7	7	2	4	1	28	85	1.3	250	0.13	0.19	1.0	Trace
Waffles, made from mix, enriched, egg and milk added, 7-inch diameter.	1 waffle	75	42	205	7	8	3	3	1	27	179	1.0	170	0.11	0.17	0.7	Trace
Wheat, puffed, added nutrients.	1 cup	15	3	55	2	Trace	—	—	—	12	4	0.6	0	0.08	0.03	1.2	0
Wheat, shredded, plain	1 biscuit	25	7	90	2	1	—	—	—	20	11	0.9	0	0.06	0.03	1.1	0
Wheat flakes, added nutrients.	1 cup	30	4	105	3	Trace	—	—	—	24	12	1.3	0	0.19	0.04	1.5	0
Wheat flours:																	
Whole-wheat, from hard wheats, stirred.	1 cup	120	12	400	16	2	Trace	1	1	85	49	4.0	0	0.66	0.14	5.2	0
All-purpose or family flour, enriched:																	
Sifted	1 cup	115	12	420	12	1	—	—	—	88	18	3.3*	0	0.51*	0.30*	4.0*	0
Unsifted	1 cup	125	12	455	13	1	—	—	—	95	20	3.6*	0	0.55*	0.33*	4.4*	0
Self-rising, enriched	1 cup	125	12	440	12	1	—	—	—	93	331	3.6*	0	0.55*	0.33*	4.4*	0
Cake or pastry flour, sifted.	1 cup	96	12	350	7	1	—	—	—	76	16	0.5	0	0.03	0.03	0.7	0

Fats, oils

Food	Measure																
Butter:																	
Regular, 4 sticks per pound:																	
Stick	½ cup	113	16	810	1	92	51	30	3	1	23	0	3,750†	—	—	—	0
Tablespoon (approx. ⅛ stick).	1 tablespoon	14	16	100	Trace	12	6	4	Trace	Trace	3	0	470†	—	—	—	0
Pat (1-inch square by ⅓-inch high; 90 per pound).	1 pat	5	16	35	Trace	4	2	1	Trace	Trace	1	0	170†	—	—	—	0
Whipped, 6 sticks or 2 8-ounce containers per pound:																	
Stick	½ cup	76	16	540	1	61	34	20	2	Trace	15	0	2,500†	—	—	—	0
Tablespoon (approx. ⅛ stick).	1 tablespoon	9	16	65	Trace	8	4	3	Trace	Trace	2	0	310†	—	—	—	0
Pat (1¼-inch square by ⅓-inch high; 120 per pound).	1 pat	4	16	25	Trace	3	2	1	Trace	Trace	1	0	130†	—	—	—	0
Fats, cooking:																	
Lard	1 cup	205	0	1,850	0	205	78	94	20	0	0	0	0	0	0	0	0
	1 tablespoon	13	0	115	0	13	5	6	1	0	0	0	0	0	0	0	0
Vegetable fats	1 cup	200	0	1,770	0	200	50	100	44	0	0	0	—	—	—	—	0
	1 tablespoon	13	0	110	0	13	3	6	3	0	0	0	—	—	—	—	0
Margarine:																	
Regular, 4 sticks per pound:																	
Stick	½ cup	113	16	815	1	92	17	46	25	1	23	0	3,750‡	—	—	—	0
Tablespoon (approx. ⅛ stick).	1 tablespoon	14	16	100	Trace	12	2	6	3	Trace	3	0	470‡	—	—	—	0
Pat (1-inch square by ⅓-inch high; 90 per pound).	1 pat	5	16	35	Trace	4	1	2	1	Trace	1	0	170‡	—	—	—	0
Whipped, 6 sticks per pound:																	
Stick	½ cup	76	16	545	1	61	11	31	17	Trace	15	0	2,500‡	—	—	—	0
Soft, 2 8-ounce tubs per pound:																	
Tub	1 tub	227	16	1,635	1	184	34	68	68	1	45	0	7,500‡	—	—	—	0
	1 tablespoon	14	16	100	Trace	11	2	4	4	Trace	3	0	470‡	—	—	—	0
Oils, salad or cooking:																	
Corn	1 cup	220	0	1,945	0	220	22	62	117	0	0	0	—	—	—	—	0
	1 tablespoon	14	0	125	0	14	1	4	7	0	0	0	—	—	—	—	0
Cottonseed	1 cup	220	0	1,945	0	220	55	46	110	0	0	0	—	—	—	—	0
	1 tablespoon	14	0	125	0	14	4	3	7	0	0	0	—	—	—	—	0
Olive	1 cup	220	0	1,945	0	220	24	167	15	0	0	0	—	—	—	—	0
	1 tablespoon	14	0	125	0	14	2	11	1	0	0	0	—	—	—	—	0

*Iron, thiamin, riboflavin, and niacin are based on the minimum levels of enrichment specified in standards of identity promulgated under the Federal Food, Drug, and Cosmetic Act.

†Year-round average.

‡Based on the average vitamin A content of fortified margarine. Federal specifications for fortified margarine require a minimum of 15,000 I.U. of vitamin A per pound.

Table of food composition—cont'd

Food, approximate measure, and weight (in grams)		Water (%)	Food energy (kcal.)	Protein (gm.)	Fat (gm.)	Fatty acids Saturated (total) (gm.)	Fatty acids Unsaturated Oleic (gm.)	Fatty acids Unsaturated Linoleic (gm.)	Carbohydrate (gm.)	Calcium (mg.)	Iron (mg.)	Vitamin A value (I.U.)	Thiamin (mg.)	Riboflavin (mg.)	Niacin (mg.)	Ascorbic acid (mg.)
Peanut	1 cup	220	0	1,945	220	40	103	64	0	0	0	—	0	0	0	0
	1 tablespoon	14	0	125	14	3	7	4	0	0	0	—	0	0	0	0
Safflower	1 cup	220	0	1,945	220	18	37	165	0	0	0	—	0	0	0	0
	1 tablespoon	14	0	125	14	1	2	10	0	0	0	—	0	0	0	0
Soybean	1 cup	220	0	1,945	220	33	44	114	0	0	0	—	0	0	0	0
	1 tablespoon	14	0	125	14	2	3	7	0	0	0	—	0	0	0	0
Salad dressings:																
Blue cheese	1 tablespoon	15	32	75	8	2	2	4	1	12	Trace	30	Trace	0.02	Trace	Trace
Commercial mayonnaise type:																
Regular	1 tablespoon	15	41	65	6	1	1	3	2	2	Trace	30	Trace	Trace	Trace	—
Special dietary, low-calorie.	1 tablespoon	16	81	20	2	Trace	Trace	1	1	3	Trace	40	Trace	Trace	Trace	—
French:																
Regular	1 tablespoon	16	39	65	6	1	1	3	3	2	0.1	—	—	—	—	—
Special dietary, low-fat with artificial sweeteners.	1 tablespoon	15	95	Trace	Trace	—	—	—	Trace	2	0.1	—	—	—	—	—
Home cooked, boiled	1 tablespoon	16	68	25	2	1	1	Trace	2	14	0.1	80	0.01	0.03	Trace	Trace
Mayonnaise	1 tablespoon	14	15	100	11	2	2	6	Trace	3	0.1	40	Trace	0.01	Trace	—
Thousand island	1 tablespoon	16	32	80	8	1	2	4	3	2	0.1	50	Trace	Trace	Trace	Trace
Sugars, sweets																
Cake icings:																
Chocolate made with milk and table fat.	1 cup	275	14	1,035	38	21	14	1	185	165	3.3	580	0.06	0.28	0.6	1
Coconut (with boiled icing).	1 cup	166	15	605	13	11	1	Trace	124	10	0.8	0	0.02	0.07	0.3	0
Creamy fudge from mix with water only.	1 cup	245	15	830	16	5	8	3	183	96	2.7	Trace	0.05	0.20	0.7	Trace
White, boiled	1 cup	94	18	300	0	—	—	—	76	2	Trace	0	Trace	0.03	Trace	0
Candy:																
Carmels, plain or chocolate	1 ounce	28	8	115	3	2	1	Trace	22	42	0.4	Trace	0.01	0.05	0.1	Trace
Chocolate, milk, plain	1 ounce	28	1	145	9	5	3	Trace	16	65	0.3	80	0.02	0.10	0.1	Trace
Chocolate-coated peanuts	1 ounce	28	1	160	12	3	6	2	11	33	0.4	Trace	0.10	0.05	2.1	Trace
Fondant; mints, uncoated; candy corn.	1 ounce	28	8	105	1	—	—	—	25	4	0.3	0	Trace	Trace	Trace	0
Fudge, plain	1 ounce	28	8	115	4	2	1	Trace	21	22	0.3	Trace	0.01	0.03	0.1	Trace

Food	Measure	g	Water	Food energy	Protein	Fat	Fat (sat.)	Fat (oleic)	Fat (linoleic)	Carbohydrate	Calcium	Iron	Vitamin A	Thiamine	Riboflavin	Niacin	Ascorbic acid
Gum drops	1 ounce	28	12	100	Trace	Trace	—	—	—	25	2	0.1	0	0	Trace	Trace	0
Hard	1 ounce	28	1	110	0	Trace	—	—	—	28	6	0.5	0	0	0	0	0
Marshmallows	1 ounce	28	17	90	1	Trace	—	—	—	23	5	0.5	0	0	Trace	Trace	0
Chocolate-flavored syrup or topping:																	
Thin type	1 fluid ounce	38	32	90	1	1	Trace	Trace	Trace	24	6	0.6	Trace	0.01	0.03	0.2	0
Fudge type	1 fluid ounce	38	25	125	2	5	3	2	Trace	20	48	0.5	60	0.02	0.08	0.2	Trace
Chocolate-flavored beverage powder (approx. 4 heaping teaspoons per ounce):																	
With nonfat dry milk	1 ounce	28	2	100	5	1	Trace	Trace	Trace	20	167	0.5	10	0.04	0.21	0.2	1
Without nonfat dry milk	1 ounce	28	1	100	1	1	Trace	Trace	—	25	9	0.6	—	0.01	0.03	0.1	0
Honey, strained or extracted	1 tablespoon	21	17	65	Trace	0	—	—	—	17	1	0.1	0	Trace	0.01	0.1	Trace
Jams and preserves	1 tablespoon	20	29	55	Trace	Trace	—	—	—	14	4	0.2	Trace	Trace	0.01	Trace	Trace
Jellies	1 tablespoon	18	29	50	Trace	Trace	—	—	—	13	4	0.3	Trace	Trace	0.01	Trace	1
Molasses, cane:																	
Light (first extraction)	1 tablespoon	20	24	50	—	—	—	—	—	13	33	0.9	—	0.01	0.01	Trace	—
Blackstrap (third extraction)	1 tablespoon	20	24	45	—	—	—	—	—	11	137	3.2	—	0.02	0.04	0.4	—
Syrups:																	
Sorghum	1 tablespoon	21	23	55	—	—	—	—	—	14	35	2.6	—	—	0.02	Trace	—
Table blends, chiefly corn, light and dark	1 tablespoon	21	24	60	0	0	—	—	—	15	9	0.8	0	0	0	0	0
Sugars:																	
Brown, firm-packed	1 cup	220	2	820	0	0	—	—	—	212	187	7.5	0	0.02	0.07	0.40	
White:																	
Granulated	1 cup	200	Trace	770	0	0	—	—	—	199	0	0.2	0	0	0	0	0
Granulated	1 tablespoon	11	Trace	40	0	0	—	—	—	11	0	Trace	0	0	0	0	0
Powdered, stirred before measuring	1 cup	120	Trace	460	0	0	—	—	—	119	0	0.1	0	0	0	0	0

Miscellaneous items

Food	Measure	g	Water	Food energy	Protein	Fat	Fat (sat.)	Fat (oleic)	Fat (linoleic)	Carbohydrate	Calcium	Iron	Vitamin A	Thiamine	Riboflavin	Niacin	Ascorbic acid
Barbecue sauce	1 cup	250	81	230	4	17	2	5	9	20	53	2.0	900	0.03	0.03	0.8	13
Beverages, alcoholic:																	
Beer	12 fluid ounces	360	92	150	1	0	—	—	—	14	18	Trace	—	0.01	0.11	2.2	—
Gin, rum, vodka, whiskey:																	
80-proof	1½ fluid ounces jigger	42	67	100	—	—	—	—	—	Trace	—	—	—	—	—	—	—
86-proof	1½ fluid ounces jigger	42	64	105	—	—	—	—	—	Trace	—	—	—	—	—	—	—
90-proof	1½ fluid ounces jigger	42	62	110	—	—	—	—	—	Trace	—	—	—	—	—	—	—
94-proof	1½ fluid ounces jigger	42	60	115	—	—	—	—	—	Trace	—	—	—	—	—	—	—
100-proof	1½ fluid ounces jigger	42	58	125	—	—	—	—	—	Trace	—	—	—	—	—	—	—
Wines:																	
Dessert	3½ fluid ounces, glass	103	77	140	Trace	0	—	—	—	8	8	—	—	0.01	0.02	0.2	—
Table	3½ fluid ounces, glass	102	86	85	Trace	0	—	—	—	4	9	0.4	—	Trace	0.01	0.1	—

Table of food composition—cont'd

Food, approximate measure, and weight (in grams)		Water (%)	Food energy (kcal.)	Protein (gm.)	Fat (gm.)	Fatty acids			Carbohydrate (gm.)	Calcium (mg.)	Iron (mg.)	Vitamin A value (I.U.)	Thiamin (mg.)	Riboflavin (mg.)	Niacin (mg.)	Ascorbic acid (mg.)
						Saturated (total) (gm.)	Unsaturated									
							Oleic (gm.)	Linoleic (gm.)								
Beverages, carbonated, sweetened, nonalcoholic:																
Carbonated water	12 fluid ounces 366	92	115	0	0	—	—	—	29	—	—	0	0	0	0	0
Cola type	12 fluid ounces 369	90	145	0	0	—	—	—	37	—	—	0	0	0	0	0
Fruit-flavored sodas and Tom Collins mixes.	12 fluid ounces 372	88	170	0	0	—	—	—	45	—	—	0	0	0	0	0
Ginger ale	12 fluid ounces 366	92	115	0	0	—	—	—	29	—	—	0	0	0	0	0
Root beer	12 fluid ounces 370	90	150	0	0	—	—	—	39	—	—	0	0	0	0	0
Bouillon cubes, approx. ½ inch.	1 cube 4	4	5	1	Trace	—	—	—	Trace	—	—	—	—	—	—	—
Chocolate:																
Bitter or baking	1 ounce 28	2	145	3	15	8	6	Trace	8	22	1.9	20	0.01	0.07	0.4	0
Semi-sweet, small pieces	1 cup 170	1	860	7	61	34	22	1	97	51	4.4	30	0.02	0.14	0.9	0
Gelatin:																
Plain, dry powder in envelope.	1 envelope 7	13	25	6	Trace	—	—	—	0	—	—	—	—	—	—	—
Dessert powder, 3-ounce package.	1 package 85	2	315	8	0	—	—	—	75	—	—	—	—	—	—	—
Gelatin dessert, prepared with water.	1 cup 240	84	140	4	0	—	—	—	34	—	—	—	—	—	—	—
Olives, pickled:																
Green	4 medium or 3 extra large or 2 giant. 16	78	15	Trace	2	Trace	2	Trace	Trace	8	0.2	40	—	Trace	—	—
Ripe: Mission	3 small or 2 large. 10	73	15	Trace	2	Trace	2	Trace	Trace	9	0.1	10	—	Trace	—	—
Pickles, cucumber:																
Dill, medium, whole, 3¾ inches long, 1¼-inch diameter.	1 pickle 65	93	10	1	Trace	—	—	—	1	17	0.7	70	Trace	0.01	Trace	4
Fresh, sliced, 1½-inch diameter, ¼-inch thick.	2 slices 15	79	10	Trace	Trace	—	—	—	3	5	0.3	20	Trace	Trace	Trace	1
Sweet, gherkin, small, whole, approx. 2½ inches long, ¾-inch diameter.	1 pickle 15	61	20	Trace	Trace	—	—	—	6	2	0.2	10	Trace	Trace	Trace	1
Relish, finely chopped, sweet.	1 tablespoon 15	63	20	Trace	Trace	—	—	—	5	3	0.1	—	—	—	—	—

Popcorn. *See* Grain products.

Food	Measure	Grams	Water (%)	Food energy (cal.)	Protein (g)	Fat (g)	Saturated fat (g)	Oleic (g)	Linoleic (g)	Carbohydrate (g)	Calcium (mg)	Iron (mg)	Vitamin A (I.U.)	Thiamin (mg)	Riboflavin (mg)	Niacin (mg)	Ascorbic acid (mg)
Popsicle, 3 fluid ounce size	1 popsicle	95	95	70	0	0	0	0	0	18	0	Trace	0	0	0	0	0
Pudding, home recipe with starch base:																	
Chocolate	1 cup	260	66	385	8	12	7	4	Trace	67	250	1.3	390	0.05	0.36	0.3	1
Vanilla (blanc mange)	1 cup	255	76	285	9	10	5	3	Trace	41	298	Trace	410	0.08	0.41	0.3	2
Pudding mix, dry form, 4-ounce package.	1 package	113	2	410	3	2	1	1	Trace	103	23	1.8	Trace	0.02	0.08	0.5	0
Sherbet	1 cup	193	67	260	2	2	—	—	—	59	31	Trace	120	0.02	0.06	Trace	4
Soups:																	
Canned, condensed, ready-to-serve:																	
Prepared with an equal volume of milk:																	
Cream of chicken	1 cup	245	85	180	7	10	3	3	3	15	172	0.5	610	0.05	0.27	0.7	2
Cream of mushroom	1 cup	245	83	215	7	14	4	4	5	16	191	0.5	250	0.05	0.34	0.7	1
Tomato	1 cup	250	84	175	7	7	3	2	1	23	168	0.8	1,200	0.10	0.25	1.3	15
Prepared with an equal volume of water:																	
Bean with pork	1 cup	250	84	170	8	6	1	2	2	22	63	2.3	650	0.13	0.08	1.0	3
Beef broth, bouillon consomme.	1 cup	240	96	30	5	0	—	—	—	3	Trace	0.5	Trace	Trace	0.02	1.2	—
Beef noodle	1 cup	240	93	70	4	3	1	1	1	7	7	1.0	50	0.05	0.07	1.0	Trace
Clam chowder, Manhattan type (with tomatoes, without milk).	1 cup	245	92	80	2	3	—	—	—	12	34	1.0	880	0.02	0.02	1.0	—
Cream of chicken	1 cup	240	92	95	3	6	1	2	3	8	24	0.5	410	0.02	0.05	0.5	Trace
Cream of mushroom	1 cup	240	90	135	2	10	1	3	5	10	41	0.5	70	0.02	0.12	0.7	Trace
Minestrone	1 cup	245	90	105	5	3	—	—	—	14	37	1.0	2,350	0.07	0.05	1.0	—
Split pea	1 cup	245	85	145	9	3	1	2	1	21	29	1.5	440	0.25	0.15	1.5	1
Tomato	1 cup	245	90	90	2	3	Trace	1	—	16	15	0.7	1,000	0.05	0.05	1.2	12
Vegetable beef	1 cup	245	92	80	5	2	—	—	—	10	12	0.7	2,700	0.05	0.05	1.0	—
Vegetarian	1 cup	245	92	80	2	2	—	—	—	13	20	1.0	2,940	0.05	0.05	1.0	—
Dehydrated, dry form:																	
Chicken noodle (2-ounce package).	1 package	57	6	220	8	6	2	3	1	33	34	1.4	190	0.30	0.15	2.4	3
Onion mix (1½-ounce package).	1 package	43	3	150	6	5	1	2	1	23	42	0.6	30	0.05	0.03	0.3	6
Tomato vegetable with noodles (2½-ounce package).	1 package	71	4	245	6	6	2	3	1	45	33	1.4	1,700	0.21	0.13	1.8	18
Frozen, condensed:																	
Clam chowder, New England type (with milk, without tomatoes):																	
Prepared with equal volume of milk.	1 cup	245	83	210	9	12	—	—	—	16	240	1.0	250	0.07	0.29	0.5	Trace
Prepared with equal volume of water.	1 cup	240	89	130	4	8	—	—	—	11	91	1.0	50	0.05	0.10	0.5	—
Cream of potato:																	
Prepared with equal volume of milk.	1 cup	245	83	185	8	10	5	3	Trace	18	208	1.0	590	0.10	0.27	0.5	Trace

Table of food composition—cont'd

Food, approximate measure, and weight (in grams)		Water (%)	Food energy (kcal.)	Protein (gm.)	Fat (gm.)	Fatty acids			Carbohydrate (gm.)	Calcium (mg.)	Iron (mg.)	Vitamin A value (I.U.)	Thiamin (mg.)	Riboflavin (mg.)	Niacin (mg.)	Ascorbic acid (mg.)
						Saturated (total) (gm.)	Unsaturated Oleic (gm.)	Unsaturated Linoleic (gm.)								
Prepared with equal volume of water.	1 cup	240	90	105	3	5	3	2	Trace	12	58	1.0	410	0.05	0.05	0.5	—
Cream of shrimp:																	
Prepared with equal volume of milk.	1 cup	245	82	245	9	16	—	—	—	15	189	0.5	290	0.07	0.27	0.5	Trace
Prepared with equal volume of water.	1 cup	240	88	160	5	12	—	—	—	8	38	0.5	120	0.05	0.05	0.5	—
Oyster stew:																	
Prepared with equal volume of milk.	1 cup	240	83	200	10	12	—	—	—	14	305	1.4	410	0.12	0.41	0.5	Trace
Prepared with equal volume of water.	1 cup	240	90	120	6	8	—	—	—	8	158	1.4	240	0.07	0.19	0.5	—
Tapioca, dry, quick-cooking	1 cup	152	13	535	1	Trace	—	—	—	131	15	0.6	0	0	0	0	0
Tapioca desserts:																	
Apple	1 cup	250	70	295	1	Trace	—	—	—	74	8	0.5	30	Trace	Trace	Trace	Trace
Cream pudding	1 cup	165	72	220	8	8	4	3	Trace	28	173	0.7	480	0.07	0.30	0.2	2
Tartar sauce	1 tablespoon	14	34	75	Trace	8	1	1	4	1	3	0.1	30	Trace	Trace	Trace	Trace
Vinegar	1 tablespoon	15	94	Trace	Trace	0	—	—	—	1	1	0.1	—	—	—	—	2
White sauce, medium	1 cup	250	73	405	10	31	16	10	1	22	288	0.5	1,150	0.10	0.43	0.5	2
Yeast:																	
Baker's, dry, active	1 package	7	5	20	3	Trace	—	—	—	3	3	1.1	Trace	0.16	0.38	2.6	Trace
Brewer's dry	1 tablespoon	8	5	25	3	Trace	—	—	—	3	17	1.4	Trace	1.25	0.34	3.0	Trace
Yoghurt. *See* Milk, cheese, cream, imitation cream; related products.																	

Appendix G | *Selected sources of reliable nutrition information*

American Dental Association
222 E. Superior Street
Chicago, Ill. 60611

The American Dietetic Association
620 N. Michigan Avenue
Chicago, Ill. 60611

American Institute of Baking
400 E. Ontario Street
Chicago, Ill. 60611

American Medical Association
535 N. Dearborn Street
Chicago, Ill. 60610

Borden Co.
350 Madison Avenue
New York, N. Y. 10017

National Academy of Sciences
National Research Council
2101 Constitution Avenue
Washington, D. C. 20418

National Dairy Council
111 N. Canal Street
Chicago, Ill. 60606

National Meat and Livestock Board
33 S. Wabash Avenue
Chicago, Ill. 60603

The Nutrition Foundation, Inc.
99 Park Avenue
New York, N. Y. 10016

Superintendent of Documents
U. S. Government Printing Office
Washington, D. C. 20402

U. S. Department of Agriculture
Washington, D. C. 20250

481

Appendix H | *Formulas of vitamins and amino acids*

FAT-SOLUBLE VITAMINS

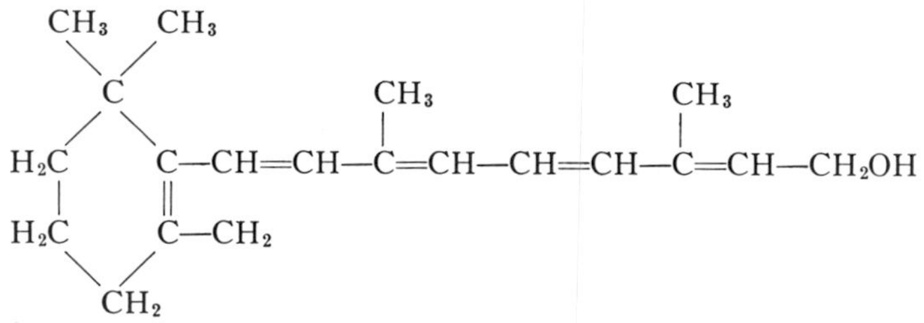

Retinol (vitamin A)

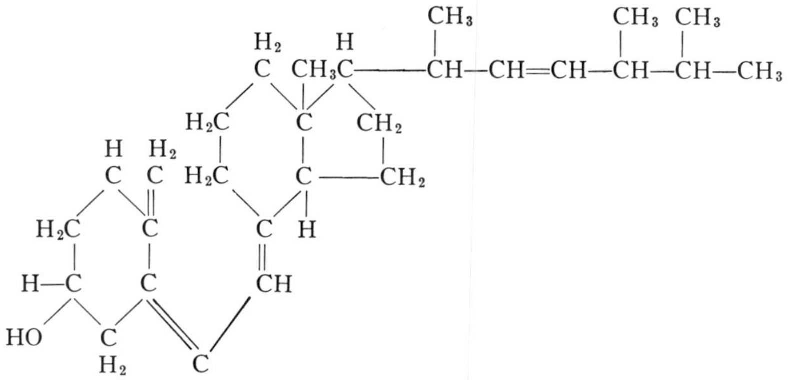

Cholecalciferol (vitamin D)

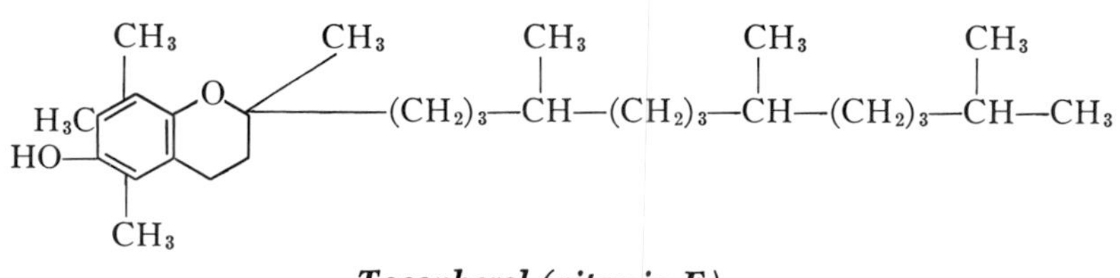

Tocopherol (vitamin E)

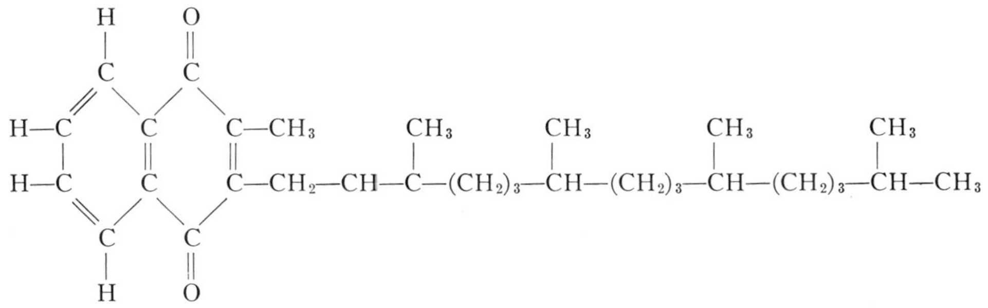

Phylloquinone (vitamin K)

WATER-SOLUBLE VITAMINS

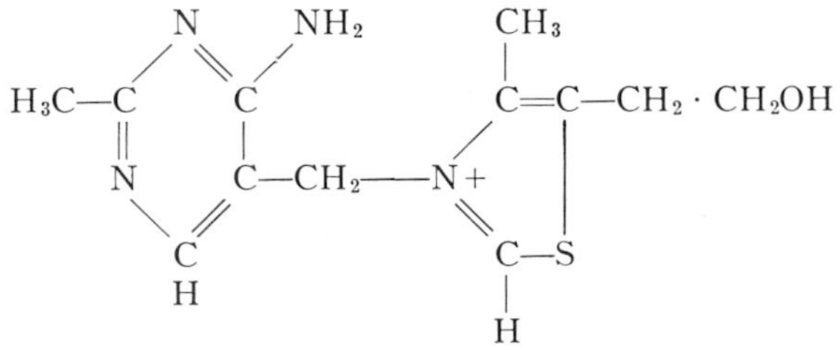

Thiamin (vitamin B₁)

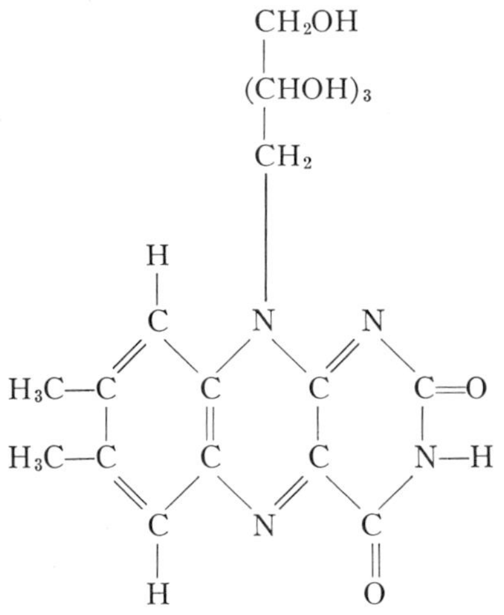

Riboflavin (vitamin B₂)

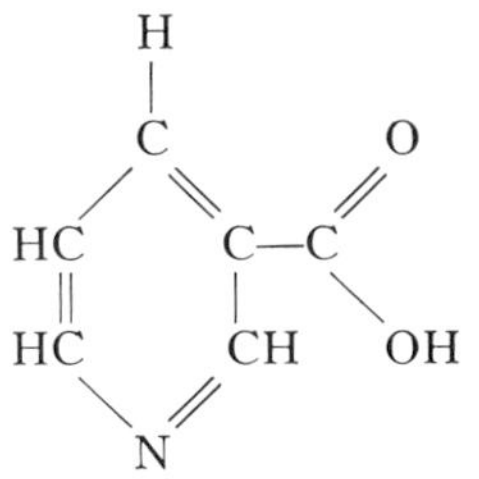

Niacin (nicotinic acid)

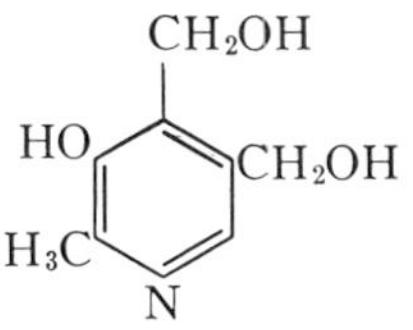

Pyridoxine (vitamin B₆)

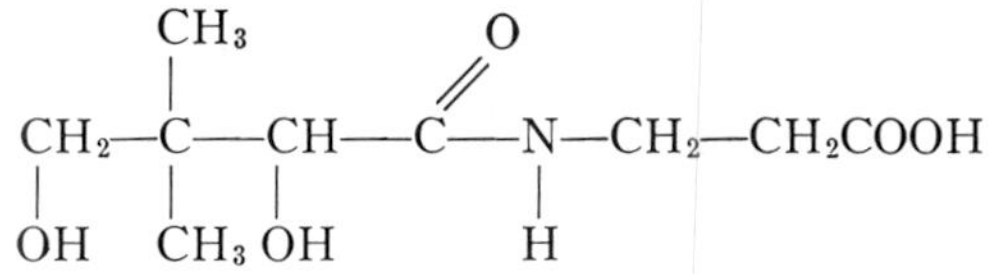

$$CH_2-\underset{\underset{CH_3}{|}}{\overset{\overset{CH_3}{|}}{C}}-\underset{\underset{OH}{|}}{CH}-\overset{\overset{O}{\parallel}}{C}-\underset{\underset{H}{|}}{N}-CH_2-CH_2COOH$$
OH

Pantothenic acid

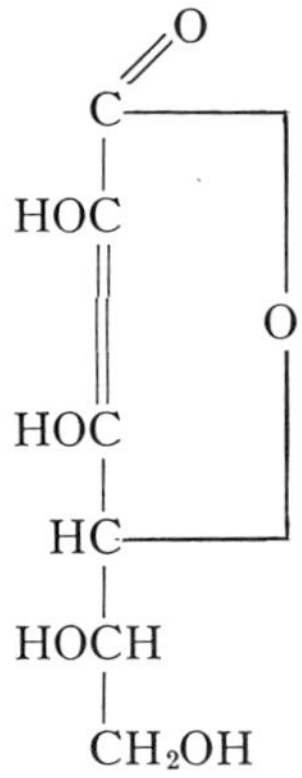

$$\overset{\overset{O}{\parallel}}{C}$$
HOC
HOC
O
HC
HOCH
CH₂OH

Ascorbic acid (vitamin C)

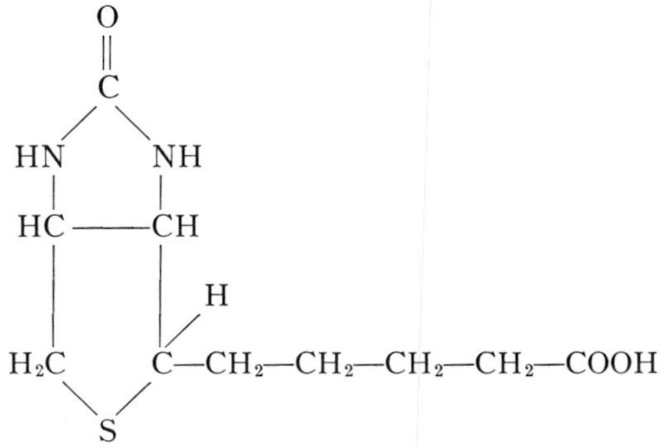

$$\overset{\overset{O}{\parallel}}{C}$$
HN   NH
HC——CH
H
H₂C   C—CH₂—CH₂—CH₂—CH₂—COOH
S

Biotin

$$HOOC-\underset{\underset{CH_2}{|}}{\overset{\overset{H}{|}}{C}}-\underset{\underset{}{\overset{\overset{H}{|}}{N}}}-\overset{\overset{O}{\parallel}}{C}$$
HOOC—CH₂

N N —NH₂
N
N
OH
H H
N—C
H

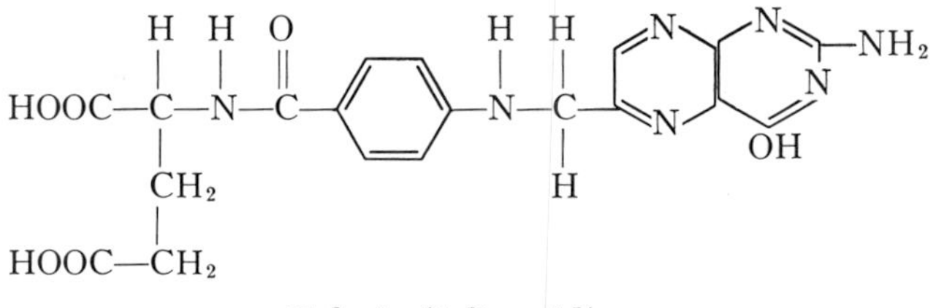

Folacin (folic acid)

Cobalamin (vitamin B₁₂)

ESSENTIAL AMINO ACIDS

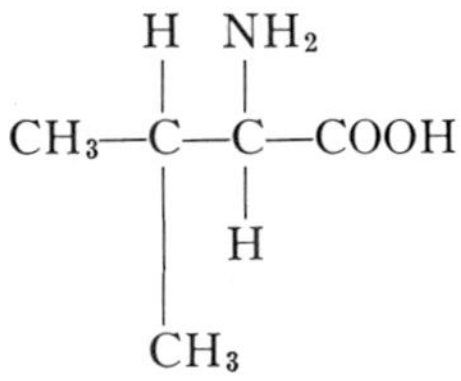

$$CH_3-\underset{\underset{CH_3}{|}}{\overset{\overset{H}{|}}{C}}-\underset{\underset{H}{|}}{\overset{\overset{NH_2}{|}}{C}}-COOH$$

Valine

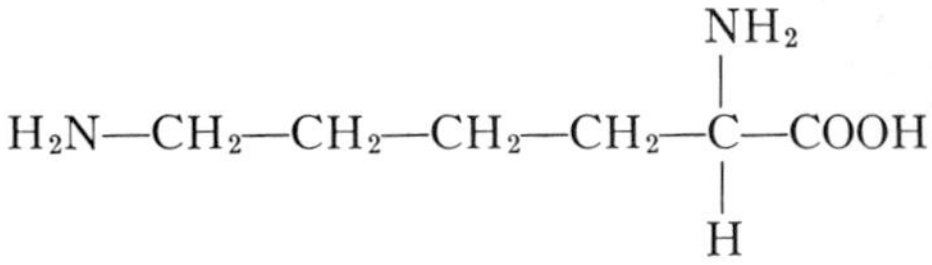

$$H_2N-CH_2-CH_2-CH_2-CH_2-\underset{\underset{H}{|}}{\overset{\overset{NH_2}{|}}{C}}-COOH$$

Lysine

$$CH_3-\underset{\underset{CH_3}{|}}{CH}-CH_2-\underset{\underset{H}{|}}{\overset{\overset{NH_2}{|}}{C}}-COOH$$

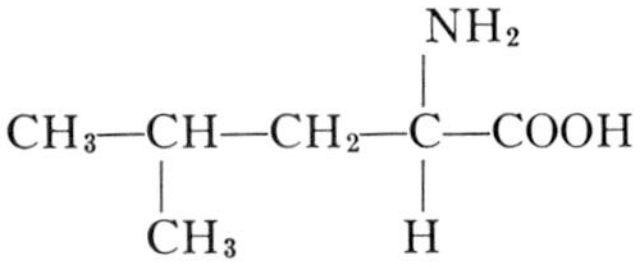

Leucine

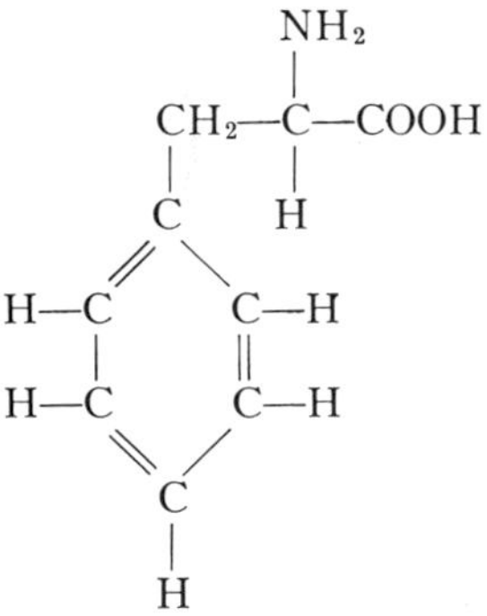

Phenylalanine

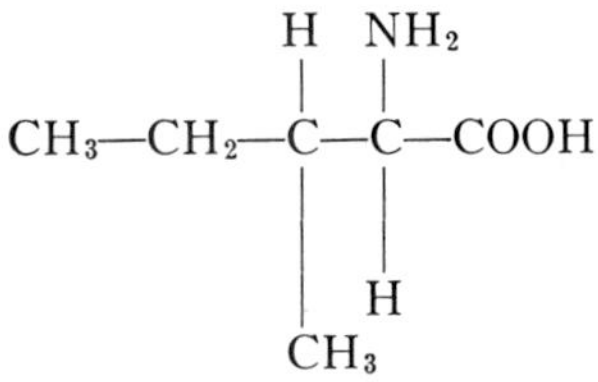

$$CH_3-CH_2-\underset{\underset{CH_3}{|}}{\overset{\overset{H}{|}}{C}}-\underset{\underset{H}{|}}{\overset{\overset{NH_2}{|}}{C}}-COOH$$

Isoleucine

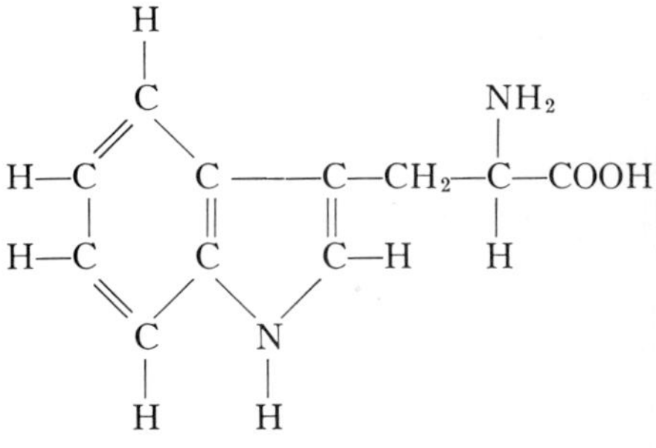

$$CH_3-\underset{\underset{OH}{|}}{\overset{\overset{H}{|}}{C}}-\underset{\underset{H}{|}}{\overset{\overset{NH_2}{|}}{C}}-COOH$$

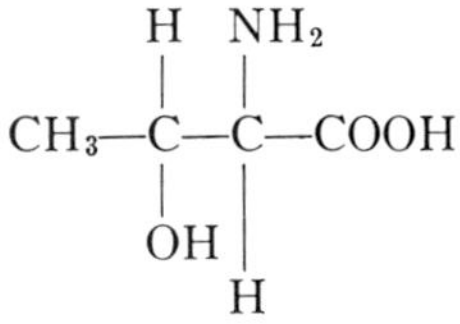

Threonine

Tryptophan

$$H_3C-S-CH_2-CH_2-\underset{\underset{H}{|}}{\overset{\overset{NH_2}{|}}{C}}-COOH$$

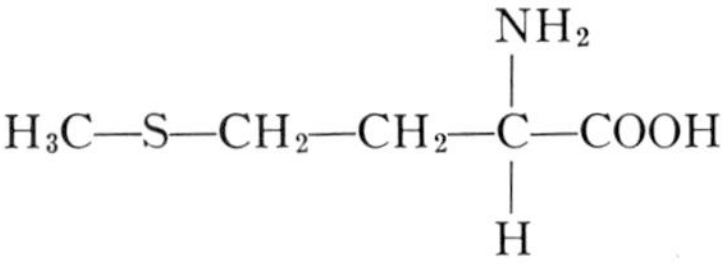

Methionine

Index

A

Abortion and low protein diets, 339
Absorption
  of alcohol, 33
  of ascorbic acid, 225-226
  of calcium, 109-113, 205-206
  of carbohydrate, 27-28
  of cobalamin, 269
  of copper, 164
  of fats or lipids, 40
  of folacin, 264
  of iodine, 151
  of iron, 140-142
  of manganese, 163
  of molybdenum, 166
  of niacin, 251-252
  in nutrient intake of aging, 386
  of nutrients, phosphorus and, 125
  of phosphorus, 126
  of protein, 57
  of riboflavin, 246-248
  of sodium, 129-130
  of thiamin, 236-237
  of vitamins; *see also* other specific vitamins
    A, 195-196
    D, 207
    E, 211
    K, 216
Acetyl CoA, 260, 277
Acetyl coenzyme A, 260, 279
Acetylcholine, 277
  formation and breakdown of, 109
  pantothenic acid and, 260
Achlorhydria, iron absorption and, 141
Acid-base balance
  mineral elements and maintenance of, 99-101
  zinc and, 161
Acidity of digestive mass, 110
Activity
  decreased, obesity and, 399-400
  energy required for, 88, 89-90
  increased, obesity and, 407
  and total energy needs, 92
Adenosine diphosphate, 125, 133
Adenosine triphosphate, 125
Adermin, 254
Adipose cells, 41, 44
Adolescence, 156, 372-375
ADP, 125, 133
Adrenal gland
  aging and, 387

Adrenal gland—cont'd
  ascorbic acid and, 224-225
  basal energy needs and, 86-87
Adrenaline
  basal metabolic rate and, 87
  protein and formation of, 56
Adulthood, nutrition from infancy to, 365-379; *see also* Nutrition from infancy to adulthood
Adults
  ascorbic acid needs for, 226
  calcium needs for, 116
  desirable weights for, 448-449
  iron needs for, 142
A/E ratio, 72
Age
  and basal energy needs, 87, 90
  and total energy needs, 92, 93
Aging, 380-392
  adequacy of diets in, 391
  defective RNA from DNA in, 381
  dietary supplements in, 391-392
  loss of cells in, 381
  nature of, 380-383
  nutrient intake in, 383-391
    digestion and absorption in, 386
    ingestion of nutrients in, 383-386
    metabolism and excretion in, 386-387
  nutritive needs in, 387-391
Alanine, 50
Albinism, copper and, 164
Albumin, plasma, 40
Alcohol, 33
Alcohol dehydrogenase, 33
Aldehyde, 16, 165
Aldehyde oxidase, 165
Aldosterone, 129, 130
Alkali, thiamin loss and, 242
Alkaline mineral elements, 99
Alkaline phosphatase, 106
  nutritional status and, 310
  during pregnancy, 327
  vitamin D and, 206
  zinc and, 161
Alliithiamin, 236
Allowances, recommended dietary; *see* Recommended dietary allowances; Requirements
Alopecia, riboflavin deficiency and, 249
Alpha-carotene, 195-196
Alpha-tocopherol, 210
Altitude, iron absorption and, 141-142

Gamma-carotene, 195-196
Gastric lipase in digestion of fats or lipids, 38-40
Gastric protease, 57
Gastrointestinal motility
  calcium absorption and, 111
  pantothenic acid and, 262
  during pregnancy, 326
Gastrointestinal tract
  vitamin A and changes in, 202
  water exchange in, 180
Genetic factors, obesity and, 401-403
Genitourinary tract changes, vitamin A and, 202
Geriatrics, 380; *see also* Aging
Gerontology, 380; *see also* Aging
Gestation, fetal weight at different ages in, 324
Glands
  activity of, basal metabolism and, 82
  adrenal
    in aging, 387
    ascorbic acid and production of hormones of, 224-225
  ductless, basal energy needs and, 86-87
  endocrine, obesity and, 403
  mammary
    fat deposits in, 329
    lactation and, 341
  parathyroid, thyroidectomy and, 158
  salivary
    of infants, 360
    thyroxin and, 155
  thyroid
    in aging, 387
    iodine and, 150
Glossitis, 249
Glucogenic amino acid, 59, 60
Gluconeogenesis, 30
Glucose, 21, 22, 23, 27, 28
  conversion of galactose to, 31
  levels of, blood, normal fasting, 22
  tolerance for, chromium and, 166
Glutamic acid, 50, 262
Glutamine, 50
Glutathione, cobalamin and, 270
Glycerides, formula for, 37
Glycerol
  chemical structure of, 35
  obesity and, 404
Glycine, 50, 51, 277
Glycogen, 24
  athletes and, 377
  water and, 177
Glycogen phosphorylase, 256
Glycogen storage disease, 32
Glyoxal, 342
Goiter, 9, 155-158
  endemic, 156, 157
  exophthalmic, 87
  in pregnancy, 333
Goitren, 154
Goitrogenic effect of cobalt toxicity, 167
Goitrogens, 154, 308
Graves' disease, 158
Ground substance, 105

Growth
  calcium and, 108
  of children, evaluation of, 312-313
  dietary protein intake for, 65
  energy needs during, 94
  fetal, rate of, 324
  iron needs and, 139
  of liver and bone marrow cells, myoinositol and, 276
  micronutrient elements and, 159
  mineral elements and, 104
  nitrogen requirements for, 62, 63
  period of, during pregnancy, 325-326
  protein as essential for, 55-56
  rate of, breast-feeding and, 349
  retarded
    riboflavin deficiency and, 249
    zinc deficiency and, 161
  standards of, for children, 446-447
  of tumors, protein and, 56
  vitamin A and, 191
Gums, changes in, in ascorbic acid deficiency, 308

H
Habits, nutritional
  improving of, 378
  and nutrient intake in aging, 383
  obesity and family food, 399
Hair, changes in, nutritional deficiencies and, 308
Harelip, riboflavin deficiency and, 249
Head Start, 426
Healing, ascorbic acid in
  of burns, 225
  of wounds, 234
Heart disease and fats or lipids, 47-48
Heat
  and basal energy needs, 87-88
  of combustion of food, 77, 79
  in destruction of thiamin, 242
  effect of, on use of dietary protein, 68
  unit of, 76
Height
  and estimation of basal energy needs, 85
  and weight tables, 312-314, 448-449
Heme, 138
Hemochromatosis, 150
Hemoglobin
  in biochemical analysis, 311
  content of, in blood, 138, 144, 148
  and functions of iron, 137-139
  levels of, 326
    deficiency of iron and, 148
    during pregnancy, 326
  manufacture of, 142
  molecule of, 137
  protein and formation of, 56
  synthesis of, pyridoxine and, 255
Hemolysis, erythrocyte, vitamin E and, 214
Hemorrhage
  neonatal, 334
  vitamin K deficiency and, 217
Hemorrhagic anemia, 149-150
Hemosiderin, 137
Heparin, 26

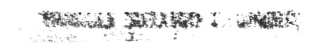

Weight; *see also* Weight control
  of body
    comparison of, in established standards, 394-395
    gain or loss in, 94-96
    in kilograms and kg.$^{3⁄4}$, 86
    metabolic, energy needs and, 90
  desirable, for height for adults, 448-449
  and estimation of basal energy needs, 85-86
  and height tables, 312-314
  of mother
    at conception, 329
    postpartum loss of, 330
    in pregnancy, 93-94, 328-329
  reduction of
    diets for, 95-96
    excessive, athletes and, 377-378
Weight control, 393-412; *see also* Weight
  fats and diets for, 42
  obesity in, 393-410
    causes of, 398-404
    classification of, 404-405
    diagnosis of, 394-395
    dietary aids and, 407-410
    disadvantages of, 396-398
    prevalence of, 395-396
    prevention of, 410
    transition diet and, 410
    treatment of, 405-407
  underweight in, 410-411

Wetzel grid, 313, 314
White House Conference on Food, Nutrition, and Health, 6
WHO, 436
Wills factor, 262
Wilson's disease, 165
Women
  adequate diet for, 296
  desirable weights for height for, 449
Work, energy required for, 88, 89-90
World food supply, 433-436
World Health Organization, 115, 436
Wound healing, ascorbic acid deficiency and, 234

X

Xanthine oxidase, 165
Xanthurenic acid, 255-256, 310
Xerophthalmia, 214, 308
X-rays
  in anthropometric data, 312, 314
  in measurement of body fat, 394
Xylose, 22

Y

Yellow enzyme; *see* Riboflavin

Z

Zinc, 160-162
  deficiency of, 159, 161
  toxicity of, 162